EXPLORING Health Care CAREERS

Editorial Staff

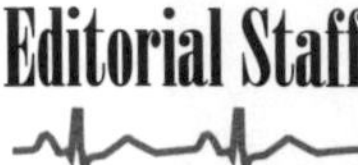

Editorial Director: David Hayes

Editors: Miriam Creeden, Irene Ferguson, Anne Paterson, Alfred Smuskiewicz, Jeffrey Tegge

Production Assistants: Joyce Lofton, Amy McKenna

Additional Editorial Assistance: Holli Cosgrove

Writers: Carole Bolster, Shawna Brynildssen, Mickey Cohen, Kelly Cronin, Patty Cronin, Tim Cronin, Deborah Douglas, Jennifer Elcano, Nic Gengler, Bonnie Griffin, Janyce Hamilton, Kathleen Hayes, Louise Howe, Sally Jaskold, Jane Lawrence, Andrew Morkes, Kathryn Quinlan, Tim Schaffert, Elizabeth Taggart, Nancy Weatherwax

Bibliographer: David King

Book Design Based on Concepts by: Joe Grossmann, Grossmann Design & Consulting

EXPLORING Health Care CAREERS

Real People Tell You What You Need to Know

David Hayes, Editor

Ferguson Publishing Company Chicago

Exploring health care careers : real people tell you what you need to know /
[David Hayes, editor].

v. <1-   >. cm.

Includes bibliographical references and index.

Summary: Provides information about 110 careers in the health care field including job descriptions, education and licensing requirements, salary, advancement opportunities, and employment outlook.

ISBN 0-89434-217-7

1. Medicine—Vocational guidance—Juvenile literature.

[1. Medicine—Vocational guidance. 2. Vocational guidance.]

I. Hayes, David, 1955 Dec. 15-

R690.E97 1998 97-18163

610.69—dc21 CIP

AC

Printed in the United States of America

U-8

contents

VOLUME 1

neurological surgeon

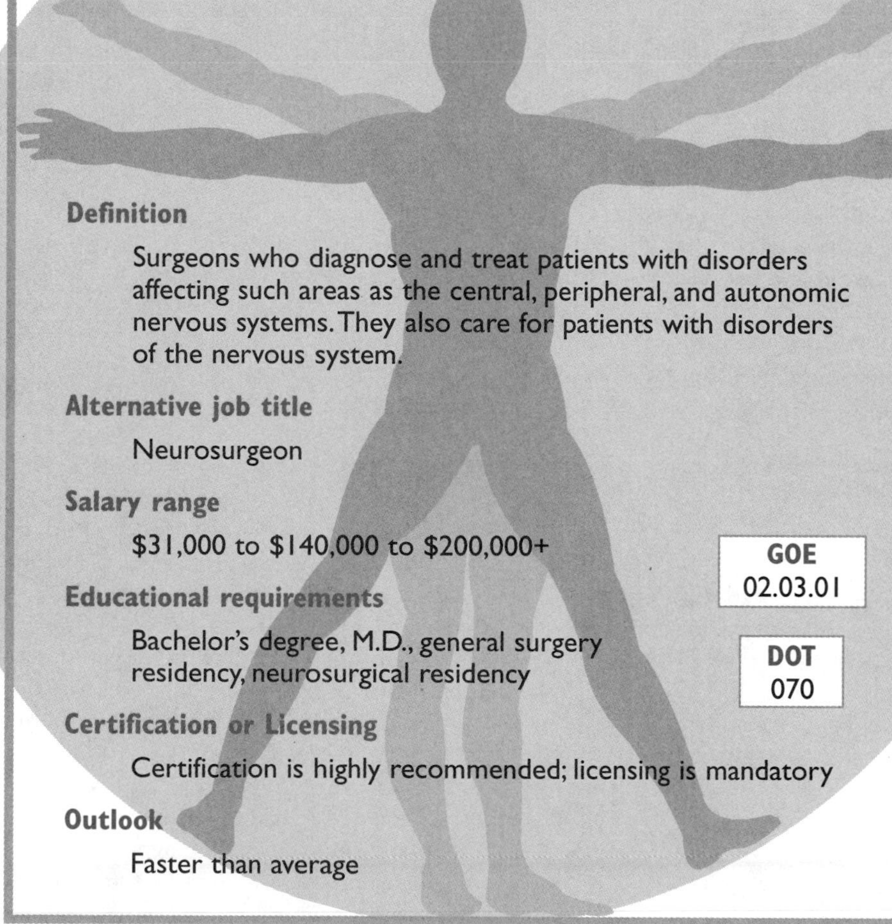

Definition

Surgeons who diagnose and treat patients with disorders affecting such areas as the central, peripheral, and autonomic nervous systems. They also care for patients with disorders of the nervous system.

Alternative job title

Neurosurgeon

Salary range

$31,000 to $140,000 to $200,000+

Educational requirements

Bachelor's degree, M.D., general surgery residency, neurosurgical residency

Certification or Licensing

Certification is highly recommended; licensing is mandatory

Outlook

Faster than average

GOE
02.03.01

DOT
070

High School Subjects

Biology
Chemistry
English
Mathematics
Physics

Personal Interests

Helping people
Problem solving
Using your hands
Working with technology

Crushed and bloody, the victim was rushed into the emergency room as paramedics shouted out vital statistics. Two trucks had collided, and this trucker was the victim in the worst condition. Dr. Sherry Apple looked down at the man she was helping to wheel into the operating room. One eye dangled from its socket. His rib cage was smashed, his arms and legs were broken, his skull cracked, and his brain visibly protruding. Unbelievably, he was still conscious. She whispered some words of encouragement to him. "What's your name?" he asked her.

"Sherry," she answered softly.

"No," he said. "What's your handle? Your CB name?"

Dr. Apple was more than a little taken aback. How did he know that she had a CB? "Dr. Fruit Loops," she said. "It's what the kids in the surgical ward call me." The man seemed to calm down almost instantly.

"I know," he said. "We talked all the way to Louisville. It's me," he whispered. "Woodpecker."

Dr. Apple sucked in her breath sharply, but made no other comment, as the man passed out. A nurse took over at the gurney and Dr. Apple went to scrub and gown herself.

Months before, while she was driving from Georgia to Kentucky for interviews for a neurosurgical residency, she'd almost fallen asleep at the wheel. A kindly and talkative trucker named Woody Key had saved her life by first honking at her when her car began to swerve, and later by talking to her over the CB to help keep her awake during the long drive. When she had said goodbye, she thought that she would never see him again. Now, here he was in her operating room. And tonight it looked like he was going to need her help.

Hours later, the trucker came out of the craniotomy—a surgery to open the skull, stop the bleeding, and relieve the pressure on his brain. Dr. Apple and another neurological surgeon had worked on his head injuries, while other surgeons tried to repair the damage done to the rest of his body. He would need reconstructive surgeries to put his face back together, but he'd made it, in large part because of Dr. Apple. The knowledge that she was there, working to save his life, helped him recover.

lingo to learn

Angiogram Dye is injected into a neck or groin artery to make the smaller arteries visible to X rays. This test provides physicians with a view of the arteries going to and coursing from the brain, enabling them to determine, for example, if any are blocked. Also known as an arteriogram.

Computerized tomography A form of radiology, or X ray, which uses computers to construct two-dimensional pictures of selected body parts. Dye may be injected into a vein to obtain a better picture. Also referred to as a CT or CAT scan.

Congenital anomaly An abnormality, usually a structural one, that is present at birth.

Degenerative disease An illness in which the structure of a tissue or its function deteriorates.

Electroencephalogram (EEG) A procedure that uses electrodes attached to the scalp to record the brain's continuous electrical activity.

what does a neurological surgeon do?

A board-certified *neurological surgeon* diagnoses, evaluates, and treats patients with disorders affecting the central, peripheral, and autonomic nervous systems—which include the brain, meninges (any of the three membranes that envelope the brain and spinal cord), skull, spinal cord, pituitary gland, and nerves—and their supporting structures and vascular supply. This specialist provides both nonsurgical and surgical care, depending upon the nature of the injury or illness. Neurological surgery also includes the operative and nonoperative management, diagnosis, evaluation, treatment, critical care, and rehabilitation of patients with disorders of the nervous system.

Within the broader specialty of neurological surgery, there are three subdivisions, or subspecialties: brain; spine; and peripheral nerve and muscles. Any accident that injures the head, spinal cord, or nerves might require neurosurgical treatment. As a result, neurological surgeons treat a wide variety of illnesses and conditions. For example, a patient who suffers a serious stroke may have neurosurgery to increase the blood supply to areas of the brain and spinal cord. In order to restore normal circulation to the brain, neurological surgeons frequently remove the arteriosclerotic debris that clogs neck arteries. Children, born with a deformed brain or spinal cord, or suffering from poor spinal fluid circulation, are helped by neurosurgery that corrects these problems. Perhaps the most common problem neurological surgeons treat is the neck or lower back pain that can spread to the arms and hands. A ruptured disc can cause this type of pain. Slipped discs and pinched nerves, on the other hand, may be treated non-surgically, with bed rest, braces, physical therapy, or a combination of these methods.

Many people often confuse the work of *neurologists* and *neurological surgeons.* Of the two professions, however, only neurological surgeons are allowed to perform the complex neural surgeries. Patients usually see neurological surgeons in two different situations. In the first instance, if a patient is admitted to an emergency room with traumatic injuries, the emergency room physician will ask that a neurological surgeon evaluate the patient. Cases such as these are called acute care, because the patient requires immediate attention and might possibly need surgery. In the second instance, neurological surgeons see patients who have been referred to them by neurologists. Ideally, a neurologist evaluates all non-acute care patients and, if the neurologist believes a patient has problems that can be best treated through surgery, she or he will refer the patient to a neurological surgeon.

Neurological surgeons work with many of the same problems as neurologists, such as epilepsy, peripheral nerve diseases, and tumors. But unlike the neurologist, the neurological surgeon becomes involved with non-acute care patients usually when nonsurgical treatments, such as medication, have failed or are inadequate to correct or reduce the problem. Because of their specialized surgical talents and skills, neurological surgeons spend most of their time in the operating room. Some of their time, however, is devoted to clinic, rounds, consultations, conferences, and teaching responsibilities.

what is it like to be a neurological surgeon?

"There are some specialties where you make decisions based on lots of information—this isn't one of them," states Dr. Frances Conley, Chief of Neurosurgery at the Palo Alto Veterans Administration Medical Center, and a professor of Neurosurgery at Stanford University School of Medicine, in San Francisco, California.

If this sounds strange and more than a little intimidating, consider that neurological surgeons routinely operate on bundles of nerves the size of hairs, that they expertly wield lasers near the fragile stem of the spinal cord, and that they systematically cut through the rock-hard skull that protects our brains to remove tumors buried in the delicate gray matter. In short, they work on the most sensitive areas of the human body, areas that are responsible for both our most basic and advanced functions. Neurological surgeons work on three major areas of the nervous system: the brain, the spine, and the peripheral nerves and muscles. Any accident that injures the head, spinal cord, or nerves may require neurosurgical treatment. Although many specialize in one of the three areas, neurological surgeons are trained to treat illnesses and conditions that run the gamut of neurological injuries.

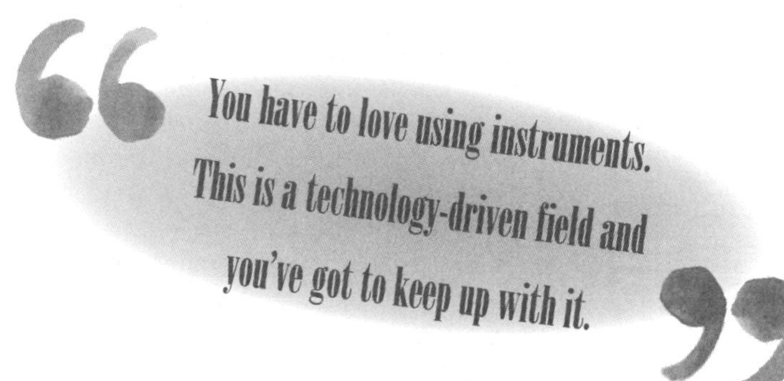

Patients often come to the neurological surgeon in bad shape, and it is up to the neurological surgeon to determine the best course of action. "A typical case," says Dr. Conley, "is a patient who is brought to the emergency room. He has a bruise on his forehead, he's awake, but not talking, and he has a left-sided weakness. Where is the injury? Did he have a fall? Does he have a blood-clot as a result of the fall?" The ER physician brings the neurological surgeon in to evaluate the patient and see if surgery is, in fact, the way to go. Based on training and experience, the neurological surgeon must act quickly and decisively, whether that means ordering advanced tests, consulting with a neurologist, or performing emergency surgery. If the fall was less serious or, for some other reason, the patient had been taken to a clinic instead of the emergency room, he would probably have seen a neurologist. Depending upon the diagnosis, a consultation with a neurological surgeon might then follow.

Neurological surgeons use several diagnostic procedures to determine whether or not the patient is functioning normally, especially in terms of cranial nerve function. To determine if there are any problems, neurological surgeons check the patient's balance, reflexes, motor skills, and cognitive abilities. The doctor needs to answer such questions as: Is the patient's speech slurred? Can the patient see? Can the patient hear? The answers may indicate a problem, but not necessarily the source of the problem. Neurological surgeons use simple logic combined with a vast knowledge of neural anatomy and physiology to begin solving the problem behind a patient's complaint of pain or abnormal function. Based on their conclusions, they may also order a number of tests to try to pinpoint the source and location of the problem or to rule out other possibilities.

Among the tests a neurological surgeon may request for a patient are computerized tomography or computer-assisted tomography (also referred to as a CT or CAT scan), electroencephalogram (EEG), and magnetic resonance imaging (MRI). These tests may then help the neurological surgeon to determine whether surgery is an option. If the tests indicate that a surgical procedure is the best solution, the neurological surgeon schedules the surgery.

more lingo to learn

Electromyogram (EMG) A test that measures and records electrical activity from the muscles and nerves. It is often used in cases involving pain, numbness, tingling, or weakness.

Magnetic resonance imaging (MRI) An advanced way of making images of what is inside the brain. For this test a patient lies still in a small chamber for approximately thirty minutes while a very strong magnet passes over the brain.

Myelogram A test in which dye is injected into the spinal canal, making the structure clearly visible to X rays. The test is often used to diagnose patients with neck or back pain, or suspected spinal tumors.

Neurosonography A test that uses ultra high-frequency sound waves to analyze blood flow, most often in stroke victims.

Children present specific challenges to neurological surgeons. Dr. Alexa Canady, a pediatric neurological surgeon, is Chief of Neurosurgery at Children's Hospital of Michigan and Vice-Chairman of Neurosurgery at Wayne State University in Detroit, Michigan. Every day she treats infants and children with a variety of neurological problems and disorders, including brain tumors, traumatic head injuries, congenital spinal problems, abnormal skull development, epilepsy, and hydrocephalus (excessive fluid in the brain). Her patients may have been born with these problems, or they may have been brought to the emergency room after, for example, being hit by a car. "Basically, I see anyone with a neurological problem with a possible surgical solution," she says. Dr. Canady enjoys her work, especially the fact that children are her patients. She explains, "The patients in the adult neurosurgery wing are terrified. It's serious and somber. The children's unit is completely different. Kids don't know enough to be terrified. Their parents might be—but they're not. So, the atmosphere is lighter, more playful." She adds, "I also like the spectrum of diseases in pediatric neurosurgery. I like working with congenital problems versus degenerative problems."

Neurological surgeons spend most of their day in the operating room, and that day begins early. "I get up at 5:00 AM and go for a run for thirty minutes to an hour. I'm at the hospital by 7:15 and operating by 7:30," says Dr. Conley. "I'm usually in the OR all day." As in every surgical specialty, each neurological surgeon determines the atmosphere in the operating room. One may prefer a tense, energetic mood to keep the medical team on their toes during the procedure, while another may prefer a more serene, calm setting. "It's very individual," says Dr. Conley, who prefers a relaxed atmosphere and has classical music playing during her surgeries. Dr. Canady, while she does not ask that music be playing, also enjoys what she calls, "a calm, focused, but fairly informal atmosphere."

As with any surgery, neurological surgery carries a great deal of risk. There is, however, a great deal of variety in the surgeries. Dr. Conley admits that it would drive her crazy if she had to perform the same procedure over and over again, day in and day out. Neurological surgeries often require the surgeon to be innovative in terms of surgical technique or even instrumentation. Sometimes, the creative part of the surgery is how the neurological surgeon accesses the surgical site. Other times the creative part is how the actual repair work is conceived and executed. Still other times, the creative moment of the surgery comes in devising a unique tool that will allow a neurological surgeon to attempt something that has never been done successfully before. "You do have a lot of manual creativity, particularly with spine work. You really devise things ad hoc." Dr. Conley loves the wide range of challenges that her work presents. "Backs, necks, carotid arteries, the front and back of the brain—it's diverse."

Dr. Kline, Head of the Department of Neurosurgery at the Louisiana State University Medical Center in New Orleans, Louisiana, is one of the world's leading peripheral nerve specialists. "I see patients, take histories, sort through the injuries, and determine what can be surgically repaired," he says. He further subdivides his specialty into three areas. A large group of patients comes to him with lacerations, stretches, and lesions on the brachial plexus, the nerves running to the arm, forearm, and hand.

Another group of patients comes to him with what are called spontaneous entrapments. Basically, a spontaneous entrapment is when a nerve becomes trapped and compressed, which causes a great deal of pain for the patient. The solution is straight forward—make more room for the nerve. The surgical remedy, however, is complex. To provide more room, Dr. Kline first identifies the precise location of the compressed nerve using electrical studies. Carpal tunnel syndrome is the most common nerve compression problem. In a patient with carpal tunnel, the nerve into the hand thickens and rubs against a ligament in the wrist. A segment of the ligament is cut to decompress the nerve and create more space.

The third category of nerve problems that Dr. Kline treats is tumors. They can grow in or next to nerves, affecting muscles and sensation. Many nerve injuries damage the entire length of the nerve, in which case a nerve graft becomes necessary. Seventy percent of Dr. Kline's patients come from outside of Louisiana. "Many are referrals from other neurosurgeons or neurologists," he says, "Difficult cases that they want me to take a look at. Other patients have just heard of me and feel like I'm their last hope."

Dr. Kline spends his days in his office, seeing patients, or at the hospital making rounds, or in surgery. Likewise, on clinic days, Dr. Conley sees scheduled patients, patients referred to her by other physicians, patients on the hospital wards, and any drop-in patients in ER. Dr. Conley, Dr. Canady, and Dr. Kline all teach, and many of their responsibilities involve teaching and working with residents, who usually accompany them on their rounds. These surgeons also supervise clinical presentations and conferences. "I usually operate four days a week," says Dr. Canady. "Mondays, I'm in my office, seeing patients, other days—I'm teaching or running clinics. Craniofacial clinics, for example, and tumor board, where we review all the tumor cases."

To be a successful neurological surgeon you should

- Have a great deal of stamina
- Be decisive and capable of making quick decisions
- Enjoy doing detailed and fine work
- Have a superb grasp of neural anatomy and physiology
- Know your limitations

have I got what it takes to be a neurological surgeon?

Neurological surgery is one of the most demanding of the medical specialties. Those who enter the field will be challenged emotionally, physically, and intellectually. High levels of stress, long hours, and difficult, complex cases are among the drawbacks to working as a neurological surgeon. Patients requiring neurosurgical attention are usually quite ill. Often, a surgical procedure is possible, but it may not be successful. "You need to know your limitations," explains Dr. Conley. "You frequently have to tell families there's nothing more to do, or there isn't a surgical solution."

Neurological surgeons work long hours, and on those days that they have surgeries scheduled, they usually spend the entire day on their feet in the operating room. Surgeries can take an hour or two, or they can last for much longer. "You need stamina," says Dr. Conley. "A surgery can last anywhere from an hour to fifteen hours." Dr. Canady says her longest surgery lasted twenty-three hours. "That's very unusual," she says. "It was a surgery to correct a malformation of the child's brain." Ordinarily, Dr. Canady says she works fourteen-hour days.

In addition to long days filled with surgeries, neurological surgeons are also on call several nights a week, depending on such factors as the number of neurosurgical cases there are or the number of other neurological surgeons on staff at the hospital or clinic where they work. Dr. Kline, for example, is on call every fourth weekend; while Dr. Canady is on call every third night during the week. When it comes to their own patients, neurological surgeons are on call twenty-four hours a day.

Neurological surgeons must also deal with the stress of handling complex, difficult cases. "It's harder to help people with this type of surgery than with any other," explains Dr. Kline. "There are limits to what you can do, but the complexity appeals to me." Part of the complexity of the cases comes from the delicate nature of neurological surgery and the sensitive areas of the body on which it is performed.

The instruments and technology used in neurological surgery also add to the complexity. "You have to love using instruments," Dr. Kline stresses. "This is a technology-driven field and you've got to keep up with it." In addition to understanding and interpreting the tests mentioned earlier, such the CT scan or MRI, neurological surgeons routinely use electrodes, recording machines, microscopes, and micro-instruments. "Occasionally, I use a laser," says Dr. Conley. She goes on to list some of her instruments. "I use air-driven power tools to remove and cut through bone, special soft-tissue instruments and, if necessary, I may create a tool." Throughout their careers, neurological surgeons constantly learn new techniques and the instruments that support them. "How to use them and when to use them," Dr. Kline adds.

A sense of humor comes in handy in most professions. Surgeons, however, seem to thrive on joking banter, both in and out of the operating room. Prospective neurological surgeons should be aware of this propensity for sharp humor. Those who work with surgeons usually learn to put up with the cutting remarks or decide to work elsewhere. One explanation may be that with the stress, long hours, and emotionally taxing cases, these specialists develop thick skins in order to deal with their work. At the very least, Dr. Canady believes humor keeps her grounded.

how do I become a neurological surgeon?

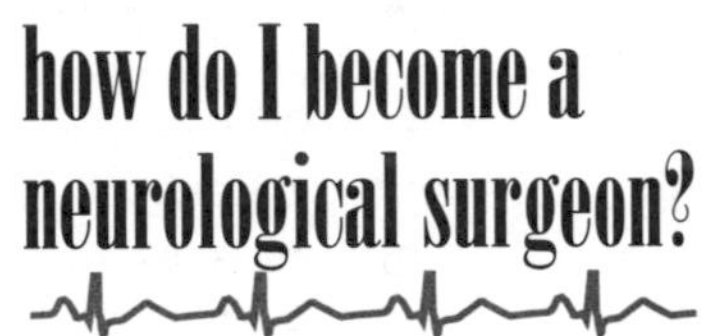

education

Science and the medical field appealed to Dr. Apple even when she was a child. Although she did not originally plan to become a neurological surgeon, the brain seemed to fascinate her from a very early age. "I won a science fair in the second grade for a project on the brain," she says with a chuckle. "So, I guess it was in my future."

High School

If you are interested in pursuing a medical degree, a high school education emphasizing college preparatory classes is a must. Science courses, such as biology, chemistry, and physics, are necessary, as are math courses. These classes will not only provide you with an introduction to basic science and math concepts, but also allow you to determine your own aptitude in these areas. Since college will be your next educational step, it is also important to take English courses to develop your researching and writing skills. Foreign language, social science, and computer classes will also help make you an appealing candidate for college admission as well as prepare you for your future undergraduate and gradu-

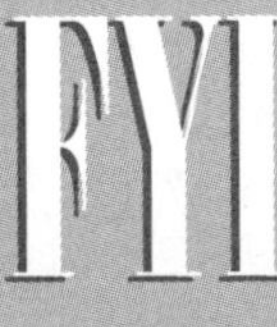

Only 71 women have been certified by the ABNS since its incorporation in 1940. In total, the ABNS has certified 4,442 neurological surgeons, approximately 3,250 of whom are actively practicing today. Over 1000 residents are training in accredited programs in the United States and Canada; 85 of these residents are women.

ate education. As a high school senior you may want to consider applying to colleges or universities that are also associated with a medical school. High school guidance counselors should also be able to provide you with information about such schools.

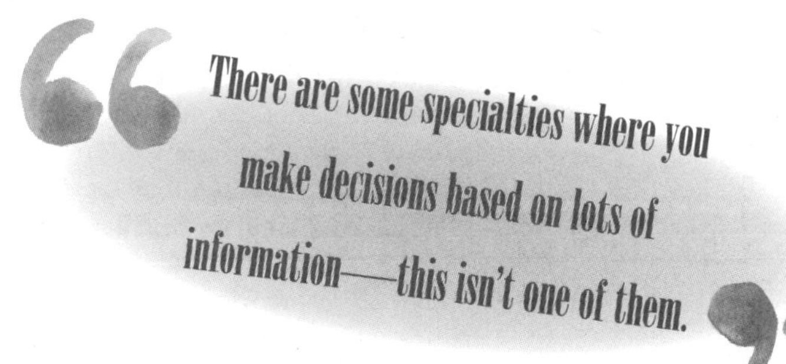

Postsecondary Training

Following high school, the next step on your educational path to be a neurological surgeon is to earn a bachelor's degree from an accredited four-year college or university. Suggested premedical courses include physics, biology, and organic and inorganic chemistry. Courses in English, mathematics, and the social sciences, are also highly recommended.

After receiving an undergraduate degree, your next step is to apply to and be accepted by a medical school. Admission is competitive, and applicants must undergo a fairly extensive and difficult admissions process that takes into consideration grade point averages, scores on the Medical College Admission Test (MCAT), and recommendations from professors. Most students apply to several schools early in their senior year of college. Only about one-third of the applicants are accepted.

In order to earn the degree doctor of medicine (M.D.), a student must complete four years of medical school study and training. For the first two years of medical school, students attend lectures and classes and spend time in laboratories. Courses include anatomy, biochemistry, physiology, pharmacology, psychology, microbiology, pathology, medical ethics, and laws governing medicine. They learn to take patient histories, perform routine physical examinations, and recognize symptoms.

In their third and fourth years, students are involved in more practical studies. They work in clinics and hospitals supervised by residents and physicians and they learn acute, chronic, preventive, and rehabilitative care. They go through what are known as rotations (brief periods of study) in such areas as internal medicine, obstetrics and gynecology, pediatrics, dermatology, psychiatry, and surgery. Rotations allow students to gain exposure to the many different fields within medicine.

Upon graduating from an accredited medical school, physicians must pass a standard examination given by the National Board of Medical Examiners. Most physicians complete an internship, also referred to as a transition year. The internship is usually one year in length, and helps graduates to decide what their area of specialization will be.

Following the internship, the physicians begin what is known as a residency. Physicians wishing to pursue the specialty of neurosurgery must first complete a residency in general surgery. Per requirements set down by the Accreditation Council for Graduate Medical Education (ACGME) and the Royal College of Physicians and Surgeons of Canada, general surgery residents must complete a five-year program that is broad-based and leads to either continued study and training in general surgery or to entering a training program in another surgical specialty.

Throughout the general surgery residency, residents are supervised at all levels of training, with the attending surgeon ultimately responsible for the patient's care. Residents begin their training by assisting on and then performing basic operations, such as the removal of an appendix or a hernia repair. As the residency years continue, residents gain responsibility through teaching and supervisory duties. Eventually the residents are allowed to perform complex operations independently.

Neurological surgery residency programs, which follow the general surgery residency, are comprised of sixty months (five years) of specialized training, following fundamental clinical skills. Of those sixty months, at least thirty-six months must be spent in clinical neurosurgery, of which twelve months are served with senior clinical responsibilities.

Residents in neurosurgery study the basic neurosciences, neuropathology, neuroradiology, research and other related disciplines. During their residency years, residents in neurological surgery are required to maintain a record of the operative procedures they complete. This record will be used later, when they seek board certification.

certification or licensing

Licensing is a mandatory procedure in the United States. It is required in all states before any doctor can practice medicine. In order to be licensed, doctors must have graduated from medical school, passed the licensing test of the state in which they will practice, and completed their residency.

Certification is not mandatory but is highly recommended. The American Board of Neurological Surgery (ABNS), formed fifty-five years ago, has the responsibility of certifying neurological surgeons who graduate from accredited programs in the United States.

During their training, and as part of the ABNS certification process, residents in neurological surgery take the written Primary Examination, which covers fundamental clinical skills plus the basic neurosciences. After successfully completing the residency in neurological surgery, each candidate makes a formal application to the ABNS for the oral examination and certification.

Prior to making this application, the residents must spend two years in practice. Along with the application, the ABNS requires that each candidate submit letters of support from the director of his or her residency program and fellow physicians, as well as letters detailing the candidate's hospital privileges from each hospital where the candidate cares for patients. In addition, data on all hospital patients treated by the candidate over a period of twelve months must be reviewed and approved by the ABNS.

Finally, the candidate takes the last step in the certification process—three hours of oral examination by ABNS directors. Once all these steps have been met and approved by the ABNS, the candidate is certified as a Diplomate of the ABNS. The requirements of residency programs take into account these requirements, so that they can best prepare residents for the certifying examinations.

scholarships and grants

Scholarships and grants are often available from individual institutions, state agencies, and special-interest organizations. The book *Dollars for College: Medicine, Dentistry, and Related Fields* by Ferguson Publishing Company is an excellent source for this information. Many students finance their medical education through the Armed Forces Health Professions Scholarship Program. Each branch of the military participates in this program, paying students' tuitions in exchange for military service. Contact your local recruiting office for more information. The National Health Service Corps Scholarship Program also provides money for students in return for service. Another source for financial aid, scholarship, and grant information is the Association of American Medical Colleges. Remember to request information early for eligibility, application requirements, and deadlines.

Association of American Medical Colleges
2450 N Street, NW
Washington, DC 20037
TEL: 202-828-0400
WEBSITE: http://www.aamc.org
Specific information on financial aid programs can be found at:
WEBSITE: http://www.aamc.org/stuapps/finaid

Ferguson Publishing Company
200 West Madison, Suite 300
Chicago, IL 60606
TEL: 312-580-5480

National Health Services Corps Scholarship Program
U.S. Public Health Service
1010 Wayne Avenue, Suite 240
Silver Spring, MD 20910
TEL: 800-638-0824

who will hire me?

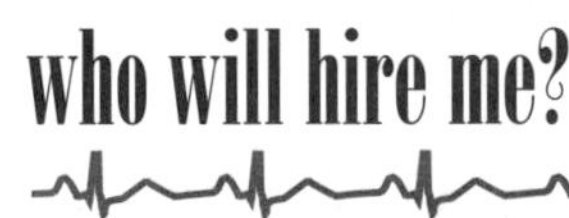

There are few solo practitioners of neurological surgery. Most neurological surgeons enter into private practice with a partner or a small group. Those working at medical schools, private clinics, and hospitals are part of larger groups of neurological surgeons.

where can I go from here?

Research and teaching are two options for the neurological surgeon. Many neurological surgeons combine the two with a private practice. Advancements in this field generally consist of ascending through the ranks of physicians and surgeons to head a department or a hospital. Many neurological surgeons aspire to become the Chief of Neurosurgery, but appointment to this position is extremely competitive.

what are the salary ranges?

Salaries for residents vary from about $30,000 to $42,000 a year. Salaries will vary depending on the kind of residency, the hospital, and the geographic area.

According to surveys by the American Medical Association, annual income for surgeons in the mid-1990's ranged from approximately $140,000 to $300,000, with the median income at about $200,000. These figures are for all surgeons, and incomes may vary from specialty to specialty. Other factors influencing individual incomes include type and size of practice, hours worked per week, geographic area, and professional reputation.

what is the job outlook?

The health care industry is thriving and the employment of physicians in almost all fields is expected to grow faster than the average for all occupations through the year 2005.

Neurological surgery is so specialized and highly competitive that there will always be a demand for the special skills and expertise of the neurological surgeon. As technology continues to increase and procedures are developed that enable previously inoperable cases to be successfully resolved through surgery, the case load will also rise.

how do I learn more?

professional organizations

Following are organizations that provide information on the profession of neurological surgeon. The Association of Women Surgeons publishes *Pocket Mentor—A Manual for Surgical Interns and Residents*, a guide for women in the surgical specialties.

American Association of Neurological Surgeons
22 South Washington Street
Suite 100
Park Ridge, IL 60058
TEL: 847-692-9500
WEBSITE: http://www.aans.org

Association of Women Surgeons
414 Plaza Drive
Suite 209
Westmont, IL 60559
TEL: 630-655-0392

bibliography

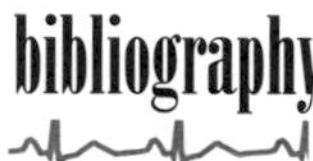

Following is a sampling of materials relating to the professional concerns and development of neurological surgeons.

Books

Allen, Marshall B., and Ross H. Miller. *Essentials of Neurosurgery: a Guide to Clinical Practice*. New York, NY: McGraw-Hill, 1994.

Apuzzo, Michael, editor. *Neurosurgery for the Third Millennium*. Park Ridge, IL: American Association of Neurological Surgeons, 1992.

Black, Peter M., and Eugene Rossitch. *Neurosurgery: an Introductory Text*. New York, NY: Oxford University Press, 1995.

Flitter, Marc. *Judith's Pavilion: the Haunting Memories of a Neurosurgeon.* South Royaltron, VT: Steerforth Press, 1997.

Greenblatt, Samuel H., T. Forcht Dagi, and Mel H. Epstein. *A History of Neurosurgery*. Park Ridge, IL: American Association of Neurological Surgeons, 1996.

Grossman, Robert G., and Christopher M. Loftus, editors. *Principles of Neurosurgery*, 2nd edition. Philadelphia, PA: Lippincott-Raven, 1997.

Jennett, Bryan, and Kenneth W. Lindsay. *An Introduction to Neurosurgery*, 5th edition. Newton, MA: Butterworth-Heinemann, 1994.

Tindall, George N., Paul R. Cooper, and Daniel L. Barrow. *The Practice of Neurosurgery*. Baltimore, MD: Williams & Wilkins, 1995.

Vertosick, Frank T., Jr. *When the Air Hits Your Brain: Tales of Neurosurgery*. New York, NY: Norton, 1996.

Wilkins, Robert, editor. *Neurosurgical Classics*, 2nd edition. Park Ridge, IL: American Association of Neurological Surgeons, 1992.

Periodicals

Journal of Neurosurgery. Monthly. Presents medical articles relating to neurosurgery and allied specialties. American Association of Neurological Surgeons, 1224 W. Main Street, Suite 450, Charlottesville, VA 22903, 804-924-2702.

Neurosurgery. Monthly. Explains techniques and devices, plus pertinent research in neuroscience. Congress of Neurological Surgeons, Williams & Wilkins, 428 E. Preston Street, Baltimore, MD 21202, 410-528-4000, 800-638-6423.

neurologist

Definition

Neurologists diagnose and treat patients with diseases and disorders affecting such areas as the brain, spinal cord, peripheral nerves, muscles, and autonomic nervous system.

Salary range

$31,000 to $117,000 to $147,000+

Educational requirements

Bachelor's degree, M.D., one year study in internal medicine, three years in an accredited neurological residency program.

Certification or Licensing

Certification is highly recommended; licensing is mandatory

Outlook

Faster than average

GOE
02.03.01

DOT
070

High School Subjects

Biology
Chemistry
English
Mathematics
Physics
Social sciences

Personal Interests

Helping people
Problem solving
Working with technology

Bad examples sometimes teach important lessons. During her residency training Dr. Janet Jankowiak learned from just such an example. One Monday morning she was with a group of residents on neurological service. The attending physician led the group to the room of a patient who had been brought into the trauma unit over the weekend. Although the trauma physicians and nurses had desperately tried to save the patient's life, only machines now kept the woman technically alive. By law, the neurological service unit had to perform specific tests to determine whether or not the patient was brain dead. The woman's family waited in an area nearby, and as the residents approached they could see the family members huddled together in prayer.

A nurse walked up to the attending physician and said in low tones, "The family has waited all night to speak with the neurologist. I promised I'd let them know when you got here."

Although he nodded, the attending physician made no move toward the area with the family members. Instead, he continued on into the patient's room and began leading the residents through the series of perfunctory tests. When they finished, he signed the patient's chart, indicating the woman was brain dead. Then, without so much as a glance over his shoulder, he silently lead the surprised residents down a back stairway, away from the grieving, confused family.

"I was so appalled by the whole thing, I actually can't believe I experienced it," Dr. Jankowiak says. "But it taught me the importance of understanding what people need from me, as a doctor and as a person." Today as a neurologist at a major hospital, Dr. Jankowiak works hard to address her patients' individual concerns as well as to treat their illnesses.

lingo to learn

Cerebral spinal fluid analysis Under local anesthesia, fluid is drawn from the spinal column and then analyzed. The test is often crucial in making the diagnosis of a bleeding disorder, tumor, or infection of the brain or spinal cord. Also referred to as a spinal tap.

Computerized tomography A form of radiology, or X ray, which uses computers to construct two-dimensional pictures of selected body parts. Dye may be injected into a vein to obtain a better picture. Also referred to as a CT or CAT scan.

Electroencephalogram (EEG) A procedure that uses electrodes attached to the scalp to record the brain's continuous electrical activity.

Electromyogram (EMG) A test that measures and records electrical activity from the muscles and nerves. It is often used in cases involving pain, numbness, tingling, or weakness.

Evoked potentials A test that records the brain's electrical responses to visual, auditory, and sensory stimuli. They are useful in evaluating and diagnosing symptoms of dizziness, numbness, and tingling, as well as some visual problems.

what does a neurologist do?

A *neurologist* evaluates, diagnoses, and treats patients with diseases and disorders impairing the function of the brain, spinal cord, peripheral nerves, muscles, and autonomic nervous system, as well as treating the supporting structures and vascular supply to these areas. A neurologist conducts and evaluates specific tests relating to the analysis of the central or peripheral nervous system.

In addition to treating such neurological disorders as epilepsy, neuritis, brain and spinal cord tumors, multiple sclerosis, Parkinson's disease, and stroke, neurologists treat muscle disorders and pain, especially headache. Also, illnesses, injuries, or diseases that can adversely affect the nervous system, such as diabetes, hypertension, and cancers, are treated by neurologists.

Neurologists see patients in two capacities—as a consulting physician, or as the patient's principal physician. A neurologist works as a consulting physician when asked by a patient's primary care physician to consult on a case as, for example, when a patient has a stroke or shows signs of mental confusion. As a consulting physician, the neurologist conducts a neurological evaluation and evaluates mental, emotional, and behavioral problems to assess whether these conditions are treatable. The neurologist also works with psychiatrists, psychologists, or other mental health professionals as necessary.

A neurologist is the principal physician for patients with such illnesses as Parkinson's disease or multiple sclerosis. A neurologist working as the principal physician, for example, might evaluate a patient who has suffered several inexplicable seizures. The neurologist might use the results of a CT scan and an encephalogram to diagnose the patient with epilepsy. To manage this disorder, the neurologist might prescribe medications, such as antiepileptic drugs. If the patient tolerates the medications well, the neurologist might see the patient every three to six months, maybe only once a year.

Sometimes, a primary care physician believes a consultation with a neurologist might benefit a patient. In this case the primary care physician would refer the patient to a neurologist for what is called a neurological consultation. A neurological consultation is a review of the patient's medical history, a physical examination, and tests of vision, strength, coordination, reflexes, and sensation. These tests help the neurologist to determine whether the source of the patient's problem is within the nervous system. Further tests may be necessary to confirm the diagnosis and determine specific treatment.

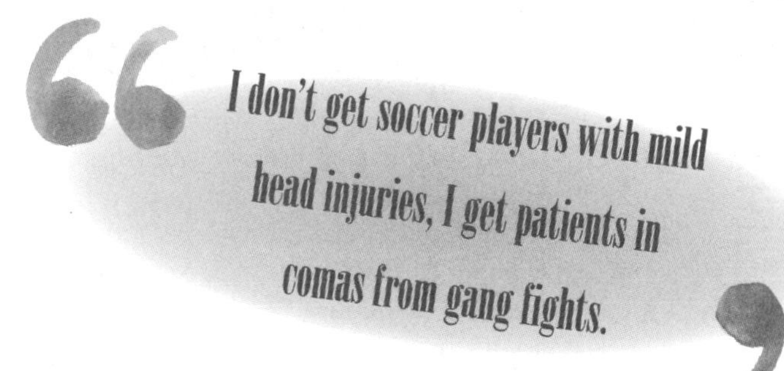

what is it like to be a neurologist?

"The nervous system gives you specific symptoms to let you know what's wrong," says Dr. Jack Whisnant, Director of the Mayo Cerebrovascular Clinical Research Center, in Rochester, Minnesota. "In other areas of medicine, discomfort doesn't necessarily indicate the precise problem." It has often been said that neurology is as close as clinical medicine comes to obeying scientific principles of biology. "Symptoms and functions are very closely related in neurology," says Dr. Whisnant. "You have to understand the anatomy and physiology of the brain and the spinal cord."

The close relationship between symptoms and functions signifies the importance of the neurologist's evaluation of the patient. Taking the history and performing a physical examination combine to provide the neurologist with the answers to important questions. "The history helps you determine the process, and the exam tells you where the problem is located," Dr. Whisnant says. As part of the physical examination, the neurologist performs reflex tests; examines the patient's ability to walk, balance on one foot, or other movements; and analyzes the patient's strength, vision, and sensation.

"The distribution of abnormalities throughout the body can tell you where the problem is," explains Dr. Whisnant. "The nervous system tells you what's going on," he emphasizes. "So, it's extremely important to detail the onset and the evolution of the problem—when the symptoms stopped or subsided, for example."

Dr. Janet Jankowiak works at an inner-city hospital in Boston, where she specializes in rehabilitating patients with strokes, geriatric dementia (mental deterioration caused by aging), traumatic brain injuries, and behavioral neurological problems. Almost all of her patient evaluations begin with a mental status examination in which she gauges how alert and attentive her patients are. She runs them through a series of tests, checking such things as their attention span, language skills, and memory. For example, she might ask a patient to show her how to use a hammer or to name in order the days of a week. If the patient has trouble remembering what a hammer is or the names and order of days, it could be an indication of damage to the frontal lobes.

Diagnostic neurology reveals the patient's condition, but this is only one side of the job; managing the case is the flip side. Practicing neurologists often have the responsibility for managing the acute- and long-term care and rehabilitation of their patients. Since 1994, Dr. Jankowiak has been the Director of Brain Injury Rehabilitation at Jewish Memorial Hospital and Rehabilitation Center (JMHRC). "Seventy percent of traumatic brain injuries are to young men in their early twenties—men in the prime of their lives, really—who are victims of motor vehicle accidents, assaults, gun shot wounds." Dr. Jankowiak works with her patient's family to get the patient into rehab. "Getting through to these patients and convincing them of the necessity of rehabilitation is often difficult in these circumstances. Most of these patients say they don't need help or rehabilitation," says Dr. Jankowiak. "And they usually have a host of other problems that complicate things." These problems range from alcoholism and drug use to poverty to physical abuse. According to Dr. Jankowiak, however, if the patient leaves the hospital without help, his or her problems could multiply. "Often, these patients have short-term memory problems. If a patient has a job, he could lose it in the days following his head injury because he just can't remember things. A housewife can't divide her attention between tasks because that part of her brain has suffered some damage."

It's no wonder, then, that part of Dr. Jankowiak's job involves identifying the social issues that complicate her patients' lives and then trying to get her patients to agree to some modification of those issues for the betterment of their own health. Sometimes, she can get her patients into group homes, but the odds are usually against her patients scoring triumphant recoveries. Often, they revert to the drugs or alcohol or physical abuse that, in turn, leads them back into situations in which they sustain more damaging injuries. "You just do the best you can," says Dr. Jankowiak. "You try and help them modify their behavior."

Dr. Whisnant's specialty is stroke patients. Strokes are caused by abnormalities in the brain's blood vessels. According to Dr. Whisnant, strokes generally occur in one of two manners. Either the force of blood coursing through the arterial wall causes the wall to break, and blood leaks (hemorrhages) through the breach, or the blood vessel itself is obstructed (occluded) and the tissue dies. The dead tissue is also called an infarction. Strokes occur more frequently in older patients, but younger patients, even children, can experience strokes. Neurologists can usually identify a stroke easily by the patient's complaint of a sudden onset of paralysis on one side. Often, the paralysis is complicated by compromised vision and aphasia (loss of speech and language). Amazingly, for all the damage it has wreaked, the stroke might not alter the patient's consciousness at all.

"A stroke is severe at the outset, but it can subside," Dr. Whisnant says. "It can do its maximum damage in a second." More often, he explains, the stroke evolves for a short period of time, usually several hours. In more rare cases, the stroke may evolve over a period of a few days. In severe cases, the patient typically goes to the hospital or urgent-care center where a neurological surgeon evaluates him or her. With a more mild stroke, the patient often delays the visit to his or her physician or neurologist for up to a week or more. Dr. Whisnant says that although patients usually know something is wrong, if the symptoms seem mild enough to ignore for a bit, patients usually do ignore them. Unfortunately, this can jeopardize their recovery. "It's so important that they be evaluated, because strokes can be prevented," stresses Dr. Whisnant. "We have preventative medications and surgical procedures to prevent strokes. There are drugs to dissolve clots and promote recovery, but they must be administered within the first three hours of the stroke's occurrence."

Among the most common surgical remedies is the carotid endarterectomy. In this procedure an angiogram (a radiographic image of blood vessels) is taken to show exactly where the artery narrows due to the accumulation of plaque. Neurological surgeons then surgically remove the plaque from the arterial wall. Preventative medications, like surgery, carry their own set of risks. For example, thrombolitic drugs (drugs that cause the break up of a blood clot) that have the potential to prevent strokes or reverse paralysis are not appropriate for all patients because they can increase the risk of hemorrhage. These drugs have been through clinical trials and received Federal Drug Administration (FDA) approval, but their practical application hasn't yet been perfected. "The clinical trials are complete," Dr. Whisnant says, "but they're still evolving." He goes on to

more lingo to learn

Magnetic resonance imaging (MRI) An advanced way of making images of what is inside the brain. For this test a patient lies still in a small chamber for approximately thirty minutes while a very strong magnet passes over the brain.

Myelogram A test in which dye is injected into the spinal canal, making the structure clearly visible to X rays.

Neurosonography A test that uses ultra high-frequency sound waves to analyze blood flow, most often in stroke victims.

Seizure A sudden attack often characterized by altered consciousness and convulsions.

explain that using drugs like these requires a team of doctors working together to monitor the application of the drugs.

Dr. Whisnant is at ease discussing the research side of neurology for good reason. Since 1975 he has been the Director of the Mayo Clinic's Cerebrovascular Clinical Research Center, dividing his time between practicing neurology and working in neurological research—specifically, population-based epidemiology. He recently retired from diagnostic neurology to devote himself, full time, to his research. "The primary goal of my research has been to discover what causes diseases, or chronic disease epidemiology," explains Dr. Whisnant. Epidemiology is the record of the natural history of a disease. His work focuses on the epidemiology of strokes in Rochester County, Minnesota—a comparison of factors that influence the occurrence of strokes in patients within that defined area. "The records for Rochester County begin in 1907, but the most important data begins in the 1950s," Dr. Whisnant says. His duties as director of the clinical research center include planning studies, supervising data collection and abstract writing, and conducting statistical analysis of as many as 1,500 patients in order to determine the outcomes and what influenced those outcomes. Dr. Whisnant still teaches neuroscience at the Mayo Medical School. Before he retired from practice, he took rounds in the morning with the resident staff and saw patients individually on an outpatient basis in the afternoons.

To be a successful neurologist, you should

- Be a good clinician
- Be able to listen and communicate well
- Be patient and detail-oriented
- Enjoy helping and working with people
- Have good hand-eye coordination and manual dexterity

have I got what it takes to be a neurologist?

Dr. Jankowiak doesn't mince words when describing the rigors and frustrations of her job. "I work in an inner city hospital," she says, "with the kind of patients Medicaid and Medicare doesn't want to pay for. I don't get soccer players with mild head injuries, I get patients in comas from gang fights. Many don't make it. Those who do come around, generally have a whole host of other problems to complicate their rehabilitation—alcoholism, drug use, abusive behavior."

Each day presents a new challenge, whether it is cutbacks due to managed care, insurance companies refusing to pay for an expensive test for an indigent patient, or patients who refuse to be helped. Granted, not all neurologists practice in the inner city, but most do have a variety of cases. Because they treat patients who have suffered injuries to the head, neurologists need to have a calm and soothing presence with patients who may be experiencing alternating emotions, including confusion and anger. Many of Dr. Jankowiak's patients are older and have geriatric dementia. "Very often, I spend a lot of time reassuring them that they're not crazy," she says. "They realize something is wrong, but they don't want to admit it and they don't want to be treated like children. In fact, the closer you get to the areas of their deficits, the more angry and defensive they get. Sometimes, you have to struggle to remember that each person is different, and will require from you something different than the last patient. It can be very difficult. You need the patience of a saint." Dr. Jankowiak adds, "You do as much as you can—but you have to realize there are limits. Still, it's not always easy to let go."

"You need to be able to treat your patients with a great deal of compassion. You have to try and preserve the dignity of each patient. People always seem amazed when I manage to reach through to a patient with dementia. It's like learning another language. You don't always have to know the words to get your point across." She uses a common analogy to illustrate her point. "I like to see the glass as half full, rather than seeing the glass as half empty. I always ask myself, 'what can we do to expand their lives?'"

In addition to compassion, neurologists need a mind capable of sifting through a lot of data for specific details. "You need an interest in relating to people and sorting out diseases," advises Dr. Whisnant. "People who are very compulsive about details are attracted to neurology," he adds. "It's a demanding specialty, and medical students aren't easily attracted to it because it seems too complicated. You do need a broad base of knowledge, but neurology looks to be more complicated than it really is."

While Dr. Jankowiak acknowledges that neurology is a challenging speciality, she believes young doctors considering a specialty should not be intimidated by the field. "If you like it and have the passion to do it—do it," she says. "You really need the passion. Just don't lose sight of what uniqueness you bring to the job."

Both Dr. Whisnant and Dr. Jankowiak agree that the field is incredibly exciting. "Talk about a frontier," says Dr. Jankowiak. "Neurology truly is a pioneering field."

how do I become a neurologist?

education

High School

If you are interested in pursuing a medical degree, a high school education emphasizing college preparatory classes is a must. Science courses, such as biology, chemistry, and physics, are necessary, as are math courses. These classes will not only provide you with an introduction to basic science and math concepts, but also allow you to determine your own aptitude in these areas. Since college will be your next educational step, it is also important to take English courses to develop your researching and writing skills. Foreign language, social science, and computer classes will also help make you an appealing candidate for college admission as well as prepare you for your future undergraduate and graduate education. Some colleges and universities that also have medical schools have accelerated programs for students who are certain that they want at attend medical school. High school seniors who are sure of their desire to pursue a medical degree may wish to look carefully at these programs. These programs typically reduce or consolidate the number of years spent as an undergraduate and, thereby, speed up entrance into medical school. Often, the programs refer to the number of years in their title. For example, a six- or seven-year med student is actually enrolled in two or three years, respectively, of undergraduate school, plus the requisite four years of medical school. Special restrictions and qualifying requirements apply, so students interested in this option should contact the school early on in the application process. High school guidance counselors should also be able to provide you with information and direction.

Postsecondary Training

If you are not entering an accelerated program following high school, the next step on your educational path to be a neurologist is to earn a bachelor's degree from an accredited four-year college or university. Suggested premedical courses include physics, biology, and organic and inorganic chemistry. Courses in English and the humanities, mathematics, and the social sciences are also highly recommended.

After receiving an undergraduate degree, you must then apply and be accepted to medical school. Admission is competitive and applicants must undergo a fairly extensive and difficult admissions process which considers grade point averages, scores on the Medical College Admission Test (MCAT), and recommendations from professors. Most students apply to several schools early in their senior year of college.

In order to earn the degree doctor of medicine (M.D.), a student must complete four years of medical school study and training. For the first two years of medical school, students attend lectures and classes and spend time in laboratories. Courses include anatomy, biochemistry, physiology, pharmacology, psychology, microbiology, pathology, medical ethics, and laws governing medicine. They learn to take patient histories, perform routine physical examinations, and recognize symptoms.

In their third and fourth years, students are involved in more practical studies. They work in clinics and hospitals supervised by residents and physicians and they learn acute, chronic, preventive, and rehabilitative care. They go through what are known as rotations (brief periods of study) in such areas as internal medicine, obstetrics and gynecology, pediatrics, dermatology, psychiatry, and surgery. Rotations allow students to gain exposure to the many different fields within medicine and to learn firsthand the skills of diagnosing and treating patients.

Dr. Jankowiak decided to go to medical school in France and attended the L'Universite Louis Pasteur de Strasbourg, Faculte de Medecine. Taking science courses in French

in-depth

Repetitive head injuries

Nationally, repetitive head injuries account for a large chunk of the traumatic brain injury cases, many of which come from sports-related incidents. "Football players, boxers," Dr. Janet Jankowiak ticks them off a mental list, "and, believe it or not, soccer players, who constantly butt the ball with their heads. What used to be considered a mild concussion, may not be so mild after all." She explains, "It used to be that a loss of consciousness was the standard for keeping players from going back into the game. Fortunately, there is a new grading system for checking out players before they return to the field. It's a lot easier to keep players off the field with the new system, and thus prevent further damage to their brains."

Repetitive blows to the brain damage it in subtle ways that have not-so-subtle repercussions down the line. "Strange, violent, and socially inappropriate behavior may be attributable to head injuries. Patients with a history of these sort of injuries tend to have impaired insight and judgment and lose all inhibitions. They get themselves into situations that can only lead to further damage. It's a vicious cycle," says Dr. Jankowiak.

As Director of Brain Injury Rehabilitation at Jewish Memorial Hospital and Rehabilitation Center (JMHRC) in Boston, Massachusetts, Dr. Jankowiak is all for preventative measures that would safeguard against damage to the brain. "The most prominent injury is to the frontal lobes," she warns. "This is the part of the brain that is responsible for organization, planning, insight—for what makes you a human being," she says forcefully. "So, wear your seat belt at all times, keep infants and small children in the back seat, and when you're riding your bike, wear your helmet." She adds, "I biked all over France without a helmet, and then I did my first rotation in neurology. I never rode a bike without a helmet again." Also, the helmet has to be worn correctly for it to do any good. "It should cover the entire forehead," she instructs. "On most people, the helmet is back too far, leaving the frontal lobes vulnerable to injury."

was difficult, she says, but worthwhile. "Science saved me," she admits. "My French wasn't so good, back then."

Upon graduating from an accredited medical school, physicians must pass a standard examination given by the National Board of Medical Examiners. Graduates of non-U.S. medical schools must pass the examinations administered by the Educational Commission for Foreign Medical Graduates (ECFMG).

Most physicians complete an internship, also referred to as a transition year. The internship is usually one year in length, and helps graduates to decide what will be their area of specialization.

Following the internship, physicians usually begin what is known as a residency. Those physicians who choose to specialize in neurology must first complete a full year of training in internal medicine in a program approved by the Accreditation Council for Graduate Medical Education (ACGME). Then, the physician must enroll in an accredited, three-year neurology residency program. As an alternative to this prescribed training, the physician may complete four years of training in an ACGME-approved neurology program. These residency programs provide supervised neurology experience in both hospital and ambulatory (outpatient) settings. Educational conferences and research training are also part of a neurology residency.

"Look for a mentor to give you feedback and encouragement," Dr. Whisnant suggests.

He had already chosen internal medicine as his specialty and entered the residency that would move him one step closer to becoming a neurologist, but he credits a professor with whom he worked as being the real force behind his decision. “One of my mentors, the Chair of the department, nurtured me through my rotation in neurology. He was an excellent teacher who gave a lot of attention to me and my learning,” explains Dr. Whisnant. “He influenced me by his care of patients, but even more than that, he took the time to nurture me as an individual, rather than treating me as just another resident rotating through.”

Often, residents learn quickly what they don’t want to do, which helps them narrow down their interests. “I knew I didn’t want to be in acute care,” says Dr. Jankowiak. “I respect and admire those who can withstand all that stress, but I didn’t like the emergency room. I didn’t want to be on the spot all the time. I like to mull things over, sit back and think about a problem.”

certification or licensing

Upon completion of residency training, neurologists may seek certification from the American Board of Psychiatry and Neurology (ABPN). To be eligible for certification, qualified applicants must have: an unrestricted state license to practice medicine; completed the required years of residency training; and successfully passed both a written (Part I) and oral (Part II) examination, as administered by the ABPN.

Licensing is a mandatory procedure in the United States. It is required in all states before any doctor can practice medicine. In order to be licensed, doctors must have graduated from medical school, passed the licensing test of the state in which they will practice, and completed their residency.

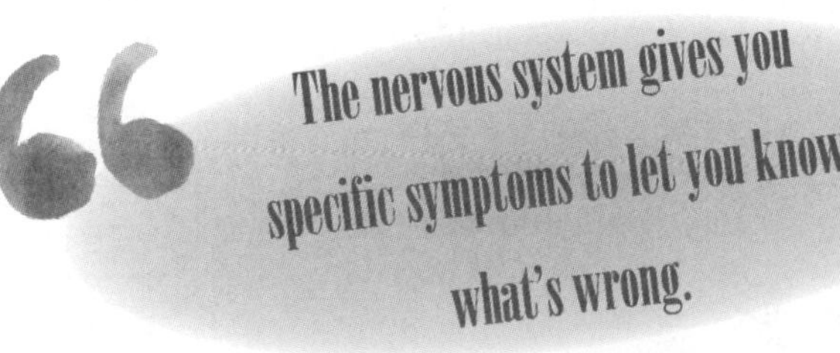

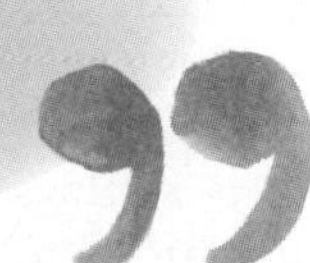

scholarships and grants

Scholarships and grants are often available from individual institutions, state agencies, and special-interest organizations. The book *Dollars for College: Medicine, Dentistry, and Related Fields* by Ferguson Publishing Company is an excellent source for this information. Many students finance their medical education through the Armed Forces Health Professions Scholarship Program. Each branch of the military participates in this program, paying students’ tuitions in exchange for military service. Contact your local recruiting office for more information. The National Health Service Corps Scholarship Program also provides money for students in return for service. Another source for financial aid, scholarship, and grant information is the Association of American Medical Colleges. Remember to request information early for eligibility, application requirements, and deadlines.

Association of American Medical Colleges
2450 N Street, NW
Washington, DC 20037
TEL: 202-828-0400
WEBSITE: http://www.aamc.org
Specific information on financial aid programs can be found at:
WEBSITE: http://www.aamc.org/stuapps/finaid

Ferguson Publishing Company
200 West Madison, Suite 300
Chicago, IL 60606
TEL: 312-580-5480

National Health Services Corps Scholarship Program
U.S. Public Health Service
1010 Wayne Avenue, Suite 240
Silver Spring, MD 20910
TEL: 800-638-0824

who will hire me?

Positions are available in general and subspecialty neurology in academic teaching institutions and group practice, military, health maintenance organizations (HMOs), and solo practice in urban and rural areas. Subspecialization in new and emerging areas include neuroimmunology, neuromuscular disorders, instrumental brain and nervous system monitoring, neurooncology, rehabilitation, and geriatric neurology.

There are also many opportunities in academic neuroscience and clinical and basic research in neurology for MD investigators. Neuroscience is the most rapidly-expanding field in all of medical research and, as a result, research and teaching positions should be plentiful, well into the year 2005 and beyond.

where can I go from here?

Neurologists can advance in their field by heading departments and chairing committees, by assuming administrative and/or supervisory positions, and by increasing their standing in the field by publishing articles in respected medical journals, such as *JAMA*, or *Neurology*.

Research is a vital part of neuroscience, and neurologists who are interested in research can advance their careers by running research projects and neurological studies. Pharmaceutical companies also need trained researchers to head their research in neurological science.

Participating in committees and professional organizations and societies can also help neurologists make valuable connections that may one day lead to other jobs. In addition, Dr. Jankowiak recommends getting involved in medical politics. "I believe it's important to be politically involved. You can't just sit back and complain without trying to make a difference." Dr. Jankowiak started a faculty and administration organization called "Forum for Positive Change" to address issues in medicine. She also volunteers for the American Academy of Neurology, helping them publicize the role of the neurologist and the field.

what are the salary ranges?

The national average salary for first-year residents in the mid-1990's was approximately $31,000. That average increased to $41,800 by the final residency year. Salaries will vary depending on the kind of residency, the hospital, and the geographic area.

According to the Medical Group Management Association, a 1995 report based on data from the previous year indicates that the median salary for neurologists with one to two years of experience was approximately $117,000. Neurologists practicing for between three to seven years averaged annual salaries of about $147,000. Those neurologists with between eight and seventeen years of experience earned an average annual salary of approximately $171,000. These figures are only a guide. Individual salaries will vary depending on such factors as type and size of practice, geographic area, and professional reputation.

what is the job outlook?

The health care industry is thriving and the employment of physicians in almost all fields is expected to grow faster than the average for all occupations through the year 2005. In particular, the specialty of neurology should increase. In the United States, neurologic illnesses make up 15 to 20 percent of all general medical care. As effective therapies are developed for more neurologic diseases, and some diseases, such as Alzheimer's, increase in prevalence, the demand for neurologists will increase.

how do I learn more?

professional organizations

Following are organizations that provide information on the certification and profession of neurologist.

American Academy of Neurology, Member Services
2221 University Avenue SE, Suite 335
Minneapolis, MN 55414
TEL: 612-623-8115
WEBSITE: http://www.aan.com

The American Board of Psychiatry and Neurology, Inc.
500 Lake Cook Road, Suite 335
Deerfield, IL 60015
TEL: 847-945-7900

bibliography

Following is a sampling of materials relating to the professional concerns and development of neurologists.

Books

Beran, Roy. *Neurology for General Practitioners*. New York, NY: McGraw-Hill, 1996.

Curtis, Brian A. *Neurosciences: the Basics*. Baltimore, MD: Williams & Wilkins, 1990.

Gilroy, John. *Basic Neurology,* 3rd edition. New York, NY: McGraw-Hill, 1996.

McLeod, James, and others. *Introductory Neurology,* 3rd edition. Cambridge, MA: Blackwell Science, 1995.

Ward, Christopher D. *Outline of Neurology.* New York, NY: Butterworth-Heinemann, 1992.

Weiner, William J., and others. *Neurology for the Non-Neurologist,* 3rd edition. Philadelphia, PA: Lippincott-Raven, 1994.

Periodicals

Annals of Neurology. Monthly. Contains articles on research and clinical advances, brief communications, neurological progress, and editorials. American Neurological Association, Little, Brown, Medical Journals, 34 Beacon Street, Boston, MA 02108, 617-859-5500.

Journal of Comparative Neurology. Weekly. Presents articles about the anatomy and physiology of the nervous system. Wiley Journals, 605 Third Avenue, New York, NY 10058, 212-850-6645.

Neurology. Monthly. Reports, discussions, case findings, and clinical findings on current research and developments in neurology. Covers neurological symptoms of diseases, diagnostic methods, and treatments. Advanstar Communications, Inc., 7500 Old Oak Boulevard, Cleveland, OH 44130, 215-826-2839.

Seminars in Pediatric Neurology. Quarterly. Covers topics of current importance in the field of pediatric neurology. W.B. Saunders Co., Curtis Center, 3rd Floor, Independence Square West, Philadelphia, PA 19106, 215-238-7800.

nuclear medicine technologist

Definition

Nuclear medicine technologists work with patients and physicians to diagnose and treat certain conditions with radioactive drugs. They prepare and administer dosages, operate cameras that record images of the drug as it passes through or stays in parts of the body, and keep careful records for review by the supervising physician.

Salary range

$28,000 to $35,000 to $42,000

Educational requirements

High school diploma; completion of training program in either a hospital, community college, or four-year college or university

Certification or licensing

Certification by one of two national organizations is required in most jobs; about half of all states require a state license as well.

Outlook

Faster than average

GOE
10.02.02

DOT
078

High School Subjects

Algebra
Biology
Chemistry
Physics

Personal Interests

Anatomy
Computers
Physiology
Social services
Team sports

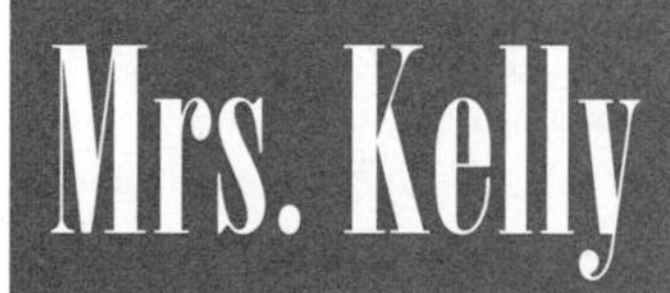

sits on the edge of her chair in the waiting room, fingering an outdated *People* magazine. She looks nervous. Behind the door of room 119, Tim Dunn, who has just finished a half-hour quality control test on his cameras, scans his patient list.

Soon Tim enters the waiting room. "OK, Mrs. Kelly. I'm Tim, and I'll be running a few tests. How're you feeling today?"

Mrs. Kelly smiles apologetically. "My back hurts a lot now, and I'm pretty tired. My doctor thought I should get checked. Is this dangerous?"

Tim has seen Mrs. Kelly's medical record. He knows that she had her right breast removed for cancer three years ago, and that the cancer may have metastasized (spread) to her bones.

"Well, Mrs. K., I'm sorry to hear you're not at your best. This test is a good way to find out why your back hurts. I'm going to inject a radioactive substance into your bloodstream to see how it is absorbed by your bones. It won't hurt, and it'll expose you to only about as much radiation as a chest X ray."

After the injection, Tim notices Mrs. Kelly take a deep breath and then sigh. "It'll take a while for this substance to get into your bones, so you can go do some errands. Let's see, it's 9:00 now, so I'll see you just before lunch. I think there's a haddock special in the hospital cafeteria, so you can treat yourself afterwards."

At 11:30, Mrs. Kelly is waiting. Tim greets her again, "Come on in, Mrs. K. You'll just get up on this table here. No, you don't have to wear a johnny, just take off your watch and your earrings. Your test will take about forty-five minutes. We're going to take pictures of your whole body from head to toe."

Later, Tim reshoots the abdominal area, which was blurry on the first pass, and prints out on film several views for the nuclear medicine physician to examine. By then he suspects what he cannot tell Mrs. Kelly: that her breast cancer has spread to her lower spine. The diagnosis will be relayed to her oncologist (cancer doctor), who will tell Mrs. Kelly what to expect from this new turn in her disease.

lingo to learn

Cancer A general term for many diseases that are characterized by uncontrolled, abnormal growth of cells, which can spread through the bloodstream to other parts of the body.

Gamma ray Electromagnetic radiation put out by an element going through radioactive decay, having the energy of thousands or even millions of electron volts.

Nuclear medicine The area of medical technology and knowledge based on using radioactive elements to identify and treat certain diseases.

Radiation The energy that is emitted from atomic elements when their nuclei break up.

Radioactivity A characteristic that certain elements (such as radium and strontium) have that makes their atomic nuclei disintegrate and thus emit alpha, beta, and/or gamma rays.

Radium A shiny radioactive element that is used in the treatment of cancer.

what does a nuclear medicine technologist do?

Radiation has long been used to diagnose and treat many illnesses. Doctors use radiography (X-ray imaging) to penetrate the soft tissues of the body to reveal on film a crack in a bone, for example, or a tumor in an organ. Nuclear medicine technology is also used for diagnosing and treating illness and disease, but, unlike radiography, with nuclear technology a patient is given radioactive drugs, either by injection or by drinking liquid or taking a pill. The progress of the radioactive substance through the body is recorded by special cameras or scanners, and the functions of body systems are thus documented.

Nuclear medicine imaging is used to diagnose several types of diseases and disorders of major organs such as the bones, heart, brain, lungs, liver, and kidneys. Sometimes the technology is used on specimens from a patient, such as blood or urine, to detect and measure small amounts of hormones or drugs. At other times, the technology is used for therapy; for example, to destroy abnormal thyroid tissue that may have migrated throughout the body. In some instances, radioactive strontium is administered to ease the pain of terminally ill patients with bone cancer.

Nuclear medicine technologists are involved primarily with patient care, under the direction of physicians, although they usually set their own schedules. They prepare dosages of radioactive drugs to give to patients, explain procedures to patients and reassure them that the procedures are safe, position patients for imaging, and operate the gamma-ray-detecting equipment and scanner. They make sure the images of the target organ are clear and understandable and then process the images. Technologists sometimes have to rescan certain areas to get a better diagnosis. Nuclear medicine technologists also work in the lab, applying radioactive drugs to specimens from patients to detect certain drugs or hormones.

Radioactive substances are under the control of either the federal Nuclear Regulatory Commission or a state agency, depending on where the hospital or clinic is located. Because they work with radioactive substances, nuclear medical technologists must follow strict procedures and keep complete and accurate records. Technologists are responsible for the inventory, storage, and use of these substances, and the correct disposal of radioactive waste. The technologists are exposed to very little radiation themselves and use lead shields to reduce their risk. They also wear badges that measure radiation while they are in a radiation area.

The administrative duties that these technologists must perform include keeping records of patients and the scanned images, keeping track of the radioactive drugs delivered to the office for use with patients, and overseeing other staff members. Some technologists are responsible for scheduling and assigning tasks for other colleagues.

what is it like to be a nuclear medicine technologist?

Nuclear medicine technologists usually work in hospitals, although employment in clinics and outpatient facilities is becoming more common. They work closely with other professionals in the field, especially radiologic (X-ray) technicians and nuclear medicine physicians.

Tim Dunn, who works at Maine Medical Center, the largest hospital in his state, sees a lot of Mrs. Kellys. He also sees patients like Mr. Sanders, who is forty-two, slightly overweight, and has just quit smoking for the third time. Mr. Sanders is coming in for a cardiac-function test. He will walk and jog on a treadmill until he is exhausted and can't run any more. Then Tim will inject a radioactive substance into one of Mr. Sanders's veins, have him lie on a stretcher, and take pictures of his heart action as revealed by the substance passing through his blood vessels. After forty-five minutes in the lab, Mr. Sanders will be able to leave the hospital but will have to come back after three hours so that Tim can take more pictures to see in what way his heart function returns to a resting state.

Most routine nuclear medicine tests are done during the daytime hours, Monday through Friday, although some hospitals and clinics may have daytime weekend hours as well. In addition, technologists are often on call for emergencies on a rotating basis with their colleagues.

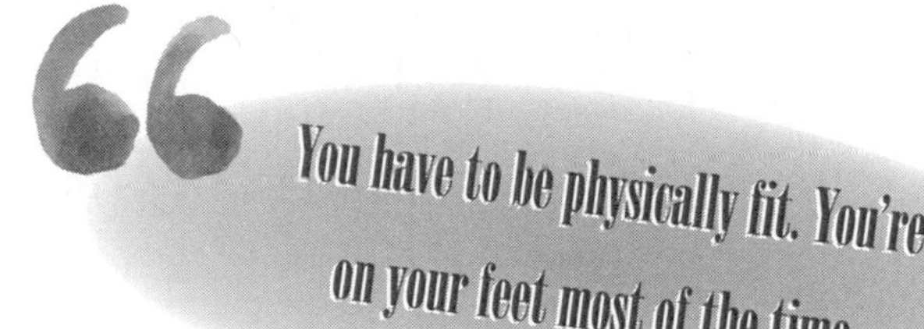

Tim has been at this job for three years. "You set your own schedule. You need to know how long each test takes, how often the images must be recorded, and so on, so that you can make the most efficient use of your time. . . . Oh, and you have to be physically fit. You're on your feet most of the time. Sometimes, if you can't get an orderly, you have to lift patients up onto the table. Maura, who was hired about when I was, works out a couple of days a week at least, to keep her back in shape."

Some crucial aspects of the job may appear routine, such as checking all the diagnostic equipment every day, recording all the information about each test in the patient's record, and keeping track of all the radioactive drugs administered. "My friend Shaun, who works in a smaller hospital north of here, has to do a lot of paperwork because his department is so small. I guess I'm lucky to be in a big hospital, since we have a unit secretary who does the everyday chores," says Tim.

On the other hand, the technologist must be prepared for emergencies. "Just last Monday," says Tim, "another technologist came running into my room and said that her heart patient had just arrested [had a heart attack] right after his stress test. I called in a code and started CPR [cardiopulmonary resuscitation]. Someone else gave him the oxygen bag. When the code team got there they said I was doing just fine, so I kept it up until they got the paddles on him. Whew! I don't want to do that every day. The guy's fine, just got out of surgery with a triple bypass. Boy, I'm glad I insisted I learn CPR!"

have I got what it takes to be a nuclear medicine technologist?

Nuclear medicine technologists must, above all, be good with people. According to Tim,

"First of all, patients are worried about their diagnosis. Some of them suspect that their cancer may have come back or that their heart is in bad shape. You have to be compassionate about their illness, and the pain and fear they are experiencing. Then too, you have the nuclear tag. You need to reassure people that they won't be harmed by radioactivity."

"I was a high school hockey player and can't stress enough the importance of being on a team. You have to work together with the doctors and other technologists. You need to be able to communicate clearly. Part of this is keeping up with your paperwork, so that every member of the team understands what tests the patient had, what the results were, and so forth."

"A person going into this field should have taken physics, biology, and chemistry in high school, and advanced math. I like algebra, and think it relates to this job. I wasn't too fond of calculus, but I don't think that it's a crucial subject," asserts Tim. A good understanding of anatomy and physiology is essential when taking the training.

In some hospitals, nuclear medicine technologists must concoct radioactive drugs out of the raw materials. They need to have good attention to detail, be able to follow procedures, and have math skills adequate enough to understand the relationship of the patient's weight to drug dosage.

A familiarity with computers and an ability to do visual analysis (that is, to see certain patterns) are important as well. "I never thought that the art history course I loved in college would be so useful," states Tim.

To be a successful nuclear medicine technologist, you should

- Communicate well with people, being especially compassionate about their health
- Be able to analyze visual material
- Understand mathematical concepts
- Have the capacity and knowledge to perform CPR
- Know how to be organized and to keep accurate records
- Be relatively physically fit

how do I become a nuclear medicine technologist?

Tim majored in biology in college. "Without a graduate degree," he says, "I couldn't find a job using my major. Then I heard that a fellow graduate had gone into the field as a technologist. Soon after that, I was waiting tables and found out that the wife of one of the regular customers was a nuclear medicine technologist. On her suggestion I toured a local hospital, liked it, and applied to their program."

education

High School

All programs in nuclear medicine technology require a high school diploma. There is no way to apprentice or get hands-on experience without postsecondary education. High school courses in biology, physics, chemistry, and algebra are important for a nuclear medicine technologist. As in Tim Dunn's case, having been involved in a team sport is surprisingly helpful. And, as with many careers, volunteer work (in this case, perhaps in social service) provides valuable learning experiences.

Postsecondary Training

There are a number of ways to become a nuclear medicine technologist, depending on prior education and previous medical work experience. Some training programs are based in hospitals, some are offered in technical colleges, and some are a part of four-year colleges. Students can earn either a certificate, an associate's degree, or a bachelor's degree. All programs that are accredited by the Committee on Allied Health Education and Accreditation (CAHEA) prepare students for entry-level positions in hospitals and clinics.

More than one hundred programs nationwide offer instruction and clinical internship in nuclear medicine technology. These programs can be found mostly on the East Coast, in the Midwest, and on the far West Coast. Most programs are open to a small number of students per year (six to twenty-four), although some are larger. They range in length from one to four years, depending on the qualifications of the student entering.

The curriculum includes courses in anatomy, physiology, nuclear physics, mathematics, chemistry, and computer science. Students also study psychology and sociology, medical terminology, and medical ethics. Course work involves learning the use of the cameras, the nature of radioactive drugs, and federal laws and procedures on handling radioactive materials.

Students usually spend time in hospitals while they are completing their academic course work. This allows them to practice imaging techniques with patients as well as acquaint themselves with laboratory work. According to Tim, it is very important to make sure there is enough clinical training in a program. "I've seen some recent graduates who are really not well prepared to deal with patients."

The professional program is very demanding and competitive, given the small number of openings within most programs. Anyone thinking of this career should talk with program directors at several schools about what will be required of them.

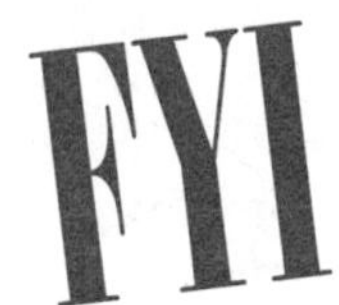

Female Mentor

Manya (Marie) Sklodowska is part of the history of nuclear technology and medicine. Manya learned to read at the age of four and had a remarkable memory. When she was sixteen she won a gold medal and many other awards from the Russian school she attended in her native Poland. She became a teacher and also took part in the "floating university," which was forbidden by the Russians who had control of Poland at the time; she secretly read in Polish to women workers.

Manya, a brilliant scientist, eventually went to Paris, and her marriage to Pierre Curie began a partnership that would lead them to major scientific discoveries. Marie Curie coined the term *radioactivity*, which is the phenomenon that occurs when invisible radiation is emitted from the atoms of certain elements, such as radium. In 1911 she was awarded the Nobel Prize in chemistry for her work in isolating pure radium, which kills diseased cells. Marie Curie was a pioneer, dedicated to science as well as the pursuit of personal goals.

certification or licensing

In some instances, completion of a training program is sufficient for an entry-level position. However, many such positions, especially in hospitals, are open only to those who become registered or certified, by either the Nuclear Medicine Technology Certification Board (NMTCB) or the American Registry of Radiologic Technologists (ARRT). The certification exams are offered two or three times a year by the NMTCB and the ARRT (there are close to forty NMTCB centers and more than one hundred ARRT locations nationwide). The tests can be taken three times. Any candidate who fails the third time has to complete more course work and can retake the tests. Those who pass certification exams may use the title of either Certified Nuclear Medical Technologist (CNMT) or Radiologic Technologist in Nuclear Medicine (RTN), depending on the certifying organization.

Many states require state licensure as well as national certification. These states will accept national certification from either the NMTCB or the ARRT. To maintain a license, the technologist must take a certain number of hours of CEUs (continuing education units). For example, Tim has to take twenty-four credits every two years. These courses are available in day-long workshops as well as in weekend programs. Sometimes, such accredited courses are offered by pharmaceutical companies that run workshops presenting new diagnostic techniques and tools within the hospital.

scholarships and grants

Individual schools may have their own financial aid programs, so you should talk with a counselor in the financial aid office of wherever you are applying. Stipends (which are like allowances given with scholarships) are offered in a small number of institutions, especially in California.

Related Jobs

Nuclear medicine technologists are like radiologic technologists in that they operate diagnostic imaging equipment. The U.S. Department of Labor classifies nuclear medicine technologists under the headings Occupations in Medical and Dental Technology (DOT) and Nursing, Therapy, and Specialized Teaching Services: Therapy and Rehabilitation (GOE). Others in medical and dental technology occupations include biochemistry technologist, cytogenetic technologist, medical radiation dosimetrist, radiologic technologist, Holter scanning technician, and radiation-therapy technologist. Others working in therapy and rehabilitation include dialysis technicians, respiratory therapists, and occupational therapists.

who will hire me?

Hospitals are still the primary employer of nuclear medicine technologists, although clinics, doctors' offices, and research institutions employ 15 percent of them.

Various regional nuclear medicine journals advertise job openings, as do publications geared toward radiologic and nuclear medicine technologists. Some colleges have placement services, and students who have trained in a hospital program may find work at that hospital.

Tim got his job indirectly because of his excellent performance as a student. "One of my fellow students heard that there was an opening here and he applied. The hospital asked the director of my school program for a recommendation for this person, which the director felt he was not in position to give. However, he warmly recommended me instead. I came to interview, and here I am."

where can I go from here?

Staff technologists who do well in their jobs and who have education beyond the associate's degree may advance to become *chief technologist* in their department. More experienced technologists may wish to instruct others in nuclear medicine technology.

As mentioned earlier, some technologists work for pharmaceutical companies, where they conduct research that is aimed at improving laboratory procedures or imaging techniques. Those who like sales may wish to work for such a company selling pharmaceuticals, computers, or other nuclear medicine equipment. Others who enjoy hands-on education may become *applications specialists*, traveling around the country helping hospital departments learn to use new computer equipment.

what are the salary ranges?

Salaries vary according to level of experience and management responsibilities. According to a survey conducted by the University of Texas Medical Branch, the average minimum

Advancement Possibilities

Chief nuclear medicine technologists supervise the technologists; write and revise procedures and safety policies, and make sure that they are followed; and train staff in how to operate specific equipment.

Nuclear medicine equipment sales representatives sell medical equipment and supplies to doctors, hospitals, medical schools, and retail establishments.

Research technologists assist engineers in developing new and improved methods to treat people with nuclear medicine.

in-depth

Nuclear Imaging

Nuclear imaging is one way of diagnosing problems not easily detected by X rays. In nuclear imaging, the patient swallows, inhales, or is instilled or injected with a radioactive isotope, which acts like a marker or tracer. The isotope goes directly to where problem is and is then located by a special camera, which produces an image.

Two uses of nuclear imaging are the bone scan and the bone density test. These tests are more sensitive than X rays and can often identify a problem months before it shows up on the X ray. They are used when the X rays come back normal, but symptoms persist.

In the bone scan the patient receives an injection of a bone-seeking nuclide in a vein. Scanning begins two to four hours later. Either the entire body or just the part concerned is imaged. Injuries, infections, and tumors can all be located with this technique.

The bone density test is used to diagnose osteoporosis, the decrease in bone density that is the major cause of fractures in the elderly. The patient lies on a table while two L-shaped devices (an emitter above the table and a detector below the table) pass over him or her. The emitter emits energy and the detector detects it. Because the energy has to go through the patient's body before it is detected by the detector, the amount that the body absorbs is an indication of the patient's bone density. This procedure is called absorptiometry.

salary for a nuclear medicine technologist was about $28,000 a year. The overall median salary was about $35,000. Those at the top end of the pay scale earned on average about $42,000 a year.

what is the job outlook?

The long-range outlook for nuclear medicine technologists is good, especially since the population is aging and nuclear medicine is employed in diagnosing many diseases of the elderly. Current projections indicate more than one thousand openings annually through the year 2005, which is three hundred more per year than are currently graduating in the field.

On the other hand, noninvasive imaging technologies (those that don't involve penetration of the skin, as with injections), such as magnetic resonance imaging (MRI), may supplant nuclear medicine for certain tests because they don't involve radioactivity. Also, cost-cutting measures by hospitals may lead to the merging of nuclear medicine departments. These factors could cause employment opportunities in nuclear medicine technology to level off.

how do I learn more?

professional organizations

Following are organizations that provide information on nuclear medicine technologist careers, accredited schools, and possible employers.

American Board of Nuclear Medicine
900 Veteran Avenue
Los Angeles, CA 90024
TEL: 310-825-6787

American College of Nuclear Medicine
PO Box 175
Landisville, PA 17538
TEL: 717-898-6006

American Registry of Radiological Technologists
1255 Northland Drive
St. Paul, MN 55120
TEL: 612-687-0048
WEBSITE: http://www.arrt.org

Nuclear Medicine Technology Certification Board
2970 Clairmont Road, Suite 610
Atlanta, GA 30329
TEL: 404-315-1739

The Society of Nuclear Medicine
Technologist Section
136 Madison Avenue
New York, NY 10016
TEL: 212-889-0717

bibliography

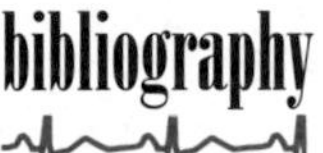

Following is a sampling of materials related to the professional concerns and development of nuclear medicine technologists.

Books

Mundy, Wanda M., and Gregory Passmore, editors. *Curriculum Guide for Nuclear Medicine Technologists,* 2nd edition. Reston, VA: Society of Nuclear Medicine, 1992.

Murphy, Wendy, and Jack Murphy. *Nuclear Medicine.* New York, NY: Chelsea House, 1994.

O'Conner, Michael K., editor. *The Mayo Clinic Manual of Nuclear Medicine.* New York, NY: Churchill Livingstone, 1996.

Smith, Ronald R. *Nuclear Medicine Technologist.* San Jose, CA: R & E Research Associates, 1993.

Wagner, Henry N. Jr., Zsolt Szabo, and Julia W. Buchanan, editors. *Principles of Nuclear Medicine,* 2nd edition. Philadelphia, PA: W.B. Saunders Co., 1995.

Periodicals

Nuclear Medicine and Biology. Bimonthly. Technical articles covering the application and interpretation of radionuclides. Pergamon Press, Inc., 660 White Plains Road, Tarrytown, NY 10591, 914-524-9200.

Nuclear Medicine Annual. Annual. Raven Press, 1185 Avenue of the Americas, New York, NY 10036, 212-930-9500.

nurse anesthetist

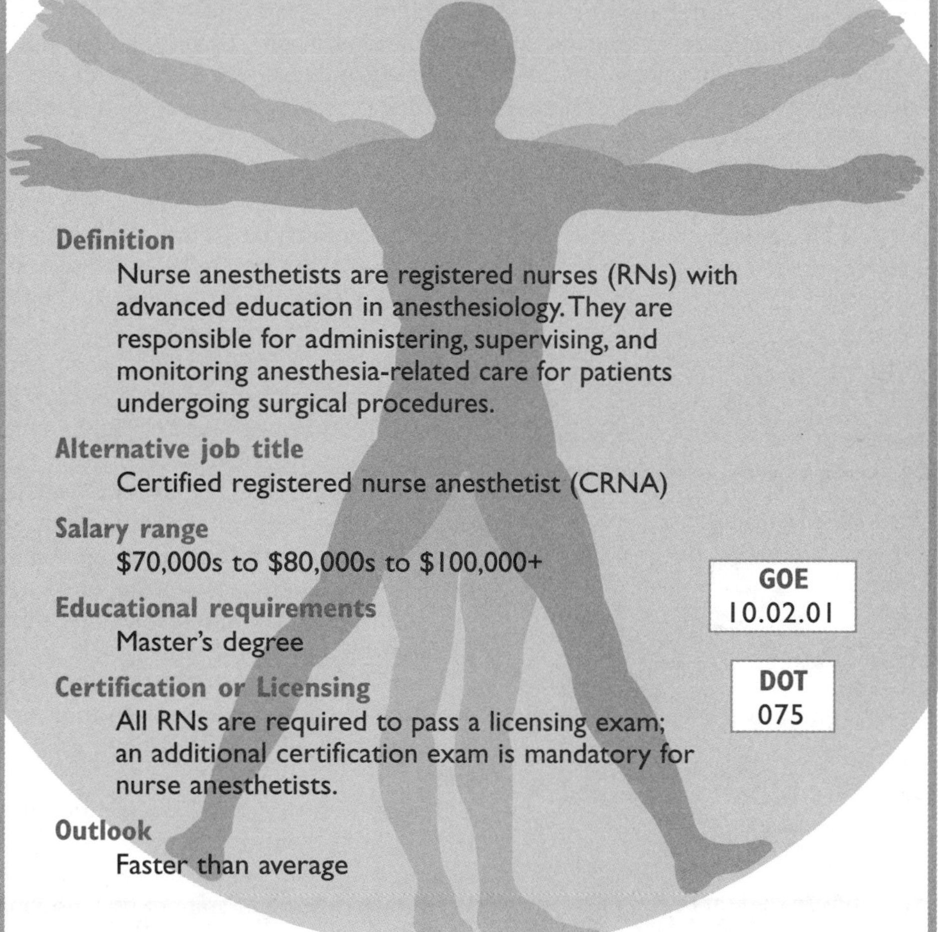

Definition

Nurse anesthetists are registered nurses (RNs) with advanced education in anesthesiology. They are responsible for administering, supervising, and monitoring anesthesia-related care for patients undergoing surgical procedures.

Alternative job title

Certified registered nurse anesthetist (CRNA)

Salary range

$70,000s to $80,000s to $100,000+

Educational requirements

Master's degree

Certification or Licensing

All RNs are required to pass a licensing exam; an additional certification exam is mandatory for nurse anesthetists.

Outlook

Faster than average

GOE
10.02.01

DOT
075

High School Subjects

Biology
Chemistry
Physics
Mathematics
English

Personal Interests

Helping people
Medical technology
Health care

"Good," Andy said, looking at the clock. "It's not yet 6:30 and I'm on schedule." Andy Griffin, a nurse anesthetist, had checked the anesthesia machine and made sure that the oxygen meter and monitoring devices were working properly. He had laid out the tubes and other essentials that would be used in the first operation of the day—the removal of a middle-aged man's diseased gall bladder.

Andy picked up the patient's chart and carefully reviewed it. By 7 AM, he would be greeting the patient in the holding room to begin the process of administering general anesthesia.

what does a nurse anesthetist do?

Nurse anesthetists, also known as *certified registered nurse anesthetists* (CRNAs), are registered nurses with advanced training in anesthesiology. Reliable methods of putting a patient to sleep were first developed in the 1840s when the discovery of ether anesthesia revolutionized surgery. Before that time, when surgery offered the only possible chance of saving a person's life (if a gangrenous leg had to be amputated, for example), all that the surgeon could do was to offer alcohol or opium to deaden the pain and then saw off the limb as fast as possible before the patient went into shock.

Anesthesiologists are physicians who completed a residency in anesthesiology and passed medical board exams in that specialty. Before World War II, only seven anesthesiology physician residency programs were available; in 1942, there were 17 nurse anesthetists for every anesthesiologist. During the first half of the century, medical students and physicians were often trained by nurse anesthetists in anesthesiology techniques.

Approximately 26 million anesthetic procedures are carried out annually in U.S. medical facilities; more than 65 percent of these are administered by nurse anesthetists. In 85 percent of rural hospitals, nurse anesthetists are the only anesthesia providers.

Contemporary anesthesiology is far more complicated than in the early days when an ether- or chloroform-soaked cloth or sponge was held up to the patient's face. In advance of surgery, a nurse anesthetist takes the patient's history, evaluates his or her anesthesia needs, and forms a plan for the best possible management of the case (often in consultation with an anesthesiologist). The nurse anesthetist also explains the planned procedures to the patient and answers questions. On the morning of the operation, the nurse anesthetist administers an intravenous (IV) sedative to relax the patient.

Usually a combination of several anesthetic agents is administered by the nurse anesthetist to establish and maintain the patient in a controlled state of unconsciousness, insensibility to pain, and muscular relaxation. Muscular relaxant drugs prevent the transmission of nerve impulses to the muscles to ensure that involuntary movements by the unconscious patient will not interfere with the surgery. Some general anesthetics are administered by inhalation through a mask and tube—the most common are nitrous oxide, halothane, enflurane, and isoflurane. Others are administered intravenously. Because the muscular relaxants prevent patients from breathing on their own, the nurse anesthetist has to provide artificial respiration through a tube inserted into the windpipe.

Throughout the surgery, the nurse anesthetist monitors the patient's vital signs (blood pressure, respiration, heart rate, and temperature) by watching the video and digital displays. The nurse anesthetist is also responsible for maintaining the patient's blood, water, and salt levels and from moment to moment read-

lingo to learn

Analgesics Pain-relieving medications.

Epidural Local anesthesia administered by injection into the space just outside the dural sac that surrounds the spinal cord.

Holding room Room just outside the operating room where the patient is prepared for surgery.

Infiltration Local anesthesia administered by injection directly into the surgical area.

IV Intravenous; refers to anesthetics or any other substance administered through a vein.

Nerve block Local anesthesia administered by injection near the nerves that control sensation in the surgical area.

Spinal Local anesthesia administered by injection into the dural sac that surrounds the spinal cord, resulting in loss of sensation in the entire body below that point in the spinal cord.

Tertiary health care The high-tech specialized diagnosis and treatment available only at large research and teaching hospitals.

Topical Local anesthesia administered by applying a drug to the surface of a mucous membrane that absorbs it; a method often used for surgery on the eye, nose, or throat.

justing the flow of anesthetics and other medications to ensure optimal results. After surgery, nurse anesthetists monitor their patients' return to consciousness and watch for complications; they may also be involved in postoperative pain management.

General anesthesia is not necessary for all surgical procedures. Nurse anesthetists also work on cases in which they provide various types of local anesthesia—topical, infiltration, nerve-block, spinal, and epidural or caudal.

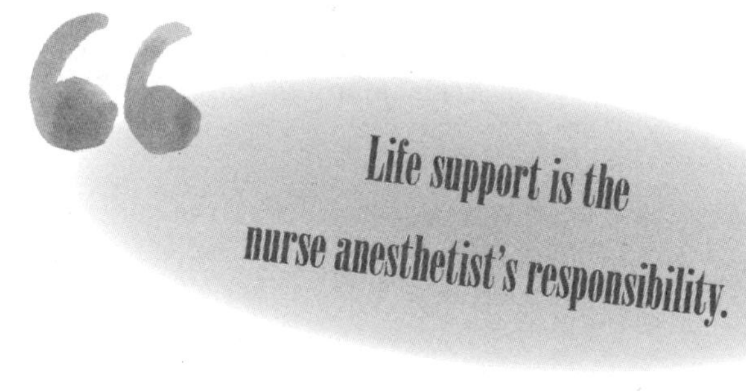

what is it like to be a nurse anesthetist?

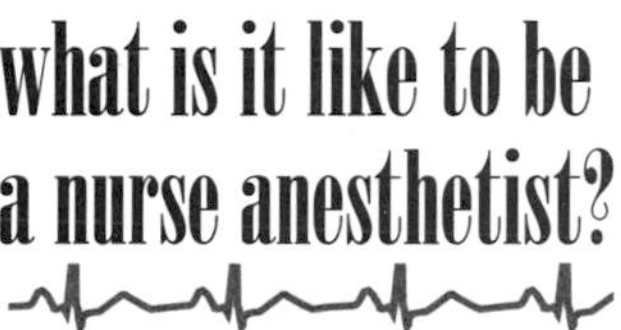

Andy Griffin sometimes tells people that the existence of the nurse anesthetist is "one of the best-kept secrets in the United States." He discovered nurse anesthetists during a summer job as an operating room assistant (orderly) during his undergraduate days. Andy already knew he was interested in pursuing a career in a medical field, and watching the work of nurse anesthetists in the operating room made him recognize what a challenging job that would be.

After receiving his bachelor's degree in nursing and becoming a licensed R.N., Andy worked for two years in a hospital intensive care unit (ICU) before beginning a master's degree program in anesthesiology. Although he is still a few months away from graduation at the Middle Tennessee School of Anesthesia, he has already worked as nurse anesthetist on nearly 700 cases. After graduation, he will be working for an anesthesia group that has contracts with three Nashville hospitals—St. Thomas, Baptist, and Centennial.

Today would be fairly typical, thought Andy. After the 7:30 AM gall bladder, there would be several other surgical patients. Occasionally, one complicated operation would take all day; recently he was on an open-heart operation that lasted from 7:30 AM to 3:00 PM.

It might be a typical day, but there are never any merely "routine" cases. At every moment of the surgery, Andy has to be vigilant—watching the dials on the equipment, adjusting the levels of anesthetic agents being administered (some phases of the operation required deeper anesthesia than others), and monitoring the patient's respiration. During the first month or so of his master's program, Andy had learned the basic facts of anesthesia—the various anesthetic agents available and how to calculate dosage on the basis of the patient's weight. The next 2½ years were spent learning how to anticipate problems; he had to learn what to do in the 5 percent of cases that do not go as planned.

Sometimes, for example, it turns out to be impossible to maintain an airway without performing a tracheotomy (an incision in the throat to insert a breathing tube into the windpipe, or trachea). "The surgeon stays with the surgery," Andy explained. "Life support is the nurse anesthetist's responsibility." At the hospitals where Andy works, an anesthesiologist who is responsible for monitoring four to six operating rooms at the same time is available for consultation in a crisis.

As the surgeon begins closing the incision, Andy simultaneously reduces the anesthesia in order to bring the patient back to consciousness. After the surgery, Andy pulls out the breathing tube as soon as the patient is alert enough to respond to his or her name. When patients are stable, which usually means awake and breathing independently, Andy turns them over to the recovery room nurse.

Carole Rietz is a nurse anesthetist and clinical nurse specialist in Vanderbilt University Hospital's pediatrics division. She works with children and adolescents; her patients range in age from premature infants to eighteen-year-olds. She occasionally has patients over the age of eighteen whose special needs make it most appropriate for them to be treated in pediatrics.

Since Carole shares responsibility with anesthesiologists for the care of her patients before, during, and after surgery, she must be skilled in the use of airways, ventilators, IVs, blood- and fluid- replacement techniques, and postoperative pain management.

Some children come to the hospital for one-time operations, such as a tonsillectomy, appendectomy, or hernia repair. Those with long-term medical problems may need to return for surgery and/or other treatment on a regular basis. Many of Carole's patients are children with serious chronic illnesses; some are premature infants with complicated health problems requiring a series of surgeries. Carole works closely with physicians in various pediatric subspecialties (anesthesiology, oncology, orthopedics, urology, and others) and with clinical nurse specialists to ensure the best possible care for each child.

Communicating with children and their parents is an important part of Carole's job. Providing the best possible physical care for patients is obviously essential, yet psychological and social needs are also vital. Vanderbilt tries to provide a nonthreatening hospital environment with approachable staff members. Children and parents can take tours of the facility, where the equipment and medical procedures being planned for the child are explained. Parents need to be trained as primary caregivers in the home, especially in cases of long-term health problems. "If the mother is comfortable, then that feeling of confidence is transferred to the child," explains Carole.

It is essential to answer children's questions at the appropriate age level. A four-year-old with cancer or failing kidneys is still a four-year-old with a child's perspective. Caregivers need to be constantly aware that children do not think like adults.

FYI

Approximately 26 million anesthetic procedures are carried out annually in U.S. medical facilities—and more than 65 percent of these are administered by nurse anesthetists. In 85 percent of rural hospitals, nurse anesthetists are the only anesthesia providers.

Carole stresses the importance of giving children choices, whenever possible, to help them feel that they have some say in what is happening to them. They may choose a breathing mask in one of several flavors, or they may bring a favorite toy with them into the operating room. If the child will be returning frequently to the hospital, Carole tries to arrange for care from the same providers each time—to avoid the anxiety of having to meet new staff members on every visit.

Carole especially appreciates the team-oriented, problem-solving approach to health care. After more than 30 years in nursing, Carole strongly believes that health care providers must take an active role in fighting for their patients to prevent the "business perspective" from taking over medicine.

have I got what it takes to be a nurse anesthetist?

Nurse anesthetists must have the ability to concentrate intently for lengthy periods. They are responsible for keeping the anesthetized patient alive, which requires careful attention to every detail. They need to be critical thinkers who can analyze problems accurately and swiftly, make decisions, and take appropriate action. All nurses need the ability to remain calm during emergencies; the operating room can be an especially stressful environment.

Research studies of anesthesia-related problems have demonstrated that most could have been avoided if the anesthesia provider had monitored the patient's condition more vigilantly. The *Journal of the American Medical Association* published new guidelines called the Harvard Minimal Monitoring Standards on Anesthesia Care in 1986. More recently, the American Association of Nurse Anesthetists issued even more detailed monitoring standards.

Nurse anesthetists also need to be efficient in their time management. "The surgeons have to be kept happy by having the patients moved along quickly without long delays between cases," was the way one nurse anesthetist put it. If a nurse anesthetist is slow in finishing one case and setting up for the next, the surgeon may be reluctant to work with that individual again.

how do I become a nurse anesthetist?

To be a successful nurse anesthetist you should

- Be able to analyze and solve problems quickly
- Be able to handle stressful situations
- Be able to remain calm in emergencies
- Have strong powers of concentration

education

High School

To become a nurse anesthetist, you must first be a registered nurse. Anyone who is interested in a nursing career needs to take a college-preparatory course in high school that gives a good foundation in the laboratory sciences. You need to take biology, chemistry, physics, and mathematics. If your high school offers advanced biology or a human physiology course beyond the introductory biology class, these would be good choices for electives. English classes and other courses that develop communication skills are also important.

High school would be a good time to test your interest in nursing by getting some hands-on experience. There may be opportunities for volunteer work or a part-time job at a hospital, community health center, or nursing home in your community. You might also talk with people in various nursing fields or join a Future Nurses Club.

Postsecondary Training

There are three ways to become a registered nurse—a two-year associate's degree program at a junior or community college, a three-year hospital nursing school program, or a bachelor's-degree program (BSN) at a college or university nursing school. Sometimes persons who already have a bachelor's degree in another field enter nursing through a master's-level program (MSN) rather by earning another bachelor's degree. All programs combine classroom education and actual nursing experience. Part-time or summer jobs in health care offer additional opportunities for exploring the nursing field.

The bachelor's- or master's-degree route is strongly recommended since a nurse with less than a BSN has few opportunities for advancement. All applicants to nurse anesthetist programs are required to have at least a bachelor's degree. (The other advanced-practice nursing fields—nurse practitioner, clinical nurse specialist, and nurse midwife—also expect applicants to have a bachelor's degree before beginning specialized training.)

Undergraduate nursing programs include courses in biology, microbiology, human anatomy and physiology, psychology, nutrition, and statistics. Some classes in humanities and social sciences are also required in BSN programs. After completing the nursing degree, it is necessary to pass a national licensing exam; only then are you registered nurse.

There are over ninety accredited nurse anesthesia programs in the United States. They last twenty-four to thirty-six months and nearly all offer a master's degree. There are also a few clinical nursing doctorate programs for nurse anesthetists. (Beginning in 1998, the few programs that were offering only a certificate in anesthesiology will be required to offer at least a master's degree.) Applicants to nurse anesthetist programs must have at least one

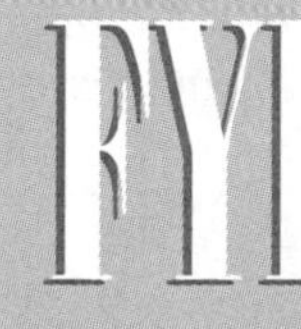

FYI

For centuries, alcohol, opium, mandrake, hemp, and herbane were given orally or by inhalation during surgery or childbirth. The Indians of Peru chewed the leaves of the coca plant—from which cocaine is derived—and used their saliva to reduce local pain during surgery.

in-depth

The first nurse anesthetist was Sister Mary Bernard, who practiced in Pennsylvania in the 1870s. The first school of nurse anesthetists was founded in 1909 at St. Vincent Hospital in Portland, Oregon. Since then, many schools have been established, including the famous Mayo Clinic Anesthesia Program.

During World War I, America's nurse anesthetists were the major providers of care to the troops in France. They also trained the French and British nurses and physicians in anesthesia procedures.

Prior to World War II, anesthesia was considered a nursing specialty. In 1942, there were 17 nurse anesthetists in the United States for every anesthesiologist.

The nurse anesthesia specialty was formally created on June 17, 1931, when the American Association of Nurse Anesthetist (AANA) held its first meeting.

year of experience as an RN in an intensive care unit; many have considerably more. The admissions process is competitive. Andy Griffin recently estimated that the average undergraduate grade point average of the students at the Middle Tennessee School of Anesthesia was about a 3.5 on a 4.0 scale.

Students enrolled in nurse anesthetist programs take classes in pharmacology (the science of drugs and their uses), anatomy and physiology, pathophysiology (the physiology of disease), biochemistry, chemistry, and physics. Students also acquire hundreds of hours of anesthesia-related clinical experience in surgery and obstetrics.

certification or licensing

Nurse anesthetists are required to pass national certification exams after completing their educational program. The certification process was initiated by the American Association of Nurse Anesthetists in 1945. All states recognize certified registered nurse anesthetist status. Nurse anesthetists are not required to work under the supervision of an anesthesiologist, although some licensing laws do stipulate that they must work with a physician.

scholarships and grants

There are many sources of financial aid (grants, scholarships, loans, and other forms of assistance) for students in nursing fields. The best way to begin is by consulting the financial-aid office of the educational institution you plan to attend.

Other possible aid sources include the Nurses' Association in your state, the National Student Nurses' Association, nursing honor societies, state departments of education, the federal government, private agencies, civic and alumni associations, and the U.S. military.

You may be eligible for scholarship aid designated for members of specific racial/ethnic groups. Some nursing-scholarship sponsors require recipients to work for their agency for a specified length of time after receiving the degree; generally this means professional employment at full salary. The National League for Nursing publishes an annual guide, *Scholarships and Loans for Nursing Education*.

If you are already an RN employed by a health care agency and want to return to graduate school, your employer may provide full or partial tuition reimbursement.

who will hire me?

Many nurse anesthetists are employed by hospitals or outpatient surgery centers (this would include dental and podiatry work as well as same-day surgery). Others are in group or independent practice and provide services to hospitals and other health care centers on a contract basis. Some work for the U.S. Public Health Services. Most rural hospitals rely on nurse anesthetists as their only providers of anesthesia. Nurse anesthetists are eligible to receive direct Medicare reimbursement (under the 1986 Omnibus Budget Reconciliation Act).

The U.S. military also employ nurse anesthetists. In every twentieth-century war, nurse anesthetists were the major providers of anesthesia care, especially in forward-positioned medical facilities. In the Vietnam War, there were three nurse anesthetists for every physician anesthetist.

Because the high-quality, cost-effective anesthesia service provided by nurse anesthetists is widely acknowledged, more and more health care institutions are eager to employ them.

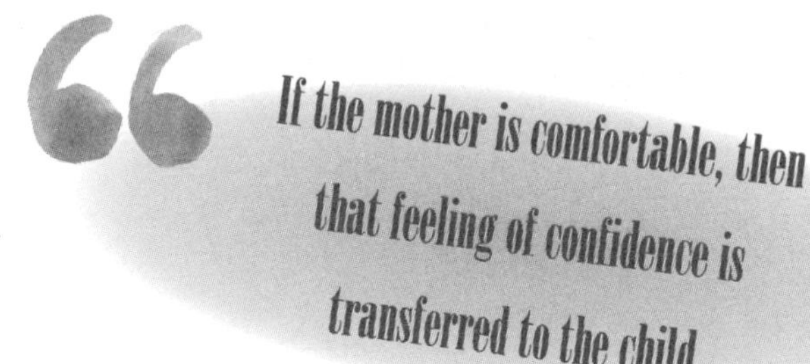

where can I go from here?

Experienced nurse anesthetists can earn over $100,000 a year. Those who want new professional challenges beyond direct practice might consider teaching or administrative positions or involvement in research for improved or specialized anesthesia equipment and procedures. Some nurse anesthetists choose to acquire other advanced-practice nursing qualifications so they can be involved in a wider range of nursing activities. Doctoral programs for nurse anesthetists are expected to expand in the near future.

what are the salary ranges?

Nurse anesthetists are probably the highest paid nursing specialists. Salaries range from the $70,000s to the $80,000s to over $100,000 for experienced nurse anesthetists. The average annual salary is in the $80,000s. Anesthesiologists, by contrast, average over $220,000.

what is the job outlook?

The job outlook for nurse anesthetists is excellent. A 1990 study concluded that 30,000 new nurse anesthetists would be needed by 2000 and over 35,000 by 2010. To meet this goal, there would need to be 1,800 new nurse anesthetists graduating each year through 2000 and 1,500 each year for the next decade. In 1993, only about 900 nurse anesthetists graduated—barely half the number required to keep up with projected demands.

Another 1990 study predicted that a greater use of nurse anesthetists could result in nationwide savings of $1 billion annually by 2010. Ten nurse anesthetists can be educated for the cost of educating one anesthesiologist. In addition to the much higher annual cost of educating an anesthesiology resident, the total educational process for producing a nurse anesthetist (including undergraduate and graduate work) is on average four years shorter.

how do I learn more?

professional organizations

To learn more about a career as a nurse anesthetist, contact the following:

American Association of Nurse Anesthetists
222 Prospect Avenue
Park Ridge, IL 6008
TEL: 708-692-7050

National League for Nursing
350 Hudson Street
New York, NY 10014
TEL: 212-989-9393
WEBSITE: http://www.nln.org

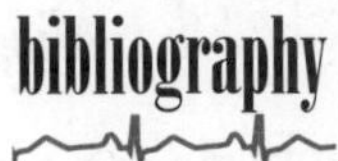

Following is a sampling of materials relating to the professional concerns and development of nurse anesthetists.

Books

Chitwood, Linda B. *Overview of Anesthesia for Nurses*. South Easton, MA: Western Schools, 1992.

Gerbasi, Francis R., editor. *Nurse Anesthesia: PreTest Self-Assessment and Review.* New York, NY: McGraw-Hill, 1996.

McIntosh, Laura W., editor. *Essentials of Nurse Anesthesia.* New York, NY: McGraw-Hill, 1996.

Waugaman, Wynne R., and Scot D. Foster. *Certification Review in Nurse Anesthesia,* 2nd edition. New York, NY: Appleton & Lange, 1997.

Periodicals

C R N A: the Clinical Forum for Nurse Anesthetists. Quarterly. Updates on clinical advances, and abstracts with commentary on recent literature in the field. W.B. Saunders Co., Curtis Center, 3rd Floor, Independence Square West, Philadelphia, PA 19106, 215-238-6445.

Imprint. 5 per year. Practical journal for people interested in nursing careers. January issue is devoted to career planning. National Student Nurses Association, 555 W. 57th Street, New York, NY 10019, 2122-581-2211.

nurse assistant

Definition

Nurse assistants care for patients in hospitals and nursing homes under the supervision of nurses.

Alternative job titles

Nurse or nursing aide

Nursing assistant

Orderly

Salary range

$11,900 to $12,800 to $14,600

Educational requirements

High school diploma; completion of training program in either a community college or vocational school

Certification or Licensing

Voluntary for hospitals

Mandatory for nursing homes

Outlook

Faster than average

GOE
10.03.02

DOT
355

High School Subjects

Biology
English
Health
Sociology

Personal Interests

Helping people
Personal health
Teaching

Hurrying about to answer call lights; helping nursing home residents get showered, dressed, and off to breakfast; taking residents to the bathroom; it had been a hectic morning and now Dorothy Reeve must make a bed. It may not seem like much, but the resident is bedridden and fragile, and can't be moved about much. Dorothy will leave the resident in the bed while making it; she'll work slowly and carefully, a contrast from the fast action that's been required of her all morning.

First Dorothy draws the curtain to protect the resident's privacy. "Are you comfortable, Mrs. Lanning?" she asks, adjusting the pillow and raising the bed. When she's certain that the resident is at ease and unexposed, she lowers the side rail and begins to make up half the bed. She then raises the side rail again and helps the resident to the other side of the bed to finish. Before leaving, she checks again with Mrs. Lanning to make certain she's comfortable and has everything she needs. Mrs. Lanning responds with a smile and she squeezes Dorothy's hand. Dorothy leaves the room with the certainty that her tasks, though small and routine, are important to the residents and the home.

what does a nurse assistant do?

Though the job title suggests someone who assists nurses, *nurse assistants* actually perform many duties independently; in some cases, they become more closely involved with patients or nursing home residents than do registered nurses. Nurse assistants work under the supervision of nurses and perform tasks that allow the nursing staff to perform their primary duties effectively and efficiently.

Nurse assistants perform basic nursing care in hospitals and nursing homes. Male nurse assistants are perhaps better known as orderlies. Working independently and alongside nurses and doctors, nurse assistants help move patients, assist in patients' exercise and nutrition, and see to the patients' personal hygiene. They bring the patients their meal trays and help them to eat. They push the patients on stretchers and in wheelchairs to operating and X-ray rooms. They also help to admit and discharge patients. Nurse assistants must keep charts of their work for review by nurses.

Most nurse assistants work in nursing homes, tending to the daily care of elderly residents. They help residents with baths and showers, meals, and exercise. They help them in and out of their beds and to and from the bathroom. They also record the health of residents by taking body temperatures and checking blood pressures.

Because the residents are living within such close proximity to each other, and because they need help with personal hygiene and health care, a nurse assistant also takes care to protect the privacy of the resident. It is the responsibility of a nurse assistant to make the resident feel as comfortable as possible. Nurse assistants may also work with patients who are not fully functional, teaching them how to care for themselves, educating them in personal hygiene and health care.

The work can be strenuous, requiring the lifting and moving of patients. Nurse assistants must work with partners, or in groups, when performing the more strenuous tasks, so that neither the nurse assistant nor the resident is injured. Some requirements of the job can be as routine as changing sheets and helping a resident with phone calls, while other requirements can be as difficult and unattractive as assisting a resident with elimination and cleaning up a resident who has vomited.

Nurse assistants may be called upon by nurses and physicians to perform the more menial and unappealing tasks, but they also have the opportunity to develop meaningful relationships with residents. Nurse assistants work closely with residents, often gaining their trust and admiration. When residents are having personal problems, or problems with the staff, they may turn to the nurse assistant for help.

Nurse assistants generally work a forty-hour work week, with some overtime. The hours and weekly schedule may be irregular, however, depending on the need of the care institution. An assistant may have one day off in the middle of the week, followed by three days of work, then another day off. Nurse assistants are needed around the clock, so beginning assistants may be required to work late at night, or very early in the morning.

lingo to learn

Ambulatory care Serving patients who are able to walk.

Acute care Providing emergency services and general medical and surgical treatment for acute disorders rather than long-term care.

Asepsis Methods of sterilization to ensure the absence of germs.

Gerontology A branch of medicine that deals with aging and the problems of the aged.

Neonatal Pertaining to newborn children.

Pediatrics A branch of medicine concerned with the development, care, and diseases of babies and children.

what is it like to be a nurse assistant?

Dorothy Reeve works in the Medicare wing of a ninety-resident nursing home in Petaluma, California. "I clock in at 7:00 AM," she says, "and I hit the floor." She works under the supervision of registered nurses and LVNs (licensed vocational nurses), as well as therapists (physical, occupational,and speech). But mostly she performs her own set of daily responsibilities. Dorothy starts by getting three or four residents out of bed and helps them to start their day. Getting a patient out of bed sometimes requires a mechanical lift. "The lift," Dorothy explains, "supports their weight under a sling and they are lifted like an engine from a car." Also, Dorothy works with another nurse assistant who helps with lifting and feeding. "There are twenty-one residents on our wing when full," she says. By taking turns with a partner each nurse assistant can take breaks as well as keep watch over residents in the wing.

"I give the person a shower if it's scheduled," she says, "and I get them dressed if they are unable to dress themselves." The residents have set schedules and many must be up at certain times for physical therapy and other appointments. Once her residents are dressed, they are brought out to the dining hall for breakfast. Breakfast is served from 8:00 AM until around 9:00 AM.

"We have to be done with our morning care by 11:00 AM," she says. In addition to getting patients ready for the day, Dorothy must attend to call lights; call lights are the way residents signal the nurse assistants for help. "You have to make sure that the call lights are answered within three minutes," Dorothy says. "It's the law." Call lights usually have accompanying noises to alert the assistant. "You have to constantly be aware of the sounds that are normal and be alert for the sounds that are not." The call lights are typically going off throughout the morning, and through breakfast and lunch.

Dorothy also takes the residents' vital signs and reports any abnormal readings. She says, "You really have to know your residents individually to know if they're feeling up to par."

When caring for a resident, privacy is important. "We have to make sure that when the residents are receiving personal care," Dorothy says, "that the privacy curtains are pulled and no one can see in. We make sure the door is firmly shut and the drapes are pulled closed for the resident's dignity."

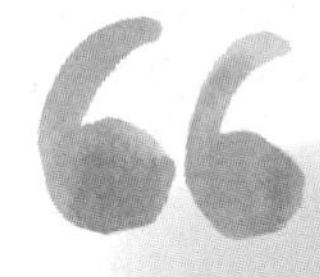

In some cases, we care givers are the only family they have now.

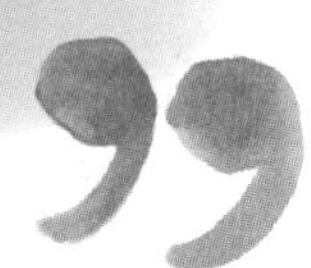

After helping patients with their morning routines and appointments, then helping them with their lunch, Dorothy takes some of the residents to the bathroom and helps them down for a rest. "Then I get all my information together for legal charting," she says. "The charts we keep are legal documents and when we sign our name we are liable for all the information we chart. If there are any legal questions at sometime in the future we had better know why we charted what we did. The state inspectors look at our charting and the RNs get a lot of their information from our viewpoint and from what we chart." Dorothy spends thirty minutes or more preparing the day's chart. To assist in chart preparation, she records her work throughout the day so she doesn't have to try to remember everything she did for each individual resident.

Dorothy's day is usually complete at 3:00 PM, though she occasionally works overtime. She is paid for 37.5 hours a week and works a rotating schedule; this means she works three or four days, then has two days off, followed by another three or four days of work.

have I got what it takes to be a nurse assistant?

A nurse assistant must care about the work and the patients and must show a general understanding and compassion for the ill, disabled, and the elderly. Because of the rigorous physical demands placed on a nurse assistant, you should be in good health. Also, the hours and responsibilities of the job won't allow you to take many sick days. Along with this good physical health, you should have good mental health, as well. The job can be emotionally demanding, requiring your patience and stability. You should also be able to take orders and to work as part of a team.

Though the work can often be rewarding, a nurse assistant must also be prepared for the worst. "When I first started," Dorothy says, "I had the illusion that the patients would be just like my grandmother was at the time...baking, sewing, alert." But she almost quit after the first week. "The residents hit, they screamed, they fell down. You had to feed them their meals and they could not shower themselves." But, after her training, Dorothy came to appreciate the work and to care about the residents. "I like people," she says, "and I love to take care of them. I like to see them smile. In some cases, we care givers are the only family they have now." Dorothy also appreciates the steadiness of the work and the certainty that experienced nurse assistants will always be in high demand.

how do I become a nurse assistant?

Dorothy has worked in nursing homes for more than thirteen years. She completed high school and has had earned some junior college credits. She has also completed a state-required training program and received certification. Dorothy found the training process to be overwhelming at first. "There's so much to remember," she says. "And you need to learn everything quickly so that you can work on your own."

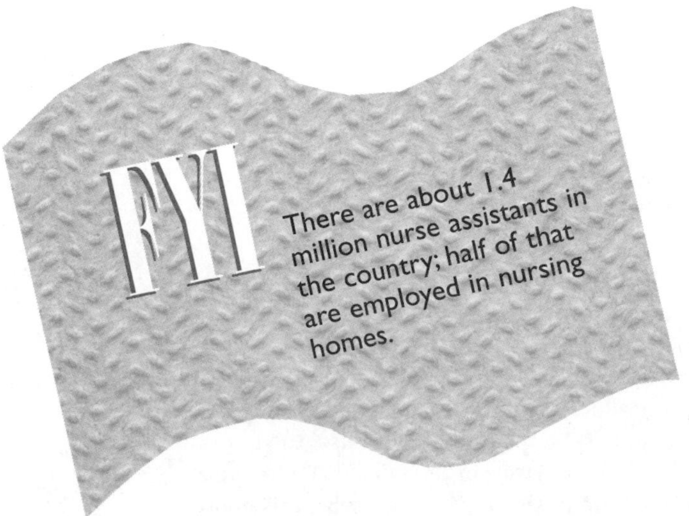

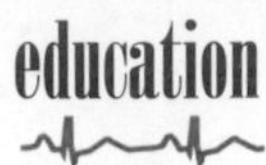

High School

Communications skills are valuable for a nurse assistant, so take English, speech, and journalism courses. Science courses, such as biology and anatomy, will also prepare you for future training. Because a high school diploma is not required of nurse assistants, many high school students are hired by nursing homes and hospitals for part-time work. Job opportunities may also exist in a hospital or nursing home kitchen, introducing you to diet and nutrition. Also, volunteer work can familiarize you with the work nurses and nurse assistants perform, as well as introduce you to some medical terminology.

Postsecondary Training

Nurse assistants are not required to have a college degree but may have to complete a short training course at a community college or vocational school. These training courses, usually instructed by a registered nurse, teach basic nursing skills and prepare students for the state certification exam. Nurse assistants typically begin the training courses after getting their first job as an assistant, and the course work is incorporated into their on-the-job training.

Many people work as nurse assistants as they pursue other medical professions; someone interested in becoming a nurse or a paramedic may work as an assistant while taking courses. A high school student or a student in a premedical program may work as a nurse assistant part-time before going on to medical school.

certification or licensing

Nurse assistants in hospitals are not required to be certified but those working in nursing homes must pass a state exam. The Omnibus Budget Reconciliation Act (OBRA) passed by Congress in 1987 requires nursing homes to hire only certified nurse assistants.

Dorothy says, "Certification took almost six months of training and class work. California has very strict guidelines." OBRA also requires continuing education for nurse assistants, and periodic evaluations.

who will hire me?

Half of all nurse assistants work in nursing homes. Other places where they are employed include hospitals, halfway houses, retirement centers, and private homes. Dorothy started working as a nurse assistant when she was twenty-one years old. "I had two children to support," she says, "and this field has always interested me because I've always liked older people. And they offered to pay me as I learned." Dorothy heard about the job through a friend and visited the nursing facility directly and filled out an application. She began training in 1984; she worked for the same nursing facility for a year, then worked in a few other homes in the area over the following few years. She then returned to the place where she trained and has stayed there for nine years. It is typical for nurse assistants to try different facilities after receiving training.

Because of the high demand for nurse assistants, you can apply directly to the health care facilities in your area. Most will probably have a human resources department that advertises positions in the newspaper and interviews applicants.

where can I go from here?

One of the things Dorothy appreciates about her work is that it allows her to perform many of the tasks and duties of a nurse. "Some day I would like to get my nursing degree," she says. But she emphasizes that she is very happy in her current position. "I would like the extra training, but I don't want to just push pills and sit behind a desk and not get to know the residents like I do now." Dorothy would also be interested in trying her work in a different setting, like a hospital.

For the most part, there is not much opportunity for advancement within the job of nurse assistant. To move up in a health care facility requires additional training. Some nurse assistants, after gaining experience and learning medical technology, enroll in nursing programs, or may even decide to pursue medical degrees.

A nursing home requires a lot of hard work and dedication so nurse assistants frequently burn-out, or quit before completing their training. Others may choose another aspect of the job, such as working as a home health aide. Helping patients in their homes, these aides see to the client's personal health, hygiene, and home care.

To be a successful nurse assistant you should

- Be a compassionate person
- Be in good health
- Be able to perform some heavy lifting
- Have a great deal of patience
- Take orders well
- Be a good team player
- Be emotionally stable

what are the salary ranges?

Although the salaries for most health care professionals vary by region and population, the average hourly wage of nurse assistants is about the same across the country. Midwestern states and less populated areas, where a large staff of nurse assistants may be needed to make up for a smaller staff of nurses and therapists, may pay a little more per hour.

On the low end, nurse assistants make around $4.80 per hour; the average hourly wage is at about $5.50. Experienced nurse assistants make up to $7.10 per hour.

what is the job outlook?

There will continue to be many job opportunities for nurse assistants. Because of the physical and emotional demands of the job, and because of the lack of advancement opportunities, there is a high turnover rate of employees. Also, health care is constantly changing; more opportunities open for nurse assistants as different kinds of health care facilities are developed. Business-based health organizations are limiting the services of health care professionals and looking for cheaper ways to provide care. This may provide opportunities for those looking for work as nurse assistants.

Government and private agencies are also developing more programs to assist dependent people. And as the number of people seventy years of age and older continues to rise, new and larger nursing care facilities will open.

how do I learn more?

professional organizations

American Health Care Association
1201 L Street, NW
Washington, DC 20005
TEL: 202-842-4444

American Nursing Assistants Association
35526 Grand River, suite 225
Farmington Hills, MI 48335

bibliography

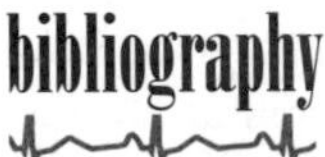

Following is a sampling of materials relating to the professional concerns and development of nurse assistants.

Books

Casey, Margaret, editor. *How to Be a Nurse Assistant: Career Training in Long Term Care*. St. Louis, MO: Mosby, 1994.

Frazier, Marjorie, G., and Barbara A. Vitale. *Long-Term Practice: Skills for the Certified Nursing Assistant.* Boston, MA: Little, Brown, 1995.

Frederickson, Keville. *Opportunities in Nursing*, revised edition. Lincolnwood, IL: VGM Career Horizons, 1995.

Hegner, Barbara R., and Esther Caldwell. *Nursing Assistant,* 6th edition. Albany, NY: Delmar, 1992.

Polski, Arlene, and Judith P. Warner. *Saunders Fundamentals for Nursing Assistants*. Philadelphia, PA: W.B. Saunders Co., 1994.

Periodicals

Imprint. 5 per year. Practical journal for people interested in nursing careers. January issue is devoted to career planning. National Student Nurses Association, 555 W. 57th Street, New York, NY 10019, 212-581-2211.

Nursing Notes. Annual. Covers educational and professional and semiprofessional nursing information. Includes employment opportunity listings. American Nursing Assistant's Foundation, 35526Grand River Avenue, Suite 225, Farmington Hills, MI 48335

nurse-midwife

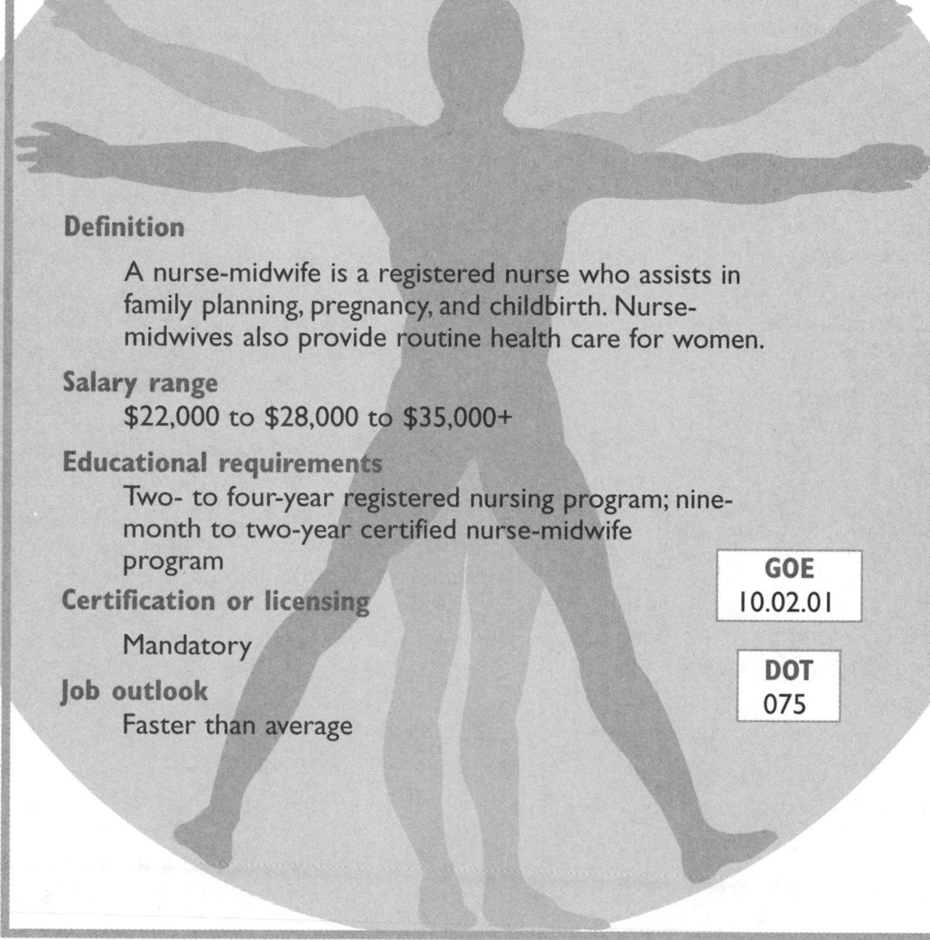

Definition

A nurse-midwife is a registered nurse who assists in family planning, pregnancy, and childbirth. Nurse-midwives also provide routine health care for women.

Salary range

$22,000 to $28,000 to $35,000+

Educational requirements

Two- to four-year registered nursing program; nine-month to two-year certified nurse-midwife program

Certification or licensing

Mandatory

Job outlook

Faster than average

GOE
10.02.01

DOT
075

High School Subjects

Biology
Chemistry
English
Philosophy
Psychology

Personal Interests

Children
Helping people
Peer counseling
Women's rights

The young woman found out last month that she was pregnant. It would be her second child. When she was pregnant the first time, three years ago, she was seeing an obstetrician for her prenatal care. She also had the obstetrician deliver her baby.

But she wanted to do things differently this time. Last time, she felt that she didn't receive the emotional support she needed from her doctor. And with all the pain-killing drugs she was given during delivery, she almost felt as if she weren't in the room when her baby was born.

So this time she decided she was going to have a nurse-midwife give her prenatal care and deliver her baby. It would be a natural pregnancy and a natural childbirth. And now, after meeting with Deborah Woolley, her nurse-midwife, she knew she had made the right decision.

what does a nurse-midwife do?

Midwifery, the act of assisting at childbirth, has been practiced around the world for thousands of years. But in the United States, pregnancy and childbirth are often considered technical medical procedures best left in the hands of physicians known as obstetricians and gynecologists. Midwifery has traditionally been frowned upon by both the medical community and the public.

Since the 1960s, however, this attitude has been changing as more women insist on "natural" methods of giving birth. *Nurse-midwives,* officially known as *certified nurse-midwives,* have generally become accepted as respected members of health care teams involved with family planning, pregnancy, and childbirth. A number of studies have even indicated that babies delivered by nurse-midwives are less likely to experience low birth weights and other health complications than babies delivered by physicians.

Most nurse-midwives work at hospitals or at family planning clinics or birthing centers affiliated with hospitals. Some nurse-midwives operate independent practices providing home birth services.

Nurse-midwives examine pregnant women and monitor the growth and development of fetuses. Typically, a nurse-midwife is responsible for all phases of a normal pregnancy, including prenatal care, assisting during labor, delivering the baby, and providing follow-up care. A nurse-midwife always works in consultation with a physician, who can be called upon should complications arise during pregnancy or childbirth. Nurse-midwives can provide emergency assistance to their patients while physicians are called. In most states, nurse-midwives are authorized to prescribe and administer medications. Many nurse-midwives provide the full-spectrum of women's health care, including gynecological exams.

An important part of a nurse-midwife's work is concerned with the education of patients. Nurse-midwives teach their patients about proper nutrition and fitness for healthy pregnancies, and about different techniques for labor and delivery. Nurse-midwives also council their patients in the postpartum period—that is, after birth—about breast feeding, parenting, and other areas concerning the health of mother and child. Nurse-midwives provide counseling on several other issues, including sexually transmitted diseases, spousal and child abuse, and social support networks. In some cases, counseling extends to patients' family members.

Not all midwives are certified nurse-midwives. Most states recognize other categories of midwives, including *certified* (or *licensed) midwives* and *lay* (or *empirical) midwives.*

Certified midwives are not required to be nurses in order to practice as midwives. They typically assist in home births or at birthing centers, and are trained through a combination of formal education, apprenticeship, and self-education. Certified midwives are legally recognized in 29 states, which offer licensing, certification, or registration programs. Certified midwives perform most of the services of nurse-midwives, and they generally have professional relationships with physicians, hospi-

lingo to learn

Catching Babies An informal term used to describe the act of assisting in the delivery of an infant.

Cesarean section A surgical procedure to deliver a baby through an incision in the abdomen. The procedure is named after Julius Caesar, who was supposedly born in this way.

Episiotomy An incision made between the vagina and anus to provide more clearance for birth.

Gynecologist A physician who specializes in the diseases and routine health care of the reproductive systems of women.

Natural childbirth A term used to emphasize pregnancy, labor, and childbirth as natural processes. In natural childbirth, pain-reducing and labor-inducing drugs either are not used or are used conservatively.

Obstetrician A physician who specializes in childbirth and in prenatal and postpartum care.

Pap smear A procedure in which cells are collected from the cervix; the cells are then examined under a microscope for signs of cancer.

Prenatal Before childbirth.

Postpartum After childbirth.

tals, and laboratories to provide support and emergency services.

Lay midwives usually obtain their training by apprenticing with established midwives, although some may acquire formal education as well. Lay midwives are midwives who are not certified or licensed, either because they lack the necessary experience and education or because they pursue nontraditional childbirth techniques. Many lay midwives practice only as part of religious communities or specific ethnic groups. Lay midwives typically assist only in home birth situations. Some states have made it illegal for lay midwives to charge for their services.

The rest of this article will concern itself only with certified nurse-midwives.

"Midwifery's focus is on improving conditions for women and their families. In a way, midwifery is a radical departure from the old way of looking at pregnancy."

what is it like to be a nurse-midwife?

Deborah Woolley has been a registered nurse since 1975, and has been practicing as a nurse-midwife since 1983. She currently practices at the University of Illinois Hospital, where she also serves as the director of the university's Nurse-Midwifery Educational Program. For Deborah, midwifery offered her the opportunity to have a positive impact on women's health care and childbirth experiences. "I started out as a nurse assigned to the labor and delivery unit. But I became frustrated with the type of care the women were getting," Deborah says. "You'll find that a lot among midwives. Most of the midwives I talk to can point to an event that was the straw that broke the camel's back,as it were—when they realized that they wanted to have more influence over the experience the woman is having. Midwifery's focus is on improving conditions for women and their families. In a way, midwifery is a radical departure from the old way of looking at pregnancy."

Deborah typically arrives at the hospital at 7:00 AM and spends the first hour or more seeing patients in postpartum—that is, women who have given birth the day or night before. At about 8:30, Deborah goes down to the clinic to begin seeing other patients. "I work a combination of full days and half days during the week. On a half day, I'll see patients for four hours and work on paperwork for one hour. On a full day, I'll see patients for eight hours and work on paperwork for two hours," Deborah says. "But that doesn't mean I always leave exactly at five o'clock. At the clinic, we see everyone who shows up."

After Deborah meets a new patient, she'll spend an hour or so taking the patient's medical history, examining her, and getting her scheduled into the prenatal care system. "I also ask about a patient's life. I spend time with the patient and try to get to know her and what's going on in her life. It makes a big difference in the care she's provided. I think one of the things that makes midwives so effective is that they really get to know their patients." Deborah points to one patient to highlight this. "One of my patients was a woman who was having her third child. This woman had always been good about keeping her appointments. Then she stopped coming in. I knew something had to be wrong. So I called people at different agencies, and they helped me track her down. It turned out that she had moved, and she wasn't doing well. We were able to get her back into the system and make sure she had a healthy baby."

Educating her patients is another part of the care Deborah provides. In fact, Deborah believes that education is one of a midwife's most important responsibilities. "I spend a lot of time teaching things like nutrition, the process of fetal development, and basic parenting skills. I'll refer patients to Lamaze classes. I'll also screen patients for family problems, such as violence in the home, and teach them how to get out of abusive situations," Deborah says. "In other words, I'll teach a patient anything she needs to know if she's pregnant. I try to empower women to take charge of their own health care and their own lives."

Apart from seeing patients, Deborah is also responsible for maintaining patients' records. "I have to review lab results and ultrasounds, and fill out birth certificates—things like that. I also have to make sure I have correct addresses on my patients," Deborah says. "There's a lot of writing involved, too. I have to document everything that I do with patients, including what I've done and how and why I've done it."

have I got what it takes to be a nurse-midwife?

"Speaking as both a midwife and someone who teaches midwives, I think there's one area that seems most difficult for some nurses who get into this profession," Deborah says. "That's making the leap from just being a physician's 'assistant' to having the autonomy of a midwife. As a midwife, you take on more responsibilities for the patient, and that means you have to be prepared to accept the consequences of the decisions you make. There is no more saying, 'I was only following orders,' if something goes wrong. Some nurses find that very stressful. But it's also part of what attracts a lot of us to this field. We really have a lot more direct influence on the quality and nature of our patients' care."

Midwifery is still not accepted by some physicians and other health care providers. "We don't get the slack that docs do," Deborah says. "A lot of people take a doctor's word as law. But a good midwife needs to know her business. She has to have a lot of information at the top of her head—things like statistics, data, and procedures—and she needs to know exactly where that information comes from. This is because people still challenge a midwife's knowledge. And while a lot of obstetricians and gynecologists accept us, there are still many who don't. So you must be confident and poised when working with doctors."

Midwives share both in the joys of childbirth and in the tragedies. "The birth of children is supposed to be fun," Deborah says, "but the reality is that people also die. And in childbirth, when it goes bad, it goes really bad. I've had to hold babies while they die, and I've had to comfort mothers whose babies have died. This is especially difficult for midwives because they become so involved in their patients' lives. So anyone considering midwifery needs to be aware of this part of it, too. But again, most of us become midwives because of the real impact we can have on our patients and their childbirth experiences. It's a great job if you love it. And there really are many more ups than downs."

Giving her patients a sense of empowerment is one of the most important and most satisfying parts of Deborah's career. "Of course I love 'catching' [delivering] babies," Deborah says. "There's nothing as much fun as that. But over the course of my career I've gained more perspective, and I see now that that's not really where a midwife can make the most difference. The biggest part of what I do is to help women learn the stuff they need to make their own lives better. I've learned to ask a woman what she needs, and then to help her get it. The best is when I'm assisting a woman who's giving birth, and she looks up into my eyes and says, 'I did it.'"

Trying to empower patients can be very difficult. "There is a lot of frustration," Deborah acknowledges. "You're dealing with a lot of political and socioeconomic realities, like poverty, violence, and neglect, and this can become overwhelming at times. There's so

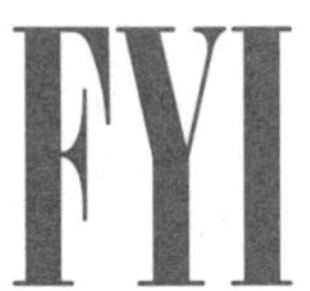

Childbirth Is Natural

The practice of midwifery is many thousands of years old. In most cultures around the world, births are usually attended to by midwives rather than physicians. The United States is one of the few countries where births are usually physician-delivered in hospital settings.

Hospitals began to replace homes as the places of birth early in the 20th century. At the same time, the use of drugs to reduce pain and induce labor became commonplace. In addition, cesarean sections, in which the uterus is cut open for childbirth, increased in frequency.

Though this approach to childbirth undoubtedly decreased infant mortality in the United States, many people began to criticize it during the 1960s. The main criticism was that modern medicine was robbing women of the feelings and sensations associated with childbirth. The natural childbirth movement increased the popularity of midwifery.

Today, midwifery, as practiced by professional nurses who work in consultation with physicians, is generally accepted by the medical establishment.

much that needs to be done, and it's frustrating to recognize that you can't do it all. And these are aspects that cut across all levels of society. It's not just something that you face in a city hospital. It's in the suburbs and in rural areas, too." For Deborah and many midwives, however, this challenge is part of what brought them to this career. "As a midwife," Deborah says, "you have an impact not only on the birth experience, but also on all of a patient's life."

To be a successful nurse-midwife, you should

- Enjoy working with people
- Be independent and able to accept responsibility for your actions and decisions
- Have strong observation, listening, and communication skills
- Be confident and composed

how do I become a nurse-midwife?

education

High School

A high-school student should begin preparing for a career in midwifery by emphasizing science courses. "I'd advise a high-school student to take heavy science," Deborah says. Those science courses may seem inapplicable at the time, but as you move into nursing you'll see how useful they actually are."

A prospective midwife needs to gain a broad range of education and experience. "A midwife is just as people-focused as she is science-focused," Deborah says. "So take courses in English, language, philosophy, psychology, and sociology. Language and communication skills are especially necessary because you'll be responsible for maintaining detailed reports on what you do with patients, and you'll be communicating information with patients, doctors, nurses, and insurance companies."

Deborah advises students to gain as much work experience as possible. "They should volunteer at hospitals, especially at facilities where they can work with adolescents. They can also become involved in peer-to-peer counseling." These experiences can make a difference in gaining admission into a midwifery program.

Postsecondary Training

All nurse-midwives begin their careers as registered nurses. In order to become a registered nurse, one must graduate from either a four-year bachelor's degree program in nursing or a two-year associate's degree program in nursing. After receiving a degree, a registered nurse applies for admission into an accredited certificate program in nurse-midwifery or an accredited master's degree program in nurse-midwifery.

A student with an associate's degree in nursing is eligible for acceptance into a certificate program in nurse-midwifery. A certificate program requires nine to twelve months of study. In order to be accepted into a master's degree program in nurse-midwifery, a student must have a bachelor's degree in nursing. A master's degree program requires sixteen to twenty-four months of study. Some master's degree programs also require one year of clinical experience in order to earn a degree as a nurse-midwife. In these programs, the prospective nurse-midwife is trained to provide primary care services, gynecological care, preconception and prenatal care, labor delivery and management, and postpartum and infant care.

Procedures that nurse-midwives are trained in include performing physical examinations, Pap smears, and episiotomies. They may also repair incisions from cesarean sections; administer anesthesia; and prescribe medications. Nurse-midwives are also trained to provide counseling on such subjects as nutrition, breastfeeding, and infant care. Nurse-midwives learn to provide both physical and emotional support to pregnant women.

certification or licensing

After graduating from a nurse-midwifery program, nurse-midwives are required to take a national examination administered by the American College of Nurse-Midwives (ACNM). Those who have passed this examination are licensed to practice nurse-midwifery in all fifty states. Each state, however, has its own laws and regulations governing the activities and responsibilities of nurse-midwives.

who will hire me?

Deborah Woolley earned a bachelor's degree in nursing and then began her career as a nurse at a labor and delivery unit in a Texas hospital. While working, she attended graduate school and received a master's degree in maternal child nursing. She then came to Chicago, where she began training as a nurse-midwife. "After earning my nurse-midwifery degree," Deborah says, "I heard there were openings at Cook County Hospital here in Chicago. So I applied for a job there. What I liked about Cook County was that they continued to train me while I was working. They gave me assertiveness training and training in urban health issues."

Hospitals are the primary source of employment for nurse-midwives. Approximately 85 percent of the more than 6,000 nurse-midwives in the United States work in hospitals. Most of the remaining nurse-midwives work in family planning clinics (including Planned Parenthood centers) and other health care clinics and agencies. Some nurse-midwives operate their own clinics and birthing centers, while others work independently and specialize in home birth deliveries.

where can I go from here?

With experience, a nurse-midwife can advance into a supervisory role or into an administrative capacity at a hospital, family planning clinic, birthing center, or other facility. Many nurse-midwives, like Deborah Woolley, choose to continue their education and complete Ph.D. programs. With a doctorate, a nurse-midwife can do research or teaching. "I spent four-and-a-half years at Cook County while I was working on my Ph.D.," Deborah says. "From there I was recruited to Colorado to head up the midwifery unit at a hospital there. After six years as a director in Colorado, I learned that the director's position here at UIC was open, and I jumped at the chance to come back to Chicago."

what are the salary ranges?

Nurse-midwives are among the highest paid of nursing professionals. The average salary for an experienced nurse-midwife is around $38,000 per year. The most experienced nurse-midwives, including those in supervisory, director, and administrative positions, can earn more. Starting salaries for beginning nurse-midwives range from $22,000 to $28,000 per year, depending on the place of employment; those working for large hospitals tend to earn more than those working for small hospitals, clinics, and birthing centers. Salaries also vary according to the region of the country; according to urban, suburban, or rural setting; and according to whether the employing facility is private or public.

Nurse-midwives generally enjoy a good benefits package, although these too can vary widely. Most nurse-midwives work a forty-hour week. The hours are sometimes irregular, involving working at night and on weekends. This is partly due to the fact that the timing of natural childbirth cannot be controlled.

what is the job outlook?

The number of nurse-midwifery jobs is expected to grow faster than the average for all occupations through 2005, as nurse-midwives gain a reputation as an integral part of the health care community. Currently, there are more positions than there are nurse-midwives to fill them. This situation is expected to continue for the near future.

There are two factors driving the demand for nurse-midwives. The first factor is the growth of interest in natural childbearing techniques among women. The number of midwife-assisted births has risen dramatically since the 1970s. Some women have been attracted to midwifery because of studies that indicate natural childbirth is more healthful for mother and child than doctor-assisted childbirth. Other women have been attracted to midwifery because it emphasizes the participation of the entire family in prenatal care and labor.

The second factor in the growing demand for nurse-midwives is economic in nature. As society moves toward managed care programs and the health care community emphasizes cost-effectiveness, midwifery should increase

in-depth

Breastfeeding—benefits and bothers

Midwifery supports the practice of breastfeeding over bottle-feeding. Human milk contains antibodies that protect infants from infections, and breastfeeding strengthens the psychological bond between mother and child.

However, problems sometimes develop with breastfeeding. A breast may become engorged with milk, preventing the infant from sucking properly. In addition, nipples can become sore and cracked, and infections and abscesses can develop in the breasts.

Lactation consultants are health care professionals who help prevent and solve breastfeeding problems. They work in hospitals, public health centers, and private practices. The International Board of Lactation Consultant Examiners certifies lactation consultants. Among the people certified as lactation consultants are many nurse-midwives, dieticians, physicians, and social workers.

Information about becoming a lactation consultant can be obtained from the International Lactation Consultant Association, 200 N. Michigan Ave., Suite 300, Chicago, IL 60601; Tel: 312-541-1710.

in popularity. This is because the care provided by nurse-midwives costs substantially less than the care provided by obstetricians and gynecologists. If the cost advantage of midwifery continues, more insurers and health maintenance organizations will probably direct patients to nurse-midwives for care.

how do I learn more?

professional organizations

Following are organizations that provide information on nurse-midwife careers, accredited schools, and employers.

American College of Nurse-Midwives
818 Connecticut Ave., NW, Suite #900
Washington, DC 20006
TEL: 202-728-9860
WEBSITE: http://www.acnm.org

Midwives Alliance of North America
P.O. Box 175
Newton, KS 67114
TEL: 316-283-4543

bibliography

Following is a sampling of materials relating to the professional concerns and development of nurse-midwives.

Books

Bennet, V. Ruth, and Linda K. Brown, editors. *Myles Textbook for Midwives,* 12th edition. New York, NY: Churchill Livingstone, 1993.

Croft, Jennifer. *Careers in Midwifery*. New York, NY: Rosen Group, 1995.

Davis, Elizabeth. *Heart and Hands: a Midwife's Guide to Pregnancy and Birth.* Berkeley, CA: Celestial Arts Publishing Co., 1995.

Hobbs, Leslie. *The Independent Midwife: a Guide to Independent Midwifery Practice.* New York, NY: Butterworth-Heinemann, 1993.

Oakley, Anne, and Susanne Houd, editors. *Helpers in Childbirth: Midwifery Today.* Bristol, PA: Taylor & Francis, 1990.

Weaver, Pam, and Sharon K. Evans. *Practical Skills Guide for Midwifery: a Tool for Midwives and Students.* Bend, OR: Morningstar Publishing, 1994.

Periodicals

Journal of Nurse-Midwifery. Bimonthly. Includes the presentation of current knowledge in the fields of nurse-midwifery, parent-child health, obstetric, well-woman gynecology, family planning, and neonatology. American College of Nurse-Midwives, Elsevier Science, Inc., 655 Avenue of the Americas, New York, NY 10010, 212-989-5800.

Midwifery Today and Childbirth Education. Quarterly. Directed to professionals and non-professionals alike; balances technical articles with personal accounts and photography to present a wide range of options and perspectives on current birth care issues. Jan Tritten, Box 2672, Eugene, OR 97402, 503-344-7438.

Special Delivery. Quarterly. Discusses midwifery alternatives in birth, parenting, and early childhood education. Association of Labor Assistants and Childbirth Educators, Informed Birth and Parenting, Box 382724, Cambridge, MA 02238, 617-441-2500.

nurse practitioner

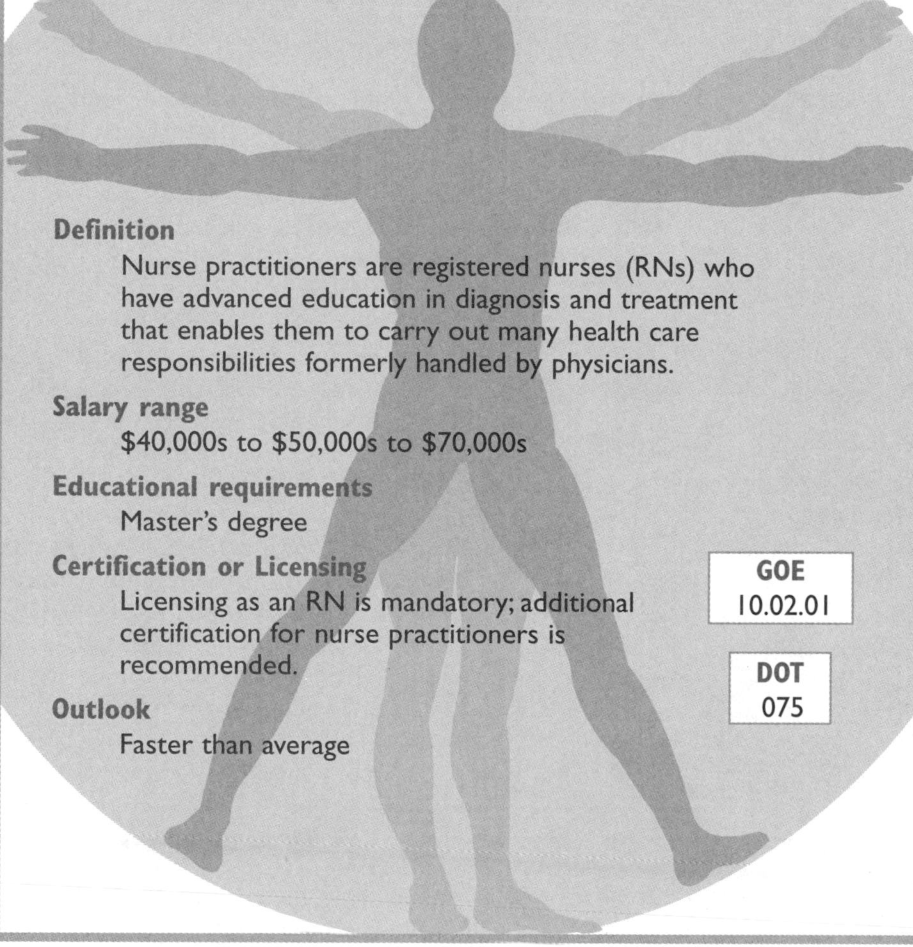

Definition

Nurse practitioners are registered nurses (RNs) who have advanced education in diagnosis and treatment that enables them to carry out many health care responsibilities formerly handled by physicians.

Salary range

$40,000s to $50,000s to $70,000s

Educational requirements

Master's degree

Certification or Licensing

Licensing as an RN is mandatory; additional certification for nurse practitioners is recommended.

Outlook

Faster than average

GOE
10.02.01

DOT
075

High School Subjects

Biology
Chemistry
English
Mathematics

Personal Interests

Working with people
Helping people
Health care
Accepting challenges

In working with college students, Harvey Bennett says it is essential to establish rapport. "You need to be a good listener and make it clear that confidentiality will be respected," he explains.

Harvey, the head nurse practitioner at Vanderbilt University's Student Health Service, spends much of his work day seeing students with a variety of health complaints. An average of 150 students visit the Health Service each day, with problems ranging from colds and sore throats to alcohol-related problems or eating disorders.

Careful assessment of each case is important. Most of the time, it turns out that one of the Center's six nurse practitioners can handle the problem without calling in a staff physician.

what does a nurse practitioner do?

Nurse practitioners provide health care in a wide range of settings, generally focusing on primary care, health maintenance, and prevention of illness. They carry out many of the medical responsibilities traditionally handled by physicians. They do physical exams, take detailed medical histories, order lab tests and X rays, and recommend treatment plans.

lingo to learn

Acute Describes a disease or symptom that begins suddenly and does not last long.

Advanced practice nurses Nurses with advanced education that enables them to take on many responsibilities formerly carried out by physicians; nurse practitioners, clinical nurse specialists, certified nurse midwives, and certified registered nurse anesthetists are classed as advanced-practice nurses.

Chronic Describes a disease or condition that develops gradually and often remains for the rest of the person's life, such as glaucoma.

Clinical Pertaining to direct, hands-on medical care; from the Greek word for "bed."

LPN Licensed practical nurse—an individual trained in basic nursing who usually works under the supervision of a registered nurse.

PAP smear A test that examines cells (taken during a pelvic exam) to detect cancers of the cervix.

Protocol A written plan (prepared in advance) that details the procedures to be followed in providing care for a particular medical condition.

RN Registered nurse—a professional nurse who has completed an approved course of study and passed the National Council of Licensing Examination.

Wellness A dynamic state of health in which a person moves toward higher levels of functioning—a term often used by nurse practitioners.

The nurse practitioner role developed in the 1960s in response to the shortage of physicians and the need for alternative health care providers, especially in remote rural areas. Harvey Bennett was attracted to the profession during its early years because he valued its goal—to keep people out of the hospital by providing good primary and preventive care.

As a result of their advanced training, nurse practitioners are qualified to work more autonomously than staff nurses. In 1986, a study carried out by the U.S. Congress Office of Technology Assessment found that "within their areas of competence, nurse practitioners provide care whose quality is equivalent to that of care provided by physicians." In preventive care and communication with patients, nurse practitioners were found to excel doctors. By 1992, there were approximately 30,000 nurse practitioners in the United States, and the number is continuing to increase rapidly.

A nurse practitioner's exact responsibilities depend on the setting in which she or he works and the field of specialization chosen. A nurse practitioner may work in close collaboration with a physician at a hospital, health center, or private practice office or, as in the case of a rural health care provider, may have only weekly telephone contact with a physician. Nurse practitioners may not function entirely independently of a physician, although the degree of consultation required varies from state to state. As Harvey points out, it is important for nurse practitioners to develop the judgment to recognize when an illness or injury is beyond their level of competence.

Most nurse practitioners have a field of specialization. The commonest specialty (and the broadest in its scope) is *family nurse practitioner* (FNP). Family nurse practitioners, who are often based in community health clinics, provide primary care to people of all ages—assessing, diagnosing, and treating common illnesses and injuries. Their interactions with patients have a strong emphasis on teaching and counseling for health maintenance. Nurse practitioners recognize the importance of the social and emotional aspects of health care, in addition to the more obvious physical factors.

Nurse practitioners in other specialties perform similar tasks, though working with different age groups or with people in school, workplace, or institutional settings. *Pediatric nurse practitioners* (PNPs) provide primary

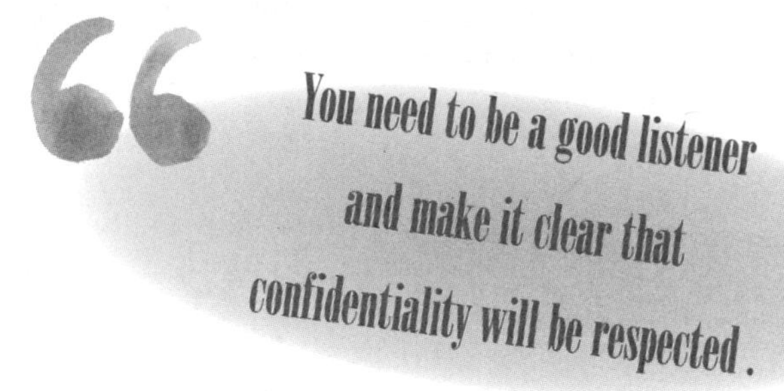

health care for children (infants through adolescents). Developmental assessment is an important part of the pediatric nurse practitioner's responsibilities: Is this child within the norms of physical and social growth for his or her age group? *Gerontological nurse practitioners* work with older adults. They are often based in nursing homes.

School nurse practitioners work in school settings and provide primary health care for students in elementary, secondary, or higher education settings. *Occupational health nurse practitioners* focus on employment-related health problems and injuries. They work closely with occupational health physicians, toxicologists, safety specialists, and other occupational health professionals to identify potential dangers and to prevent work-related illness or injury. *Psychiatric nurse practitioners* work with people who have mental or emotional problems.

Women's health care nurse practitioners provide primary care for women from adolescence through old age. In addition to handling overall primary care, they do Pap smears and breast exams, provide information on family planning and birth control, monitor normal pregnancies, and offer treatment and counseling for gynecological problems and sexually transmitted diseases. Some nurse practitioners are also certified in midwifery.

In most states, nurse practitioners are allowed to write certain prescriptions, but a physician's signature is often required to validate the prescription.

what is it like to be a nurse practitioner?

Harvey Bennett has been a nurse practitioner in Vanderbilt's Student Health Service since 1984. He is certified as a family nurse practitioner. Though he is qualified to provide primary care to persons of all ages, in his present position his practice is confined to the Vanderbilt student population—undergraduates who are generally 18 to 22 and graduate and professional students who may be in their 20s, 30s, and 40s.

After completing the nurse practitioner program at Vanderbilt, Harvey spent six years working as a family nurse practitioner based in rural health clinics in Alabama and Georgia. Each clinic was staffed by a nurse practitioner; there was a physician "somewhere in the county." During his Georgia years, the nearest good hospital was 35 miles away. The shortage of doctors and hospitals meant that the nurse practitioners formed long-term relationships with the people they served and had the satisfaction of knowing that they were making a difference in people's lives. It also meant that they were likely to have people knocking on the door in the middle of the night with a medical emergency. In both Alabama and Georgia, Harvey found a high level of acceptance from patients, but in Alabama there was considerable hostility to nurse practitioners from the medical establishment. During the Reagan administration, clinic funding was cut back, so Harvey returned to Nashville.

At Student Health, Harvey spends most of his time seeing students who have come in with health problems. He takes a history from each patient, does a physical, and orders lab tests (if indicated). Treatment is based on a protocol developed by the nurse practitioners and doctors; as long as the complaint can be handled within the protocol, the nurse practitioner works without consulting the doctor.

In assessing each case, it is essential to find out whether the reported symptoms may actually reflect a more serious underlying problem. For example, in many cases, students suffering from depression come to the Center complaining of headaches, stomach pains, or fatigue.

Teaching and counseling are important parts of the job. College students are at a formative age, and Harvey tries to make a positive impact on their daily health habits. Health topics he discusses with them include alcohol and tobacco use, diet, seat-belt use, and the need to wear bicycle safety helmets. Students often need assistance in making the connection between the symptoms they are experiencing and their behavior (such as smoking or excessive consumption of alcohol). In addition to seeing patients, Harvey, as head nurse practitioner, is also responsible for scheduling and quality control.

Another area of specialization is gerontological nursing care. Kay Grott spent about seven years as a gerontological nurse practitioner in several Tennessee nursing homes. She first encountered this specialty in a junior-year seminar during her undergraduate nursing program at East Tennessee State University. At that time, the lack of appropriate health care for older adults had become a focus of public concern, and Kay decided that she wanted to contribute to solving the problem.

At first, she planned to become a clinical nurse specialist with a concentration in gerontological care, but one of her instructors urged her to become a nurse practitioner instead; he pointed out that nurse practitioners were assuming an increasingly important role in the health care industry. Receiving her M.S. from the Medical College of Virginia, Kay found the nurse- practitioner role to be a "good fit."

As a nurse practitioner at a nursing home, Kay was the person responsible for coordinating her patients' total care. She was the liaison between the patient's family, the physician, and the other health care providers. Good communication skills are essential, as well as being comfortable working with older people; that part was easy for Kay, who grew up in an extended multigenerational family. Her work included taking detailed medical histories of each patient, performing physical exams, ordering lab tests and X rays, and monitoring chronic illnesses It is also important to monitor the patient's progress under the treatment plan drawn up by the health care team. Some typical medical problems are Alzheimer's disease, Parkinson's disease, cardiac conditions, and COPD (Chronic Obstructive Pulmonary Diseases).

Working with people approaching the end of life, Kay often had to deal with issues of death and dying. Sometimes that meant helping to make people's last months as peaceful and comfortable as possible instead of pursuing an aggressive treatment plan.

A nurse practitioner employed at a nursing home is not always involved in direct patient care. At one point, Kay worked as director of nursing. In that position, she succeeded in raising the nursing home's standards of care to meet new federal standards introduced in the late 1980s.

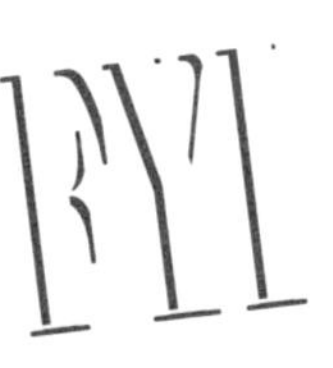

The nurse practitioner role developed in the 1960s in response to the shortage of physicians and the need for alternative health care providers.

have I got what it takes to be a nurse practitioner?

A nurse practitioner needs to enjoy working with people and to be strongly committed to making a positive difference in people's lives. Nurse practitioners must develop excellent communication skills. Being a good listener is essential, as is the ability to encourage people to answer questions about personal matters that they may find it difficult to talk about. Anyone going into a health care field needs to have patience and flexibility and the ability to remain calm in an emergency.

Since nurse practitioners work more independently than nurses traditionally do, it is important for them to develop the capacity to take active responsibility in health care situations. At the same time, they must have the judgment to identify those situations that are beyond their competence and to call in a physician or other specialist.

Because the nurse practitioner role is strongly focused on health maintenance and prevention, a person considering becoming a nurse practitioner should find teaching and counseling at least as satisfying as dramatic medical interventions.

A nurse practitioner has to be prepared for the possibility of friction with professional colleagues. The nurse-practitioner profession is still new, and some physicians are uncomfortable with it; some display hostility to the idea of nurses functioning in autonomous roles. The nurse practitioner seems to be perceived as a threat by some physicians. Relations with staff nurses can also be a problem for nurse practitioners at times, because some staff nurses resent taking orders from anyone except a doctor. Some patients who have never encountered a nurse practitioner before may be concerned about "just seeing the nurse instead of the doctor." All these situations need to be handled in a mature and professional way.

The problems involved in dealing with insurance companies are also a major source of stress for many nurse practitioners. Although the nurse practitioner is widely recognized as a cost-effective provider of health care, insurance regulations make it difficult for them to receive direct reimbursement.

To be a successful nurse practitioner you should

- Be strongly committed to making a positive difference in people's lives
- Have patience and the ability to remain calm in an emergency
- Find teaching and counseling as satisfying as dramatic medical interventions
- Be able to identify those medical situations where it is necessary to call in a physician

how do I become a nurse practitioner?

education

High School

Future nurse practitioners should take a well-balanced college preparatory course in high school, with a good foundation in the sciences. Obviously, biology, chemistry, and physics are important courses. If your high school offers anatomy and physiology as a follow up to the basic biology course, that would be a good elective. You also need to take courses in the humanities and social sciences. Classes that improve communication skills are especially helpful for anyone going into a people-oriented field like nursing.

The high school years are also a good time to start getting some hands-on experience in health care. Try doing volunteer work at a local hospital, community health center, or nursing home. There are probably nurse practitioners in your community who would be glad to discuss their work with you and let you follow them around for a few days to observe.

Postsecondary Training

You need to be a registered nurse (RN) before you may become a nurse practitioner. There are three ways to become an RN: an associate's degree program at a junior or community college, a diploma program at a hospital school of nursing, or a bachelor's-degree program at a college or university. All programs combine classroom study and clinical experience in hospitals and other health care settings.

The bachelor's degree is generally necessary for anyone who wants to go on for the additional training (usually at the master's-degree level) required to become a nurse practitioner. A student who begins nursing study in an associate's degree or diploma program may transfer into a bachelor's-degree program later. Students with an undergraduate major other than nursing may also enter nursing-degree programs, although they may need to fulfill some additional prerequisites. (Harvey Bennett has an undergraduate degree in engineering. After serving in the Navy in the Vietnam War, he decided that he wanted to find a different profession.)

In nursing school, students study the theory and practice of nursing, taking such courses as human anatomy and physiology, psychology, microbiology, nutrition, and statistics. Students in bachelor's-degree programs also study English, humanities, and social sciences. After finishing their educational program, students must pass a national examination in order to be licensed to practice nursing in their state and to use the initials "RN" after their name.

A master's degree is usually required to become a nurse practitioner. Programs last one to two years and provide advanced study in diagnostic skills, health assessment, pharmacology, clinical management, and research skills. Classroom work is combined with "hands-on" clinical practice. Usually the student begins with generalist work and later focuses on preparation for a specific nurse practitioner specialty. Admission to good nurse practitioner programs is very competitive.

certification or licensing

Every state requires RNs to pass the National Council Licensing Examination before they are allowed to practice in that state. Some states require continuing education for license renewal.

National certification exams for nurse practitioners are available and strongly recommended by professional organizations, although not every state requires nurse practitioners to have national certification.

scholarships and grants

There are numerous sources of financial assistance for people studying nursing at both the undergraduate level and advanced levels. The Nurses Association in your state, the National Student Nurses' Association, nursing honor societies, state departments of education, the federal government, private agencies, civic and alumni associations, and the U.S. military are all possible sources of scholarships.

There may be scholarship aid targeted for members of specific racial/ethnic groups. The National League for Nursing publishes an annual guide, *Scholarships and Loans for Nursing Education.* Students should be aware that some scholarship sponsors require recipients to work for their agency for a certain length of time after graduation, generally at full salary.

If you are already an RN employed by a health care agency and you want to take graduate courses to prepare to become a nurse practitioner, you may be eligible for tuition assistance or reimbursement from your employers.

In addition to the sources mentioned above, you should consult the financial-aid office of the educational institution you plan to attend. When applying for any sort of financial aid, always be sure to begin the process in time to get your paperwork in by the deadline.

who will hire me?

Nurse practitioners are employed in hospitals, clinics, physicians' offices, community health centers, rural health clinics, nursing homes, mental health centers, educational institutions, student health centers, nursing schools, home health agencies, hospices, prisons, industrial organizations, the U.S. military, and other health care settings. In the states that allow nurse practitioners to practice independently, self-employment is an option.

The particular specialty you pursue is obviously is a major factor in determining your employment setting. Another important factor is the degree of autonomy you desire. Nurse practitioners in remote rural areas have the most autonomy, but they must be willing to spend a lot of time on the road visiting patients who are unable to get to the clinic, to be on call at all hours, and to make do with less than optimal facilities and equipment.

The placement office of your nursing school is a good place to begin the employment search. Contacts you have made in clinical settings during your nurse practitioner program are also useful sources of information on job opportunities. Nursing registries, nurse employment services, and your state employment office have information about available jobs. Nursing journals and newspapers list openings. If you are interested in working for the federal government, contact the Office of Personnel Management for your region. Applying directly to hospitals, nursing homes, and other health care agencies is also an option for nurse practitioners.

where can I go from here?

Nurse practitioners have many avenues for advancement. After gaining experience, they may move into positions that offer more responsibility and higher salaries. Some choose to move into administrative or supervisory positions in health care organizations or nursing schools. They may become faculty members at nursing schools or directors of nursing at a hospital, clinic, or other health agency.

Some advance by doing additional academic and clinical study that gives them certification in specialized fields. Those with an interest in research, teaching, consulting, or policymaking in the nursing field would do well to consider earning a Ph.D. in nursing. In the early 1990s, there were thirty-three doctoral-degree programs in nursing in the United States, and that number seems likely to increase.

what are the salary ranges?

In 1996, nurse practitioners' salaries ranged from the low $40,000s to over $70,000, with the national median estimated to be from the upper $40,000s to the low $50,000s. Geographical location and experience are factors in salary levels. Nurse practitioners must often expect to work long and inconvenient hours, especially if they are in rural practice.

what is the job outlook?

The job outlook for nurse practitioners is excellent, since the nurse practitioner is being increasingly recognized as a provider of the high-quality yet cost-effective medical care that the nation's health care system needs. More and more, people are recognizing the importance of preventive health care, which, of course, is one of the nurse practitioner's greatest strengths. All nurse practitioner specialties are expected to continue growing. There should be an especially strong demand for gerontological nurse practitioners, as the percentage of the U.S. population in the over-sixty-five age group increases. The Midwest and the South are expected to be the areas of greatest growth in demand for nurse practitioners.

Nurse practitioner organizations are working to promote legislation that will increase the degree of autonomy available to nurse practitioners and make it easier for them to receive insurance company reimbursement. This should make the profession an even more attractive route of advancement for RNs.

At the same time, it is important for those entering the profession to have realistic expectations. Some nurse practitioners report increasing frustration with recent cutbacks in the health care industry that make it difficult to persuade insurance companies to approve for reimbursement the treatment plans considered necessary by health care professionals. Problems with insurance companies and current restrictions on autonomy lead to burnout and disillusionment for some nurse practitioners, who emerged from their master's-degree programs with idealistic goals for their profession.

how do I learn more?

professional organizations

For additional information about a career as a nurse practitioner, contact the following:

American Academy of Nurse Practitioners
Capitol Station, LBJ Building
P.O. Box 12846
Austin, Texas 78711
TEL: 512-442-4262

National Alliance of Nurse Practitioners
325 Pennsylvania Avenue SE
Washington, DC 20003
TEL: 202-675-6350

bibliography

Following is a sampling of materials relating to the professional concerns and development of nurse practitioners.

Books

Becker, Betty G., and Dolores T. Fendler. *Vocational and Personal Adjustments in Practical Nursing*, 7th edition. St. Louis, MO: Mosby, 1993.

Burns, Catherine E., and others. *Pediatric Primary Care: a Handbook for Nurse Practitioners*. Philadelphia, PA: W.B. Saunders, 1996.

Camenson, Blythe. *Nursing*. Lincolnwood, IL: VGM Career Horizons, 1995.

Fondiller, Shirley H., and Barbara J. Nerone. *Nursing: the Career of a Lifetime*. New York, NY: National League for Nursing, 1995.

Frederickson, Keville. *Opportunities in Nursing Careers,* revised edition. Lincolnwood, IL: VGM Career Horizons, 1995.

Heron, Jackie. *Exploring Careers in Nursing,* revised edition. New York, NY: Rosen Group, 1990.

Kelly, Lucie Y., and Lucille A. Joel. *The Nursing Experience: Trends, Challenges, and Transitions,* 3rd edition. New York, NY: McGraw-Hill, 1996.

Kurzen, Corrine R. *Contemporary Practical Vocational Nursing,* 3rd edition. Philadelphia, PA: Lippincott-Raven, 1996.

Newell, Robert, editor. *Developing Your Career in Nursing.* New York, NY: Cassell, 1996.

Sherman, Margie. *Your Opportunities in Nursing.* Salem, OR: Energeia Publishing Co., 1994.

Yannes-Eyels, Mary. *Mosby's Comprehensive Review of Practical Nursing,* 11th edition. St. Louis, MO: Mosby, 1995.

Periodicals

American Academy of Nurse Practitioners Journal. Quarterly. Captures what's happening in clinical practice, management, education, research, and legislation. Slack, Inc., 6900 Grove Road, Thorofare, NJ 08086, 609-848-1000.

Imprint. 5 per year. Practical journal for people interested in nursing careers. January issue is devoted to career planning. National Student Nurse Association, 555 W. 57th Street, New York, NY 10019, 212-581-2211.

Nurse Practitioner: the American Journal of Primary Health Care. Monthly. Offers articles of interest to primary health care nurses. Elsevier Science, 655 Avenue of the Americas, New York, NY 10010, 212-989-5800.

Nursing: the World's Largest Nursing Journal. Monthly. Articles offer how-to, step-by-step approaches to clinical situations. Springhouse Corp., 111 Bethlehem Pike, Box 908, Springhouse, PA 19477, 215-646-8700, 800-346-7844.

obstetrician/gynecologist

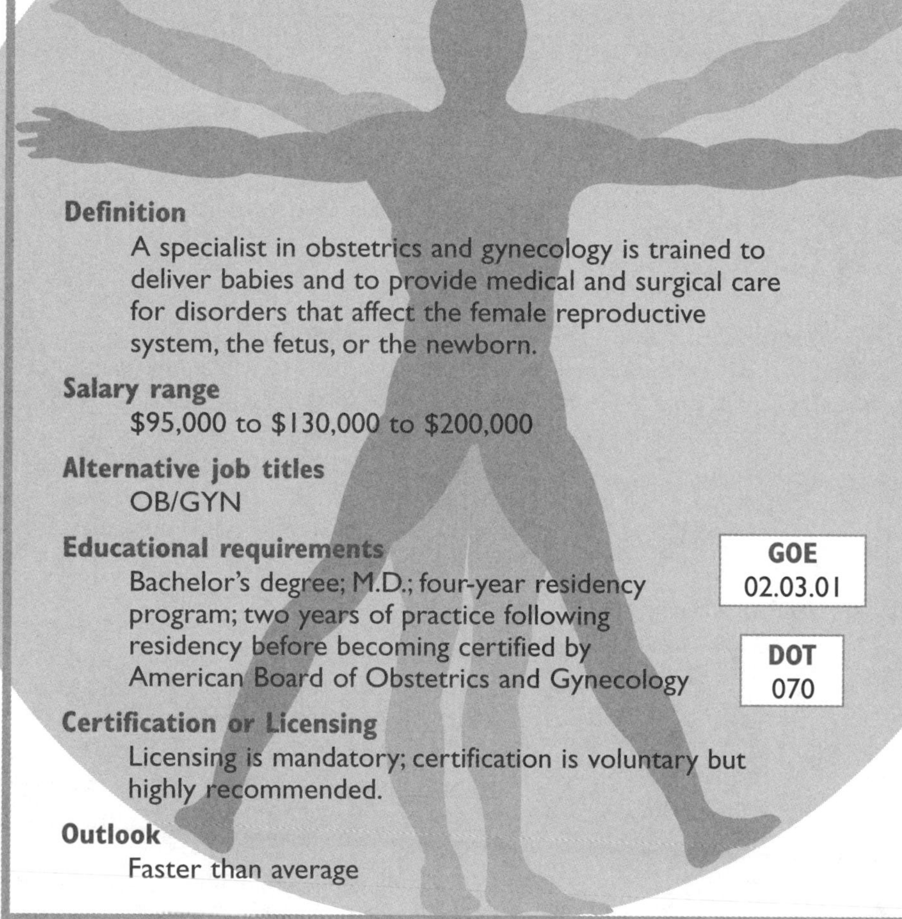

Definition

A specialist in obstetrics and gynecology is trained to deliver babies and to provide medical and surgical care for disorders that affect the female reproductive system, the fetus, or the newborn.

Salary range

$95,000 to $130,000 to $200,000

Alternative job titles

OB/GYN

Educational requirements

Bachelor's degree; M.D.; four-year residency program; two years of practice following residency before becoming certified by American Board of Obstetrics and Gynecology

Certification or Licensing

Licensing is mandatory; certification is voluntary but highly recommended.

Outlook

Faster than average

GOE
02.03.01

DOT
070

High School Subjects

Biology
Chemistry
Computer Science
English
Health
Math

Personal Interests

Babies
Helping others
Science
Women's health

Handel's Water Music is playing softly in the background. The lights are dim and a voice says gently, but firmly, "Okay—now, push."

The pregnant woman lying on the bed in the birthing room has broken into a fine sweat, but she nods at her obstetrician's command. Her face screws up with determination and she tries to concentrate on pushing, but the epidural shot the obstetrician gave her an hour ago has kicked in and she has little feeling below her waist.

"Come on, now, Gretchen. You've got to try and push, 'cause this baby of yours wants to say hello." Gretchen's obstetrician looks over at Gretchen's sister, Ida. "See if you can help her focus."

Ida takes her sister's hand and begins taking Gretchen through a focusing exercise. Although this is Gretchen's fourth baby, it's the first time she's had an epidural. Suddenly, Gretchen breaks into laughter as she struggles to push.

The obstetrician looks beneath the drape that covers Gretchen's legs. She smiles broadly and gives the thumbs up sign. Gretchen gives another push, and again breaks into laughter.

"Keep laughing," smiles Linda, "every time you laugh, the baby's head comes further out."

what does an obstetrician/gynecologist do?

Obstetrician/gynecologists provide medical and surgical care for disorders that affect the female reproductive system, the fetus, or the newborn.

lingo to learn

Cervix The narrow outer end of the uterus. As the time of delivery of a baby approaches, the cervix dilates, or opens, to allow the baby to pass through the uterus, into the birth canal, and out of the woman's body.

Cesarean birth In a cesarean birth a surgical incision of the walls of the abdomen and uterus allows for the safe delivery of the baby. Also called a cesarean section, or a c-section.

Epidural Anesthesia administered into the spinal cord that numbs the pelvic area of a woman in labor.

Pap smear A method for the early detection of uterine cancer. The method involves the staining of exfoliated uterine cells using a special technique which differentiates diseased tissue. Also called a Pap test.

Speculum A medical instrument used to separate the walls of a body cavity for examination.

STD An acronym for sexually transmitted disease. Among the most common are such diseases as AIDS, herpes, gonorrhea, syphilis, and chlamydia.

They care for and treat women before, during, and after childbirth. They commonly serve as consultants to physicians who practice in other areas of medicine.

The specialty of obstetrics and gynecology can be divided into two parts. Obstetrics focuses on the care and treatment of women before their pregnancy, during their pregnancy, and after the child is born. Gynecology is concerned with the treatment of diseases and disorders of the female reproductive system. Because the areas overlap, the specialties are generally practiced together. Preventative measures and testing make up a large part of an obstetrician/gynecologist's practice.

Obstetrician/gynecologists provide many different types of health services to women, from prenatal care to Pap tests to screening tests for sexually-transmitted diseases (STDs) to breast exams and birth control. With specialization, the obstetrician/gynecologist's practice may focus on pregnant patients, cancer patients, or even infertile patients.

The subspecialties of obstetrics and gynecology are critical care medicine, gynecologic oncology, maternal-fetal medicine, and reproductive endocrinology. A *critical care medicine obstetrician/gynecologist* has received additional training in order to manage aspects of the critically ill patient. This specialist works in the hospital's intensive care unit (ICU) with various specialists to utilize recognized techniques for vital life support and to care for a patient with a critical illness. A *gynecologic oncologist* is trained in the comprehensive management of patients with cancers that affect the female reproductive system. A gynecologic oncologist works in an institutional setting in which all forms of cancer therapy are available to the patient. Comprehensive management includes diagnostic and therapeutic procedures that are necessary for the total care of patients with cancer, or its resulting complications.

A *specialist in maternal-fetal medicine* cares for, and consults on, patients with high-risk pregnancies. This specialty requires advanced knowledge in the medical and surgical complications of pregnancy, and their effect on both the mother and the fetus. This specialty also requires expertise in the most current diagnostic and treatment techniques that are used in the care of patients with high-risk pregnancies. Finally, a *reproductive endocrinologist* or an REI specialist is an obstetrician/gynecologist who has been trained in the management of the complex problems relating to reproductive endocrinology and infertility.

Patients usually see obstetrician/gynecologists in one of several settings: in a private solo or group practice; in an institutional clinic at a large hospital or university; or in a public health agency clinic that is active in preventive health care.

Regardless of the setting, the routine is the same. The patient schedules an appointment, arrives early to fill out the necessary paperwork that will contribute to the patient's history, and then meets with the physician. The obstetrician/gynecologist first takes the patient's history and listens as the patient describes the problem, or the reason for the visit. The second part of the visit is the examination, and the type and extent of the exam depends upon the purpose of the visit. While the general area of the examination is pretty much the same (vaginal area, cervix, ovaries, and uterus), the prenatal exam of a pregnant woman in her eighth month would differ from the gynecologic exam of a woman with a yeast infection. The obstetrician/gynecologist might use an instrument called a speculum to better observe the condition of the vagina and its walls, and to see the shape of the cervix. If the obstetrician/gynecologist felt it were necessary, he or she might schedule the patient for tests or X rays. The obstetrician/gynecologist then explains to the patient what the disorder is and the treatment he or she recommends.

Disorders that obstetrician/gynecologists commonly treat include yeast infections, pelvic pain, endometriosis, infertility, and uterine and ovarian cancer. An obstetrician/gynecologist prescribes medicines or other therapies, and if necessary, schedules and performs surgery.

When an examination and test indicates that a patient is pregnant, an obstetrician/gynecologist sets up regular appointments with the patient throughout the pregnancy. These visits make up a crucial part of any woman's prenatal care, helping her learn about her pregnancy, nutrition and diet, and activities that could adversely affect the pregnancy. In addition, during these visits the patient is examined to see that the pregnancy is progressing normally. Later in the pregnancy, the frequency of visits increase, and they become important in determining a birthing strategy, and any alternative plans. An obstetrician/gynecologist will deliver the baby and care for the mother and child after the delivery.

At these prenatal appointments, the physician listens to the baby's heartbeat and examines its position within the mother's uterus. An obstetrician/gynecologist also checks the mother's health and well-being, since these can directly affect the baby's health. For example, if the mother is depressed and ill, she may not be eating regularly or well, and her poor diet could harm the baby's development. An obstetrician/gynecologist treats any difficulties that may occur in the mother or the unborn child.

To be a successful obstetrician/gynecologist , you should:

- Be a good clinician
- Be an extremely good communicator, capable of putting patients at ease
- Have good hand-eye coordination and manual dexterity
- Enjoy working with and helping people

When labor begins, an obstetrician/gynecologist meets the patient at the hospital, examines her, and periodically checks on her to see that the labor is progressing. Labor can last anywhere from several minutes to several days; the obstetrician/gynecologist supervises the labor, and makes decisions based on the health of the mother and unborn child, as well as on previous discussions the obstetrician/gynecologist has had with the patient. For example, some women want to experience as little discomfort as possible. To accommodate those wishes, the patient and the obstetrician/gynecologist discuss the option of having anesthetics administered, such as an epidural. Other women consider the pain and discomfort a natural part of the labor and delivery process, and they would ask that no anesthetics be administered. In the event of a serious problem, an obstetrician/gynecologist may have to overrule the wishes of the patient in the interests of the collective health of patient and child.

During delivery, an obstetrician/gynecologist may work with an anesthesiologist or nurse anesthetist who administers anesthetics to the patient. The obstetrician/gynecologist might use his or her hands to guide the baby's head through the mother's vagina, or birth canal, or he or she might use forceps. The desired position of the baby for delivery is head first, but sometimes the position of the baby requires a feet-first delivery. If the baby is ready to be delivered, but for some reason cannot pass through the birth canal, the obstetrician/gynecologist performs what is known as a cesarean delivery, also referred to as a cesarean section. This involves making an incision on the woman's abdomen, surgically removing the baby from the uterus, removing the placenta, and then closing the incisions with sutures. In a normal, vaginal delivery, an obstetrician/gynecologist waits until the woman expels the placenta (or afterbirth), and then he or she ties and cuts the umbilical cord.

After delivery, an obstetrician/gynecologist visits the mother in the hospital to make sure she is recovering well. In the event the obstetrician/gynecologist has performed a cesarean section delivery, he or she checks the closing sutures to make certain they are healing and are not infected. Six weeks after delivery, the mother goes back to the obstetrician/gynecologist for a checkup. Throughout the pregnancy, delivery, and postdelivery period, an obstetrician/gynecologist keeps a detailed medical record on the patient.

what is it like to be an obstetrician/gynecologist?

Dr. Carol Cook describes herself as a typical obstetrician/gynecologist. She is in a large single specialty group practice with seven other obstetrician/gynecologists. "We bridge the office practice typical of internists, with the surgical practice of a general surgeon," she explains. "I see a lot of women for routine checkups," she says. "I would say that around 30 percent of my cases are yearly checkups."

"We see pregnant women on the OB side, and gynecological disorders on the GYN side," says Dr. Cook. "There aren't any subspecialists in our group. If I have a patient who's pregnant with triplets, I'll call my person in Maternal-Fetal Medicine, and I'll say, 'let's do it together.' The same goes for a patient with uterine cancer. I'll call the Gyn-Onc specialist."

Dr. Cook is usually in her office by 8:00 AM every day. "Today, my eight o'clock was an OB patient," she says. "She's thirty-eight weeks along, and she came in with her two-year old and her husband. Her first delivery she had elsewhere, and it was a nine-and-a-half pound baby by c-section," Dr. Cook explains. "This time, she wants to deliver vaginally, if at all possible." Dr. Cook describes her examination of the patient. "I check the size of the cervix. It was two centimeters, getting what we call, 'ripe.' She's almost ready to give birth," says Dr. Cook. "Remember, she's already at thirty-eight weeks. Thirty-seven to forty-two weeks is term." Dr. Cook pauses and then continues. "Then, I see how big the baby is—I do this every visit—by checking the fundal height. Fundis is latin for 'top of the uterus.' It felt pretty good-sized, so she's probably going to have another nine pounder. At any rate, I check the baby's heart tones, and then we discuss what we're going to do. Because she wants to deliver vaginally, we talked it over and decided to wait until forty weeks, and then we'll probably induce." Dr. Cook explains that c-sections are harder to recover from than vaginal births, so many women try and deliver the baby on their own, without surgery.

On the flip side of the coin—the gynecological side of her practice—Dr. Cook sees patients with a wide range of problems. Typical gynecological problems that she treats include urinary tract and yeast infections, pelvic pain, infertility, and cervical, uterine, and ovarian cancer. Although she never hesitates to call a specialist in the particular area. "I want my patient to have the best care, and that means getting the person involved who spent extra time studying that particular area, whether that's an REI specialist or a Gyn-Onc."

Another type of patient Dr. Cook treats is the older patient who is in menopause. The onset of menopause can have distressing symptoms such as interruption of sleep, extreme moodiness, night sweats, and hot flashes, among others. "Some women have such bad symptoms, they can't function," Dr. Cook explains. Menopausal women have the choice of taking hormone replacement therapy (HRT), usually a combination of progesterone and estrogen, to counteract and/or mitigate the symptoms of

FYI

During the 1930's Dr. George Papanicolaou found that cervical cancer could be detected by studying cells from a woman's genital tract. This led to the development of the Pap test, now a routine gynecological procedure used to detect cervical cancer. According to the American Cancer Society, the Pap test, along with regular gynecological check-ups, has reduced deaths caused by cervical cancer by 70 percent over the past forty years.

severe menopause. According to Dr. Cook, there are actually some advantages to being on HRT. "Women on HRT have less heart disease. When women are in menopause, though, and without HRT, their risk of heart attack is equal to that of men. Women are also at risk of osteoporosis. HRT can help [lower the risk] we believe."

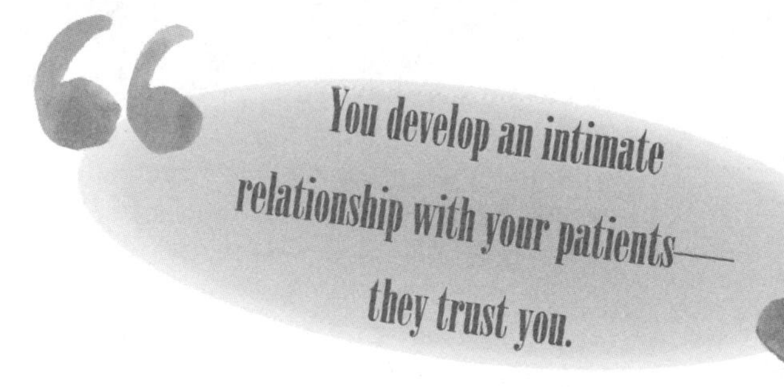

have I got what it takes to be an obstetrician/gynecologist?

Obstetrician/gynecologists, like all physicians, should enjoy helping and working with people. Most of their time is spent with patients, talking to them and listening to their histories and problems. Because of the intimate nature of the profession, they may also end up with a more complete picture of their patients personal lives than most other physicians ever obtain. "I'm a people person," says Dr. Cook. "I really enjoy communicating with my patients. But I also enjoy surgery. Ob/Gyn is a nice mix of both." She often finds that her rapport with her patients makes them more likely to use her as a sounding board for other medical questions. "I do a lot of primary care," says Dr. Cook. "But, according to my insurance, I'm not designated as such, so I can't do it officially. Still, you develop an intimate relationship with your patients—they trust you—and ask you things they might not ask another physician. So I get asked for a lot of medical advice."

Communication skills are essential to all physicians, but especially to an obstetrician/gynecologist. The intimate nature of both the patient's condition and the examination, requires that an obstetrician/gynecologist be able to put the patient at ease while asking questions of an intimate nature.

Obstetrician/gynecologists work long, irregular hours. They may be paged at any moment to rush to the hospital to deliver a baby or handle a medical emergency. On a typical day, an obstetrician/gynecologist might have to travel from his or her office to the hospital several times in one day. An obstetrician/gynecologist might start the day by reviewing patient charts at the office and then head to the hospital to perform surgery and make rounds. After returning to the office, an obstetrician/gynecologist might see patients during the afternoon, and then finish the day by updating medical records, phoning patients, and reading journals to keep up with new developments in the field.

It is still possible for an obstetrician/gynecologist to have a relatively normal life outside of the world of obstetrics and gynecology. Unlike a trauma surgeon, the obstetrician/gynecologist knows which obstetrics patients of his or hers are likely to deliver, and which gynecological patients are at risk of some emergency.

how do I become an obstetrician/gynecologist?

education

High School

High school students should prepare for a future in medicine by taking courses in biology, chemistry, physics, algebra, geometry, and trigonometry. Courses in computer science are a must, as well, since the computer is changing the way medicine is communicated and shared by busy medical professionals. Also important are courses such as English or speech, that foster good communication skills, which will be needed by any prospective physician.

Postsecondary Training

University or college courses that may help prepare prospective medical students for medical school, are math, biology, chemistry, anatomy, and physics, as well as courses in the humanities, such as English composition. Many students wishing to attend medical school will follow a premed program of study, which includes many science courses. Prospective medical school students usually take the Medical College Admission Test (MCAT) in their junior or senior year. This test is required to apply to medical schools.

Admission to medical school is competitive and applicants must undergo an extensive admissions process which considers grade point averages, scores on the MCAT, and recommendations from professors. Most premedical students apply to several schools early in their senior year of college. Competition is stiff; only about one-third of the applicants are accepted.

In order to earn an M.D., a student must complete four years of medical school study. For the first two years, students attend lectures and classes and spend time in laboratories. Courses include anatomy, biochemistry, physiology, pharmacology, psychology, microbiology, pathology, medical ethics, and laws governing medicine. They learn to take patient histories, perform routine physical examinations, and recognize symptoms.

In their third and fourth years, students are involved in more practical studies. They work in clinics and hospitals supervised by residents and physicians and they learn acute, chronic, preventive, and rehabilitative care. They go through what are known as rotations, or brief periods of study in a particular area, such as internal medicine, obstetrics and gynecology, pediatrics, psychiatry, and surgery. Rotations allow students to gain exposure to the many different fields within medicine and to learn firsthand the skills of diagnosing and treating patients.

Upon graduating from medical school, physicians must pass a standard examination given by the National Board of Medical Examiners. Most physicians complete an internship. The internship is usually one year in length, and helps graduates to decide what will be their area of specialization.

Following the internship, physicians begin what is known as a residency. Physicians wishing to pursue the surgical specialty of obstetrics-gynecology must first complete a minimum of four years in residency, thirty-six months of which must be entirely in obstetrics and gynecology, with a one-year elective.

After completing a residency in obstetrics and gynecology, a specialist in obstetrics and gynecology may pursue additional training to subspecialize in critical care medicine, gynecologic oncology, maternal-fetal medicine, and reproductive endocrinology.

certification or licensing

All physicians must be licensed by their state to practice medicine legally. Certification by the American Board of Obstetrics and Gynecology (ABOG) is highly recommended.

In the last months of the obstetrician/gynecologist's residency, he or she takes the written examination given by the ABOG. Candidates for certification take the final oral examination after two or more years of practice. Candidates must have successfully passed the written portion of the certifying exam before they are eligible to take the oral portion.

scholarships and grants

Scholarships and grants are often available from individual institutions, state agencies, and special-interest organizations. The book *Dollars for College: Medicine, Dentistry, and Related Fields* by Ferguson Publishing is an excellent source for this information. Many students finance their medical education through the Armed Forces Health Professions Scholarship Program. Each branch of the military participates in this program, paying students' tuitions in exchange for service in the military. Contact your local recruiting office for more information on this program. The National Health Service Corps Scholarship Program also provides money for students in return for public service. Another source for financial aid, scholarship, and grant information is the Association of American Medical Colleges. Remember to request information early for eligibility, application requirements, and deadlines.

Association of American Medical Colleges
2450 N Street, NW
Washington, DC 20037
TEL: 202-828-0400
WEBSITE: http://www.aamc.org
Specific information on financial aid programs can be found at:
WEBSITE: http://www.aamc.org/stuapps/finaid

Ferguson Publishing Company
200 West Madison, Suite 300
Chicago, IL 60606
TEL: 312-580-5480

National Health Services Corps Scholarship Program
U.S. Public Health Service
1010 Wayne Avenue, Suite 240
Silver Spring, MD 20910
TEL: 800-638-0824

in-depth

Cesarean Birth

Cesarean birth is a major surgical procedure requiring some form of anesthesia. There are two basic types of cesarean birth techniques—cervical and classical. The cervical type involves making a horizontal or vertical incision in the lower uterus. Classical cesarean involves making a vertical incision in the main body of the uterus. Today, the horizontal cervical type is by far the most common method of cesarean birth.

There are several reasons for a physician to choose to deliver a baby via cesarean. The most common is *dystocia,* a catch-all term meaning "difficult labor." There are three different conditions that lead many doctors to indicate dystocia: abnormalities of the mother's birth canal; abnormalities in the position of the unborn child in the uterus; and significant abnormalities in uterine contractions. Another cause for cesarean birth is fetal distress—when the unborn child develops a markedly abnormal heart rate, endangering the health of the child.

The procedure of making an incision into the abdominal area to facilitate childbirth can be traced back nearly 5,000 years, to ancient Egypt. There are various theories concerning the source of the name. One states that the name dates back to 715 BC, when a set of Roman laws, the *Lex Caesare,* mandated the surgical removal of an unborn child upon the death of the mother. Another theory traces the name to the story that Julius Caesar was born using this procedure.

Cesarean birth was generally used as a last resort until the 1970s. With the refinement of surgical techniques, improved fetal monitoring equipment, the rise of malpractice lawsuits, and the development of new antibiotics, use of cesarean birth technique has increased rapidly—tripling from 5 to 16.5 percent of all births from 1970 to 1980. There has been some controversy surrounding the increased use of this technique, with some who believe that it is used too frequently. Today, about 23 percent of all births in the United States occur via cesarean.

who will hire me?

Most obstetrician/gynecologists are in private solo or group practice, although some work for public health agencies, women's organizations, and university hospitals and clinics. Obstetrician/gynecologists who work for public health agencies and clinics are active in preventive health care and work in these settings as administrators, consultants, or planners.

A growing number of physicians are partners or salaried employees of group practices. Organized as medical groups, these physicians can more easily afford expensive medical equipment, insurance costs, and other business expenses.

where can I go from here?

Advancement opportunities for an obstetrician/gynecologist comes by way of acquiring more skill and knowledge and increasing the size of the practice. Going back to school to learn a subspecialty is one way of advancing; however, it also means a serious investment, both of time and finances. Involvement in professional organizations and societies may lead to committee appointments and chairs, which are markers of respect by one's peers.

what are the salary ranges?

The national average salary for first-year residents in the mid-1990's was approximately $31,000. That average increases to $41,800 by the final residency year. Salaries will vary depending on the kind of residency, the hospital, and the geographic area.

According to surveys by the American Medical Association, practitioners of internal medicine in the mid-1990's had a salary range of approximately $95,000 to $200,000. The median income was about $130,000. These figures are for all doctors of internal medicine, and income for obstetrician/gynecologists may vary from these numbers. Other factors that influence annual income include size and type of practice, hours worked per week, professional reputation of the individual, and the geographic location.

what is the job outlook?

The general population is aging, and health care needs increase dramatically with age. The health care industry, in general, is doing exceptionally well, despite the claims of managed care critics to the contrary. The employment of physicians in almost all fields is expected to grow faster than the average for all occupations through the year 2005. Salaries, however, are predicted to drop somewhat, due to managed care.

Specifically, the demand for obstetrician/gynecologists hasn't abated. The specialty is shifting from a male-dominated field to a female-dominated field; of the medical students planning to enter obstetrics and gynecology, 60 percent are now women.

how do I learn more?

professional organizations

Following are organizations that provide information on the profession of obstetrician/gynecologist.

American Board of Obstetrics and Gynecology (ABOG)
2915 Vine Street
Dallas, TX 75204
TEL: 214-871-1619

American College of Obstetricians and Gynecologists (ACOG)
409 12th Street SW
Washington, DC 20024
TEL: 202-638-5577
WEBSITE: http://www.acog.com

American Gynecological and Obstetrical Society
UVA Health Science Center
Box 387
Charlottesville, VA 22908
TEL: 804-923-9937

bibliography

Following is a sampling of materials relating to the professional concerns and development of obstetrician/gynecologists.

Books

Beckmann, Charles R., and others. *Obstetrics and Gynecology*, 2nd edition. Baltimore, MD: Williams & Wilkins, 1995.

Gant, Norman, and F. Gary Cunningham. Basic *Obstetrics and Gynecology*. New York, NY: Appleton & Lange, 1993.

Nolan, Thomas E. *Primary Care for the Obstetrician and Gynecologist.* New York, NY: Wiley, 1996.

Periodicals

American Journal of Obstetrics and Gynecology. Monthly. American Gynecological and Obstetrical Society, Mosby, 11830 Westline Industrial Drive, St. Louis, MO 63146, 314-872-8370, 800-325-4177.

Contemporary Ob-Gyn. Monthly. Sets the standards for women's health. Includes practical advice by leading authorities in the ob-gyn field. Medical Economics, Five Paragon Drive, Montvale, NJ 07645, 800-526-4870.

Female Patient: Practical Ob-Gyn Medicine. Monthly. Total health for women. Excerpta Medica, Inc., Core Publishing Division, 105 Raider Boulevard, Belle Mead, NJ 08503, 908-874-8550.

Obstetrical and Gynecological Survey. Monthly. Reviews articles of important obstetrical and gynecological articles from nearly 100 U.S. and international journals. Williams & Wilkins, 428 E. Preston Street, Baltimore, MD 21202, 410-528-4000, 800-638-6423.

occupational safety and health worker

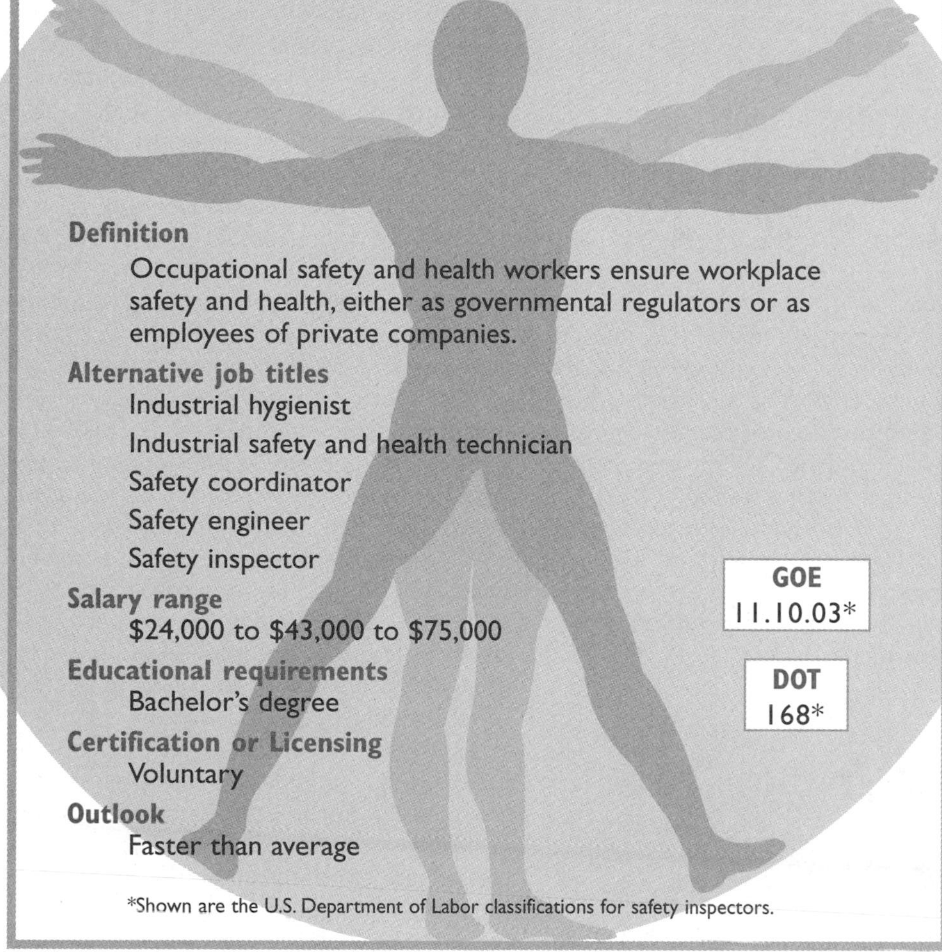

Definition
Occupational safety and health workers ensure workplace safety and health, either as governmental regulators or as employees of private companies.

Alternative job titles
Industrial hygienist
Industrial safety and health technician
Safety coordinator
Safety engineer
Safety inspector

Salary range
$24,000 to $43,000 to $75,000

Educational requirements
Bachelor's degree

Certification or Licensing
Voluntary

Outlook
Faster than average

GOE
11.10.03*

DOT
168*

*Shown are the U.S. Department of Labor classifications for safety inspectors.

High School Subjects

Algebra
Biology
Chemistry
English
Speech
Trigonometry

Personal Interests

Health
Working with people
Science
Puzzles

Inspections always required Chuck to be at the office early. This inspection, for a paper recycling plant, was generated by an employee complaint. He checked his paperwork and equipment one last time and headed to his car for the drive to the site. He expected to be gone all day.

When he arrived, he went through the ritual of showing his identification and announcing the inspection. The management was surprised, but cooperated. Chuck explained that he would take air samples, talk confidentially with employees, and tour the plant looking for possible hazards. Once he had explained the procedure he began the inspection.

From his interviews Chuck learned that the employees had been telling management for years about health concerns they had. People complained of nausea, headaches, and dizziness, but nothing had been done. Finally, someone filed a complaint with the Occupational Safety and Health Administration (OSHA). By the time he finished, it was late afternoon. He talked briefly with managers about what he had found. He could not be sure until his samples came back from the lab, but experience lead him to believe that the problem was excess carbon monoxide, a deadly and debilitating gas.

what does an occupational safety and health worker do?

Occupational safety and health workers are responsible for preventing accidents and illnesses related to the workplace environment. They work in industries like construction, steel making, automobile manufacturing, and insurance to identify and eliminate potential causes of worker injuries. In the government sector, *safety inspectors* and *industrial hygienists* work to see that companies are following laws governing employee safety and health.

Only since the late 19th century has an attempt been made to protect the lives of people who work in factories, mines, building sites, and offices. Little effort was made before then to protect workers. Even in the first half of this century, common wisdom held that there would be one death for each million dollars spent on construction. The building of the Golden Gate Bridge (1933-37) was a landmark in the progress of safety engineering. Through experimentation with new safety equipment and techniques and rigorous enforcement of work rules, there were no deaths for the first three years of construction. Overall, deaths on this very dangerous project were cut by two-thirds.

Safety and health workers not only save lives, but money as well. By eliminating lost work days, workers compensation claims, expensive lawsuits, and by lowering insurance premiums, companies can improve their profitability and competitiveness.

There are a number of different job descriptions that fall under safety and health work. *Safety engineers* try to eliminate conditions and practices that lead to accidents on the job. In construction and demolition they write safety plans for specific projects that reflect the unique nature of each job. They ensure that safety equipment like hard hats, safety shoes, and eye protection are worn. Safety engineers inspect work sites to see that rules concerning safety digging trenches, excessive dust (which causes breathing problems) and the operation of heavy equipment, are followed. In the trucking industry, *safety coordinators* deal with things like driver fatigue, proper loading and lifting, and equipment maintenance. Safety inspectors are employed by public utilities (gas, electric, etc.), and must have an understanding of electrical safety, proper climbing equipment and techniques, and fire prevention and fighting. All of these people investigate accidents when they occur and write recommendations for preventing future accidents.

Some occupational safety and health workers are employed by insurance companies or as consultants in the field of risk management. Claims resulting from accidents and illness cost the insurance industry many millions of dollars every year. Insurance companies employ experts to recommend ways of preventing costly accidents to their policyholders. These experts may specialize in fire prevention, safety engineering, or industrial hygiene.

Safety and health workers in government service are responsible for enforcing a broad range of laws and regulations governing every-

lingo to learn

Abatement date The date set by OSHA, after inspecting a facility and issuing a citation, when required modifications to correct a violation must be completed.

Repetitive Motion Injuries Injuries caused by doing the same task all day, as data entry or assembly line workers might do. These injuries can be very serious and are a growing source of insurance claims.

Site-Specific Safety Plan A safety plan for construction projects that take special dangers or unusual conditions into account.

Trench Safety Each year, workers are killed when improperly supported trenches collapse. Safety engineers help prevent these accidents by making sure excavations are braced.

thing from mine safety to the amount of fresh air someone working in a office must have. Inspectors investigate accidents and complaints. They cite infractions and levy fines, and sometimes testify in judicial proceedings. They work with private industry in an advisory role, too, educating and advising companies about their rights and responsibilities under the law.

In addition to their on-site inspection or laboratory work, occupational safety and health workers must do a great deal of recordkeeping and paperwork. They must complete worker compensation, insurance, and hospitalization forms after accidents in addition to any internal documentation that may be required. OSHA requires that a running tabulation of workplace injuries be maintained and displayed.

what is it like to be an occupational safety and health worker?

Chuck Wilson is an industrial hygienist for OSHA, working out of the Chicago-North office in Des Plaines, Illinois. He is responsible for seeing that workplaces do not have excessive lead, carbon monoxide, silica (tiny particles of sand), asbestos, or any other potentially dangerous substances. The story related above is just one of his inspections. It was a paper recycling company. "They used twenty propane-powered forklifts," he recalls. Tests showed that there was four times the legal exposure to carbon monoxide, which accounted for the headaches and nausea experienced by the employees. "The company had to improve ventilation in the plant and get the trucks serviced more frequently," he says, "but they cooperated. They even requested a reinspection after they made their changes."

The experience at the recycling plant is representative of what Chuck's job is usually like. Inspecting, taking samples, issuing citations where necessary, and occasionally reinspecting. "The inspector is the one who makes the decision on whether a reinspection is needed," Chuck explains. "Requesting a reinspection is pretty unusual." Chuck usually works alone, but there is support available if needed.

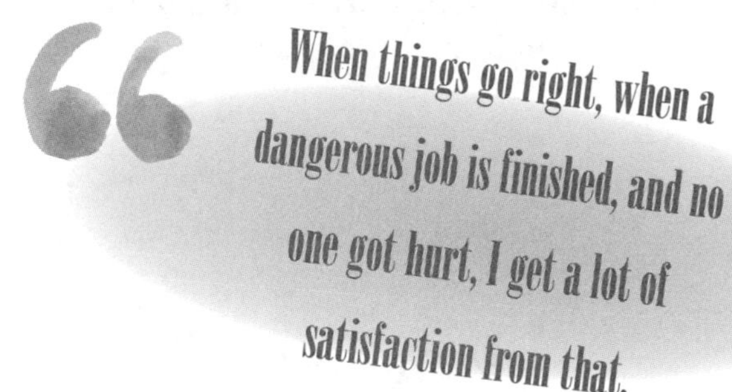

Chuck is assigned an inspection by his office supervisor. "Usually they [the assigned inspections] start as employee complaints," he says, "but we can also get referrals from other inspectors who might have been through a particular place." Once he is assigned to a case, he has to prepare. "I try and find out as much as possible about the company and the industry," Chuck says. On the day of the inspection, he calibrates his equipment, because accuracy of the devices is critical to an accurate assessment. He arrives at the site unannounced so that he gets a true picture of the situation as it has been maintained. "Most of the time, companies cooperate," he says. "Occasionally, a big company will insist I get a warrant, which takes a couple of days. They use the time to take care of as many violations as they can, to limit their penalty."

Once inside, there are specific steps he follows to ensure the inspection is done properly and the rights of companies are respected. "I explain what is going to happen first," he says. After he briefs management, Chuck conducts a walk-through to check for obvious violations, conducts confidential interviews with employees, and takes samples for later testing. "I can usually finish my inspections in one day," he says. Back in the office Chuck writes a narrative of the inspection (explaining exactly what went on during the investigation), prepares samples for shipment to laboratories, writes citations for any violations noted, and once again calibrates his equipment. Between the research prior to inspection and the quantity of paperwork after an it, Chuck does not get as many inspections done as he would like. "My goal is two inspections per week," he says, "but I don't always make it."

Tim Lally is a safety supervisor for National Wrecking Company of Chicago. Demolition is very hazardous work. Tim's job is to make it less dangerous. He investigates accidents when they occur but his biggest responsibility is pre-

To be a successful occupational safety and health worker you should

- Be articulate and have the ability to speak persuasively
- Be able to interact with a variety of people
- Have a good understanding of science and technology
- Be willing to work outdoors or in dangerous environments at times
- Have a strong commitment to creating safe work environments
- Have knowledge of a variety of industries

venting accidents from happening at all. "You have to play 'devil's advocate'," he explains. "What's the worst thing that could happen here? Then you try and prepare for it." He spends about half of his time doing on-site inspections; the other half is spent on paperwork, in transit, or in meetings.

For many of National's jobs, there are site-specific safety plans that must be written. Whatever task he is performing, Tim must be able to show that what he is doing is having an impact. "You have to justify what you do," he says. "You have to show management how you are improving productivity or profitability. It's a struggle sometimes, but they know that the costs of one bad accident can wipe out the profits from the next three or four." There is a lot of paperwork—insurance forms, doctors' office reports, accident reports, and government forms. During his on-site inspections, Tim talks to everyone from laborers to the job foremen. After all, it is they who will suffer if something goes wrong. Speaking about how safety initiatives are received by the workers, Tim has this to say. "The laborers, the equipment operators, they want to do the right thing. Everything comes down to the foremen, though. If they work with you, it makes the job much easier."

have I got what it takes to be an occupational safety and health worker?

Safety and health is first and foremost a communication job. Occupational safety and health workers must be able to speak persuasively to every type of person from top-level management to laborers. They must be confident and articulate. They must be able to think creatively to devise safety plans for changing circumstances. They must also have a good understanding of science and technology. Some types of safety and health work, such as fire prevention engineering, demand even greater technical proficiency. Since safety and health work is frequently outside, workers must be willing to endure bad weather and sometimes dangerous conditions.

Chuck has a science background, and he frequently uses his background skills in biology and chemistry. "There are some complex formulas for calculating the final exposures [to airborne contaminants]," he says. "You have to be comfortable with the technical aspects." Using his authority as an inspector took some getting used to. "At first, you're really eager, but you're nervous, too," Chuck recalls. "Walking into some huge company and telling them that they are about to be inspected was difficult. It's easy now, with experience."

There are many inspections waiting to be conducted at any given time, and unfortunately, not all of them are based on legitimate complaints or problems. "It's frustrating when people make phony complaints just to get back at their employers," Chuck says. "They are a waste of time. We end up not getting to the legitimate complaints as soon as we should, and that means people are in danger."

Tim's safety work requires him to be critical sometimes. "I get tired of finding fault," he says. "People perceive safety people as the bad guy." He addresses this misconception by trying to recognize the good things workers and supervisors do as well as criticize their errors. Managers can be difficult to deal with, especially when they feel that safety restrictions are cutting into the bottom line by requiring additional expenditures to fix problems or prevent possible ones. "Sometimes you have to convince guys that have been doing a job one way for years that they have to change," Tim says. Despite the headaches, Tim finds his work very rewarding. "When things go right, when a dangerous job is finished, and no one got hurt, I get a lot of satisfaction from that," Tim says. "I'm making the company safer. I'm helping people continue to enjoy the things they take for granted."

how do I become an occupational safety and health worker?

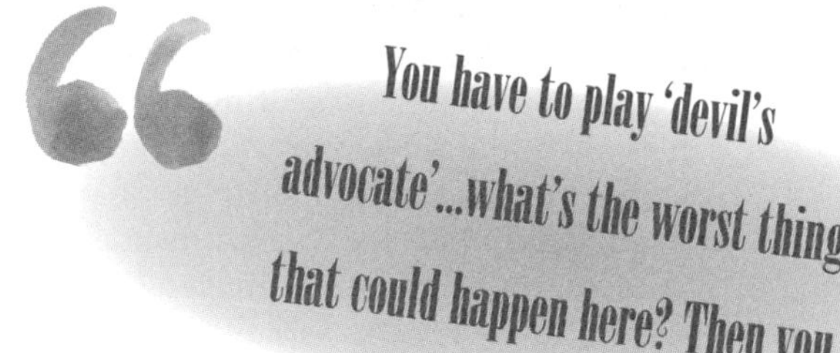

education

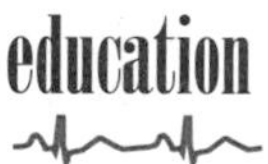

Occupational safety and health work requires at least a bachelor's degree. For most positions, safety engineering, safety management, or industrial hygiene degrees are preferred, but biology, chemistry, chemical engineering, or electrical engineering degrees are also possible routes into the field.

High School

High school students interested in safety and health work should take courses in biology, chemistry, algebra, and trigonometry. Written and oral communications are very important, so speech and English composition are helpful. Practical experience in industrial hygiene for high school students might be difficult to find, but for those interested in safety work in the construction industry, there are often summer construction jobs available. Tim Lally worked in construction and the experience has helped him understand what can and cannot be done on a job site. "Having worked in construction increases your credibility," he says.

Postsecondary Training

Neither Chuck nor Tim planned on careers in safety when they went to college. Chuck majored in biology and minored in chemistry before taking a job doing biological research for the Veterans Administration. Tim was studying communications when he decided to change majors to safety management. "I took a safety class to satisfy an elective requirement, and I really liked it," he remembers. There are more than one hundred schools offering degrees in safety and health related specialties. Some schools offer safety courses as part of their engineering programs but many have separate departments.

Many companies try to combine safety, industrial hygiene, and environmental management (preventing contamination of air, ground water, etc.) into a single position. People having experience or education in more than one area, a bachelor's degree in safety engineering and a minor in environmental engineering, for example, are more attractive to employers than those with a single specialty.

certification or licensing

Certification is voluntary. There are two types of occupational safety and health certification. The Board of Certified Safety Professionals offers a program to become a Certified Safety Professional (CSP). The American Board of Industrial Hygienists offers certification as a Certified Industrial Hygienist (CIH). Both require a combination of experience and education plus passing a comprehensive exam.

internships and volunteerships

Interning is a good way to gain experience and network for a job. Many large firms offer internships. College placement offices and trade publications are good places to look for openings.

who will hire me?

Chuck made a drastic career change, going from lab researcher to industrial hygienist, but his employer, the Federal Government, stayed the same. "It's a good career," he says, speaking of government service. "The benefits are excellent." Government agencies like OSHA are among the largest employers of safety and health workers. Heavy industries (e.g. steel making, motor vehicle manufacturing, oil refining), construction, and insurance, are also major employers of occupational safety and health workers. Companies advertise openings in industry trade journals or in journals devoted to safety engineering. Large companies often hire safety workers directly. Smaller companies may hire safety consultants who work on a contract basis. Some insurance companies offer industrial hygiene or safety reviews to their clients as a way of lessening the risk of a major claim from a serious accident.

where can I go from here?

Chuck is a GS12, a change of three pay grades from when he first came to OSHA. "GS13 and 14 are where you start to see people getting management positions," Chuck says. As positions in other offices become available, government employees are free to apply for them. This opens up possibilities for advancement for those willing to relocate. Outside government service, there is no single path of promotion that safety workers follow. Successful safety professionals can head company safety programs for several different facilities, or move from a branch office to the home office. Tim has advanced through several companies to the position he now holds as head of the National Wrecking Company's safety program.

Advanced degrees in areas such as business or law are helpful for moving into safety management or other executive positions. Those who wish to work for themselves become consultants once they have sufficient experience.

what are the salary ranges?

Salaries for beginning safety engineers start at about $24,000 per year, with experienced nonmanagers making about $43,000 per year. Managers and those with the most experience and advanced degrees may make up to $75,000 per year. Government service pays slightly less than private industry.

what is the job outlook?

Job growth for safety and health workers is expected to be stronger than average. Companies are finding it necessary to have safety and health workers on staff, even in difficult economic times, because the costs of accidents are simply too high. As mentioned above, those with more than one area of expertise will be the most marketable. As the workforce continues to become less industrial, there will be an increasing need for people specializing in things like repetitive motion injuries and in ensuring safe office environments.

how do I learn more?

professional organizations

Following are organizations that provide information on careers in occupational safety and health and certification requirements.

American Board of Industrial Hygienists
4600 West Saginaw
Suite 101
Lansing, MI 48917
TEL: 517-321-2638
WEBSITE:
http://www.midtown.net/~hcg/pro_abih.html

Board of Certified Safety Professionals
208 Burwash Avenue
Savoy, IL 61874
TEL: 217-359-9263
WEBSITE: http://www.bcsp.com/

For information on training and education requirements for the Occupational Safety and Health Administration (OSHA) contact:

OSHA Training Institute, Office of Training and Education
1555 Times Drive
Des Plaines, IL 60018
TEL: 847-297-4810

bibliography

Following is a sampling of materials relating to the professional concerns and development of occupational safety and health workers.

in-depth

Sick Building Syndrome

You find yourself complaining at work about the frequency of headaches, nausea, fatigue, and the inability to concentrate. Many of your co-workers have similar complaints. This might be a sign of a "sick building."

Sick building syndrome can have a variety of causes, all having to do with indoor air quality. Some of these are:

Poor ventilation of vapors of cleaning compounds, solvents, or other chemicals

The presence of carbon monoxide because of the proximity of building air intakes to vehicular traffic, a source of carbon monoxide.

Vapors emitted from new carpet, fresh paint, or photocopy machines.

Poorly designed heating and cooling systems.

Molds or fungi found in humidification systems.

The World Health Organization estimates that nearly a third of all new or renovated buildings may contain polluted air.

Books

Brimson, Terence J. *The Health and Safety Survival Guide: a Comprehensive Handbook for Managers*. New York, NY: McGraw-Hill, 1995.

Cox, Sue, and Tom Cox. *Safety, Systems, and People*. Newton, MA: Butterworth-Heinemann, 1996.

Erickson, Paul A. *Practical Guide to Occupational Health and Safety*. San Diego, CA: Academic Press, 1996.

LaDon, Joseph, editor. *Occupational Health and Safety,* 2nd edition. Itasca, IL: National Safety Council, 1993.

Weeks, James L., and others, editors. *Preventing Occupational Disease and Injury*. Washington, D.C.: American Public Health Association, 1991.

Periodicals

Applied Occupational and Environmental Hygiene. Monthly. Articles of interest to the occupational and environmental safety and health professional. American Conference of Governmental Industrial Hygienists, Inc., Elsevier Science, Inc., 655 Avenue of the Americas, New York, NY 10010, 212-633-3990.

Chilton's Industrial Safety and Hygiene News. Monthly. News of safety, health and hygiene, environmental, fire, security, and emergency protection equipment. Chilton Co., One Chilton Way, Radnor, PA 19089, 215-964-4028.

Industrial Hygiene News. 7 per year. Information on occupational health and high technology safety. Rimbach Publishing, Inc., 8650 Babcock Boulevard, Pittsburgh, PA 15237, 412-364-5366.

Job Safety and Health Quarterly. Quarterly. Features articles on job safety and health topics and contains current information on OSHA activities. U.S. Occupational Safety and Health Administration, Department of Labor, Frances Perkins Building, Room S2315, 200 Constitution Avenue, NW, Washington, DC 20210, 202-523-8148.

Occupational Hazards. Monthly. News on industrial safety, occupational health, environmental control, insurance, first aid, medical care, and hazardous material control. Penton Publishing, 1100 Superior Avenue, Cleveland, OH 44114-2543, 216-696-7000.

Occupational Health and Safety Letter:...Towards Productivity and Peace of Mind. Biweekly. News for workplace managers on maintaining staff safety; includes Americans with Disabilities Act regulations. Business Publishers, Inc., 951 Pershing Drive, Silver Springs, MD 20910-4464, 301-587-5300.

Safe Worker. Monthly. On-the-job safety information for non-supervisory personnel. National Safety Council, 1121 Spring Lake Drive, Itasca, IL 60143, 708-775-2281.

Safety and Health: the International Safety, Health, and Environmental Magazine. Monthly. For occupational safety, health, and environmental professionals. Provides extensive coverage of international safety, health, and environmental issues, including occupational health, traffic safety, environmental health, and industrial hygiene. National Safety Council, Periodicals Department, 1121 Spring Lake Drive, Itasca, IL 60143, 708-775-2285.

occupational therapist

Definition

Health care professionals who use "occupation," or purposeful activity, to help people with physical, developmental, or psychological disabilities relearn or maintain the abilities necessary for independent and satisfying lives.

Alternative job titles

OTR (occupational therapist, registered)

Salary range

$34,400 to $42,245 to $53,000

Educational requirements

Bachelor's degree in occupational therapy or bachelor's degree followed by an eighteen month program or bachelor's degree plus master's degree

Certification or Licensing

Certification is mandatory; licensing is mandatory in some states

Outlook

Much faster than average

GOE
10.02.02

DOT
076

High School Subjects

Biology
Physics
Psychology
Statistics

Personal Interests

Cooking
Design and construction
Helping people
Sewing
Using your hands

Chocolate chips bursting from a recently opened package lie on the counter. Two children, Josh and Ariel, are bustling about the specially designed kitchen facility. With great concentration, Josh measures a cup of flour into a large bowl. Ariel slowly adds a teaspoon of baking soda. Both leave a trail of ingredients in their wake, but Karen Jacobs, who is supervising the exercise, ignores the mess. "That's great work," she says with enthusiasm. "What do we add next?"

The harmony of this scene is suddenly disrupted, as Ariel snatches an egg carton from Josh's hands. "I want to put the eggs in," Ariel says belligerently.

Karen intercedes, gently putting a hand on the girl's arm. "Ariel, how would you feel if Josh had taken the egg carton away from you?"

The girl shrugs, but continues to clutch the egg carton tightly. "I wanna do it," she mumbles.

"Well, let's think about this problem," says Karen. "Both you and Josh want to add the eggs to the dough. The recipe says we need two eggs to make the cookies. Can you think of a solution that will make both of you feel good?"

Reluctantly, Ariel answers, "We can both put one egg in the bowl, I guess."

Karen Jacobs smiles. "That's a good idea," she says. As an occupational therapist, Karen uses activities such as baking cookies, carving pumpkins, or planting flowers to help children with developmental disabilities develop important social skills, such as cooperation and compromise.

"Occupational therapy takes a very holistic approach to working with people," explains Karen. "We work with the individual's—and the family's—physical, emotional, spiritual, and social context to help enhance the client's quality of life. When I work with children, I try to develop real-world exercises that will be fun and rewarding for children, while helping them develop necessary skills. To bake cookies, for instance, the children have to develop a plan for accomplishing the task by breaking it down into steps. They have to measure ingredients, which requires cognitive and small motor skills, and they have to cooperate. These are important skills that can help a person with a developmental disability succeed in an employment situation and live more independently."

Later, Ariel and Josh proudly place the warm cookies they have made on a small plate to share as they discuss the morning's activity with Karen. "I try to develop activities that will enable the children to feel a sense of accomplishment," Karen comments. "Occupational therapists also help clients, of every age, enhance their self esteem."

lingo to learn

Assistive technology Simple or complex tools that are designed to aid or increase the skills of a person with physical or mental limitations.

Ergonomics The design and placement of tools and equipment so that people can interact with these items at the maximum level of efficiency and safety.

Fine motor skills The fine or precise use of coordinated movements such as for writing, buttoning, and tying shoelaces.

Gross motor skills The use of large muscle groups to coordinate body movements such as for walking, balance, and throwing.

Psychosocial development The normal and orderly development of trust, autonomy, identity, and intimacy. A person begins this psychological and social development in infancy. Psychosocial dysfunction results from abnormal or arrested development.

Role playing Exercise in which a simulated situation, such as confronting someone with a disagreement, is acted out in order to give the participants an understanding of their emotions, appropriate behavior, and possibilities for resolution.

what does an occupational therapist do?

An *occupational therapist* uses everyday activities to help clients learn or relearn the skills necessary to care for themselves and to live more satisfying lives. Professionals in this field strive to help clients become as independent as possible in home, school, and work environments. Unlike physical therapists, who concentrate on helping clients regain physical functions, occupational therapists address the psychological and social dimensions, as well as the physical implications, of their clients' disabilities.

Frequently occupational therapists work closely with other health care providers, such as physicians, nurses, psychiatrists, speech therapists, physical therapists, and social workers. Together these professionals develop an appropriate treatment strategy for each client. Occupational therapists are trained to consider the client's needs, interests, potential, and likes and dislikes when establishing a treatment program. To succeed, treatment programs must be tailored to each client's personal circumstances.

Occupational therapists work with people, of all ages, who face a wide variety of challenges, including physical, developmental, or psychological disabilities. Some therapists, like Karen, work with children with physical or developmental challenges, helping them develop gross and fine motor skills, cognitive-perception skills, and psychosocial abilities. Others work with individuals who have become physically disabled through illness or injury. Occupational therapists also work with people who are recovering from work-related injuries, people recovering from substance abuse problems, elderly individuals, and premature infants.

Those who work with people who have disabilities concentrate on helping their clients learn, or relearn, basic daily skills, such as bathing, dressing, and eating. A client who has lost a limb may need to learn how to use a prosthetic device, such as an artificial leg. A client who has suffered a severe spinal cord injury may need to learn how to use a wheelchair or how to eat and dress with limited use of his or her hands. Once clients have mastered these fundamental skills, the occupational therapist helps them develop the skills necessary to care for a home and family, pursue an education, or maintain employment.

Occupational therapists who work in mental health or rehabilitation facilities help individuals who suffer from addiction, depression, eating disorders, or stress-related disorders regain self-confidence and prepare to resume control of their lives. These therapists may engage clients in role-playing exercises or in activities designed to reinforce planning and time-management skills.

Many occupational therapists work in nursing homes, helping older clients adapt to changes in their abilities due to advancing age. A client whose mobility is limited, for example, might need to learn to use a walker and to grip the handrail in the bathroom. An individual with arthritic hands may benefit from activities that emphasize manual dexterity, such as typing or knitting. Occupational therapists also help elderly individuals maintain physical and cognitive abilities through activities designed to exercise clients' muscles and stimulate their minds.

A growing number of occupational therapists today offer home health care services. By visiting clients at home, therapists are able to design real-world activities that can enhance clients' self sufficiency. These therapists can also help clients adapt their homes to their abilities. Many practitioners apply the concepts of ergonomics to make both the home and work environment more "user friendly."

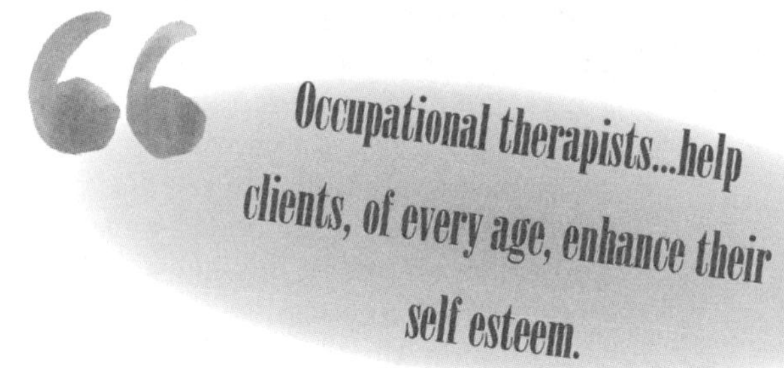

In addition to providing therapy, occupational therapists must maintain records of information about client evaluations, progress reports, staff notes, daily treatment notes, billing statements, and discharge notices. Many also supervise certified occupational therapy assistants (COTA) and act as consultants or advisors to local or state agencies. For those who pursue advanced degrees, teaching and research positions are also available.

what is it like to be an occupational therapist?

Karen, who is a clinical associate professor of occupational therapy at Boston University, in Boston, Massachusetts, is in her office by 7:30 AM, sipping tea as she reviews her lecture notes. At 8:00, Karen hurries to a nearby classroom to deliver a lecture on occupational therapy principles and their application to diverse client groups. Karen draws on her past experiences as a practicing occupational therapist to illustrate the theories and to keep the students focused on the purpose of the profession, which is to help people who are experiencing physical, emotional, or mental challenges.

At 10:30, Karen supervises a clinical laboratory class in which students are designing and constructing assistive technology. One student is building a portable "Wheel of Fortune" game to help clients who are recovering from strokes improve their vocabulary and memory. Another is cutting out pieces of cardboard that will be used as the foundation for a candy house. By frosting the house and decorating it with candy pieces, children who have cerebral palsy will enhance their fine motor skills. "Be careful not to choose candy pieces that are too small, Laela," says Karen. "It's very important to enable the children to experience success."

Over lunch, Karen grades student papers and works on one of the many papers she is preparing for publication. At 1:00, she takes two undergraduate students to the William Carter School, a Boston public school for young people with severe learning disabilities. "I believe in giving students exposure to community practice very early in their academic experience," says Karen.

At the William Carter School, Karen's occupational therapy students work with children who have cerebral palsy, seizure disorders, hearing and visual impairments, communication difficulties, and impaired mobility. Karen helps her students lead activities that will encourage the children to develop or enhance important skills. One student helps a child who has difficulty brushing his teeth build a very simple model airplane. While doing something he enjoys, the child is enhancing his fine motor skills. Karen works very closely with her students, and with their clients, to design the best therapeutic strategy for each child.

At 3:00, Karen meets with a graduate student to discuss the progress he has made on his dissertation. At 4:30, she delivers a presentation for several registered nurses at a local hospital. "Occupational therapists work closely with other health care providers," Karen explains. "It's important for the entire health services team to understand the important role occupational therapy can play in accelerating a patient's recovery."

In the evening, Karen spends several hours with her family before preparing lecture notes for the following day.

Because Karen is a professor as well as an occupational therapist, her typical day may be very different from that of an occupational therapist who works in a public school system, a hospital, or a mental health facility. According to Mary Foto, an occupational therapist in California who specializes in industry issues, it is almost impossible to generalize about how occupational therapists spend their days. "This is an extremely diverse field," she explains.

Mary owns a consulting company that helps employers establish return-to-work programs for employees who were injured on the job. Because she works with adults who have employment-related injuries, Mary's job is very different from Karen's. A typical day for Mary might include several appointments with recovering patients and visits to employment sites to implement preventative practices.

"We treat injured employees like injured athletes," says Mary. "Instead of focusing on the injury, we focus on doing exercises that will help the injury heal quickly. We emphasize overall fitness to reduce recovery time and to prevent future injuries. We also do quite a bit of preventative education. At one large grocery chain, for instance, we trained employees to stretch before each shift. By stretching out their muscles before they begin lifting inventory, the employees have dramatically reduced their number of injuries."

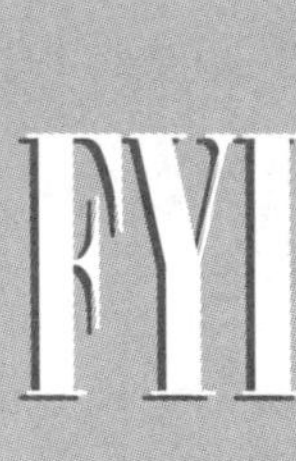

Did you know there are a number of jobs related to occupational therapist?

The U.S. Department of Labor classifies occupational therapists with other workers in therapy and rehabilitation positions.

Related jobs include:

athletic trainers
creative art therapists
dialysis technicians
kinesiotherapists
physical therapists
speech therapists

have I got what it takes to be an occupational therapist?

Wherever they work, occupational therapists spend most of their time interacting with clients and with other health care providers, so it is very important that they enjoy working with people. Excellent communications skills are also a must. "Academic skills are important," says Karen Jacobs, "but they're no substitute for the ability to establish a rapport with clients."

Because most occupational therapists work with clients who are recovering from an injury or illness or learning to live with a disability, they must also be extremely compassionate and patient individuals. "Occupational therapy practitioners should be motivated by an intense desire to help people," Karen observes.

Creativity is also an essential characteristic for people entering this profession. Occupational therapists must plan interesting exercises to help clients develop necessary skills. These activities must be designed to meet the unique needs of each client. Creativity also helps occupational therapists design adaptive aids. "As occupational therapists," Karen explains, "we often create adaptive equipment out of inexpensive, readily available materials. For example, I teach my students to make assistive technology out of three layers of cardboard glued together. We use cardboard carpentry to create adaptive puzzles for children to assemble and even portable bowling alleys that help clients develop hand-eye coordination. Any experience a person has with design, construction, or sewing will be useful in this profession."

Like other health care providers, occupational therapists must maintain meticulous records for each client. Organization, attention to detail, and good problem-solving skills are essential to becoming a successful occupational therapist.

To be a successful occupational therapist, you should

- Be able to establish a rapport with a wide variety of people
- Be creative and enjoy working with your hands
- Be patient and supportive of those working with disabilities
- Be able to keep accurate and extensive records

how do I become an occupational therapist?

education

High School

High school students who are interested in entering this field should take as many science courses as possible. Biology and physics are extremely important. Chemistry is useful, but not essential. Statistics courses, if available, can be extremely helpful. Any courses that will help a student understand human behavior, such as basic psychology and sociology, are also useful.

Postsecondary education

Although you can choose from several educational paths to become an occupational therapist, you must complete a bachelor's degree. One option is to enter a school that offers a bachelor's degree in occupational therapy. Typically in these programs the first two years are filled with taking required classes. The last two years are then concentrated on classes designed for the occupational therapy degree.

A second educational option is to enter a post-bachelor's degree program. These programs are designed for people who have already received an undergraduate degree in an area besides occupational therapy. These programs concentrate on occupational therapy courses and generally take eighteen months to complete.

A third option is to enroll in a master's degree program. Master's degree programs are also designed for people who have not received bachelor's degrees in occupational therapy. Master's degree programs generally take two to two-and-a-half years to complete. This wide range of educational choices reflects the diversity of people entering the profession. Some people begin working in occupational therapy right after college; others have earned a previous degree and worked in other fields before deciding to pursue a career in occupational therapy. Each brings his or her own unique experience to the field.

Course work at the college level typically includes basic anatomy, physiology and neurophysiology, kinesiology, statistics, psychology, and several occupational therapy practice areas, such as group dynamics, psychosocial dysfunction, and development dysfunction.

certification or licensing

After completing the course work and internships, occupational therapy students must successfully complete the National Certification Examination of the National Board For Certification in Occupational Therapy. Passing this exam is the final step in becoming an Occupational Therapist, Registered (OTR). This certification must be renewed every five years. Many states also require OTRs to obtain a state license to practice.

scholarships and grants

The following organization provides information on scholarships for students of occupational therapy. Write early for information on eligibility, application requirements, and deadlines.

American Occupational Therapy Foundation
PO Box 1725
Rockville, MD 20849

internships and volunteerships

Karen Jacobs encourages individuals who are considering occupational therapy as a career to take every opportunity to volunteer. "Volunteering is an excellent way to find out if occupational therapy is a good match with your skills and personality," says Karen. "I advise prospective occupational therapy students to work with a broad range of clients—from children with developmental disabilities to adults who are ill or aging —to find out whether they are comfortable working with people with disabilities and whether they have the necessary empathy."

Some occupational therapy programs require prospective students to participate in related volunteer activities prior to admission. College or university admissions counselors should be able to provide this information.

> Occupational therapists work closely with other health care providers...it's important for the entire health services team to understand the important role occupational therapy can play in accelerating a patient's recovery.

who will hire me?

Karen Jacobs began her career as a prevocational occupational therapist at school for very young children with disabilities. Prior to earning her Ed.D. and becoming and associate professor at Boston University, Karen also served as a job placement coordinator at a vocational high school and as a consultant for industry, hospitals, schools systems, nursing homes, and rehabilitation centers. Her experience is not unusual. Professionals within this diverse field may choose from a myriad of career opportunities.

At present, 32 percent of occupational therapists work in general, psychiatric, and pediatric hospitals. Another 19 percent work in public school systems. Others work in rehabilitation hospitals or centers, colleges and universities, home health agencies, nursing homes, and in private practice. Still others work in industry, community agencies, or as private practitioners.

The American Occupational Therapy Association publishes a weekly list of job postings and provides networking opportunities. Most occupational therapy academic programs also offer job placement services.

where can I go from here?

Occupational therapists may advance to management positions that require them to supervise other occupational therapists and occupational therapist assistants. Therapists who earn advanced degrees, like Karen Jacobs, can also pursue academic careers.

"One of the most exciting things about my job is that I have the opportunity to influence my profession," says Karen. "The students I teach this year will be my colleagues next year."

what are the salary ranges?

Entry level salaries for occupational therapists range from $30,000 to $35,600. The average starting salary is $34,400. Therapists with more experience earn between $42,000 and $45,000 and those in management earn an average annual salary of $53,000. Salaries vary, however, depending on the therapist's area of expertise. Industry occupational therapists may earn higher than average salaries, while the salaries of therapists in public school systems may be below average.

Therapists who are employed by government facilities, public agencies, or schools usually receive full benefit packages that include health insurance, sick pay, and vacation. Self-employed therapists and those who run their own businesses must provide their own benefits.

what is the job outlook?

According to the U.S. Bureau of Labor Statistics, occupational therapy is one of the most rapidly growing fields in the country. In fact, the Bureau predicts that there will be a 60 percent increase in the number of occupational therapists by the year 2005. This is a rapidly developing field.

In the past, most occupational therapists worked in hospitals. Today, occupational therapists work in industry, school systems, nursing homes, and mental health facilities, as well as in the traditional hospital setting. Many therapists also work in outpatient clinics, sheltered workshops (such as for the mentally disabled or those who have suffered from abuse), and community health agencies. Changes in our health care system are creating new opportunities in home health care and private practice. The aging of our population has also created an increased demand for occupational therapists who work with older clients.

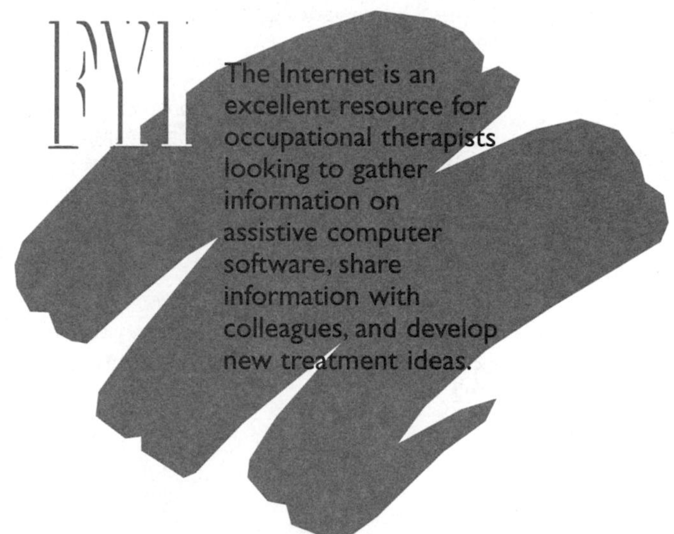

how do I learn more?

professional organizations

The following organization provides information on occupational therapy careers, accredited schools, and employers.

The American Occupational Therapy Association, Inc.
4720 Montgomery Lane
PO Box 31200
Bethesda, MD 20824
TEL: 301-652-2682
WEBSITE: http://www.aota.org/

bibliography

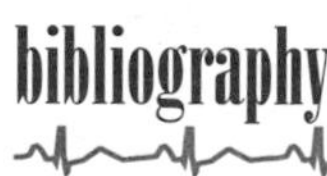

Following is a sampling of books and periodicals relating to the professional concerns and development of occupational therapists.

Books

Abbott, Marguerite, and others. *Opportunities in Occupational Therapy.* Lincolnwood, IL: VGM Career Horizons, 1995.

Brown, Margaret F. *Careers in Occupational Therapy.* New York, NY: Rosen Group, 1989.

Franciscus, Marie-Louise, Marguerite Abbott, and Zona R. Weeks. *Opportunities in Occupational Therapy Careers*. Lincolnwood, IL: VGM Career Horizons, 1994.

Punwar, Alice J. *Occupational Therapy: Principles and Practice,* 2nd edition. Baltimore, MD: Williams & Wilkins, 1993.

Periodicals

American Journal of Occupational Therapy. 10 per year. American Occupational Therapy Association, Inc., Box 21220, Bethesda, MD 20824, 301-652-2682.

Occupational Therapy Forum. Weekly. Covers new methodology, equipment, research trends, and practical and philosophical aspects of the profession. Forum Publishing, Inc., 251 W. Dekalb Pike, Suite A-115, King of Prussia, PA 19406, 215-337-0381.

Occupational Therapy in Health Care: a Journal of Contemporary Practice. Quarterly. Haworth Press, Inc., 10 Alice Street, Binghamton, NY 13904, 607-722-5857, 800-342-9678.

Occupational Therapy Week. Monthly. American Occupational Therapy Association, Inc., Box 21220, Bethesda, MD 20824, 301-652-2682.

occupational therapy assistant

Definition

Occupational therapy assistants aid people with mental, physical, developmental, or emotional limitations using a variety of activities to improve basic motor functions and reasoning abilities. Under the supervision of registered occupational therapists, occupational therapy assistants help plan, carry out, and evaluate rehabilitation programs designed to regain patients' self-sufficiency and to restore their physical and mental functions.

Salary range

$23,000 to $26,000 to $29,000

GOE
10.02.02

Educational requirements

High school diploma; two-year associate's degree, or a one-year certificate program, plus supervised clinical experience

DOT
076

Certification or licensing

Mandatory

Outlook

Much faster than average

High School Subjects

Auto shop
Physics
Applied mathematics
English
Algebra
Geometry
Electrical shop

Personal Interests

Working with your hands
Learning how things work
Electronics
Computers

The aroma of grilled cheese sandwiches, toast, and scrambled eggs may linger in the air when Corrine Shields is at work. Dishes may sit in the sink waiting to be rinsed, but Corrine is not a cook or a dishwasher. She is a certified occupational therapy assistant and she's in the kitchen in order to watch over rehabilitation patients.

Her goal is to teach them skills so that they can regain muscle tone, improve mental abilities, and become more self-sufficient. "By practicing basic living skills," Corrine says, "patients learn to care for themselves once again." Therapeutic activities such as working in the kitchen help rehabilitate patients. "Besides building up their bodies," Corrine says, "it's my job to watch out for their cognitive needs as well. For example, performing the "simple" task of making toast can be difficult for stroke victims.

"As they move about the kitchen, I evaluate how well they handle safety concerns. I note how well they follow directions and how well they are able to sequence their actions in order to succeed."

When problems arise, Corrine works with her supervisor, a registered occupational therapist, to tailor adaptive strategies for each patient's needs. "It's challenging work," says Corrine. "No two patients are alike. It takes a very creative person to be a good occupational therapy assistant."

what does an occupational therapy assistant do?

Before World War I, there were no occupational therapists or occupational therapy assistants. One consequence of modern warfare is a huge rise in the number of soldiers who survived combat, but were disabled, both mentally and physically. These veterans needed special support and training in order to learn to live with the effects of their injuries. Occupational therapy developed in response to the need for services that returned self-sufficiency and mental health to soldiers. Today, occupational therapy deals with a wide variety of patients.

Occupational therapy assistants work in hospitals, mental health facilities, hospices, substance abuse programs, schools, nursing homes, rehabilitation centers, clinics, and in private physicians' practices. They may work with children or with adults. They may work with developmentally disabled persons or with victims of accidents or illnesses. Many patients benefit from working with occupational therapy assistants, including people with arthritis, cancer, sports-related injuries, hand trauma, amputation, head or spinal cord injuries, strokes, burns, developmental disabilities, and mental illnesses.

Occupational therapy is not the same as physical therapy. Physical therapy helps people with disabilities or injuries regain movement and is mainly concerned with the well-being of patients' bodies. Occupational therapy also deals with physical rehabilitation, but it goes further and includes concern for the psychological and social effects of disabilities and injuries. The goal of occupational therapy is more than restoring physical mobility. Occupational therapy seeks to help patients develop skills that will allow them to re-enter the workplace and care for themselves at home.

Occupational therapy assistants work under the supervision of registered occupational therapists. In general, occupational therapists are responsible for developing programs while occupational therapy assistants are responsible for carrying out the programs.

Often occupational therapy assistants work more directly with individual patients than do occupational therapists. Occupational therapy assistants teach people with permanent functional disabilities how to use special equipment. For example, a person with a spinal cord injury needs to learn how to get around in a wheelchair. A stroke victim may have lost the use of one hand and has to learn how to put on shoes using a long-handled shoe horn. People with cerebral palsy or muscular dystrophy require special adaptive devices that allow them to feed themselves. Computers and computer-related equipment help speech impaired patients to talk or amputees to walk. Learning to use such complicated equipment takes time, patience, and the support of occupational therapy assistants.

Occupational therapy assistants may work with people with mental disorders. These disor-

lingo to learn

ADL (Activities of daily living) Basic functions (showering, dressing, cooking, eating, going to the bathroom) that the average person performs every day, independently or with the aid of adaptive equipment, such as a sock-aid or a long-handled shoe horn.

Adaptive equipment Tools, aids, or devices that persons with reduced or limited mobility use to hold, reach, steady, or pick up objects.

Reacher Long-handled implement with a trigger mechanism that "pinches" or "scissors" together to allow the user to grab onto items, such as objects on a high shelf.

Sub-acute care short-term care facility that patients visit prior to going home in order to learn strengthening and endurance exercises, as well as activities of daily living.

ders may be developmental or the result of emotional disturbances. They may also be a result of drug or alcohol abuse, or eating disorders.

The goal of occupational therapy assistants working with this population is to provide strategies to cope with the tasks of daily life, reduce stress, and increase productivity. For instance, when substance abusers leave their rehabilitation programs, they need new skills in order to avoid unproductive behaviors that might lead to relapses. Recovering alcoholics, for example, benefit from practice with time management and budget preparation. Occupational therapy assistants help them develop these skills and avoid repeated substance abuse.

Working with developmentally disabled persons presents a different kind of challenge. Basic personal skills such as hygiene, dressing, or eating may require attention. Occupational therapy assistants observe the level at which the person functions and, after consultation with registered occupational therapists, implement plans to increase self-sufficiency.

Occupational therapy assistants help developmentally disabled persons learn to ride the school bus or take public transportation to work. They help disabled persons learn to do household chores such as cooking and cleaning.

Some occupational therapy assistants work in schools. Along with registered occupational therapists, they assess student needs and provide ways to increase active participation in the school day. For example, a child recovering from cancer therapy may need the desk modified to make sitting more comfortable. Another student needs a special splint in order to hold a pencil better. Other children benefit from game-type activities that improve balance and increase both gross and fine motor coordination.

One branch of occupational therapy seeks to return injured workers to their jobs. Occupational therapy assistants help these people resume, as closely as possible, their original working roles. If necessary, they also provide strategies, therapies, or adaptive equipment to modify individual work situations.

what is it like to be an occupational therapy assistant?

Corrine Shields works at St. Joseph's Hospital in Tucson, Arizona. Her primary area is outpatient services, but she may "float" to work in acute care, rehabilitation, or intensive care. A typical day begins with rehabilitation therapy for transitional care patients. Transitional care is a facility within the hospital for people with cerebral-vascular trauma, or stroke.

To be a successful occupational therapy assistant, you should

- Enjoy working with people
- Have an associate's degree from an accredited college
- Be willing to work under supervision
- Have good manual dexterity and be physically fit
- Be flexible and creative

Corrine sees these patients once a day, Monday through Friday. She works with them using a variety of exercises. For instance, practice making lists is valuable for people with short-term memory loss. Other people need tasks to improve hand-eye coordination. Some patients need help with balance. To help one patient, Corrine has the patient stand beside an elevated table and play a game of cards with her. Another patient, recovering from a different type of injury but who also needs help restoring balance, stands on a foam mat and plays a more active ball exercise.

A big part of Corrine's morning is spent with patients who require assistance with the activities of daily living. She helps these people learn, or re-learn, how to dress and feed themselves, use the telephone, and write messages. She may also teach them how to safely move from a reclining position on a bed to a sitting position in a chair.

In the afternoon Corrine works in the outpatient clinic with people who require a variety of therapeutic strategies. For example, patients who have had hip replacement surgery need exercises to improve their upper body strength. Pulmonary patients sometimes panic when they are unable to "catch their breath." High levels of anxiety can slow the healing process. Corrine helps pulmonary patients recognize approaching anxiety and finds ways to circumvent it when possible.

Some people with perceptual difficulties benefit from visual activities. Corrine sets up a peg board and asks them to complete a design following a pattern on a graph. By observing their progress, she can determine how well the patients are able to follow directions. She notes how they correct errors and evaluates their general problem solving abilities.

Patients with cognitive disabilities are taken into the kitchen and asked to perform a basic task such as making scrambled eggs. Corrine watches how well they follow directions and how well they sequence the many steps needed to cook. If patients start to make mistakes, Corrine is there to correct them. She also reminds patients how to work safely within the kitchen.

The kitchen is also a great place to teach new skills to arthritis patients, people with hand injuries, or amputees who are learning to use artificial limbs. Occupational therapy assistants teach these people how to reduce their activity levels to basic movements, conserve their range of motion, and save energy.

Between patients, Corrine makes notes on medical charts, describing that day's activities. She consults with her supervisor, a registered occupational therapist, and discusses future patient care. Sometimes she meets with other hospital staff.

Nancy Morris works in a nursing home. Since she works exclusively with an older population, her job is slightly different from Corrine's. She observes residents and, when needed, devises adaptable equipment. For example, older people sometimes lose their full range of motion and cannot easily bend down to put on their shoes; so Nancy teaches them how to use long-handled shoe horns. "Reachers," a long handle with grippers that open and close, help mobility-impaired seniors pull on their clothing and dress themselves. Other people grow weaker as they grow older and find it difficult to feed themselves. The solution may be something as simple as creating a weighted eating utensil.

"Our goal as occupational therapy assistants," says Nancy, "is to keep nursing home residents as independent as possible, for as long as possible." Some of her work is similar to what goes on in the hospital. For instance, Nancy helps nursing home residents learn how to stay safe while using the bathroom. If necessary, she raises the level of the toilet seat by using special equipment. She checks to see that there is a grab bar in the shower and advises how to use it. She discusses transfer techniques for getting in and out of the bathtub safely.

have I got what it takes to be an occupational therapy assistant?

"I'm a people person," says Corrine. "Being an occupational therapy assistant is a good profession for a people person. I get to work directly with patients and not worry about paperwork as much as an occupational therapist has to." A good occupational therapy assistant is a good observer. "You have to be able to pick up on things," says Corrine, "and watch for subtle emotional signs that telegraph how the patient is really feeling. You have to establish rapport with the both the patient and the nursing staff. You need to observe what's going on with patients' minds and bodies, seek out more information when necessary, and then, based on what you've discovered, provide the necessary service."

"You can't be squeamish about being close to people either or worry about dealing with all sorts of bodily functions," she adds. "Also, occupational therapy assistance is a physically demanding field. Sometimes you're supporting the weight of patients or helping transfer them from one place to another."

Barbara Rom, director of the Green River Community College program in Auburn, Washington, emphasizes that occupational therapy assistants should be good with their hands. "You can't be awkward," she says, "because you need to make or adapt all kinds of equipment, such as hand splints. It's a great help if you are nimble, creative, and like to make things with your hands." It's also important that you be able to write clearly and concisely. Every activity an occupational therapy assistant does is noted on medical charts. Both written and oral communication skills are important. More and more, computer literacy is also needed.

Occupational therapy assistants always work under the supervision of registered occupational therapists. In most circumstances they work as part of a team, but occupational therapy assistants are not the lead members. Flexibility is a great asset for this reason.

"The methods for delivering health care are changing," Corrine stresses. "Supervisors sometimes change, and patients and their needs change daily . . . if you're not flexible, this is not the profession for you."

how do I become an occupational therapy assistant?

Corrine Shields has worked as an occupational therapy assistant for nine years. She received her associate's degree from Fox Valley Technical College in Appleton, Wisconsin.

Course work at accredited schools is intense and thorough. Students receive a broad education, including serving a supervised apprenticeship. "The goal," Corrine says, "is to produce graduates who can function immediately as staff at whatever institution they join."

education

High School

Classes in biology, chemistry, physics, social science, health, English, and computer use are helpful to students planning to pursue a career in occupational therapy.

Postsecondary Training

Occupational therapy assistants need more than a high school diploma. There are two ways to enter the profession. Most students attend a two-year program and receive an associate of applied science degree. A few students (those with many years of experience as health care workers or with several years of education past high school) may qualify instead for one-year certificate programs. Both one-year and two-year programs include academic study as well as clinical field work.

College course work includes medical terminology, basic anatomy and physiology, gerontology and aging, construction of adaptive equipment, note taking and documentation, first aid and CPR, musculoskeletal system disorders, human development, basic health care skills, and therapeutic techniques.

certification or licensing

Most states require that occupational therapy assistants be licensed. This involves passing an exam administered by the state licensing board. Almost all employers require professional certification. Twice a year the American Occupational Therapy Certification Board administers a national test to determine certification. The test is rigorous and comprehensive.

scholarships and grants

Colleges may reserve scholarships for students pursuing health careers and make specific funds available for students wishing to become occupational therapy assistants. Certain employers, especially long-term care facilities such as nursing homes, may offer stipends to students. In exchange for agreeing to work for the facility after graduation (usually for at least one year), the facility pays a portion of the student's tuition. Each year, the American Occupational Therapy Foundation offers fifteen scholarships to currently enrolled students, based on need and class standing.

who will hire me?

Occupational therapy assistants work in a variety of institutions including hospitals, mental health facilities, hospices, substance abuse programs, schools, nursing homes, rehabilitation centers, clinics, and private physicians' practices. The majority work for hospitals or nursing homes. Since demand is great for occupational therapy assistants, employers often contact schools to inquire about recent graduates. AOTA reports that new occupational therapy assistants find their first job, on average, within two months.

where can I go from here?

Because occupational therapy assistants always work under the supervision of occupational therapists, there is not much room for advancement. Unless you are willing to return to school, obtain a four-year degree, and become an occupational therapist, the highest level that occupational therapy assistants can advance to is lead assistant. These people have more responsibility and may assist in making evaluations. They may schedule work for other occupational therapy assistants and help train students.

what are the salary ranges?

In 1994, the mean income for occupational therapy assistants beginning their careers was $23,871, according to the American Occupational Therapy Association. With three to four years experience, the mean income rose to $25,060 and with seven to nine years experience, the mean income was $26,712. Occupational therapy assistants with fifteen or more years experience had a mean income of $26,615. Some occupational therapy assistants receive salaries while others, especially those just starting out, are paid hourly wages.

Those working in day care programs and in school systems receive slightly lower incomes than those working in skilled nursing facilities, rehabilitation centers, and hospitals. Most full-time occupational therapy assistants receive standard worker benefits, including health insurance.

Occupational therapy assistants may work some nights and weekends, depending on the needs of the their facility. For example, assistants involved with schools will work more regular hours than those working in nursing homes.

what is the job outlook?

"The shortage of occupational therapy assistants is so great," says Howard Holland of the American Occupational Therapy Association, "that the U.S. Bureau of Labor predicts a 78 percent increase in the number of positions available between now and 2005. This means that students can find jobs when they graduate. Most new occupational therapy assistants report receiving at least three job offers."

Rural areas are more underserved than urban areas but demand for occupational therapy assistants is high nationwide. Since the majority of jobs available are in geriatric care, areas of the country with higher percentages of seniors experience the greatest shortages of occupational therapy assistants.

how do I learn more?

professional organizations

Following are organizations that provide information on occupational therapy assistant careers, accredited schools, and employers.

American Occupational Therapy Association
4720 Montgomery Lane
PO Box 31220
Bethesda, MD 20824
TEL: 301-652-2682
WEBSITE: http://www.aota.org

American Occupational Therapy Foundation
4720 Montgomery Lane
Bethesda, MD 20824
TEL: 301-652-6611

American Occupational Therapy Certification Board
4 Research Place, Suite 160
Rockville, MD 20850
TEL: 301-990-7979

bibliography

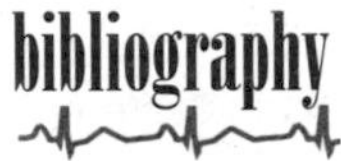

Following is a sampling of materials relating to the professional concerns and development of occupational therapy assistants.

Books

Brown, Margaret F. *Careers in Occupational Therapy.* New York, NY: Rosen Group, 1989.

Franciscus, Marie-Louise, Marguerite Abbott, and Zona R. Weeks. *Opportunities in Occupational Therapy Careers.* Lincolnwood, IL: VGM Career Horizons, 1995.

Periodicals

Advance for Occupational Therapists. Weekly. Covers news of the field of occupational therapy. Merion Publications, 650 Park Avenue West, King of Prussia, PA 19406, 215-265-7812.

Occupational Therapy in Mental Health. Quarterly. Offers timely articles for occupational therapists working in mental health clinics, psychiatric hospitals, mental health programs, and other settings. Haworth Press, Inc., 10 Alice Street, Binghamton, NY 13904, 607-722-5857.

oncologist

Definition

Oncologists are physicians who study, diagnose, and treat the tumors caused by cancer.

Salary range

$31,000 to $75,000 to $130,000+

Educational requirements

Bachelor's degree, M.D., plus specialized study in oncology

Certification or Licensing

Certification is highly recommended, licensing is required

GOE
NA*

Outlook

Faster than average

DOT
NA*

*Not Available. The U.S. Department of Labor does not classify oncologist as such, but rather classifies the oncologist's primary profession (e.g., doctor of internal medicine).

High School Subjects

Anatomy
Biology
Chemistry
Computer science
English
Mathematics

Personal Interests

Helping people
Problem solving
Reading and continuous learning
Working with people

U.S. senators and legislative aides fill the room. Dr. Harmon Eyre leans forward and speaks clearly and carefully into the microphone. He knows he has only five to ten minutes to make his point, so he chooses his words carefully. He wants these senators to support a bill levying additional tax on cigarette sales. The senators are interested in his testimony because he is the chief medical officer for the American Cancer Society. "By increasing the price of cigarettes, this bill would also decrease the annual cigarette sales and, consequently, the number of annual tobacco-related deaths," Dr. Eyre says. "Smoking is the leading cause of preventable deaths in this country. One day soon, it will be the leading cause of preventable deaths in the entire world, surpassing even infectious diseases."

what does an oncologist do?

An *oncologist* is a physician, such as a doctor of internal medicine, who specializes in the study, diagnosis, and treatment of cancerous tumors. Because cancer can affect any organ in the body, and individuals of any age, there are many different kinds of oncologists. For example, medical oncologists have studied internal medicine and treat cancer through chemotherapy. Pediatric oncologists are pediatricians who specialize in cancers that affect infants and children. Gynecological oncologists are gynecologists who specialize in cancers that attack the female reproductive organs, including the ovary, the cervix, and the uterus. Radiological oncologists treat tumors through radiation therapy. Surgical oncologists are surgeons who specialize in removing cancerous tissue to prevent its growth. There are many other subspecialties within the practice of oncology. In fact, there are almost as many different subspecialties of oncology as there are different kinds of doctors.

Before assuming his responsibilities with the American Cancer Society, Dr. Eyre practiced as a clinical oncologist. A clinical oncologist conducts clinical trials in order to identify the most successful strategies for fighting cancer. Clinical trials are studies that are conducted on consenting patients. By comparing the results of two different treatments on two groups of patients with similar symptoms, clinical oncologists are able to determine which methods are more effective in eliminating or retarding the development of cancer.

Because cancer can spread throughout the organs of the body, oncologists often work together in teams to identify the appropriate strategy for helping a patient. Many patients undergo a combination of chemotherapy, radiation therapy, and surgery to treat cancer, so it is extremely important for the physicians to coordinate the treatment process.

lingo to learn

Benign Referring to a tumor, it means noncancerous.

Cancer Any one of a group of diseases in which cells from once normal tissue grow uncontrollably and spread to different sites in the body.

Chemotherapy In the treatment of cancer, a patient is given doses of anticancer drugs that have a poisonous effect on the cancer-causing cells.

Leukemia A blood cell cancer in which abnormal blood cells accumulate in the bone marrow and blood. This cancer affects bone marrow, blood, the spleen, and other sites throughout the body.

Malignant Tending to deteriorate or cause death. When referring to a cancer it means fast growing and quickly spreading.

Radiation therapy A cancer treatment that uses a beam of radiation from X rays, cobalt, or other sources to destroy cancer cells.

Remission A period during which symptoms lessen or disappear. This is a temporary state that may become permanent.

Tumor A growth of tissue that forms an abnormal mass. Tumors can appear in any part of the body, such as the skin, bones, kidneys, or brain. Tumors may or may not be life threatening.

what is it like to be an oncologist?

Oncologists, like many physicians, must divide their time between patient consultations, medical procedures, study and publishing, and office or departmental administration. Most oncologists work far more than forty hours per week.

An oncologist may see anywhere from ten to thirty patients each day. In many of these encounters, the oncologist may have to deliver devastating information and help patients make extremely difficult choices. Oncologists must inform patients when a tumor is malignant. They must explain the various treatment options and the toxic side effects associated with the options. They must give patients realistic assessments of their chances of recovery. As patients undergo treatment, oncologists also must help them cope with the pain and discomfort that can be caused both by the disease and by some of the treatment methods.

"It is extremely important to be very direct and honest with a patient at all times," comments Dr. Eyre. "The patient must be able to have absolute trust in his or her physician."

As an oncologist, Dr. Eyre has witnessed countless tragedies. Despite these experiences, however, he considers his profession extremely rewarding. "It is immensely fulfilling to know that a patient, who might have died if his or her disease had been mismanaged, has been cured and can look forward to resuming a normal life."

According to Dr. Eyre, rewarding moments occasionally arise from terribly painful situations. "A few years ago, I treated a thirty-three-year-old man for leukemia. Before he was diagnosed with this disease, he and his wife spent all their time and energy trying to advance in their careers. His cancer caused them to reevaluate their priorities. Before he died, two and a half years after his original diagnosis, he and his wife told me that they had lived more fully during those two and a half years than they had ever lived before."

To be a successful oncologist, you should

- Be able to work with a team of medical professionals
- Be able to communicate complex scientific information clearly and concisely
- Be emotionally balanced and able to deal with unpleasant situations
- Enjoy constant learning and using technology
- Have excellent diagnostic skills

have I got what it takes to be an oncologist?

Oncologists must be extremely hard working, perceptive, and emotionally balanced individuals. They must also be voracious readers with excellent memories, as new information about the cause, prevention, and treatment of cancer is published each day. Staying current with new information also requires that the oncologist be proficient with technology, easily able to access new information through the medium of the computer. An oncologist's own researching and writing skills must be well developed, because publishing research results is an important way to advance in this profession.

"Our understanding of this disease is constantly changing," says Dr. Eyre. "We are constantly discovering new information about genetics, the immune system, and possible treatments. This job is never boring or dull."

In addition to the intellectual rigors of the job, oncologists must be prepared to accept emotional and psychological challenges. Each day, oncologists interact with people who are very ill and frightened. The oncologist must be able to maintain objectivity and composure under intensely emotional circumstances. He or she must achieve a balance between compassion and professionalism. To meet these challenges, an oncologist must be an extremely mature and emotionally stable individual. Because oncologists must explain very complex information to people who have little or no scientific background, they also must be able to communicate clearly and directly. Excellent interpersonal skills are essential. Interpersonal skills will also help the oncologist work as part of a medical team. A surgical oncologist, for example, may have to work with a medical team that includes a dietitian, a physical therapist, the original referring doctor, nurses, and other staff members.

how do I become an oncologist?

education

High School

If you are interested in a career as an oncologist, the first step is to take high school courses that are college preparatory. Science courses, such as biology, chemistry, physics, and anatomy, will help prepare you for college as well as give you the opportunity to test your ability and enjoyment in these areas. Math courses, such as algebra, geometry, and trigonometry, are also important to take. English and speech classes will help you develop your research, writing, and oral communication skills. Computer science courses give you the opportunity to gain familiarity with using this technology. Finally, courses such as social studies, government, or foreign languages will not only broaden your educational background but help to make you an appealing candidate for college admissions.

If you are certain you wish to pursue a medical career, you may want to consider entering a college or university that is associated with a medical school and offers an accelerated medical education program. In these accelerated programs, students spend either two or three years completing their undergraduate work and then spend four years at the medical school associated with that college or university. Students in accelerated programs have the advantage of finishing medical school before their peers who take the normal educational route. More information on such programs is available from high school guidance counselors. Students considering this option should look into it in their junior or early senior years.

Postsecondary Training

The next step in becoming an oncologist is to earn a bachelor's degree at an accredited college or university. Students who plan to go to medical school typically major in a science, such as biology or chemistry. Regardless of the major, however, course work should emphasize the sciences and include classes such as biology, chemistry, anatomy, and physiology. Other important classes to take include mathematics, such as calculus, English courses, ethics, and psychology classes. Volunteering or working at a hospital during your college years is also an excellent way to gain experience working in a medical setting.

To continue their education, college students in their senior year apply to medical schools. Admission to medical school is competitive and is based on a student's grade point average, scores on the Medical College Admission Test (MCAT), and recommendations from professors. Medical school lasts four years. At the end of this time the student has earned the degree doctor of medicine (M. D.). For the first two years of medical school, students attend lectures and classes and do laboratory work. Classes include biochemistry, physiology, pharmacology, psychology, and medical ethics. Students also learn to take patient histories, perform routine examinations, and recognize symptoms. In the third and fourth years, students spend time working in hospitals and clinics where they are supervised by residents and physicians. It is during this time that students go on rotations. Rotations are brief periods of study in a particular area, such as pediatrics, psychiatry, and surgery. On rotations students learn the distinctive qualities of different medical specializations and work on diagnosing and treating patients.

After graduating from medical school, physicians must pass a standard exam given by the National Board of Medical Examiners. Most physicians then complete an internship or transition year during which they decide what their area of specialization will be. Following the internship, physicians begin their residency. At this point, a doctor interested in oncology completes a residency in the area he or she has decided to specialize in. For example, someone interested in gynecologic oncology completes a four-year obstetrics and gynecology residency. Someone interested in medical oncology, on the other hand, does a residency in internal medicine. Following the residency, the doctor completes a fellowship (specialized study) in oncology. A fellowship in gynecologic oncology, for example, can take from two to four years to complete.

FYI
According to the American Cancer Society, tobacco smoke has at least forty-three cancer-causing substances. Smoking is responsible for about 83 percent of all lung cancers.

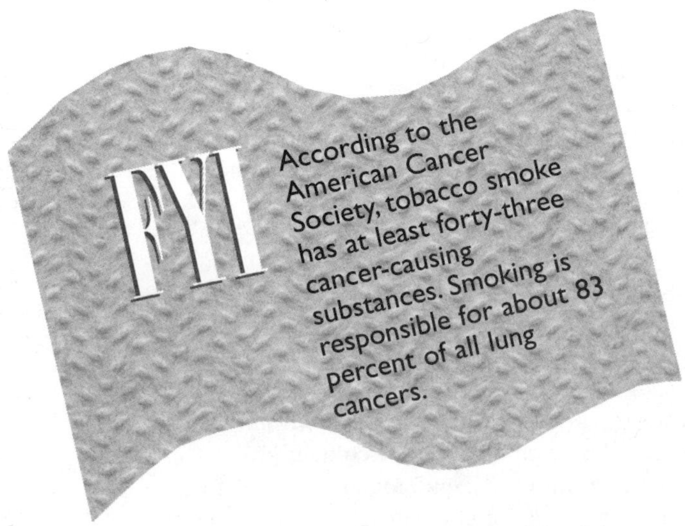

certification or licensing

All physicians must be licensed before they can practice medicine by the state in which they wish to work. In order to be licensed, doctors must have graduated from medical school, passed the licensing test of the state, and completed their residency.

Certification is not required for oncologists, but it is highly recommended. Certification for oncologists is administered by boards in their area of specialty. For example, certification for medical oncologists is administered by the American Board of Internal Medicine. Certification for gynecologic oncologists is administered by the American Board of Obstetrics and Gynecology, Inc.

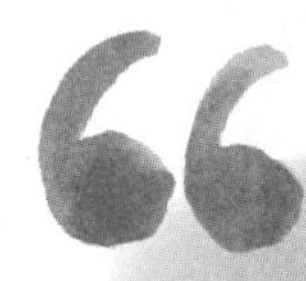

> We are constantly discovering new information about genetics, the immune system, and possible treatments. This job is never boring or dull.

scholarships and grants

Scholarships and grants are often available from individual institutions, state agencies, and special-interest organizations. The book *Dollars for College: Medicine, Dentistry, and Related Fields* by Ferguson Publishing Company is an excellent source for this information. Many students finance their medical education through the Armed Forces Health Professions Scholarship Program. Each branch of the military participates in this program, paying students' tuitions in exchange for military service. Contact your local recruiting office for more information. The National Health Service Corps Scholarship Program also provides money for students in return for service. Another source for financial aid, scholarship, and grant information is the Association of American Medical Colleges. Remember to request information early.

Association of American Medical Colleges
2450 N Street, NW
Washington, DC 20037
TEL: 202-828-0400
WEBSITE: http://www.aamc.org
Specific information on financial aid programs can be found at:
WEBSITE: http://www.aamc.org/stuapps/finaid

Ferguson Publishing Company
200 West Madison, Suite 300
Chicago, IL 60606
TEL: 312-580-5480

National Health Services Corps Scholarship Program
U.S. Public Health Service
1010 Wayne Avenue, Suite 240
Silver Spring, MD 20910
TEL: 800-638-0824

who will hire me?

Oncologists work in virtually every health-care setting. Because cancer is such a prevalent disease that takes so many different forms, oncologists are in demand in every area of medical practice. Oncologists are employed by government-funded medical facilities, private hospitals, university health centers, outpatient clinics, government agencies, pharmaceutical companies, and research laboratories.

where can I go from here?

An oncologist can advance in his or her career by becoming the head of a research or medical department. Department heads must assume extensive administrative responsibilities in addition to patient care. An oncologist also can achieve prominence in the field by publishing articles, conducting research, and participating in professional organizations, such as the American Cancer Society and the American Society of Clinical Oncology. Highly respected oncologists, such as Dr. Eyre, are asked to speak to the public and advise government bodies on health issues.

what are the salary ranges?

The national average salary for first-year residents in the mid-1990's was approximately $31,000. That average increased to $41,800 by the final residency year. Salaries vary, depending on the kind of residency, the hospital, and the geographic area.

Oncologists who have just earned certification and are beginning their practice can earn an annual salary of $75,000. With more experience, an oncologist can earn up to $130,000 per year. Oncologists who are extremely successful can earn annual salaries of $200,000 or more. Individual earnings of oncologists will vary, depending on such factors as geographic location, years of experience, professional reputation, and type of oncology practiced.

what is the job outlook?

Due to a growing and aging population, new research, changing diagnostic techniques, and new treatment possibilities, oncology is a rapidly growing field. Positions in oncology are abundant and are projected to grow at a faster than average rate into the twenty-first century.

how do I learn more?

professional organizations

Following are organizations that provide information on the profession of oncology.

American Cancer Society
1599 Clifton Road, NE
Atlanta, GA 30329
TEL: 404-320-3333
WEBSITE: http://www.cancer.org/acs.html

American Society of Clinical Oncology
225 Reinekers Lane, Suite 650
Alexandria, VA 22314
TEL: 703-299-0150
WEBSITE: http://www.asco.org

Radiation Therapy Oncology Group
American College of Radiology
1101 Market Street, 14th floor
Philadelphia, PA 19107
TEL: 215-574-3150

bibliography

Following is a sampling of materials relating to the professional concerns and development of oncologists.

Books

Calabresi, Paul, and Phillip S. Schein, editors. *Medical Oncology: Basic Principles and Clinical Management of Cancer,* 2nd edition. New York, NY: McGraw-Hill, 1993.

Casciato, Dennis A., and Barry B. Lowitz, editors. *Manual of Clinical Oncology,* 3rd edition. Boston, MA: Little, Brown, 1995.

Markman, Maurie. *Basic Cancer Medicine.* Philadelphia, PA: W.B. Saunders Co., 1997.

Murphy, Gerald P., and others, editors. *American Cancer Society Textbook of Clinical Oncology,* 2nd edition. Flushing, NY: American Cancer Society, 1995.

Pazdur, Richard, editor. *Medical Oncology: a Comprehensive Review,* 2nd edition. Huntington, NY: P R R, 1995.

Tannock, Ian F., and Richard P. Hill, editors. *The Basic Science of Oncology,* 2nd edition. New York, NY: McGraw-Hill, 1992.

Periodicals

CA–a Cancer Journal for Clinicians. Bimonthly. Covers all aspects of cancer management for clinicians in primary care, oncology, and related specialties. American Cancer Society, Inc., Lippincott-Raven Publishers, 227 E. Washington Square, Philadelphia, PA 19106, 215-238-4200.

Cancer Detection and Prevention. Monthly. International Society of Preventive Oncology, Blackwell Science Inc., 238 Main Street, Cambridge, MA 02142, 617-876-7022, 800-759-6102.

Cope: Working in Oncology. Bimonthly. Profiles professionals working in the field of oncology. Media America, Inc., Box 862268, Franklin, TN 37068, 615-790-2400.

Journal of Cancer Education. Quarterly. Addresses varied aspects of cancer education for allied health professionals. American Association for Cancer Education, Hanley & Belfus, Inc., 210 S. 13th Street, Philadelphia, PA 19107, 215-546-7293.

National Cancer Institute Journal. Semimonthly. Contains original reports, articles, reviews, and commentary on new findings in clinical and laboratory cancer research. U.S. National Cancer Institute, Information Associates Program, 9030 Old Georgetown Road, Room 213, Bethesda, MD 20814, 301-496-4907.

ophthalmic technician

Definition

Ophthalmic technicians work with ophthalmologists (eye doctors) in examining patients' eye functions. They measure vision, perform routine tests on eyes, and help to diagnose and treat eye diseases and problems.

Alternative job titles

Ophthalmic allied health professionals
Ophthalmic assistants
Ophthalmic medical technologists

Salary range

$14,000 to $28,000 to $40,000

Educational requirements

High school diploma; one to two years of formal training or on-the-job training

Certification or licensing

Highly recommended

Outlook

Faster than average

GOE
10.03.01

DOT
078

High School Subjects

Biology
Chemistry
Mathematics

Personal Interests

Helping people
Solving problems
Taking measurements
Working with mechanical instruments

Martha is sitting in the examining room with her eyes closed. "I see these shooting silver arrows going back and forth," she explains to Cathy Brown, the eye doctor's assistant. "It's like lightning bolts going on inside my brain or something. And it doesn't really stop when I open my eyes."

Cathy asks Martha more questions about how her eye problem is affecting her. Has it happened before? How long has it been going on this time? Does she experience headaches along with the "lightning bolts"?

"OK, Martha. I'm going to look at your eyes more closely." Cathy uses a pen-size flashlight to check Martha's eyelids. "There's no infection or inflammation here, so we'll do a few more things." She shines the light into one eye and then the other, noticing that both eyes constrict equally and quickly to the light. Then she checks Martha's eye muscles by covering one eye and then the other as Martha reads the eye chart. Her muscles seem to be fine.

"Martha, I want you to move forward a little; rest your chin here and your forehead here. I'm going to look into your eyes using this machine. OK. Now I'm going to blow a bit of air into your eye, so try to keep it open as wide as you can. . . . Are you still doing a lot of reading in your work? I'm thinking that maybe these shooting arrows are just a sign that you should be resting your eyes more. OK here comes the shot of air."

"The last thing I'm going to do is put some drops in your eyes to dilate your pupils. Dr. Berliner will come in to see you then, and he'll look into your eyes with a scope to see what's going on back there."

what does an ophthalmic technician do?

Cathy Brown is on her way to becoming a certified ophthalmic technician. In her job now, as an ophthalmic assistant, she performs basic eye procedures, like examining visual acuity and doing color tests. When she is ready—after having completed her formal course work studies—she will take the exam to be certified as a technician.

Ophthalmic technicians can be considered eye nurses; they help eye doctors perform their work. If you have had eye check-ups in either an optometrist's or an ophthalmologist's office, you have probably been taken care of by an ophthalmic technician. The difference between the two types of eye doctors is that the ophthalmologist works mainly with eye disease and injury; optometrists work mainly with healthy eyes that do not function properly.

Ophthalmic technicians take patient histories, perform lensometries (measure the lens of the eye), and operate various types of ocular equipment. They must be skilled in patient services such as putting on ocular dressings and shields, administering drops and ointments, and otherwise assisting patients. They must know how to work with all kinds of patients: the elderly, children, the physically disabled, and the visually disabled.

Technicians have knowledge of clinical optics, including retinoscopy, refractometry, spectacle principles, and basic ocular motility. Because contact lenses are popular vision aids, technicians have to understand the basic principles of lenses, fitting procedures, patient instruction, and troubleshooting. In addition, they should have an understanding of general medical knowledge, including anatomy, physiology, and pathology (illness and disease), and they must know CPR (cardiopulmonary resuscitation) and other first aid procedures.

The ophthalmic technician must have the same skills that assistants have, as well as knowledge of more advanced procedures. First, in taking patient histories, they ask about the "presenting complaint": why the patient has come to see the doctor. Taking the history is like interviewing the patient. What is the family history? Is there diabetes, glaucoma, or hypertension in the family? What medications is the patient taking: aspirin, steroids, birth control pills? Does the patient have allergies? And finally, if the patient wears glasses or contact lenses, how long have they worn them and how is their vision now?

Working directly with patients is the task with which the ophthalmic assistant or technician is involved the most. Many patients are elderly; they visit the ophthalmologist when they have symptoms related to eye problems, such as cataracts and glaucoma. These are the

lingo to learn

Cataract A condition that exists when the eye lens is opaque, causing loss of vision.

Cornea The part of the eyeball that covers the iris and pupil.

Dilate To administer liquid drops to the eye to cause the pupil to enlarge briefly for examination.

Glaucoma An eye disease characterized by such things as loss of vision, hardening of the eye, and a damaged optic disk.

Keratometry Measurement of the cornea.

Ophthalmology The branch of medicine dealing with the structure, functions, and diseases of the eye.

Refraction The ability of the eye to bend light so that an image is focused on the retina; a procedure performed by ophthalmic technicians to determine the eye's refractive characteristics.

Retina The membrane in the eye that allows one to see; it is connected to the brain by the optic nerve.

Retinoscopy Observation of the retina.

Visual acuity The extent to which one can see clearly.

two most common eye conditions leading to loss of sight. (When you have cataracts, it's like trying to see through a steamed-up window; vision is very blurry and opaque.) The technician will help the ophthalmologist to monitor the patient's cataracts, which develop gradually as one gets older, and then will assist the doctor when it is time for the cataracts to be removed.

Certified ophthalmic medical personnel help to bring peace of mind to both patients and the doctors with whom they work. Because ophthalmic technicians work with other professionals, there is a sense of teamwork in the office setting. Technicians are looked upon by doctors as crucial members of the team rather than just helpers. And working with patients makes the job more challenging. "Being a COT [certified ophthalmic technician] is very rewarding," another technician states. "The work is never boring or repetitious because each patient is different and there are so many skills to utilize."

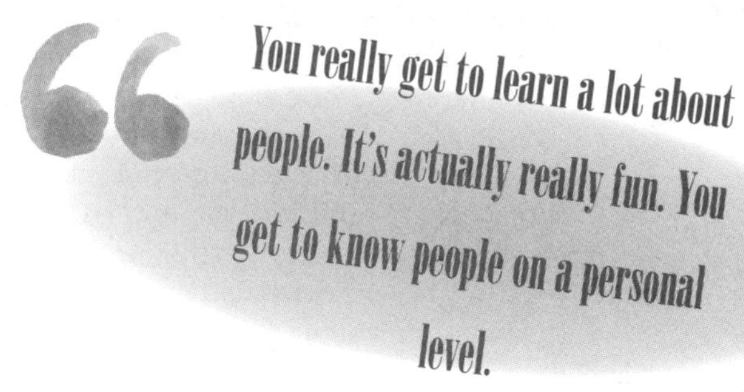

what is it like to be an ophthalmic technician?

Cathy works with ophthalmologists at Maine Eye Center, an eye-care clinic in Portland, Maine. Basically, she greets patients, settles them into examining rooms, and performs initial tests on patients' eyes. Because of her training and certification, she is qualified to take medical histories, one of the first tasks that need to be done with new patients. She asks new patients about such things as why they need an eye exam, what their family history of disease is, what their vision is like, and what types of medications, if any, they take, all the while keeping up a friendly conversation to set them at ease.

Cathy's other basic skills include measuring and recording visual acuity (that is, how sharp one's vision is). Somewhere in the doctor's office you'll probably find a Snellen chart, which shows eleven lines of progressively smaller letters, starting with the big "E" at the top and ending with "PEZOLCFTD" at the bottom. Your visual acuity is determined by how much of the chart you can read without corrective lenses. Cathy also will use color plates to test eyes for color vision.

Many ophthalmologists work in the clinic where Cathy works. Each has a different specialty, such as pediatric ophthalmology (working with children), retinal or corneal ophthalmology, ophthalmic plastic surgery, and cataracts/glaucoma. At this point in her career, Cathy assists mainly with the plastics ophthalmologist, which means that she's involved with conditions like orbital reconstruction and tearing problems. "Float" technicians are required to fill in when needed to help any one of the doctors in the office. Cathy says that this is the hardest part of the job, being skilled in just about every specialty so that you can handle any situation that comes up (be it cataracts, corneal problems, or even a simple vision test for a child).

Cathy still performs routine exams as well: checking vision, pressure, and muscle reactions and motility; doing retinoscopies and refractometries; and dilating pupils. She does a lot of patient screening, taking histories and basically talking with the patients about their eye conditions. One of the most important things she does is to reassure patients about their particular complaints. Their needs and concerns require patience and understanding.

Although much of the work is routine, every now and then an emergency comes up. Perhaps a patient comes in complaining that her vision is dark, or that she sees flashes of light. Cathy says that this should set off an alarm in the technician's mind: Is the retina attached? Is something wrong with the cornea? The patient will be screened by the ophthalmic assistant or technician, then will be examined by the ophthalmologist, and then perhaps will go to the operating room or be sent to the hospital.

Cathy feels that she has a "wonderful schedule." Her average work week is about thirty-six to forty hours, and she has Sundays and Mondays off. She is usually finished by about five in the afternoon, but she says that the ophthalmic photographers and those who work with angiograms sometimes have to stay later to wait for photos or X rays to develop.

Jeri Bloch is an ophthalmic technician who works for an ophthalmologist in California. She is skilled in the same areas as Cathy and is qualified to perform other functions as well. She fits contact lenses, plots patients' visual fields, and performs retinoscopies and refractometries. In addition, she is certified to do ophthalmic surgical assisting, for which she took special courses and exams before achieving her certification. Jeri enjoys being able to help others. The job is never boring, and she can learn something new every day. She agrees that medicine is a fascinating field.

have I got what it takes to be an ophthalmic technician?

"You definitely must have patience, especially because lots of the people you see are elderly," says Cathy. "You really get to learn a lot about people. It's actually really fun. You get to know people on a personal level."

On hectic days when you might see forty to fifty patients in one morning, "you need to be as pleasant as you can, but you have to move things along," Cathy explains. In other words, you have to be very organized. "The doctors put a lot of trust in your hands. You have to be self-motivated, use your own judgment."

Communication skills are very important, as well as keeping abreast of new technology and knowledge in the field. You should expect to attend meetings, conventions, and a yearly educational program. You need to maintain your continuing education credits within three-year cycles, so you have to be comfortable with taking tests fairly often.

Every now and then there are volunteer opportunities for technicians. For example, just recently Cathy and her colleagues volunteered at a school for the deaf. They examined the eyes of about one hundred kids, and found that it was a lot of fun. What a change from seeing mostly older patients!

To be a successful ophthalmic technician, you should

- Be able to communicate well with people
- Be able to handle hectic schedules
- Be self-motivated
- Be organized
- Know how to use your own judgment
- Not be intimidated by taking tests

how do I become an ophthalmic technician?

There are two general routes to becoming an ophthalmic technician: formal training and on-the-job training. In either case, you need to study for certification exams, take the exams (both written and performance), and continue to update your certification. According to Dr. Melvin Freeman, "Certification shows the dedication and professionalism of the employee and their dedication to the best care for patients under the ophthalmologist's guidance."

In Cathy's case, she was in a training program for ophthalmic surgical assisting when a job opened up at Maine Eye Center. She was hired as an on-the-job trainee with the obligation of going through a home-study course and ten weeks of reviewing with the resident optometrists. She eventually took her exam and was certified as an assistant. Her next step is to take courses leading to certification as a technician, which is what Jeri Bloch did after working a few years at an ophthalmologist's office in Chicago.

Cathy says that many doctors hire people to work their way up in the office, as she is doing. At one point, the doctors at Maine Eye Center needed an ophthalmic photographer but realized it was difficult to find a trained worker. They put an ad in the paper and eventually hired someone who was a skilled photographer to be trained on the job.

education

High School

Cathy recalls that it was helpful to have taken basic science and math courses in high school. She was able to take certain vocational classes in her junior and senior years, which gave her an awareness of the medical field. These classes included CPR and chemistry lab. Cathy knew that she wanted to work in a medical occupation, so she became involved in a nurses' assistant program. This, along with going on field trips and taking tours of places like hospitals, "opened doors" for her, and she became further aware of job opportunities in ophthalmology.

As with many careers, it is wise to concentrate on basic subjects like English because in this job you'll find yourself doing various administrative tasks such as writing up patient histories. You'll need to be able to communicate well, both on paper and in person. As Cathy mentioned, working for so many doctors involves teamwork and cooperation. Experience with team sports and with groups like the debate team and drama club give you opportunities to learn how to work with others.

Postsecondary Training

University degrees are not required on this career track. However, you must either (1) successfully complete an accredited ophthalmic technician's program or (2) be certified as an active ophthalmic assistant, have at least one year of full-time work experience as a certified ophthalmic assistant, and finish eighteen hours of approved continuing education credits.

The courses involved can be taken while you are working as an ophthalmic assistant, or you can enroll in a one-year full-time training program. You can expect to be quite challenged in most of your courses for this career. At this stage, classes follow a pretty standard outline and curriculum, including basic anatomy and physiology, medical terminology, medical laws and ethics, psychology, ocular anatomy and physiology, optics, microbiology, and diseases of the eye. You also learn about patient services (such as preparing ocular shields, delivering drugs, and otherwise assisting the patient), ophthalmic skills and lensometry, and instrument operation and maintenance (you have to be familiar with such equipment as ophthalmoscopes, retinoscopes, and slit lamps).

Cathy recalls her training experience as somewhat "overwhelming." But even though there was so much involved, her self-motivation influenced her to continue. She carefully watched others perform their jobs, gained the confidence to try the tasks herself, and eventually learned everything she needed for her own certification. "Everything that was presented in the courses was necessary," she says.

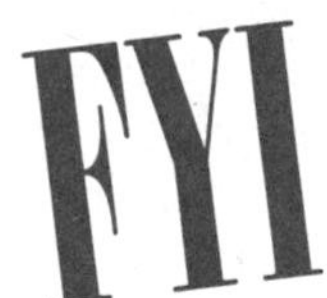

20/20: Not the TV Show!

Have you been told that you have 20/20 vision? Or do you wear glasses because you don't see 20/20? What does 20/20 vision really mean?

Well, to test your visual acuity (how well you see), the ophthalmic technician at your doctor's office will have you read the Snellen chart (you know, the one with the big "E" at the top and the tiny letters at the bottom). This chart hangs at a distance of twenty feet from the examining chair. If you can read all the letters on the chart without glasses or contact lenses, that means you have 20/20 vision. It means that you can see at twenty feet what the "optically normal" eye can see at that distance.

What if the technician tells you that you have 20/40 vision? It means that your eyes are less strong; you have to be only twenty feet away from something that the "optically normal" eye can see at forty feet. The larger the bottom number is, the weaker your visual acuity. So if you can't see the "PEZOLCFTD" at the bottom of the chart, the ophthalmic technician will probably begin fitting you for glasses!

certification or licensing

In brief, to be an ophthalmic technician you have to be certified by the Joint Commission on Allied Health Personnel in Ophthalmology (JCAHPO). The certification requirements are quite straightforward, consisting of five basic elements: (1) evidence of successful completion of education and training; (2) evidence of satisfactory work experience; (3) a current CPR certificate; (4) endorsement by a sponsoring ophthalmologist; and (5) successful completion of a skills evaluation and a written exam.

Before being certified, you may choose to first become certified as an ophthalmic assistant. Exams can be taken at a center chosen from nearly eighty locations throughout the United States and Canada. Certification exams are created by ophthalmologists and other ophthalmic medical personnel. Each written exam consists of approximately two hundred items; about 30 to 40 percent of the items are carried over from year to year. Two types of items are used on the tests: (1) single-best answer items and (2) diagrams with labels to be matched with columns of possible answers.

After becoming certified as a technician, you are required to maintain your credentials by renewing your certification periodically. It is your responsibility to apply for recertification every three years. Basically, this means that you must take a certain number of continuing education courses throughout your career. You are encouraged to take some of the credits each year, so that they add up to twenty-seven credits every three years. Accepted courses include those offered by JCAHPO at the Continuing Education Program held each year; regional courses; and self-study courses (e.g., tapes, readings, videos). The *Outlook* newsletter keeps technicians informed of more than sixteen hundred continuing education opportunities offered at various locations every year.

scholarships and grants

The Joint Commission on Allied Health Personnel in Ophthalmology selects certain students each year to receive scholarships. These students are usually enrolled in accredited education programs for ophthalmic medical personnel. The awards range on average from $1,000 to $5,000 per year per student, and they are often sponsored by grant foundations and corporations, such as the Otto Bremer Foundation, the JCAHPO Education and Research Foundation, and Vistakon (a Johnson & Johnson Vision Products Company).

Also, individual schools may have their own financial aid programs, so you should talk with a counselor at the financial aid office wherever you are applying.

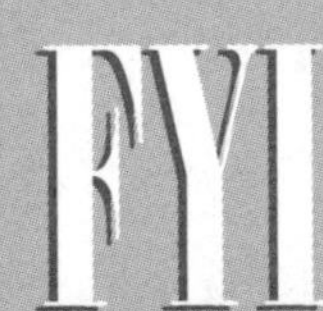

Who's Who?

What's the difference between an ophthalmologist, an optometrist, and an optician? Well, an ophthalmologist is a medical doctor, an optometrist is a doctor of optometry, and an optician is not a doctor but rather a technician.

Ophthalmologists and optometrists specialize in eye health and disease. You would need to see an ophthalmologist if you had an eye disease requiring medication or surgery or if you had a serious eye injury; you would see an optometrist if you needed contact lenses or vision therapy. Opticians, on the other hand, are qualified mainly to fill prescriptions for lenses written by the first two types of eye specialists. They make glasses, fit lenses into frames, and adjust glasses to fit a person's face (in some states, opticians can also fit contact lenses).

who will hire me?

Jeri Bloch worked as a receptionist in an eye doctor's office way back when she was in high school. Ten years later, she was still working for the same ophthalmologist, as a technician. She had worked her way up by learning on the job, taking the formal training classes, and recertifying whenever it was required. She is now thirty-five years old and still enjoys her career.

Jeri has worked in offices where there are only a few doctors; Cathy Brown, on the other hand, works with many doctors in an eye clinic. Ophthalmic technicians tend to work wherever there are ophthalmologists: doctors' offices, eye clinics, hospitals, and other medical settings.

As with other careers, if you are satisfied with the environment in which you work, you'll tend to stay there. Cathy has worked at Maine Eye Center for five years. But Jeri found that she wanted to travel and live in different places throughout the country, and she was pleased that her qualifications allowed her to do so. For example, she contacted various "headhunters" in California, and they set up interviews for her with ophthalmologists there; she accepted one of the offers and moved from Chicago to the West Coast. Because she continued to recertify her status as an ophthalmic technician and take continuing education courses, and because she had a good reputation as a responsible worker, many doctors' offices were eager to hire her.

where can I go from here?

Becoming an ophthalmic medical technologist is definitely a step up the career ladder. According to one worker, "Being a COMT [certified ophthalmic medical technologist] is a very rewarding career. There's an abundance of opportunities throughout the country." Lisa

Rovick is a COMT in a large multispecialty clinic in the Minneapolis/St. Paul area. She says that other options for advancement include going into the business side of ophthalmology, perhaps becoming a partner with the ophthalmologists at a busy office.

Other ophthalmic workers have become contractors, which means that they offer their services at various medical settings and work on a freelance basis. Education is another area of specialization. Some technicians perform in-service training and teach continuing education courses. Others work as sales representatives or researchers for manufacturers of ophthalmic equipment and pharmaceuticals.

Although it is not actually a higher-level position, *ophthalmic surgical assisting* is a special content area in which you may be examined and awarded a certificate. While taking courses in surgical assisting, Cathy decided to take a job leading to her assistant's certification; she may go back to surgical assisting in the future. On the other hand, Jeri does surgical assisting as well as technician-level tasks.

Related jobs

Ophthalmic technicians assist ophthalmologists. The skills required for being a good assistant translate quite easily to other areas of health care. Dental assistants, physician assistants, licensed practical nurses, and orthotics and prosthetics assistants all work closely with highly trained professionals in patient care.

The U.S. Department of Labor classifies ophthalmic technicians under the headings *Occupations in Medical and Dental Technology* (DOT) and *Child and Adult Care: Data Collection* (GOE). Also listed under these headings are dental hygienists, radiation therapy technologists, nuclear medicine technologists, electrocardiograph technicians, and audiometrists.

what are the salary ranges?

According to Cathy Brown, certified ophthalmic assistants in her city earn about $10 to $12 per hour; that would be about $20,800 to $25,000 a year for forty-hour work weeks. When she becomes a certified ophthalmic technician, she can expect to earn about $28,000 per year. According to the Committee on Allied Health Education and Accreditation, entry-level technicians and technologists earn about $25,000 per year.

As with many careers, salaries vary according to geographic region and job level. The Association for Technical Personnel in Ophthalmology reports that overall, ophthalmic assistant, technician, and technologist salaries range from less than $14,000 to $90,000. Earnings are higher in New England than on the West Coast, so if Cathy stays in Maine she can expect to earn more someday than Jeri did in California.

what is the job outlook?

Right now, ophthalmic workers seem to be in demand. Although in the future the health care situation could create hiring "freezes" for medical personnel, ophthalmologists currently are looking for responsible workers willing to be trained and to follow the certification process. As mentioned earlier, one of Cathy's co-workers was skilled in photography and answered a help wanted ad for an ophthalmic photographer at Maine Eye Center; she got the job and a promise of on-the-job training because of the scarcity of skilled ophthalmic photographers.

how do I learn more?

professional organizations

Following are organizations that provide information on ophthalmic technician careers, accredited schools and scholarships, and employers.

Joint Commission on Allied Health Personnel in Ophthalmology (JCAHPO)
2025 Woodlane Drive
St. Paul, MN 55125
TEL: 612-731-2944

American Academy of Ophthalmology
655 Beach Street
San Francisco, CA 94120
TEL: 415-561-8500

American Academy of Optometry
4330 East West Highway, Suite 1117
Bethesda, MD 20814
TEL: 301-718-6500

American Foundation for Vision Awareness
243 North Lindbergh Boulevard
St. Louis, MO 63141
TEL: 800-927-2382

American Optometric Association
243 North Lindbergh Boulevard
St. Louis, MO 63141
TEL: 314-991-4100

Association of Technical Personnel in Ophthalmology
c/o Peggy Yamada
306 Humboldt Road
Brisbane, CA 94005
TEL: 415-467-6304

National Association of Vision Professionals
c/o Prevention of Blindness Society
1775 Church Street, NW
Washington, DC 20036
TEL: 202-234-1010

National Eye Research Foundation
c/o Pamela Baker
910 Skokie Boulevard, Suite 207A
Northbrook, IL 60062
TEL: 847-564-4652

Vision Educational Foundation
PO Box 472305
Tulsa, OK 74147
TEL: 918-762-3947

bibliography

Following is a sampling of material relating to the professional concerns and development of ophthalmic technicians.

Books

Ahrens, Kathleen M. *Opportunities in Eye Care Careers*. Lincolnwood, IL: VGM Career Horizons, 1994.

Cassin, Barbara. *Fundamentals for Ophthalmic Technical Personnel*. Philadelphia, PA: W.B. Saunders Co., 1995.

Kanski, Jack J. *Case Presentations in Medical Ophthalmology*. Boston: Butterworth-Heinemann, 1991.

Stamper, Robert L., and Paul J. Wasson, editors. *Ophthalmic Medical Assisting: An Independent Study Course*, 2nd edition. San Francisco, CA: American Academy of Ophthalmology, 1994.

Stollery, Rosalind. *Ophthalmic Nursing*, 2nd edition. Cambridge, MA: Blackwell Science, 1997.

Zelada, A. J. A *Dispensing Optician Manual: an Introduction to Vision Care for the New Ophthalmic Technician*. Springfield, IL: C.C. Thomas, 1987.

Periodicals

Eye to Eye. Semiannual. Newsletter containing program activities of the International Eye Foundation. Eyelights, International Eye Foundation, Sibley Memorial Hospital, 7801 Norfolk Avenue, Bethesda, MD 20814, 301-986-1830.

Eyecare Business. Monthly. Directed toward vision care professionals. Viscom Publications, Inc., 50 Washington Street, Norwalk, CT 06854, 203-838-9100.

Ophthalmic Research. Bimonthly. Publishes original research on scientific aspects of ophthalmology. S. Karger Publishers, Inc., 26 West Avon Road, Box 529, Farmington, CT 06085, 203-675-7834.

Ophthalmology. Monthly. J.B. Lippincott Co., 227 East Washington Square, Philadelphia, PA 19106, 215-238-4200.

Ophthalmology Times. Biweekly. Newspaper format. Includes general news, interviews, and convention information. Advanstar Communications, 7500 Old Oak Boulevard, Cleveland, OH 44130, 216-243-8100.

ophthalmologist

Definition

An ophthalmologist is the specialist who diagnoses and treats diseases and injuries of the eye. Ophthalmologists may use drugs or surgery to treat eye diseases.

Alternative job titles

Oculist (mostly used in Great Britain)

Salary range

$31,000 to $140,000 to $200,000+

Educational requirements

Bachelor's degree; M.D.; one-year postgraduate residency in patient care; three- to four-year specialty residency in ophthalmology; optional fellowship in subspecialty.

Certification or Licensing

Mandatory

Outlook

Much faster than average

GOE
02.03.01

DOT
070

High School Subjects

Biology
Chemistry
English
Math
Physics

Personal Interests

Building models
Helping people
Problem solving
Research

The girl plopped herself down in the chair, throwing one leg casually over the arm and letting it dangle there. Her mother walked into the office a moment later with the resident in ophthalmology who was about to examine her daughter.

"Brenda, sit up straight," her mother whispered sharply to her, and rapped her daughter's knee with her knuckles. Brenda grudgingly slid her leg off the arm of the chair and sat a few inches higher, but she wasn't taking any pains to hide her displeasure in being there.

"Hi," the resident said. "My name's Tom. It's Brenda, right?" he asked the girl. She didn't answer, but leaned back on one elbow and swept a hand through the blonde bangs that fell across her eyes. She seemed to be sizing him up.

"Brenda," her mother sighed, embarrassed by her daughter's rude, indifferent behavior. The resident turned to the mother.

"Mrs. Winters, why don't you go and have a cup of coffee? We'll be fine," he assured her. She looked a little relieved and stood to go. The resident and the girl stared at one another for a brief moment before the girl blurted out, "She thinks glasses are going to help me get better grades. Phfff," the girl snorted. "I maybe can't see, but I can hear—and there's no way I'm ever going to get all that sine, cosine crap."

The resident laughed. Angered by his reaction, the girl turned her head away. He placed his hand on her arm, and shook his head. "No, no, I'm sorry. I'm laughing because I almost flunked trig, and I had 20/20 vision!" The girl looked at him skeptically. "Really, I swear," the resident answered. "Come on, let's take a look at your eyes and see what's going on." He began to examine her eyes. "Hey, you've got blue eyes under all that hair," he kidded her.

After examining her eyes, the resident wrote a prescription for lenses to help with her poor vision. Brenda returned several weeks later, a changed person—happy, almost glowing. "Dr. Weingeist, I want to thank you. I can see the stars for the first time."

lingo to learn

Blepharoplasty Plastic surgery on the eyelid, usually to remove excess or fatty tissue.

Cataract A clouding of the lens of the eye; it obstructs transmission of light to the retina.

Conjunctivitis Inflammation of the conjunctiva, the mucous membrane that lines the eyelid and covers the white of the eye.

Iritis Inflammation of the iris of the eye.

Ophthalmoscope Instrument used to view the inside of the eye, especially the retina.

Retina The delicate membrane that lines the eye. It has light-sensitive cells, called rods and cones, that change light rays into electrical impulses that are carried to the brain by the optic nerve.

Vitreous humor The clear, colorless, transparent jelly that fills the eyeball behind the lens.

what does an ophthalmologist do?

An *ophthalmologist* is the medical specialist who manages comprehensive care of the eyes. The ophthalmologist is the only practitioner who is medically trained to diagnose and treat all disorders of the eye. Ophthalmologists test the eyes and prescribe glasses or contact lenses to correct nearsightedness, farsightedness, and other visual defects. They treat eye infections and diseases, such as conjunctivitis and glaucoma, and perform surgery on the eye.

Most ophthalmologists spend approximately four days per week in the office performing routine eye examinations and screenings, and one day per week in the operating room. In a typical week, the general ophthalmologist will see, on average, a hundred patients, and perform two major surgical procedures. Cataract removal is the most commonly performed opthalmolic surgery. Other types of surgery include corneal transplants, surgery to correct glaucoma, and surgery to correct cross-eye or other eye muscle deviations. Surgery may be performed at a hospital, at a same-day ambulatory care surgical center, or in the doctor's office.

The standard ophthalmologic practice involves preventive measures as well as the treatment of patients with vision-threatening diseases, and to this end, much of the ophthalmologist's day is spent in yearly vision examinations of patients that may or may not lead to further eye exams or prescriptions for lenses.

In addition to managing local eye disorders, the ophthalmologist also works with other physicians. When examining a patient with an ophthalmoscope, the ophthalmologist studies the retina and may discover signs of diseases that involve other parts of the body, such as diabetes, atherosclerosis, and hypertension. The ophthalmologist then may be involved with another physician in the diagnosis and management of a disease, or may work as a consultant.

Like many other specialties, ophthalmology has undergone considerable subspecialization. Some ophthalmologists specialize in diseases of the cornea, conjunctiva, and eyelids. Training in this area frequently includes corneal transplant surgery and corneal surgery to correct refractive errors. The specialty of glaucoma focuses on the treatment of glaucoma and other disorders that may cause optic nerve damage. This area involves the medical and surgical treatment of both pediatric and adult patients. Other specialities include ophthalmic pathology, ophthalmic plastic surgery, and pediatric ophthalmology.

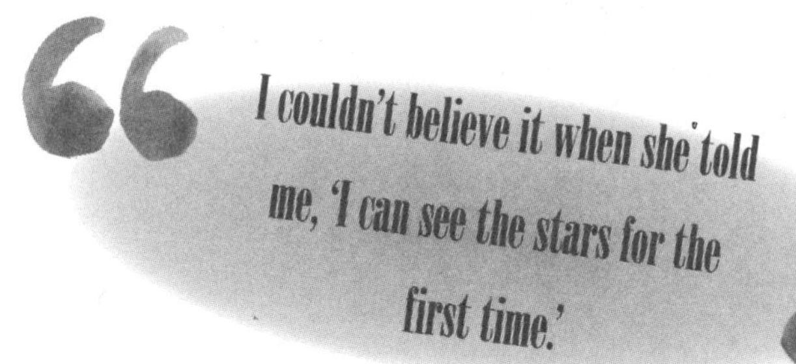

what is it like to be an ophthalmologist?

"I love what I do," says Thomas Weingeist, Ph.D., M.D., about the work he does as an ophthalmologist specializing in vitreoretinal diseases. Dr. Weingeist was the resident who helped the teenager see a starlit sky for the first time. The experience left quite an impression on him. "When that girl came in for a routine eye exam, it was like any other exam, really. I examined her, refracted her, saw she had poor vision, and wrote a prescription for glasses. I couldn't believe it when she came back and said, 'I can see the stars for the first time.' What I did for her was so simple, yet it had such an incredible impact on her life. If I had any doubts about my profession—they all vanished in that moment."

Dr. Weingeist was fortunate enough to have benefited from early exposure to the profession. His father was also an ophthalmologist. "I knew what an ophthalmologist was, and I actually spent a lot of time with him at his office. Originally, I went to graduate school to do research, but then I decided to go to medical school, afterwards. Now, my son is studying to be an ophthalmologist." Dr. Weingeist got his Ph.D. in Cell Biology at Columbia University in New York City, and then went on to the University of Iowa for his medical degree, ophthalmology residency, and fellowship in vitreoretinal diseases and surgery.

Today, Dr. Weingeist is Head of the Department of Ophthalmology at the University of Iowa, and the Director of Vitreoretinal Service. He works with patients who have age-related macular degeneration, detached retinas, and diabetic retinopathy. As part of one of the premiere research facilities in the country in ophthalmology, the departments he oversees at the University of Iowa are mainly tertiary care facilities; that is, according to Dr. Wiengeist, they are "places where patients with the hard problems go."

A typical patient who might come to Dr. Weingeist for diagnosis and treatment is one with macular degeneration—the most common cause of severe vision loss in people over sixty-five. Located in the center of our field of vision, the sensitive macula allows us to see fine details. This sharp, straight-ahead vision is necessary for driving, reading, recognizing faces, and doing close work, such as sewing. To help in the diagnosis of macular degeneration, Dr. Weingeist might use what is called an Amsler Grid—a chart that looks like simple graph paper with a dot at the center intersection. Basically, the chart is a tool for monitoring the patient's central visual field. If, while staring at the center dot, a patient sees wavy lines and blurred or dark areas of the grid, he or she most likely has some form of macular degeneration.

Another common patient complaint that Dr. Weingeist hears sounds like it has more to do with seeing flying saucers and spaceships at night on a deserted highway, than modern ophthalmology. "A lot of patients tell me they see flashing lights and floaters," says Dr. Weingeist. "My first question is usually, 'did you recently have surgery?'" The floater phenomenon is really nothing more than tiny clumps of gel or cells inside the vitreous—the clear, jelly-like fluid that fills the inside of the eye. While these objects look to the patient as if they are in front of the eye, they are actually floating inside. What the patient sees are the shadows the gel or cells cast on the retina. Floaters can have different shapes: dots, circles, lines, clouds, or cobwebs. "Actually, we ask patients that a lot, 'Do you see shadows?'" he says. As people age, the vitreous gel may start to thicken or shrink, and as it does, it can pull away from the back wall of the eye. Sometimes, the retina tears as a result of this shrinking process. Dr. Weingeist uses drops to dilate, or open, the pupils of the patient's eyes so that he can carefully examine the retina and vitreous. "We look into the patient's eye with an ophthalmoscope, checking to see if retinal detachments are causing the shadows."

Flashing lights are similar. When the vitreous shrinks, it tugs on the retina, creating a sensation of flashing lights. The flashes of light can appear on and off for several weeks, even months. The sudden appearance of light flashes could indicate that the patient's retina has been torn.

have I got what it takes to be an ophthalmologist?

"If you want to be a successful ophthalmologist, you have to love what you do," says Dr. Weingeist, "you have to become educated, give yourself a broad liberal arts background, some writing; and you have to be devoted to patient care by being honest, caring, and hardworking."

Prospective ophthalmologists should keep in mind that a typical ophthalmic practice involves the treatment of patients with vision-threatening diseases. These patients often believe (correctly or incorrectly) that they are going blind. Dealing with the prospect of vision reduction or complete loss presents a unique challenge that can be highly stressful and frustrating for both patient and physician. The ophthalmologist must be prepared to offer the patient compassion and understanding, as well as clinical expertise.

Those considering going into the field of ophthalmology should also be aware that certain visual and motor skills are necessary for effective clinical and surgical practice. Ideally, an ophthalmologist (like all surgeons), will have excellent fine motor skills, depth perception, and color vision. Any impairment of these abilities may interfere with the effective use of essential ophthalmic instruments, such as the ophthalmoscope, the operating microscope, and microsurgery instruments.

Ophthalmologists should be patient and have good communication skills, skills that come in handy when trying to set the record straight on what the profession actually does. "There's a lot of confusion about what we do. One thing I'd like to do is to clearly define the differences between an ophthalmologist and an optician and an optometrist, something that gets even trickier when you throw in the ocularist and the oculist, not to mention the Doctor of Osteopathy," Dr. Weingeist adds firmly, but good-naturedly. "A sense of humor helps, too." For a full description of the distinctions, see the sidebar article, "An eye is an eye is an eye—or is it?"

how do I become an ophthalmologist?

education

High School

"Throughout your education, you have to be a good student," advises Dr. Weingeist. "And you have to distinguish yourself." High school students should prepare for a future in medicine by taking courses in biology, chemistry, physics, algebra, geometry, and trigonometry. Courses in computer science are a must, as well, since the computer is changing the way medicine is communicated and shared by busy medical professionals.

Postsecondary Training

University or college courses that may help prepare prospective medical students for medical school and beyond, are math, biology, chemistry, anatomy, and physics, as well as courses in the humanities, such as English composition.

After receiving an undergraduate degree, the student serious about entering medical school must then apply and be accepted to one of the 141 medical schools in the United States. Admission is competitive and applicants must undergo a fairly extensive and difficult admissions process which considers grade point averages, scores on the Medical College Admission Test (MCAT), and recommendations from professors. Most premedical students apply to several schools early in their senior year of college. Only about one-third of the applicants are accepted.

In order to earn the degree, doctor of medicine (M.D.), a student must complete four years of medical school study and training. For the first two years of medical school, students attend lectures and classes and spend time in laboratories. Courses include anatomy, biochemistry, physiology, and pharmacology. They learn to take patient histories, perform routine physical examinations, and recognize symptoms.

In their third and fourth years, students are involved in more practical studies. They work in clinics and hospitals supervised by residents and physicians. They go through what are known as rotations, or brief periods of study in a particular area, such as internal medicine, obstetrics and gynecology, pediatrics, dermatology, psychiatry, and surgery. Rotations allow students to gain exposure to the many different fields within medicine and to learn firsthand the skills of diagnosing and treating patients.

Upon graduating from an accredited medical school, physicians must pass a standard examination given by the National Board of Medical Examiners. Passing this exam results in them becoming licensed to practice medicine. Most physicians complete an internship, also referred to as a transition year. The internship is usually one year in length, and helps graduates to decide what will be their area of specialization.

Following the internship, the physicians begin what is known as a residency. Physicians wishing to pursue the surgical specialty of ophthalmology, must first complete a one-year postgraduate training program in one of the following specialties: internal medicine, pediatrics, general surgery, emergency medicine, neurology, or family practice. This year of training is followed by a three-year specialty program in ophthalmology. "I enjoyed everything," Dr. Weingeist says. "I loved being a resident. Residents today do a lot of . . . complaining, but we felt lucky to get in, so we didn't complain," he says, referring to the early 70s when medical schools and residency programs were inundated with applications—the first of the baby boomers to hit graduate programs. "Every day we saw something intellectually challenging—and then we learned how to take care of those problems."

To be a successful ophthalmologist, you should:

- Be a good clinician
- Enjoy helping and working with people
- Have good hand-eye coordination and manual dexterity
- Be able to listen and communicate well

certification or licensing

To qualify for certification by the American Board of Ophthalmology (ABO) a candidate has completed the ophthalmology residency and has successfully completed both the written and oral examinations given by the board. Certification is valid for ten years, at which time the ophthalmologist must apply for recertification. While certification is voluntary, it is highly recommended. Most hospitals will not grant privileges to an ophthalmologist without board certification. HMOs and other insurance groups will not make referrals or payments without certification. Licensing is a mandatory procedure in the United States. It is required in all states before any doctor can practice medicine. An ophthalmologist is not eligible to apply for certification until he or she is licensed.

scholarships and grants

Scholarships and grants are often available from individual institutions, state agencies, and special-interest organizations. The book *Dollars for College: Medicine, Dentistry, and Related Fields* by Ferguson Publishing Company is an excellent source for this information. Many students finance their medical education through the Armed Forces Health Professions Scholarship Program. Each branch of the military participates in this program, paying students' tuitions in exchange for military service. Contact your local recruiting office for more information on this program. The National Health Service Corps Scholarship Program also provides money for students in return for service. Another source for financial aid, scholarship, and grant information is the Association of American Medical Colleges. Remember to request information early for eligibility, application requirements and deadlines.

Association of American Medical Colleges
2450 N Street, NW
Washington, DC 20037
TEL: 202-828-0400
WEBSITE: http://www.aamc.org
Specific information on financial aid programs can be found at:
WEBSITE: http://www.aamc.org/stuapps/finaid

Ferguson Publishing Company
200 West Madison, Suite 300
Chicago, IL 60606
TEL: 312-580-5480

National Health Services Corps Scholarship Program
U.S. Public Health Service
1010 Wayne Avenue, Suite 240
Silver Spring, MD 20910
TEL: 800-638-0824

who will hire me?

Ophthalmologists can choose from a variety of exciting and challenging work environments. Many ophthalmologists go into private practice, sometimes by themselves, more commonly in a small group. These small group practices are either multi-specialty practices, or single-specialty practices. Other ophthalmologists, like Dr. Weingeist, choose to work at universities and medical schools, teaching and conducting research. An academic career offers the clinical exposure of a private practice combined with the opportunity to perform more unusual surgeries.

Usually, academic careers provide the opportunity to teach, as well as handle administrative duties. The additional responsibilities of teaching and running a department are time-consuming, but rewarding. "If they paid me half of what they pay me now, I'd still do it," says Dr. Weingeist. His experience practicing ophthalmic medicine and surgery, his teaching and mentoring skills, his administrative responsibilities, and his area of specialization not only make him highly regarded by his patients, students, and peers, but also render him very employable. Prospective physicians, of all specialties, should consider every possible avenue available to them. Research, like teaching, is another option for new ophthalmologists to consider.

where can I go from here?

Ophthalmologists can advance their careers by keeping current with new technologies, medications, and techniques. Publishing articles in respected medical journals, such as *JAMA,* is another avenue for professional enhancement. Many ophthamologists combine research and teaching with a private practice. Others work as professors at universities or teaching hospitals and may advance to an administrative position, like Dr. Weingeist, who heads a university ophthalmology department.

what are the salary ranges?

The national average salary for first-year residents in the mid-1990's was approximately $31,000. That average increases to $41,800 by the final residency year. Salaries will vary depending on the kind of residency, the hospital, and the geographic area.

According to surveys by the American Medical Association, annual income for surgeons in the mid-1990's ranged from approximately $140,000 to $300,000, with the median income at about $200,000. These figures are for all surgeons, and incomes may vary from specialty to specialty. Other factors influencing individual incomes include type and size of practice, hours worked per week, geographic area, and professional reputation.

what is the job outlook?

Recent studies have predicted a national surplus of specialty care physicians, including ophthalmologists. The surplus is being driven by the trend towards managed care in the health care market. The same studies also predict a sufficient number of primary care providers, however. Geographic shortages will undoubtedly persist for all fields of medicine, including ophthalmology, as patient access to medical care will continue to be a need in rural areas and inner-city communities.

Specifically, the demand for ophthalmology, as for the other specialties, will depend on the advances of medicine and how quickly

in-depth

An eye is an eye is an eye—or is it?

The distinction between ophthalmology and optometry is a frequent source of confusion. Optometrists are often referred to as 'eye doctors' even though they don't have medical degrees. And optometrists are confused with opticians, who can't examine eyes at all, but just make the lenses. And then there are oculists and ocularists.

Here's the straight dope.

Ophthalmologists are the only specialists trained to diagnose and treat all eye and visual problems, from glasses and contact lenses to retinal surgery to corneal transplants. Ophthalmologists are physicians, doctors of medicine (M.D.) or doctors of osteopathy (D.O.) who have trained long and hard to medically and surgically care for the eyes. They complete four years of college, four years of medical school, one year of internship, three or more years of specialized medical and surgical and refractive training and experience, possibly followed by one or more years of subspecialty training. They're licensed to practice medicine and surgery. At a minimum, they train for twelve years after high school.

Optometrists are health service providers who are involved exclusively with vision problems. They are specifically trained for four years by accredited optometry colleges, but they have not attended medical school and are not medical doctors. At a minimum, they train for seven years after high school. Individual states license them to examine the eyes and to determine the presence of vision problems. They determine visual acuity and prescribe glasses, contact lenses, and eye exercises. They perform all the services that an optician performs. Some states even permit optometrists to give limited treatments of some eye conditions.

Opticians are technicians who make lenses, frames, contact lenses, and other specially fabricated optical devices from prescriptions. Opticians analyze and interpret prescriptions, determine the best lens forms for the customer, and prepare and deliver work orders for the grinding of lenses and the fabrication of eye wear. They help a client select frames and adjust eyeglasses to the client's comfort. At a minimum, they train for two years after high school.

Last, but not least, are *oculists* and *ocularists*. The former are actually ophthalmologists. In England, ophthalmologists are often called oculists. Ocularists, on the other hand, make and fit prosthetic eyes for individuals who have lost one or both of their eyes. Cosmetically, the artificial eye an ocularist makes looks like an eye, but only has an aesthetic purpose and does not function like an eye.

new procedures and techniques can be made available to the public. In the last five to ten years, ophthalmology has enjoyed more than its share of scientific and technological breakthroughs. For example, retinal laser surgery was a new procedure only ten years ago. Now, it is nearly a run-of-the-mill procedure for ophthalmologists.

In the future, the demand for ophthalmologists will also depend on the how the value of primary eye care is promoted by health insurance plans and vision care plans; many of these plans try to limit patient access to ophthalmologists, requiring so-called "gatekeeper" referrals, or the alternative services of optometrists.

how do I learn more?

professional organizations

Following are organizations that provide information on the profession of ophthalmology.

American Academy of Ophthalmology
655 Beech Street
San Francisco, CA 94109
TEL: 415-561-8500
WEBSITE:
http://www.eyenet.org/public/who/who.html

American Board of Ophthalmology
111 Presidential Boulevard, Suite 241
Bala Cynwyd, PA 19004
TEL: 610-664-1175

American Society of Contemporary Medicine, Surgery and Ophthalmology
4711 West Golf Road, Suite 408
Skokie, IL 60076
TEL: 847-568-1500
WEBSITE: http://www.social.com/health/nhic/data

bibliography

Following is a sampling of materials relating to the professional concerns and development of ophthalmologists.

Books

Albert, D. M. *Source Book of Ophthalmology*. Cambridge, MA: Blackwell Science, 1995.

Coakes, Roger L., and Patrick H. Sellors. *Outline of Ophthalmology*, 2nd edition. Newton, MA: Butterworth-Heinemann, 1995.

Newell, Frank W. *Ophthalmology: Principles and Concepts*, 7th edition. St. Louis, MO: Mosby, 1996.

Stein, H. A., and others. A *Primer of Ophthalmology: a Textbook for Students*. St. Louis, MO: Mosby, 1991.

Periodicals

International Ophthalmology Clinics. Quarterly. Covers a single, current topic in ophthalmology. Little, Brown, Medical Journals, 34 Beacon Street, Boston, MA 02108, 617-589-5500.

Key Ophthalmology. Quarterly. Surveys and abstracts of key medical literature in ophthalmology. Mosby, 11820 Westline Industrial Drive, St. Louis, MO 63146, 314-872-8370, 800-325-4177.

Ophthalmic Research. Bimonthly. Publishes original research on scientific aspects of ophthalmology. S. Karger Publishers, Inc., 26 West Avon Road, Box 529, Farmington, CT 06085, 203-675-7834.

Ophthalmology. Monthly. American Academy of Ophthalmology, Lippincott-Raven Publishers, 227 E. Washington Square, Philadelphia, PA 19106, 215-238-4200.

Seminars in Ophthalmology. Quarterly. Each issue focuses on a particular therapeutic or surgical technique. W.B. Saunders Co., Curtis Center, 3rd Floor, Independence Square West, Philadelphia, PA 19106, 215-238-7800.

optics technician

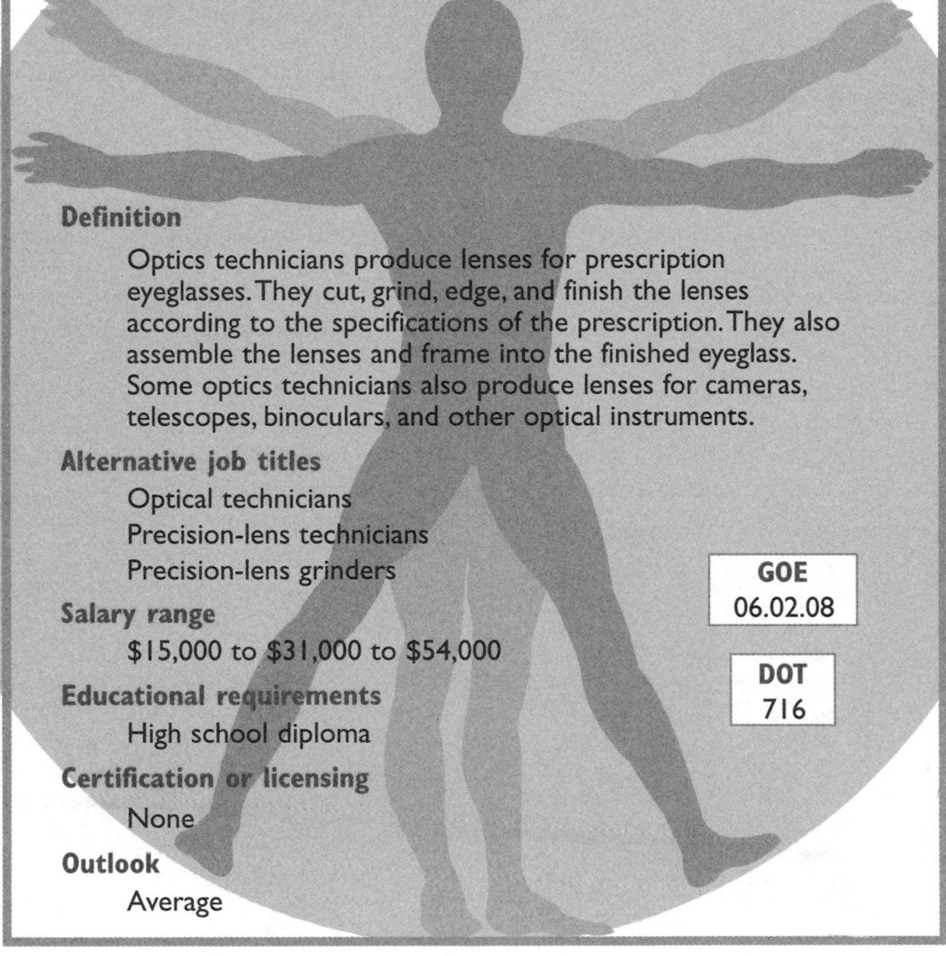

Definition

Optics technicians produce lenses for prescription eyeglasses. They cut, grind, edge, and finish the lenses according to the specifications of the prescription. They also assemble the lenses and frame into the finished eyeglass. Some optics technicians also produce lenses for cameras, telescopes, binoculars, and other optical instruments.

Alternative job titles

Optical technicians
Precision-lens technicians
Precision-lens grinders

Salary range

$15,000 to $31,000 to $54,000

Educational requirements

High school diploma

Certification or licensing

None

Outlook

Average

GOE
06.02.08

DOT
716

High School Subjects

Auto shop
Physics
Applied mathematics
English
Algebra
Geometry
Electrical shop

Personal Interests

Working with your hands
Learning how things work
Electronics
Computers

At 1:00 PM the lab at Lenscrafters is in the middle of a peak period. The store is filled with business people from the hundreds of companies in Chicago's Loop on their lunch hour eating their sandwiches, checking their watches, and waiting for their eyeglasses to be finished. Rich Crockett is circling the optical lab checking on the progress of six pairs of glasses that have to be finished within an hour.

Ron Miranda has been an optics technician for only three months, yet he must operate a handful of high tech instruments, compounds, and hand tools as proficiently as the most experienced member of the lab. If he should commit any one of many possible errors, the lens he is working on will have to be scrapped, and he will have to start the twenty-step process all over again with a new lens.

Rich is the most experienced member of the lab, so he looks over Ron's shoulder, offering valuable help and experienced tips on precision grinding. Rich glances at the clock. It will be at least another hour until there is any rest.

what does an optics technician do?

Lenses are part of so many aspects of daily, scientific, and professional life that the tremendous need for *optics technicians* to make, assemble, and maintain them is obvious. In addition, optics technicians are needed to invent new types of lenses and new uses for lenses.

Though most people think of optics technicians only as being the men and women who grind and polish the lenses for eyeglasses, there are several areas in which an optics technician may work. While an optics technician may be a part of more than one field in optics, the general areas are lens fabrication, product manufacturing, maintenance and operations, and research and development.

Lens fabrication is the area most associated with producing eyeglasses. An optics technician working in lens fabrication may have a job as any of the following: lens molder, lens blocker, lens generator, lens grinder, lens polisher, lens centerer or edger, lens coater, or lens inspector. However, the optics technician is not limited to performing only one of these jobs. Optics technicians, depending on the size and organization of the laboratory, can perform several or all of these jobs. Also, the technician may become responsible for supervising all the work done by all the technicians in these jobs.

A *lens molder* works with partially melted glass, plastic, or polycarbonate to press and form a lens blank, which is used to produce the prescribed finished lens.

A *lens blocker* places the lens blanks into blocks so that they can be held in place during the rest of the grinding and polishing.

A *lens generator* works with the instrument called the lens generator, which grinds the lens into its rough curve and thickness, and which aligns the prism-axes.

A *lens grinder* finishes shaping the lens into its prescribed curve and thickness. This may be done with machines or hand tools.

A *lens polisher* uses various compounds, pads, and machines to polish the lens so that there are no obstructions when checking the power of the lens and light refraction.

A *lens centerer* or *edger* uses the lensometer to check the degree and placement of the curves that determine the power or strength of the lens. The lens is also worked on with handstones to finish shaping the lens to fit in the frame.

A *lens coater* performs all the finishing steps in the fabrication of the lens, including the application of tints or coatings and final polishing.

A *lens inspector* checks the lens for required hardness, inspects for scratches or other defects, and ensures that all government standards have been met.

The area of product manufacturing deals mostly with fabricating lenses for use in products other than eyeglasses that use lenses. An optics technician working in this field will assemble, align, calibrate, and test optical instruments. Common products such as microscopes, telescopes, binoculars, and cameras, as well as less common, more advanced instruments, require optics technicians to install the lenses and make sure they are working properly.

lingo to learn

Aberration A condition that causes blurring, loss of clearness, or distortion of shape in the images formed by lenses or curved mirrors.

Spherical aberration Rays of light striking near the edges of the lens or mirror are brought to focus closer to the lens or mirror than are the central rays. The result is that the image of a point appears as a small disk.

Lens A curved, transparent body that bends (refracts) light rays.

Diffraction The spreading out of waves as they pass around an obstacle or go through an opening. For example, light waves are diffracted when they pass through a small sheet of glass marked with thousands of parallel lines, producing a spectrum.

Index of refraction The ratio of the speed of light in a vacuum to its speed in the particular substance being measured.

Refraction The bending of waves, such as light waves, when they pass from one substance to another. Refraction occurs because waves travel at different speeds through different substances.

Reflection The bending back of waves, such as light waves, from a surface.

Optics technicians working in maintenance and operations are responsible for any and all work needed to keep the optical instruments working. Most of the work will be done at the site where the instrument is being used. These include places such as observatories, hospitals, or even missile or satellite tracking stations. An optics technician can work with scientific cameras, large observatory telescopes, light-measuring equipment, and spectrophotometers.

Finally, an optics technician may work in the research and development area of optics, helping to develop new types of lenses and new uses for them. A researcher or developer may concentrate on surveillance equipment, security devices, measuring instruments, medical implements, and environmental tools.

what is it like to be an optics technician?

Generally, the work environment and daily tasks of an optics technician are similar throughout the entire field of optics technology. Whether one is making a pair of glasses for someone, a lens for a NASA telescope, or a crystal for a sixteenth-century museum piece, the tasks of grinding, polishing, and aligning are most always involved, and the work laboratories are clean, ventilated, and well lighted.

Rich Crockett manages an optics laboratory for Lenscrafters. Rich has been an optics technician for twenty-four years. "The size of the lab varies from place to place, and the number of tasks each technician is responsible for may be lesser or greater, but they all look pretty much the same," says Rich.

Ron Miranda has been an optics technician at Lenscrafters for only three months and sees the lab as a very new type of work environment. "I worked as a florist before coming to the lab at Lenscrafters. Here everything is so bright and clean and organized. At my other job it was completely the opposite."

Both Rich and Ron work for Lenscrafters in the heart of downtown Chicago. Because Lenscrafters provides one-hour eyeglass service, each workday is tightly filled for Rich and Ron, but it still is usually kept to an eight-hour shift. "Sometimes I have to be here from before the store opens at eight in the morning until after the store closes at seven at night because we have a problem with one of the machines, or maybe someone came in just before we closed and needs their glasses when we open the next day. Usually on those days, though, I'm so busy I don't even realize how long I've been working," Rich says.

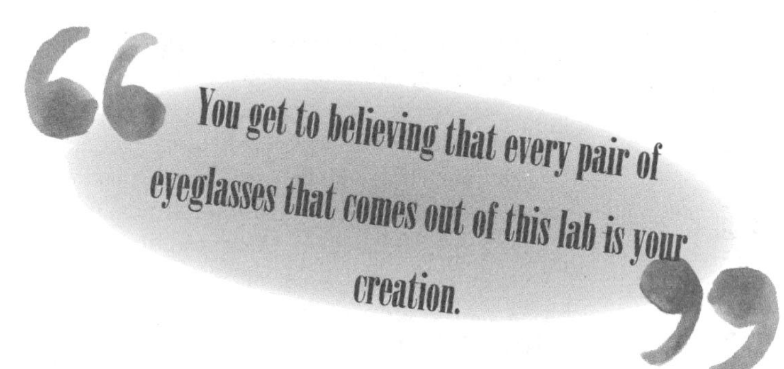

"Yeah, but sometimes you really know you've been working a long day. Still, when it's over you feel good," adds Ron. The good feeling that Ron has at the end of a longer-than-eight-hour day comes from having accomplished something very tangible. "When you're done you know you made a well-crafted product for two or three dozen people. It's not like working all day and not getting anything finished." Ron also knows that the more hours he works, the more money he makes and the more experience he earns toward becoming a lab manager himself.

The work weeks are around forty hours, and the days a technician works depend on the days the store or lab are open. Some retail eyeglass stores are open seven days a week. Some of the research laboratories are open only Monday through Friday.

Safety, efficiency, and ecology are mandatory in all optics laboratories. An optics technician works with potentially dangerous chemicals and machinery. While none of the chemicals is extremely dangerous alone or when used properly, they do pose a hazard if mixed inappropriately, and the fumes they give off are unhealthy if the work area is not ventilated. And though the machines do not threaten life and limb, the particles of glass, plastic, and other materials that are produced while grinding are very harmful to the unprotected eye.

"Everyone wears protective eye gear while in the lab, whether they are working on a lens or not. All around the lab we have emergency equipment in case a chemical gets on someone, in their eyes, or explodes. Everyone is trained thoroughly in all safety and emergency procedures. The lab is safer than most people's work places as long as all the techs are paying attention and following the rules. It only seems dangerous when everyone is busy and all the machines are making noise," says Rich.

"There are signs everywhere reminding us about safety and quality work. And in the break area there is always some literature on procedures, core values, and technical innovations," adds Ron. And, of course, the lab is so well lighted, an optics technician is never at risk of not being able to see what is being done, or read the caution signs on the walls.

have I got what it takes to be an optics technician?

Optics technicians are more than lens grinders or polishers; they are healers, fashion consultants, safety inspectors, toolmakers, and equalizers, because a pair of eyeglasses is more than just a means to correct vision. A pair of glasses is a possible remedy for headaches, a fashion statement, eye protection, an instrument to help do a job, and a chance to see the world as well as anyone. For Rich, the moment when someone puts on that first pair of eyeglasses and looks in the mirror is what makes his job great. "They look around the room and can't believe the detail they can see. Then they look in the mirror and say, 'Hey, I don't look bad at all. I look pretty darn good, in fact.' That's the best thing," says Rich.

At first glance being an optics technician looks like monotonous and hectic work. All the eyeglasses undergo the same basic process, and the production can be almost nonstop. "It can be a very high-stress job during the times when the store is filled with customers," Rich says.

in-depth

The Single Largest Mistake That's Ever Been Made in Optics . . .

The $1.5 billion Hubble Space Telescope was launched in April 1990. In June, it was discovered that it could not be focused precisely due to a spherical aberration in its 2.4-meter primary mirror. NASA's official investigation panel eventually attributed the error to "sloppiness" on the part of the optical contractor, the Perkin-Elmer Corporation of Danbury, Connecticut, where the giant lens was polished in 1980-81.

According to the NASA report, Perkin-Elmer engineers and technicians failed to heed warning signs on at least three occasions. One test that was supposed to detect bumps and irregularities involved the use of a lens that was itself 1.308 millimeter out of position. This resulted in the lens being polished very, very precisely to an incorrect shape, producing the spherical aberration. Other subsequent tests that would have revealed this crucial error were also botched because the optics techs opted for quick fixes instead of detailed investigation and correction and then acted on the assumption that other tests had checked out okay. The NASA report blamed the ultimate failure to detect the error on both itself and Perkin-Elmer, saying that officials at both organizations, overwhelmed by the massive cost overruns and schedule slippages in other parts of the project, neglected the mirror work, which seemed to be going relatively well. In short, they failed to enforce their own quality assurance procedures.

The mirror problem was finally "corrected" in December 1993 when astronauts of the space shuttle *Endeavor* spent eleven days in space mounting a new Wide Field and Planetary Camera onto the mirror. The camera was modified with a spherical aberration equal in magnitude—but opposite in sign—to the mirror, thereby bouncing corrected images back to Earth. While they were there, the astronauts also fixed other assorted Hubble problems—at an estimated cost of $692 million. The spherical aberration problem alone was estimated to have cost $86.3 million.

"You have to pay very close attention to every detail in all the steps in lens production," adds Ron. "When it gets busy, you don't have a moment to spare, but you have to take enough time to make sure that you're using the right tool and following the specifications of the prescription." Ron has, in the past, accidentally ground the lens just a little too much and had to start the whole process over. Most of the time the optics tech doesn't know for sure that the lens is right until more than halfway through production.

The attention to detail and the patience required to make a good pair of glasses can provide a sense of pride and accomplishment when it is done right. As the lab manager, Rich expects some errors. "That's how a tech learns," he says. It is because there are so many little things that can go wrong during the making of eyeglass lenses that it can really be a good feeling when a finished pair of glasses is approved by the customer.

While it is true that the new, high tech lab equipment performs a lot of detail work automatically, most of the precision work still requires a certain feel or manual dexterity on the part of the optics technician. That feel only comes with experience and ability like any craft work. "You get to believing that every pair of eyeglasses that comes out of this lab is your creation," says Rich. For example, the lens generator encloses the lens in a chamber while it grinds the lens to its prescription rough curve and thickness, and then aligns the prism-axes. The technician works entirely by feel and knowledge of the requirements for each lens. Rich likens the work on the generator to peeling a potato blindfolded.

It may take half a year to a year and a half to become proficient in all the steps. And Rich believes there is a good reason why training takes place on the job. "It takes time to learn all the machines and all the details . . . and the only way you can learn it is by doing it."

To be a successful optics technician, you should

- Have manual dexterity
- Have an aptitude for math and science
- Have the desire to learn a craft
- Work with energy and ambition
- Be patient and pay attention to detail

Rich Crockett hires the optics technicians for the Lenscrafters labs he manages. "What I am most looking for is aggressiveness. I want someone who gives it all they have in learning the skills. And I want someone who is interested in advancing in a career as an optics tech," he says. "I will train them so they will not only know every detail in making a pair of glasses for Lenscrafters, but also be thoroughly proficient in all phases of set-up, grinding, generating, aligning, polishing, and finishing."

"When they are done training after six to eighteen months, the new optics technicians will also be knowledgeable in the materials that lenses are made out of, the chemicals they are using as adhesives, polishes, and tints, and also any innovations that are being experimented with in research and development of optical goods. Then the optics technicians can move into other areas of optics with greater ease."

how do I become an optics technician?

Basically, the quickest and most popular way to become an optics technician is to apply for a position as a lab technician at a wholesale or retail lens fabricator. Most often these companies are looking for individuals whom they can train according to their own specific needs.

education

High School

Most of the lens fabrication laboratories do not insist on their optics technicians being high school graduates, but all of them prefer hiring individuals with diplomas. Almost all laboratories that specialize in research and development require a high school diploma. Because the field is becoming increasingly more competitive, those who have not finished high school will significantly reduce their chances at employment and advancement.

High school courses in mathematics, science, and shop are most useful. Optics technicians will need some knowledge of algebra, geometry, physics, chemistry, technical read-

Advancement Possibilities

Precision-lens centerers and edgers, also known as **lead technicians,** set up, operate, and train workers on the grinder and collimator to edge and bevel precision ophthalmic optical lenses, according to work order or blueprint, and center a beam of light through the lens.

Precision inspectors, also known as **optical elements inspectors** and **lens inspectors,** use precision measuring instruments to inspect precision optical and ophthalmic lenses at various stages of production and ensure that specified standards have been met.

Supervisors, also known as **inspecting supervisors** and **lens generating supervisors,** supervise and coordinate activities of workers engaged in fabricating and inspecting eyeglass, contact, and precision optical lenses. The supervisor inspects lenses for defects and adherence to specifications using devices such as polariscope, magnifying glass, protractor, and power determining instrument.

ing and writing, mechanical drawing, glass working, and photography. Most important are any courses that increase your ability to follow procedures, and shop courses that increase your manual dexterity.

Postsecondary Training

There are a few colleges and universities that offer specific training and degrees for optics technicians. An alternate method is to attend a technical institute or community college. Most of these schools offer two- or three-year programs in engineering or science. Students in one of these programs can choose courses along the way that are best suited for a career as an optics technician.

If you choose to earn a degree from a technical or community college, you should try to take courses that deal with geometrical optics, trigonometry, lens polishing, technical writing, optical instruments, analytical geometry, specification writing, physics, optical shop practices, manual preparation, mechanical drawing, and report preparation.

However, the most common route to becoming an optics technician is to finish high school and then train in an optics laboratory. These training programs are usually on-the-job and therefore provide the added benefit of income while learning. In some of the more technical or industrial labs, training is in preparation for a job with the lab and therefore provides no income until training is successfully completed. Prospective optics technicians should investigate which type of training is most useful for the area of optics they wish to enter.

certification or licensing

Certification or licensing is usually not required for optics technicians, although some states have a license requirement for optics technicians working in the area of precision lens fabrication. The licensing examinations in these states may be written, practical, or both. Prospective optics technicians should inquire at an optics laboratory in the state they wish to practice to find out about any licensing requirements.

Often, the laboratory will provide a certification upon completion of their training program. The optics technician may then be required by the lab to update their certification regularly by completing courses, seminars, conferences, written exams, practical exams, or any combination of them.

In some cases, an optics technician can take the state or national exam for certification as a licensed optics technician after they have finished training in a licensed optics laboratory.

scholarships and grants

The International Society for Optical Engineering (SPIE) offers scholarships, as do many universities, etc. Write early for information on eligibility, application requirements, and deadlines.

labor unions

Optics technicians may belong to a union, but it is not usually a requirement for employment. The major union is the International Union of Electronic, Electrical, Salaried Machine and Furniture Workers.

who will hire me?

Of the approximately 1,200,000 optics technicians in the United States in 1994, half worked in the labs of retail eyeglass stores. The vast percentage of optics technicians working in these labs is due to the growth of the one-hour eyeglass market. Stores such as Pearl Vision and Lenscrafters are located in almost every city, suburb, and town. Often there will be several such stores in one small area plus department stores with express eyeglass service. Therefore, the best bet for employment is at one of these stores. To find the store nearest you look in the phone directory under Opticians, Retail.

Ron Miranda found his first job as an optics technician at one of twenty-four Lenscrafters in the Chicagoland area. Ron had no previous experience in optics, no degree or certification, and no specific technical expertise. However, because new stores are opening all the time, the need for optics technicians is also opening up.

Those optics technicians who do not work as precision lens technicians in eyeglass fabrication labs mostly work in optical laboratories fabricating, assembling, testing, and developing lenses for other optical goods. The best way to inquire about job opportunities in these labs is to contact one of the professional organizations such as SPIE, American Optometrist Association, or the Optical Association of America.

The remaining optics technicians are employed by optometrists or ophthalmologists in their smaller labs. Once again, the way to find out more is to contact an association or check the telephone directory under Optometrists or Physicians and Surgeons.

where can I go from here?

Rich Crockett hopes to move from lab manager to district manager of seventeen stores. "The next step after I've supervised all the local stores is to move into the regional area." Rich can become a regional lab manager of all the labs in a section of a state, an entire state, or a group of states depending on the size of the state and the number of stores. This position is also called the RQC (regional quality control) because the individual must make sure that all the labs are adhering to company and governmental standards. Once optics technicians get this far they will not actually be performing any of the hands-on work, but they must possess an expertise in all the aspects of lens fabrication.

Ron Miranda is a surface technician currently. He is an optics technician who works only in the surfacing side of lens fabrication. He performs every step through lens generating. Ron would like to become the *lead technician* in a lab as soon as he has mastered all the steps. As a lead technician, Ron would supervise all the optics technicians who are performing the individual steps, and he will be responsible for ordering materials for the lab. The lead optics technician in the Lenscrafters lab is the immediate subordinate to the lab manager and therefore carries out the manager's orders concerning specifics of the lab.

what are the salary ranges?

An optics technician beginning without training may earn only minimum wage. The average salary for a technician with training but no experience is about $15,000. Those with some experience earn between $21,000 and $31,500. Senior technicians earn between $33,000 and $54,000 a year. An optics technician working in one of the more select fields of optics such as research and development for NASA may earn more than $100,000.

what is the job outlook?

Job opportunities for optics technicians are expected to increase as fast as the average for all occupations through 2005. Demand for technicians is tied directly to the demand for corrective lenses. However, the greatest need for optics technicians will come from vacancies due to technicians leaving the field of optics.

The trend is toward more Americans wearing glasses. This demographic phase is due to an ever-increasing population and a larger number of individuals middle-aged and older. Typically, middle-aged and older adults are the primary users of corrective lenses. The more people of the age likely to need corrective lenses, the greater the need for optics technicians to fabricate corrective lenses.

Another factor is the increased acceptance of eyeglasses among the public. More people realize the importance and necessity for eye care. In addition, eyewear is becoming more of a fashion item. Individuals are purchasing more than one pair of eyeglasses to have different styles for different occasions; some are even purchasing nonprescription eyeglasses purely for fashion.

how do I learn more?

professional organizations

Following are organizations that provide information on optics technician careers, accredited schools, and employers.

American Optometric Association
243 North Lindbergh
St. Louis, MO 63141
TEL: 314-991-4100
WEBSITE: http://www.aoanet.org/aoanet

American Precision Optics Manufacturers
University of Rochester
CPU Box 276386
Rochester, NY 14627-6386
TEL: 716-275-2753
WEBSITE: http://www.opticam.rochester.edu

Junior Engineering Technical Society
1420 King Street, Suite 405
Alexandria, VA 22314
TEL: 703-548-5387
WEBSITE: http://www.asee.org/jets

National Association of Vision Professionals
c/o Prevention of Blindness Society
1775 Church Street, NW
Washington, DC 20036
TEL: 202-234-1010

Optical Society of America
2010 Massachusetts Avenue, NW
Washington, DC 20036
TEL: 202-223-8130
WEBSITE: http://www.osa.org

The International Society for Optical Engineering (SPIE)
PO Box 10
1000 20th Street
Bellingham, WA 98227-0010
TEL: 206-676-3290

bibliography

Following is a sampling of materials relating to the professional concerns and development of optics technicians.

Books

Aherns, Kathleen M. *Opportunities in Eye Care Careers.* Lincolnwood, IL: VGM Career Horizons, 1994.

Brooks, Clifford W. *Essentials for Ophthalmic Lens Work.* Newton, MA: Butterworth-Heinemann, 1983.

Brooks, Clifford W. *Lens Surfacing Handbook.* Newton, MA: Butterworth-Heinemann, 1992.

Brooks, Clifford W. *Understanding Lens Surfacing Laboratory Exercises: a Laboratory Manual in Lens Surfacing.* Newton, MA: Butterworth-Heinemann, 1995.

Periodicals

Eyecare Business. Monthly. Viscom Publications, 50 Washington Street, Norwalk, CT 06854, 203-838-9100.

optometrist

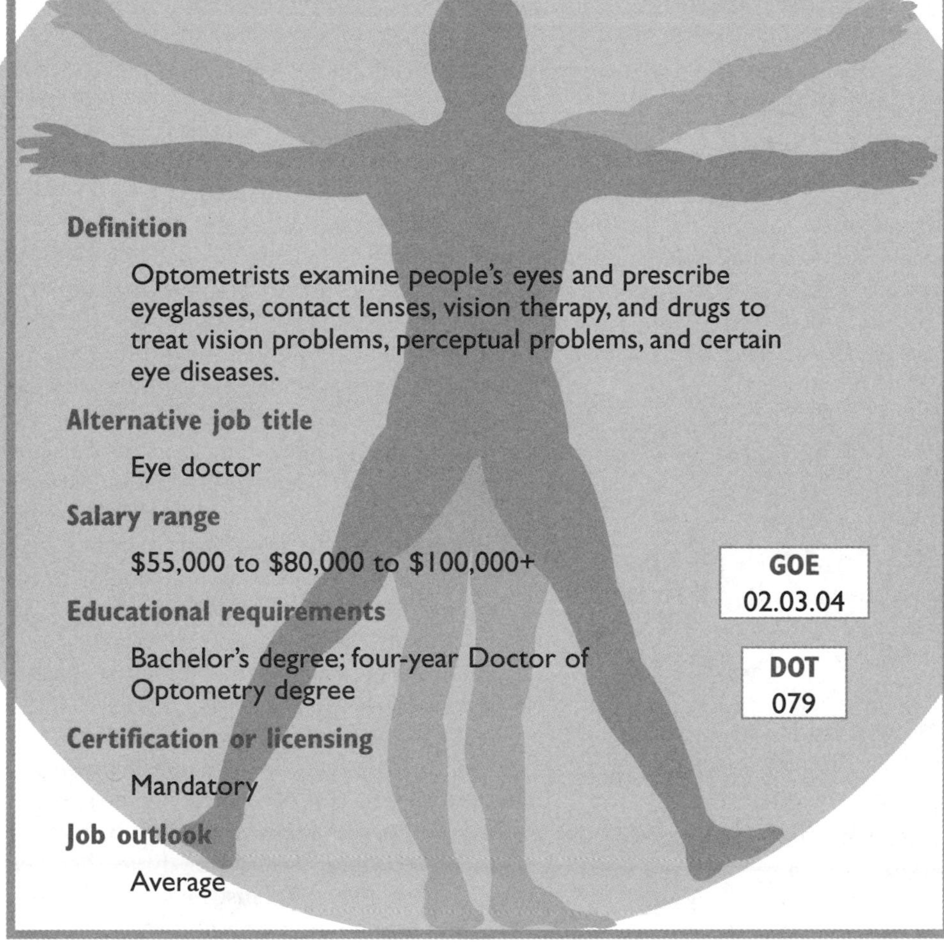

Definition

Optometrists examine people's eyes and prescribe eyeglasses, contact lenses, vision therapy, and drugs to treat vision problems, perceptual problems, and certain eye diseases.

Alternative job title

Eye doctor

Salary range

$55,000 to $80,000 to $100,000+

Educational requirements

Bachelor's degree; four-year Doctor of Optometry degree

Certification or licensing

Mandatory

Job outlook

Average

GOE
02.03.04

DOT
079

High School Subjects

Biology
Business and accounting
Mathematics
Physiology
Visual and dramatic arts

Personal Interests

Health
Helping people
Sports

Her eyes were fixed on the floor, and her head was tucked firmly against her chest. The little girl stood quietly in the pediatric head-trauma unit. Months ago, she'd been hit by a car. Since then, she hadn't raised her head.

A rehabilitation therapist stood beside her. When he saw Deborah Zelinsky, an optometrist familiar with the girl's case, he waved her over. "Hi Deb," the therapist said. He shook his head. "Still no change. We don't know if she can't raise her head or if she won't."

Deborah knelt before the girl. "Hi, Rebecca. You remember me, don't you? I'm the eye doctor lady." Deborah opened a case and took out a pair of eyeglasses. "Would you like to try these on? They're special for you."

The girl's eyes closed as Deborah fitted the glasses. "Open your eyes now, Rebecca," Deborah said gently. "It's okay."

Rebecca opened her eyes. Instantly, her head popped up. Excited, the therapist asked, "But what did you do? We've been trying to get her head up for months!"

Deborah nodded. "These glasses make things appear closer. All of a sudden the floor came rushing up at her, so she lifted her head."

Deborah smiled at Rebecca. And Rebecca, her head raised high now, smiled too.

what does an optometrist do?

More than half of the people in the United States wear glasses or contact lenses. Even if you do not wear glasses now, there is a good chance that you will require some kind of visual assistance as you get older. The health care professionals on the front lines of vision care are optometrists. *Optometrists* examine the eyes for visual ability, including depth perception, peripheral (side) vision, the ability to focus and coordinate the eyes, and the ability to see color. Optometrists use a variety of tests and instruments to examine the retina, the cornea, and other parts of the eye. During a visit to an optometrist, your eyes will be checked for their overall health.

Many people confuse a vision screening, such as one receives at school or when applying for a driver's license, with a vision examination. But unlike vision screenings, vision examinations are necessary for the health of the eyes. During an examination, an optometrist will look for conditions, including glaucoma, macular degeneration, and cataracts, that directly affect vision. An eye examination can also reveal health conditions, including diabetes and high blood pressure, that can threaten the overall health of a person.

Upon determining that a person's eyesight needs a corrective aid, an optometrist will prescribe eyeglasses or contact lenses. Often, the optometrist will then provide the patient with the glasses or contact lenses, and make certain that they fit properly. An optometrist may also prescribe medications to treat certain conditions of the eyes. When an optometrist's examination reveals the presence of a disease of the eyes or some other serious disorder, the patient will be referred to an *ophthalmologist,* a physician holding a medical degree specializing in diseases of the eye and in surgery.

Optometrists have other duties besides caring for patients. Because most optometrists work as independent practitioners, that is, they own their own offices, they are responsible for running the offices and hiring the appropriate personnel. Other optometrists work in group practices or as part of eye-wear franchises, where these responsibilities are shared.

Increasingly, optometry is concerned not only with clear vision, but also with the effects of vision on people's lives. *Developmental optometrists* provide vision therapy to people who have suffered eye injuries and to people who have such conditions as amblyopia (lazy eye) and strabismus (crossed-eyes). Developmental optometrists also provide vision therapy to people who have learning disorders and other types of disorders that may be related to perception or vision. Dyslexia and attention deficit disorder, which both adversely affect

lingo to learn

Amblyopia (lazy eye) A partial loss of vision commonly resulting from crossed-eyes. It may also result from other factors, including exposure to certain toxins.

Astigmatism An irregularity in the shape of the cornea that often causes blurred vision.

Attention deficit disorder A behavioral disorder of children that is characterized by a short attention span. It is sometimes related to vision problems.

Cataract A clouding of part or all of the lens of the eye that causes blurred or distorted vision.

Conjunctiva A mucous membrane that lines the inner surface of the eyelid and covers the white part of the eye.

Conjunctivitis (pink eye) An inflammation of the conjunctiva.

Cornea The transparent covering at the front of the eye.

Dyslexia A learning disorder in which visual signals are improperly processed by the brain.

the ability to learn, may be treated with vision therapy. In some cases, vision therapy eliminates the need for glasses. A developmental optometrist often works with other health care professionals, including neurologists, physical and occupational therapists, psychologists, and learning specialists.

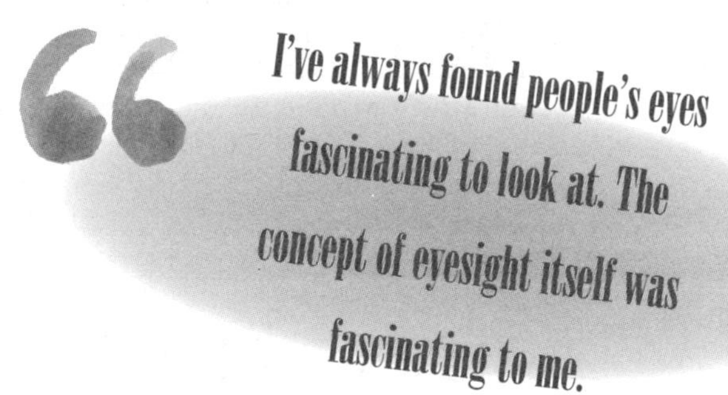

what is it like to be an optometrist?

Deborah Zelinsky has been an optometrist for twelve years. She has worked as a developmental optometrist for ten of those years. Deborah operates her own practice, called "The Mind-Eye Connection." Her practice is located in an office attached to her home in Northfield, Illinois. Deborah's interest in optometry began when she was young. "I've had a fascination with people's eyes since I was a tiny kid," she says. "I've always found people's eyes fascinating to look at. The concept of eyesight itself was fascinating to me." An experience with vision difficulties helped reinforce Deborah's choice of career. "All of a sudden, when I was eighteen or nineteen, I started seeing double," she says, "and no one could figure out why. Finally, they fitted me with bifocals, and the double vision went away."

As an independent practitioner, Deborah enjoys the freedom to set her own schedule. Generally, she sees patients four days a week, and she reserves one day a week for writing reports and pursuing her own research activities. A typical day for Deborah begins at 7:30 AM, when she reviews patient records and conducts consultations with other health care professionals over the telephone. "That part of my day usually lasts until 9:00 AM," Deborah says. "I don't start seeing patients until 10:30." Deborah is usually finished seeing patients by 5:30 PM, but one day each week she stays open until 9:00 PM to accommodate her patients' schedules.

An optometrist may see twenty or more patients each day. Each examination generally takes about twenty minutes. "But a visit with me can take one to two hours," Deborah says. "I really get involved in the patient's life. And I usually team up with other therapists involved in the patient's life and well-being."

In addition to the typical optometrist's equipment, such as lenses and prisms to measure vision, Deborah uses a variety of other instruments, such as 3-D glasses. "But my most important piece of equipment is my own brain," she says. "I develop tests and activities that go beyond the usual perception tasks, like color or depth perception. I'll test the patient's eyes in motion, because that's how we really use them. So my tests will measure things like focusing, scanning, and searching. I may use lenses that will make things seem bigger or smaller, or closer or farther, and even lenses to make the patient walk funny or hear differently. That way I can measure how the patient is using his or her eyes. A patient's eyesight is only part of what I look at."

Once Deborah identifies a problem with a patient's vision, she will explain this to the patient and discuss methods of alleviating the problem. "I might prescribe glasses, but not always," says Deborah. "When I do, they're usually part of a program of therapy exercises to help the patient learn how to better use his or her eyes. My goal is to remediate, prevent, or correct the vision problem. Many problems can be corrected completely."

Many of Deborah's patients are young children. "It's about fifty-fifty, between children and adults. I see infants sometimes. I see kids with reading problems and attention deficit disorder. I work with a lot of adults who are legally blind, and with people who have motion sickness. A lot of adults have vision or perception problems, like dyslexia, that were never diagnosed when they were young. Many of my patients are quite complicated. They may have other health problems. They may be on medications. My patients usually require hours of time and effort. It's not like general optometry at all."

Deborah's fascination with eyes has led her into research activities. "I've done some neurological research—examining vision's link with other disciplines. It's interesting to see the connection with my patients. Right now, another doctor and I are studying the various disciplines to examine the relationship between healing and vision.

have I got what it takes to be an optometrist?

A career as an optometrist offers a great deal more freedom than many other professions. "I can set my own hours," Deborah says. "And I get a chance to travel when I'm attending seminars and conventions." But in order to be successful, an optometrist must have a great deal of self-discipline and self-motivation. Knowledge of business and accounting practices is also very helpful for the independent practitioner.

more lingo to learn

Glaucoma A disease caused by the buildup of internal pressure in the fluid of the eye.

Hyperopia (farsightedness) The inability to focus on objects close by.

Iris The colored portion of the eye that opens and closes the pupil to control how much light enters the eye.

Macular degeneration An eye condition related to aging in which the portion of the retina called the macula degenerates.

Myopia (nearsightedness) The inability to see things clearly at a distance.

Prebyopia An eye condition related to aging in which the lens loses flexibility, making near vision difficult.

Strabismus (crossed-eyes) An eye disorder in which an eye is turned (or both eyes are turned) in, out, up, or down.

Optometrists should have a genuine interest in helping people, and they should be able to work well with others—both with their patients and with other vision and health professionals. Those considering careers in developmental optometry should recognize that they will often be working with people who are under stress and who have a variety of health problems. "But I can't think of any profession more fun," Deborah says. "In a way, I'm at play all day long. I look at this as a lucrative hobby. In fact, most optometrists never retire."

Working as an optometrist has proved very rewarding for Deborah. "You get the chance to help people solve problems that no one else has been able to solve. Like that little girl who wouldn't raise her head. I gave her glasses, but her problem wasn't her vision. It was her perception of what she saw. After her car accident, the signals between her eyes and her brain were mixed up. When I put the glasses on her, the floor seemed to come rushing up at her. As a response, she lifted her head. We're still discovering how intricate the relationship is between our bodies and our perception. It's nonstop new information."

Being an independent practitioner is challenging. "Running your own business gives you the freedom to choose your own future," Deborah says, "but it can be difficult. I really wish I had taken business or accounting classes in school." Opening one's own practice can be expensive, especially in purchasing equipment. Many optometrists, like Deborah, operate their offices in their own homes. "But my office and my personal space are entirely separate. In fact, the office is the largest part of my home. However, one of my long-term goals is to have a family, and having an office in my home means I'll have more time to spend with them."

how do I become an optometrist?

education

High School

A high-school student interested in pursuing a career in optometry should follow a college preparatory schedule, with an emphasis on math and science. "I was a math major. I took way more math than what was required," Deborah says. "I wish I had taken more biology classes. Microbiology would have been interesting to take." Because optometrists typically run their own businesses, it would be of benefit to the student to gain a background in business and accounting. "At school, they taught us everything about being an optometrist and nothing about running a business," Deborah says, "but that should be a requirement, too."

While it is difficult to gain practical experience in optometry, high school students can pursue certain activities that provide insight into how vision and perception work. "I've always juggled," Deborah says, "which helped me develop hand-eye coordination and gave me an awareness of 3-D space." Students can gain valuable experience working and communicating with others by finding volunteer work or part-time work at hospitals and other health care facilities. "I lived with my grandmother, which helped me understand the viewpoints of my elderly patients. I'd recommend that students try to volunteer at retirement homes for that," Deborah says.

Postsecondary Training

In order to become an optometrist, a student must first complete at least three years of undergraduate work, and then four years in a certified college or school of optometry. In addition to a general liberal arts education, a prospective optometrist should follow a course of study that includes mathematics, physics, biology, and chemistry. In order to apply for a graduate degree program in optometry, a student must take the Optometry Admission Test.

Postgraduate studies will include laboratory, classroom, and clinical work. Students can expect to study pharmacology (the science of drugs), systemic disease (disease that affects the whole body), ocular pathology (the study of eye diseases), and biochemistry (the study of the chemical processes of organisms). Practical courses include theoretical and ophthalmic optics, which discuss lenses and the use of ophthalmic glass and plastics. Students will learn how to adapt, prescribe, and fit glasses and contact lenses. They will also learn about vision therapy. The third and fourth years of an optometric degree program include clinical practice, in which students diagnose and treat the eye disorders of patients.

To be a successful optometrist, you should:

- Be interested in helping people
- Be able to work well with people
- Have good vision and coordination and some mechanical aptitude
- Be understanding of a patient's needs, and be tactful when working with patients
- Have self-discipline and the ability to motivate yourself
- Have a background in business and accounting

certification or licensing

Every state requires that optometrists be licensed in order to practice. In order to receive a license, a person must have a Degree of Optometry (OD) and pass written and practical tests. After being licensed, optometrists are required to continue their education. They must annually fulfill a specified number of course hours. Optometrists must also must pass periodic tests administered by the National Board of Examiners in Optometry and by state and regional review boards.

Optometrists interested in the field of developmental optometry can apply for fellowships in visual development. In order to be certified as a developmental optometrist, an optometrist must have at least three years of professional clinical practice, fulfill a specified number of course hours in developmental optometry, and pass an oral and written examination. Developmental optometrists must also continue their education to keep abreast of advances in the field.

who will hire me?

Deborah's first job as an optometrist was with a contact lens group in Florida. "I was fresh out of school, and I just went in for an interview," she says. "After a year of working there, I went to work for a pediatric practice. Working with kids led me into developmental optometry." Joining a group practice is a good way for a newly licensed optometrist to start out in this career, because purchasing the equipment and setting up an office can be expensive. Optometrists interested in starting up independent practices may have the best luck in rural areas, where there are generally fewer optometrists than in urban areas. Banks and other lenders are a good source for financial backing when starting up a new practice.

Most colleges and schools of optometry offer job placement assistance and will help new optometrists locate potential partnerships. They may also help new optometrists find different locations where optometrists are needed. The American Optometric Association is a professional organization that provides placement services and information on optometrists seeking to hire associates. Working as an associate with an established optometrist is a good way to develop the experience and financial resources needed before setting up an independent practice. An optometrist who starts out as an associate with an established practice may choose to eventually join the practice as a partner. Becoming a partner generally means agreeing to pay a certain amount of money to buy into the practice, and then sharing both the costs of running the business and any profits the practice produces.

An optometrist may find employment as part of a health maintenance organization (HMO), or as a member of a hospital's staff. Some optometrists join the military services or work for other government organizations, such as the Department of Veterans Affairs. After receiving a doctorate degree, an optometrist can then concentrate on research or teaching, if he or she chooses to do so.

FYI

Seeing is believing

Vision depends on light. We see objects because they reflect light in different ways. This reflected light enters the eye through the pupil, which is opened and closed by the iris to control the amount of light that reaches the lens. The lens refracts, or bends, the light onto the retina, which is a layer of nerve cells at the back of the eye. The nerve cells in the retina send signals along the optic nerve to the visual center of the brain, which processes this information and interprets what we see.

where can I go from here?

Advancement in the field of optometry typically means setting up one's own practice or becoming a partner with others in a practice. An optometrist then builds up his or her practice by adding patients. An optometrist may also decide to specialize in a particular area of optometry. Specialization generally requires the optometrist to complete an additional one-year clinical residency program in his or her chosen area of specialization. Specialties include pediatric optometry, geriatric optometry, developmental optometry, hospital-based optometry, and ocular disease. Some optometrists continue their education to receive doctorate degrees in visual science, physiological optics or neurophysiology. Some receive doctorate degrees in other areas, such as public health, health administration, health education, or health communication and information.

what are the salary ranges?

The average starting salary for a newly licensed optometrist is $55,000 per year, according to the American Optometric Association. The average income for all optometrists is about $80,000 per year. An optometrist's income varies according to whether the optometrist owns his or her own practice or works as part of a group or partnership. Income also varies depending on how many patients the optometrist treats. An established optometrist with a busy practice can earn much more than the average salary. Optometry specialists, such as developmental optometrists, also have the potential for higher earnings. In addition, an optometrist's location will affect earnings. Optometrists in rural areas generally earn less than optometrists in urban or suburban areas. Optometrists employed as salaried personnel by the government, by clinics, or by optometry groups often have higher initial earnings than optometrists who set up their own practices. However, as independent practitioners become established, their earnings typically surpass those of salaried personnel. Optometrists who are partners in established optometry groups or practices are generally considered to have the highest earning potential.

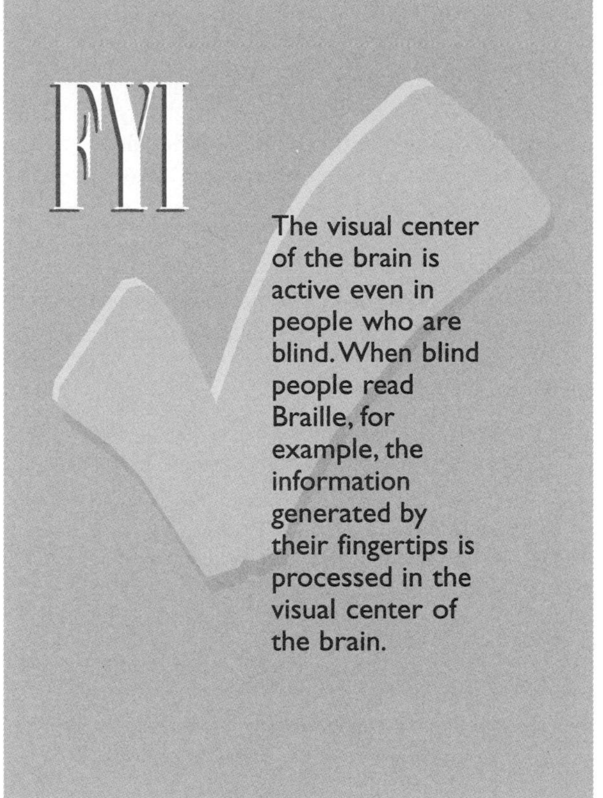

The visual center of the brain is active even in people who are blind. When blind people read Braille, for example, the information generated by their fingertips is processed in the visual center of the brain.

what is the job outlook?

Jobs in optometry are expected to grow about as fast as the average for all occupations through 2005. One factor that will affect the need for optometrists is the aging of the population. Elderly patients require many optometric services, such as treatment for presbyopia, glaucoma, cataracts, and macular degeneration. Other areas of optometry, particularly developmental optometry, are expected to grow in importance as researchers and clinicians explore the connection between vision and such disorders as dyslexia and attention deficit disorder.

Optometrists tend to continue working long after the typical retirement age. Therefore, replacement opportunities in this career are fewer than in many other health care careers. Openings for optometrists are created as optometrists retire or as optometrists leave clinic or group practices to set up their own independent practices. Two other factors that contribute to the relative scarcity of replacement opportunities are advancements in optometric equipment technology and the hiring of optometric assistants. Both factors allow current optometrists to see growing numbers of patients—thereby limiting the need for new optometrists.

how do I learn more?

professional associations

Following are organizations that provide information on optometry careers, accredited schools, and employers.

American Optometric Association
243 N. Lindbergh Blvd.
St. Louis, MO 63141
TEL: 314-991-4100
WEBSITE: http://www.aoanet.org/aoanet

Association of Schools and Colleges of Optometry
6110 Executive Boulevard
Suite 690
Rockville, MD 20852
TEL: 301-231-5944
WEBSITE: http://www.opted.org

bibliography

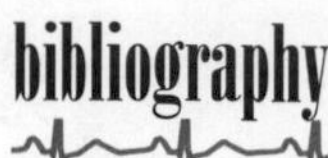

Following is a sampling of materials related to the professional concerns and development of optometrists.

Books

Aherns, Kathleen M. *Opportunities in Eye Care Careers*. Lincolnwood, IL: VGM Career Horizons, 1994.

Grosvenor, Theodore. *Primary Care Optometry*, 3rd edition. Newton, MA: Butterworth-Heinemann, 1996.

Kitchell, Frank M. *Optometry*. Lincolnwood, IL: VGM Career Horizons, 1993.

Periodicals

High Performance Optometry. Monthly. Summaries of medical and optometry journal articles about diagnosing and treating ocular disease and vision disorders. Anadem Publishing, Inc., 3620 N. High Street, Columbus, OH 43214, 514-262-2539.

Optometry and Vision Science. Monthly. Presents research and clinical findings in optometry. American Academy of Optometry, Williams & Wilkins, 428 E. Preston Street, Baltimore, MD 21202, 410-528-4000, 800-638-6423.

Optometry Clinics. Quarterly. Each issue devoted to a single topic with articles written on methods of diagnosis and management as well as practical information on latest techniques and pertinent legal issues. Appleton & Lange, Journal Division, 25 Van Zant Street, Box 5630, Norwalk, CT 06856, 203-838-4400.

orthodontist

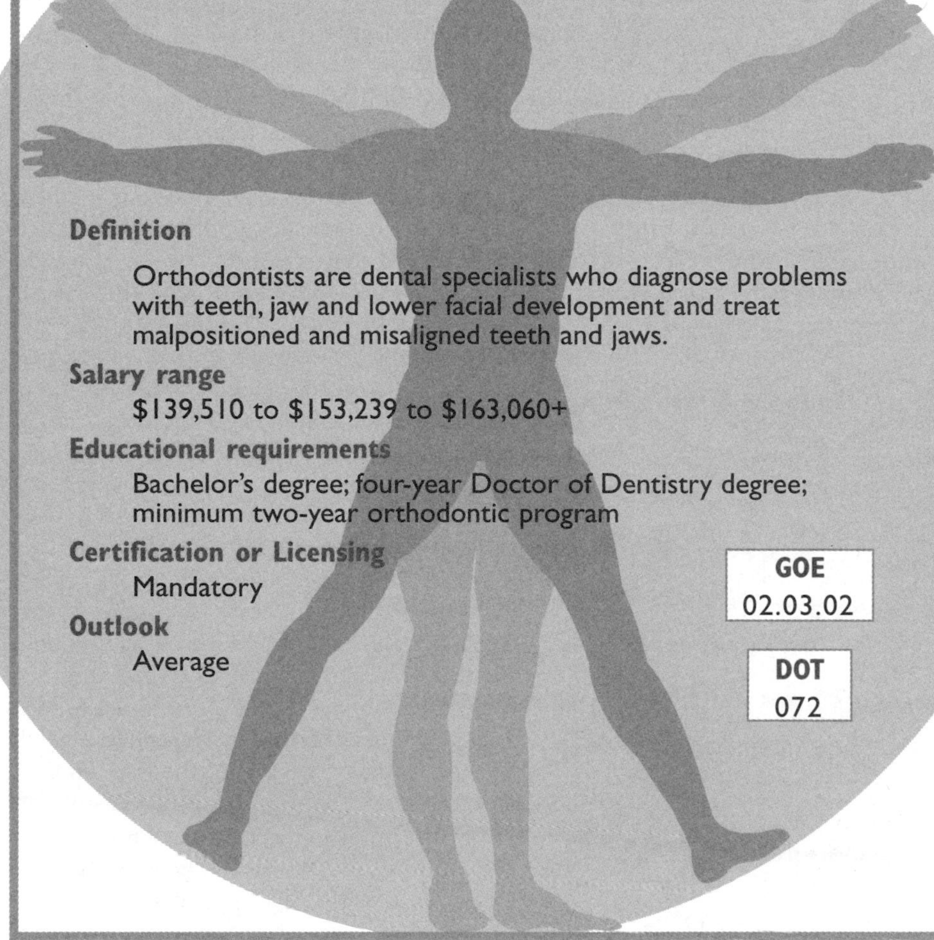

Definition

Orthodontists are dental specialists who diagnose problems with teeth, jaw and lower facial development and treat malpositioned and misaligned teeth and jaws.

Salary range

$139,510 to $153,239 to $163,060+

Educational requirements

Bachelor's degree; four-year Doctor of Dentistry degree; minimum two-year orthodontic program

Certification or Licensing

Mandatory

Outlook

Average

GOE
02.03.02

DOT
072

High School Subjects

Science
Math
Business,
Accounting,
English

Personal Interests

Exercising
Reading

"I hate my teeth," 12-year-old Kaela said loudly as she plopped onto the dental chair of Chris Carpenter, DDS, MS, PC. Her mother sat down next to her daughter and said "That's why we're seeing an orthodontist, Kaela."

"Mom, I look like Dracula," Kaela said, pointing to her teeth.

"If you've got fangs, I'd better watch my fingers in there," Dr. Carpenter joked as he walked into the exam room. As Kaela and her mother chuckled at the joke of the orthodontist, Dr. Carpenter noticed Kaela quickly covered her smile with her hand. She truly was embarrassed of her teeth.

Pulling up a stool, Dr. Carpenter sat across from Kaela. He looked her in the eye and said, "Kaela, you're not alone. Most people feel their smile could be improved. The wonder of orthodontics is that a patient can come here with an average smile or one that has problems and I can change it. Your smile has great potential. I can make it as beautiful as it can possibly be."

what does an orthodontist do?

"Ortho" means straight and "odont" means tooth. Thus, *orthodontists* improve smiles so that teeth look straight. Without orthodontic treatment, teeth can not only be crooked and crowded, but have unsightly gaps between them. People who could benefit from orthodontics includes those whose facial profile shows an overbite, underbite, "protruding lips" or even a "weak chin."

lingo to learn

Fixed appliance A device that is bonded or banded to a tooth or teeth.

Orthodontic appliance A device that influences the growth or position of teeth or position of bones.

Arch Describes the group of teeth and connecting bone of either the upper or lower jaw.

Orthodontic band A thin metal ring that is cemented to the tooth through which orthodontic attachments are secured.

Bonding Orthodontic attachments are affixed onto teeth by using an adhesive.

Dental cast A plaster replica of the patient's teeth used for diagnosis and appliance fabrication.

Crowding The resulting malpositioned teeth from inadequate room for teeth within an arch.

Elastics Rubber bands used with orthodontic appliances as a part of treatment.

Malocclusion A deviation in the normal relationship of teeth in occlusion (while biting).

Radiograph An image, usually recorded on film. It is sometimes called an "X ray."

Retainer Orthodontic appliance that maintains teeth position after corrective treatment.

People who have dental and facial irregularities often have what is termed "malocclusion," sometimes called a "bad bite." There is more than one reason for correcting a malocclusion. Sometimes it's cosmetic—to have an attractive smile, thereby improving self-esteem. Other times, however, it's for functional reasons. Crooked teeth can create speech problems, and they can also be more susceptible to decay as they are more difficult to keep clean.

Because the American Association of Orthodontists recommends that children first be evaluated by an orthodontist by age seven, some parents bring their children in for a developmental checkup on their own. Even children who have teeth that appear straight may have the beginnings of a jaw malformation. A malformation undetectable to the untrained eye now can develop into an unmistakable problem after a child becomes a teen. Other parents bring their children to the orthodontist at the suggestion of their child's general dentist, who may have suspected a dental or facial development that should be evaluated and monitored.

When the patient comes to the office, orthodontists take a complete medical and dental history to determine what is influencing health in general and teeth in particular. Next, the mouth is carefully examined to look for oral evidence of disease. The health of teeth is carefully evaluated. During the examination, an orthodontist acts like a "smile consultant," sizing up the size and shape of each tooth and the relationship between the teeth and the gums, the lips and the face. The patient's facial profile will be assessed for uniformity, symmetry, and proportion. At this time, a "before" photo of a patient's profile and smile may be taken for the patient's record. If treatment is performed, after it is completed photos will be taken again to show the "after" effects.

To make a diagnosis, the orthodontist needs to measure and evaluate relationships. To do this, casts are created from plaster by asking the patient to bite into a tray of impression material. The 3-D models made from the casts are mounted on hinges to re-enact the patient's teeth in biting motion. It's difficult for patients to hold their mouths open wide for long periods of time, so models of their teeth allow orthodontists to study the dynamics of the bite more easily and to take detailed measurements.

Orthodontists also use radiographic images such as X rays to reveal the status of tissues that can't be seen by the eye including problems inside the teeth and with the jaws, facial bones and tooth roots. X rays can help an orthodontist determine if crowded teeth would benefit from an orthodontic extraction. In other cases, certain jaw discrepancies are detected with radiographs and need correction with orthodontic appliances like braces or orthognathic (jaw) surgery.

Once a problem is diagnosed, orthodontists may give the patient an oral or written treatment plan. This plan includes the diagnosis, the recommended treatment specifics and cost estimate of treatment.

There are various types of orthodontic treatment, but almost all involve metal, plastic, or ceramic braces that are banded around, or bonded to, teeth. These braces are made up of brackets and wires that move teeth into, or hold them in, proper position. Moving teeth is a very slow process of adjusting braces slightly every three to six weeks. For a day or two after an orthodontic adjustment, patients say their teeth feel a little sore.

In the old days, braces were always metallic. Now braces can be white, clear or a color. In certain cases, orthodontists sometimes even can place "invisible braces"—those that are attached to the tongue side of the teeth.

Additional orthodontic appliances include headgear, a wire appliance that protrudes from the mouth and is fastened by a strap behind the head. Orthodontists use this approach to orthopedically slow the growth of the upper jaw. Rubber bands are another pulling force that, when changed daily by the patient, help move teeth into position.

There are many other types of orthodontic appliances, but an important one is the retainer—key in the orthodontic process. When orthodontists finish active treatment, often during two or more years, the patient comes in much less often for appointments or not at all. To make sure a new smile doesn't "relapse" into poor position, removable or permanent retainers are placed in patients' mouths at the conclusion of treatment. Removable retainers are worn at night, and sometimes during the day as well. They are removed when the patients eat and brush their teeth.

While private practitioners make up the majority of orthodontists, other orthodontists teach full- or part-time at universities, perform research at dental schools or for industry such as dental product manufacturers, work in the military as government employees, or for the U.S. Public Health Service.

what is it like to be an orthodontist?

Chris Carpenter has been an orthodontist for ten years. He is a private practitioner in a Denver orthodontic practice that employees a staff manager, a receptionist at the front desk, and four dental assistants. The office is open five days a week. Office hours are 7:00 AM to 4:30 PM and Dr. Carpenter works four days or thirty-four hours per week.

Each morning starts off with "a huddle" so that Dr. Carpenter and his staff can review the forty to sixty patients' treatments for the day and prepare as much as possible beforehand. The office has five treatment chairs. Patients are seated upon arrival and Dr. Carpenter then examines each patient, adjusts the wires, then dictates final instructions to the dental assistant. The dental assistant then completes the final aspects of the treatment and coordinates the next appointment information.

"I see patients about thirty-four hours a week. I take Wednesdays off, but I usually come into the office anyway to do all the other things involved with running a small business. I pay bills, manage staff members and do paperwork. I spend a considerable amount of time writing diagnosis and treatment plan letters with copies of radiographs to send to patients' general dentists," Dr. Carpenter said.

Other non-orthodontic responsibilities include working with insurance companies to obtain payment for procedures and overseeing the billing and collection of fees. To ensure the dental office is a safe place for employees and patients alike, Dr. Carpenter takes a regular evaluation of procedures and conditions in the office to be certain everything is in compliance with the federal Occupational Safety and Health Administration standards.

Staff members are in charge of taking inventory and ordering supplies, but orthodontists oversee the process.

Bookkeeping and accounting duties are another part of Dr. Carpenter's duties—not only for billing purposes but also for keeping track of the staff members' time cards, benefits, Social Security, and tax deductions, and for setting salaries and raises, as well.

On the practical side, Dr. Carpenter says that being an orthodontist means being organized and prepared to work efficiently so that a number of patients can be seen in one day. To accomplish this, Dr. Carpenter may review patient charts in the morning before the work day begins so that he can advise his staff at the morning meeting of the supplies needed throughout the day. Reviewing the charts helps Dr. Carpenter mentally pre-orient himself to each patient's needs, which helps him stay on schedule so that time isn't wasted during the day "catching up" with the status of each patient's treatment needs once they're in the dental chair.

Being a good time manager is a highly advantageous skill. At any one time during the day, Dr. Carpenter may have five people in dental chairs waiting for treatment and another five in his waiting room. This means efficiently going from one patient to another just to thread, tie and tighten wires and change bands. Dental assistants help immensely, as well. Dr. Carpenter may be interrupted to check their work, or to clip wires and bend them so rough edges don't irritate the patients' cheeks and lips.

Being an orthodontist is a physical challenge as well. Manual dexterity, tactility and strength are necessary assets. Fingers, hands, wrists and arms are in controlled motion within a small space throughout the day. There is little room for error. Keen vision and perception in three dimensions is needed to locate tiny openings and parts of only a few millimeters in diameter.

To prevent the back injuries that can plague orthodontists as they lean over patients all day, Dr. Carpenter tries to maintain a healthy body. He stretches during the day and exercises about three times a week. He participates in active outdoor activities such as biking or golfing and enjoys these activities throughout the year. During his two weeks of vacation a year, he is sure to golf as well.

Two years have passed since Kaela's first visit with Dr. Carpenter. Kaela, now fourteen years old, is sitting in the dental chair as Dr. Carpenter removes her braces.

"Take a look in the mirror at that gorgeous smile," Dr. Carpenter says with a grin.

Kaela looked in the hand mirror at her teeth without braces and got a bright, wide smile.

"Dr. Carpenter, thank you so much! " Kaela said, while practicing versions of her smile in the mirror. "Now I can smile without being embarrassed."

Not only did her smile look great, Kaela's posture seemed to have improved and she seemed more self-assured and confident when she spoke.

Patients who are like Kaela are the main reason Dr. Carpenter enjoys working as an orthodontist. "I think it is the most ideal profession that exists. All day long I have the opportunity to change people's lives by improving their smile. Patients are excited about the changes. Knowing that I did something that made a difference and made people happy is something that makes me happy to go to work every morning."

FYI

Orthodontics goes back to the ancient Phoenicians and Egyptians. Egyptian mummies have been found with copper bands around teeth. Researchers speculate that the teeth were pulled together with string made of animal gut. Modern orthodontics dates to 1900, when the Father of Orthodontics, Dr. Edward Angle, established a system for diagnosing orthodontic problems. His system is still used today.

have I got what it takes to be an orthodontist?

Dr. Carpenter was thoroughly trained in dental school and during his orthodontic postgraduate program he obtained a master's degree in orthodontics.

To keep abreast of advancements in orthodontics, Dr. Carpenter takes continuing education courses every year. Although some are required to maintain his dental license, others are taken because he's interested in providing the latest techniques. While most are for better skills, some are taken to improve the way he manages his practice. Business skills help keep the practice running efficiently for maximized profitability while providing highest quality results.

Says Dr. Carpenter: "The business skills and the 'people skills' are almost as important as the orthodontic treatment. Knowing how to run a business while having empathy and a genuine ability to interact well with people is critical. My success is directly related to how well I treat my patients. They need to know I truly care about their concerns."

Being a good communicator while under time pressure is critical. One moment Dr. Carpenter may be discussing the need for good cooperation with tooth brushing with an eight-year-old patient while another patient's parents are awaiting a consult on a new treatment plan while an insurance company representative is on hold about a claim misunderstanding.

"You need to be an effective communicator because you don't have the luxury of a lot of time to make your point," he added.

Always being able to control your temperament is necessary. "Having all the responsibilities of owning a practice and being your own boss is a lot of pressure. So you don't set yourself up for failure, there's no room for inflexible, perfectionist tendencies. Instead, you need to accept the fact that things will go wrong. You need to have confidence and learn from failure, whether it be with a patient, staff member, or the parent of a patient."

To be a successful orthodontist, you should

- Have dexterity for detail work
- Be self-motivated
- Have excellent eye-hand coordination
- Be able to perceive in three dimensions
- Have an "artistic eye," and be able to judge symmetry
- Maintain excellent people skills

how do I become an orthodontist?

education

High School

High school students interested in becoming an orthodontist should begin preparing for this career with a course load that emphasizes, but is not restricted to, math and science subjects. Courses such as algebra, calculus, chemistry, physics, trigonometry, biology and health are all solid baseline courses for college preparation.

Postsecondary Training

Getting admitted to dental school requires that students first complete three to four years of undergraduate college education. Maintaining a high grade point average is important while in college. Because gaining acceptance into a dental school is fiercely competitive, strong grade point averages are necessary. While a bachelor's degree is not strictly required, it is a standard that significantly heightens an applicant's chances of being admitted to a dental school.

Recommended college courses are similar to those suggested in high school. Often, students who are planning on becoming orthodontists work toward a bachelor of science degree in biology. This may involve taking math courses such as algebra, calculus, trigonometry and geometry. Science courses may include biology, anatomy, physiology, anthropology, zoology, botany, and microbiology.

On the practical side, business classes such as marketing, economics, accounting, management, and finance prepare future orthodontists for owning and operating a business.

Liberal arts courses such as psychology, sociology, English, and drama may also help a future orthodontist to become more comfortable in communicating with people. These types of classes prepare students to understand and relate to patient motivation and complex personalities.

A discussion with your college advisor, a university version of a secondary school guidance counselor, can help to identify required and suggested classes best suited for obtaining your degree and added skills for this career choice.

College students must score well on the Dental Admissions Test (DAT) before being admitted into a dental program. Doing well on the DAT helps dental schools determine whether or not students will succeed in dental school. Dental school courses are made up of advanced science, clinical and laboratory technique coursework. During the last two years of dental school, clinical treatment is emphasized and students begin supervised treatment of patients at university dental clinics. Graduates receive a Doctor of Dental Surgery (DDS) or Doctor of Dental Medicine (DMD) degree.

Formal education would end here if a student was planning on working as a general dentist. To be an orthodontist, however, takes more schooling. In fact, postgraduate programs, which are accredited by the American Dental Association Commission on Dental Accreditation, may last from two to three years.

Gaining acceptance to a postgraduate program in orthodontics is competitive. Therefore, it is critical that students maintain a high grade point average during dental school.

certification or licensing

Before newly minted dentists are allowed to practice, they must first pass a licensing examination in the state in which they are planning to practice. This test may include working on a patient. For those who wish to be orthodontic specialists, a two- or three-year postgraduate program that usually involves getting a master's degree is needed. In some states, they must also pass a specialty licensing examination.

Board certification independent of, and above and beyond that which is required for licensing, is also available through the American Board of Orthodontists (ABO). To achieve ABO diplomate status, orthodontists must file an application with the ABO, be interviewed and approved as a candidate, pass written and oral examinations, and provide written orthodontic case histories. It may take eight to ten years to gain ABO diplomate status. ABO diplomate status is sought voluntarily by orthodontists to show they've mastered excellence in their abilities.

Recalls orthodontist Dr. Carpenter: "After about two years of dental school, I became interested in orthodontics after I took a class on the subject. Following dental school, I attended a thirty-month residency in orthodontics. All in all, I went to school for ten years after high school—a big commitment, but I'd do it again if I had to. That's how much I enjoy the profession."

Orthodontists, as well as all dentists, also must plan on taking courses after they have established a practice. These continuing education courses are taken to maintain a dental license. Other educational activities include attending workshops and seminars, reading professional journals, and participating in study clubs. This helps a practicing orthodontist to acquire the most up-to-date skills and knowledge of the best materials to use.

> Now I can smile without being embarrassed.

scholarships and grants

Scholarships and grants are often available from individual institutions, state agencies, and special-interest organizations. The book *Dollars for College: Medicine, Dentistry, and Related Fields* by Ferguson Publishing Company is an excellent source for this information.Many students finance their medical education through the Armed Forces Health Professions Scholarship Program. Each branch of the military participates in this program, paying students' tuitions in exchange for military service. Contact your local recruiting office for more information on this program.

The National Health Service Corps Scholarship Program also provides money for students in return for service. Another source for financial aid, scholarship, and grant information is the Association of American Medical Colleges. Remember to request information early for eligibility, application requirements, and deadlines.

Association of American Medical Colleges
2450 N Street, NW
Washington, DC 20037
TEL: 202-828-0400
WEBSITE: http://www.aamc.org
Specific information on financial aid programs can be found at:
WEBSITE: http://www.aamc.org/stuapps/finaid

Ferguson Publishing Company
200 West Madison, Suite 300
Chicago, IL 60606
TEL: 312-580-5480

National Health Services Corps Scholarship Program
U.S. Public Health Service
1010 Wayne Avenue, Suite 240
Silver Spring, MD 20910
TEL: 800-638-0824

who will hire me?

According to the American Association of Orthodontists (AAO), there are more than 8,500 orthodontists in the United States, and more than 90 per cent of them are in private practice. There are different types of private practices, such as solo or group. Orthodontists may own their own practice or may work as an associate or a partner in another orthodontist's practice. Information about private practice opportunities is available in the *American Journal of Orthodontics and Dentofacial Orthopedics,* the scientific journal of the AAO. For those not joining an existing practice, the resources required to set up a private practice are considerable—oftentimes a bank-financed endeavor. Some orthodontists work in hospitals and dental clinics.

Other opportunities for orthodontists include teaching at university dental schools, either full-time or part-time, while also maintaining a practice. Part-time instructors sometimes are not paid, however, because there is prestige associated with university teaching and orthodontists sometimes volunteer to teach a class to build their careers. This type of activity helps capture credibility for orthodontists who plan on having a speaking career.

Some orthodontists also work in a dental school environment but choose to do research. Others perform research while testing new materials and procedures and writing about them for industry. Researchers may test new orthodontic materials or techniques by working on anything from model mouths to animals. Dogs with bad bites have even been known to get braces!

Combining one or more aspects of clinical practice, teaching, and research, some orthodontists are employed by the Federal Dental Health Services. These orthodontists may be positioned all over the country via the Air Force, Navy, Army, Veterans Hospitals, and Public Health Services. Those who work in the Pubic Health Service work with underserved populations, typically in low-income communities.

where can I go from here?

The primary career path for most orthodontists in private practice is to build a reputation for the practice with the general dentists in the surrounding community who refer the majority of the orthodontist's patients. Orthodontists who can effectively communicate with a patient's general dentist and facilitate easy coordination of treatment are more likely to be trusted by the general dentist. These practitioners are more apt to build their practices.

Involvement in orthodontic associations and study clubs may lead orthodontists to active participation in organized dental events. Some orthodontists even become officers and committee chairs of their professional associations.

After many years of working, orthodontists may slow down to part-time status or retire and teach during their retirement years.

what are the salary ranges?

The American Association of Orthodontists says that orthodontists under age thirty often have a starting salary that's double the income of other college graduates.

According to the American Dental Association Survey Center, the mean average net salary of orthodontists who are under forty is about $140,000. That's the lower end of the salary range. The mid-range salary is the mean average income; and the average annual income from the primary private practice for all orthodontists is $153,000. On the upper end of the range, orthodontists who work more than thirty-two hours a week work an average of 38.9 hours and make $163,000. (Interestingly, the average length of an orthodontic appointment is fifteen minutes; and the average number of patients treated each week by orthodontists is 147.) The average net income for orthodontists over forty years old is $ 157,000.

The location of an orthodontist's private practice may play a role in determining income, as well. Dentists in Pacific, Mountain, Northern and New England states typically have higher incomes than those in Southern states. Orthodontists in affluent and growing suburbs may have greater income potential than those in all but economically thriving parts of urban or rural areas. Specialists' incomes are also affected by how many other specialists in their area of expertise are working in the community. In an area with few or no other orthodontists, an orthodontic practice may have an edge and find it easier to obtain referrals.

what is the job outlook?

The demand for orthodontists is good to strong and is likely to remain this way. Because the motivation to receive orthodontic treatment can be cosmetic in nature, and our society values physical attractiveness, desire for these services should continue to be strong. However, because orthodontics is largely an optional procedure, problems with national economic health could impact it. Patients or their families without solid income are not likely to pursue or follow through with orthodontic treatment. However, to make the service more accessible, many offices provide financing, accept charge cards or refer the patient to financing sources where instant over-the-phone approval may be obtainable.

how do I learn more?

professional associations

Following are organizations that provide information on dental careers, accredited schools, and employees.

American Dental Association
211 E. Chicago Avenue
Chicago, IL 60611
TEL: 312-440-2500
WEBSITE: http://www.ada.org

American Association of Orthodontists
401 N. Lindbergh Boulevard
St. Louis, MO 63141-7816
TEL: 314-993-1700
WEBSITE: http://www.aaortho.org

bibliography

Following is a sampling of materials related to the professional concerns and development of orthodontists.

Books

Houston, W. J. B., and others. A *Textbook of Orthodontics,* 2nd edition. Newton, MA: Butterworth-Heinemann, 1992.

Mitchell, Laura. *An Introduction to Orthodontics*. New York, NY: Oxford University Press, 1996.

Periodicals

Functional Orthodontist: a Journal of Functional Jaw Orthopedics. Bimonthly. The AAFO, 106 S. Kent Street, Winchester, VA 22601, 703-662-2200.

I A O Straight Talk. Monthly. Contains news and concerns of association members. International Association for Orthodontics, 1100 Lake Street, Suite 240, Oak Park, IL 60301, 708-445-0320.

Journal of Clinical Orthodontics. Monthly. J C O Inc., 1828 Pears Street, Boulder, CO 80302, FAX 303-443-9355.

Seminars in Orthodontics. Quarterly. Provides authoritative and up-to-date coverage of innovative techniques, new instruments, and other products; and new uses for existing material. W.B. Saunders Co., Curtis Center, 3rd Floor, Independence Square West, Philadelphia, PA 19106, 215-238-7800.

orthopaedic surgeon

Definition

Surgeons who diagnose and treat patients with musculoskeletal disorders that are present at birth or develop later.

Alternative job titles

Orthopedic surgeon
Orthopedist

Salary range

$31,000 to $140,000 to $200,000+

Educational requirements

Bachelor's degree, M.D., minimum five years postgraduate study, optional fellowships in subspecialties

Certification or Licensing

Certification is highly recommended; licensing is mandatory

Outlook

Much faster than average

GOE
02.03.01

DOT
070

High School Subjects

Biology
Chemistry
Computer science
English
Mathematics
Physics

Personal Interests

Helping people
Problem solving
Using technology and tools
Working with your hands

"Thank you," Maria Modarelli says in Italian as she is helped into the doctor's office by the receptionist. She settles deep into the chair she has just been shown and smiles a weak smile. Maria looks around at the certificates and diplomas that decorate the walls of the Brooklyn, New York, office. Absentmindedly, she taps the rubber-capped end of her thick, polished cane against the leg of the chair. A few moments go by and she reaches down to pull a large, ornate gold watch out from the black folds of her coat. She squints at it and sighs and slips the watch back inside. Even as she sits here her left knee aches with pain.

The door to the reception area opens and the orthopaedic surgeon enters. He smiles broadly and kneels beside Maria. "Good day, Mrs. Modarelli," he says in Italian. "Where does it hurt?"

She sighs and touches her left leg. The orthopaedist, Dr. Edward Toriello, gets up and moves another chair in the room close to hers. Dr. Toriello studied medicine in Italy, and today he finds that his knowledge of Italian is an unexpected asset in dealing with a patient. Speaking in Italian in a gentle voice, he begins to tell Mrs. Modarelli how he might be able to help her with the pain in her knee. How it is possible that she might be able to move it easily again.

lingo to learn

Arthritis Inflammation of joints.

Arthroscope Fiberoptic instrument used to show the interior of a joint and to perform surgery on a joint.

Arthroscopy The process in which a joint is examined or surgery is performed using an arthroscope.

Bunion Inflammation of the bursa at the joint of the large toe.

Bursa A small, fluid-filled sac found in the area of a joint.

Bursitis Inflammation of a bursa, especially of the shoulder or elbow.

Cerebral palsy A partial or total lack of muscle control, particularly of the limbs, that results from trauma at birth or developmental defects in the brain.

Fluoroscope An instrument used for observing the internal structure of an opaque object (as the living body) by means of X rays.

Musculoskeletal Involving both the muscles and the skeleton.

Muscular dystrophy Any of a group of hereditary diseases characterized by a progressive wasting away of muscles.

Osteoporosis A condition in which bone mass decreases, causing a decrease in bone density and enlargement of spaces within the bone. This loss makes bones vulnerable to breaks and fractures. Older women are especially affected.

Scoliosis Crookedness or curvature of the spine.

what does an orthopaedic surgeon do?

Orthopaedic surgeons are concerned with the diagnosis, care, and treatment of patients with musculoskeletal disorders that are present at birth or develop later in life. These musculoskeletal problems include deformities, injuries, and degenerative diseases of the spine, hands, feet, knee, hip, shoulder, and elbow. Orthopaedic surgeons work to save and restore the form and function of the hands, feet, spine, and other structures.

In its early days, orthopaedics involved treating children with spine or limb deformities, but the specialty quickly expanded. The scope of orthopaedics today is immense. Orthopaedic surgeons treat a wide variety of diseases and conditions, from such problems as fractures, torn ligaments, and bunions to lower back pain, scoliosis, and ruptured discs to degenerative joint diseases, muscular dystrophy, and cerebral palsy.

Orthopaedic surgeons now treat patients of all ages. Orthopaedists may see children with such problems as bone tumors, hip dislocations, and growth abnormalities like unequal leg length. Orthopaedic surgeons who practice in sports medicine treat injuries to the athlete and are especially involved with knee surgeries and arthroscopic procedures (procedures using fiberoptic instruments). Orthopaedic surgeons also treat elderly patients who may have bone disorders, such as osteoporosis, or joint conditions, such as arthritis. Recently, advances in the surgical management of degenerative joint diseases have allowed orthopaedic surgeons to replace the diseased joint with a prosthetic device in a surgery known as total joint replacement. Similarly, fiberoptic scopes, or arthroscopes, which allow the orthopaedic surgeon to look inside a joint, have had an enormous impact on the diagnosis and surgical treatment of internal joint diseases. Other technological advances include microsurgery, which allows orthopaedic surgeons to replant limbs, and "space age" metal techniques that create better devices with which to repair damaged bones.

Orthopaedic surgeons use medicine and rehabilitative methods as well as surgery to treat their patients. Some disorders require surgery for correction, but others require a cast or brace and work with physical therapists, occupational therapists, and other members of a rehabilitation team. Whatever the prescribed method of treatment, orthopaedic surgeons often work closely with other health care professionals, either as the patient's primary care physician or as a consultant to other physicians.

Orthopaedic surgeons also have a large role in the organization and delivery of emergency care, working with other specialists in the management of complex trauma injuries, such as from a car accident.

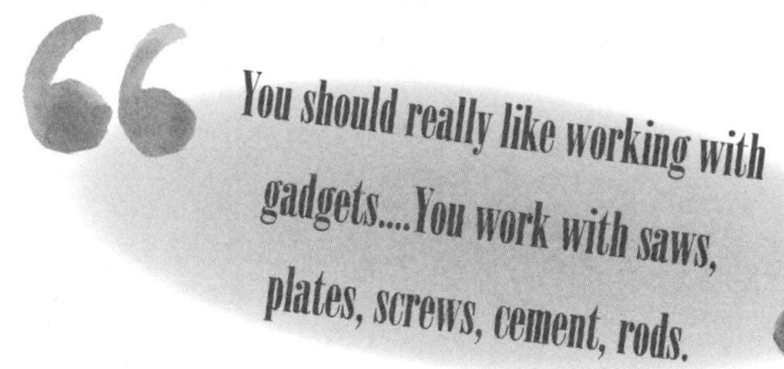

what is it like to be an orthopaedic surgeon?

"I like putting hands back together," says Dr. Diana Carr, an orthopaedic surgeon with a solo private practice in rural Florida. "I like healing sick people. We're a specialty where you can really see what we've done." She remembers as a child growing up in a very small town with no drugstore and the only hospital a long forty-five minute drive away. "When the doctor was on vacation, that was it," she says. "There wasn't anywhere to go." For as long as Dr. Carr can remember, she wanted to be the person who was the only one for miles who could help people—a doctor. She says she felt that power once when she operated on a man with a World War II injury. "The injury was as old as I was," she says. "After a radial nerve transfer, which was a new procedure at the time, he used his hand for the first time in fifty years. It felt incredible to help him do that."

Dr. Edward Toriello, Chief of the Department of Orthopaedic Surgery at Wyckoff Heights Medical Center in Brooklyn, New York, works with patients of all ages, but he tends to see more elderly patients. "They usually come in with their son or daughter. The typical elderly patient I see is healthy, overall, but with an arthritic joint, say. And this changes their whole quality of life. They want desperately to remain independent, but over the course of time—sometimes it's a short period of time, sometimes it's over a period of several months or years—they become trapped, physically. They're either housebound, or even chair bound. This can change their entire outlook and personality, making an ordinarily happy person quite bitter." Dr. Toriello is sensitive to these sorts of changes in people and takes genuine delight in helping them. "I like getting people back on their feet," he says.

As the attending orthopaedic surgeon at Catholic Medical Center in Queens, New York, Dr. Toriello also works with trauma patients. "I see patients in two areas: my office and the E.R.," he says. Most of his days, though, are spent in the office. He begins an office visit by talking with the patient, and sometimes the patient's relatives, to discover what the problem is. He takes down the patient's history and takes X rays if he thinks it necessary.

Once Dr. Toriello has come to a conclusion about the patient's case, he sits down and carefully explains the diagnosis to the patient. "I use a model to show the patient and the patient's family what I'm talking about," he says. "That's what's so great about this specialty, too. You can see it—it's not like I'm trying to describe diabetes or something intangible—it's right there, in black and white." After explaining his diagnosis, Dr. Toriello talks about the patient's options. "This is an extensive discussion," says Dr. Toriello. "Because each option has risks and advantages." He continues with an example, "A patient diagnosed with an arthritic joint has the option of doing nothing, taking meds, having arthroscopic surgery, or doing a total joint replacement." Depending on the particular characteristics of a patient's case, Dr. Toriello might recommend arthroscopic surgery. "We won't cure the arthritis," he says, "but it buys time for a lot of people. It's like light housekeeping of the joint. We wash it out, scrape or sand or shave the bone spurs. Clean it up and, hopefully, flush out some of the toxins."

Dr. Toriello wants patients to take their time deciding which option will make them feel the most comfortable. "I want them to try and figure out what's best," he says. "As much as I love surgery, you don't want to do something that won't help. After we finish talking I give them a booklet that describes what we've just talked about, and I ask them to think about it and talk it over with their families. Some are absolutely positive about wanting the surgery, in which case I might go ahead and schedule them for surgery, but most need to think it over."

In the event that a patient opts for a total joint replacement, Dr. Toriello sends them to an internist for blood work and a full checkup. "We want to determine that the patient can reasonably survive the procedure," he explains. He then sets a date for the surgery and provides the patient with information about the procedure. The morning of the surgery, Dr. Toriello meets briefly with the patient, reviews the patient's history, and notes any problems, such as allergies to medications. Most surgeries begin early in the morning, sometime between 7:30 and 8:00 AM. Dr. Toriello likes to have music playing during his surgeries. "Preferably, the blues," he adds.

The next several hours consist of cutting, sawing, and measuring. Dr. Toriello says, "During 'Take Your Daughter to Work Week' my thirteen-year old got to see a total knee replacement. She was completely impressed by all the sounds—buzzing, banging, pounding, scraping, the sucking sounds from the suction machine—she loved it." For some surgeries the patient can be awake. A spinal anesthesia allows them to remain conscious without feeling any pain. "During arthroscopic surgeries, I love it when the patient is awake. They can see what I'm doing and what the process really involves."

Following the surgery, Dr. Toriello is involved with the patient's postoperative care and recovery, including rehabilitation. With the help of a physical therapist and other members of the rehabilitation team, the patient learns how to use the joint again.

Orthopaedic Surgeons Describe Their Area of Practice

A survey by the American Academy of Orthopaedic Surgeons revealed that most surgeons considered themselves generalists. Only 23 percent considered themselves specialists and confined their practice to a special area, such as the spine, foot, or hand.

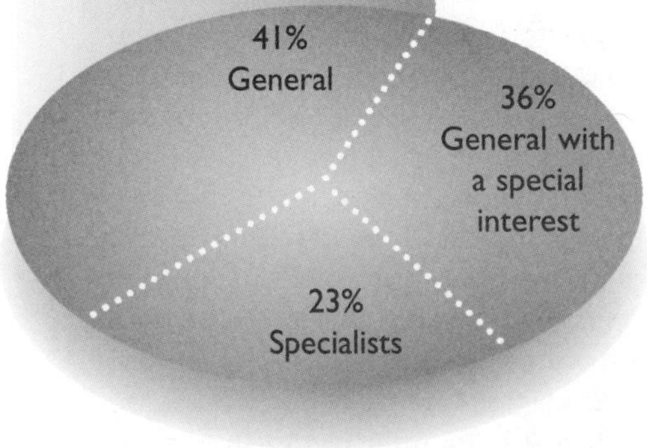

41% General

36% General with a special interest

23% Specialists

have I got what it takes to be an orthopaedic surgeon?

"You've really got to be dedicated—it's not going to be easy. Orthopaedics is a macho specialty," says Dr. Diana Carr. "You can't be thin-skinned. A sense of humor is helpful." Dr. Carr wants women to enter the field, but she wants them to realize it can be a difficult specialty. As the only woman in her orthopaedics residency and the only woman in the entire surgery department, she has toughened up and learned to use humor to deal with difficult situations.

Orthopaedic surgeons work with a wide variety of instruments, scopes, and technologies. "You should really like working with gadgets," warns Dr Toriello. "It's almost like building a room," he adds. "You work with saws, plates, screws, cement, rods." To a certain extent the work of an orthopaedic surgeon involves physical activity. "There's a lot of pulling and tugging," Dr. Toriello says. Women, however, should not worry about not being strong enough. Dr. Carr points out, "There is no reason why any woman, regardless of size, cannot successfully practice orthopaedics. The correct application of orthopaedic principles will allow reductions of fractures and dislocations by any orthopaedist." Dr. Carr finds that the real problem comes in finding tools and instruments that are properly sized. "The biggest problem I have is the size of the tools don't fit my hand. My hands are small," she says.

Stamina, more than strength, comes into play most often. One reason orthopaedic surgeons need stamina is that they wear protective lead aprons during surgeries that involve fluoroscopes. "They seem a lot heavier than their ten pounds when you're under stress. You get pretty hot," says Dr. Toriello, referring to the aprons. Fluoroscopes provide continuous X rays of the body's interior.

Orthopaedic surgeons also need stamina to last through the long surgeries. Some procedures are short and take only twenty to thirty minutes. On the other hand, a total joint replacement can take from two to three hours. And most trauma surgery on bones can take five to seven or more hours to complete. "You just keep telling yourself that no surgery can go on forever," says Dr. Toriello. "Every surgery has to end sometime."

Knowing the limits of the materials you work with is another necessary quality. As Dr. Toriello points out, technology has advanced to the point where he and other orthopaedic surgeons can use special metals that will last a long time, but in the end, nothing lasts forever. "Titanium, chromium, steel, cobalt—anything will break. It's like a coat hanger, you can keep piling clothes on one, but eventually it's going to give way. It's a race against time." An orthopaedic surgeon usually gets to help his or her patients, but there may be moments when the orthopaedic surgeon has to tell a star athlete that the days of setting record-breaking runs are over. Compassion, empathy, and understanding will help the orthopaedic surgeon to help his or her patient.

To be a successful orthopaedic surgeon, you should

- Have physical stamina
- Enjoy working with tools and technology
- Enjoy helping people
- Have good hand-eye coordination
- Be a good listener and effective communicator

how do I become an orthopaedic surgeon?

education

High School

If you are interested in pursuing a medical degree, a high school education emphasizing college preparatory classes is a must. Science courses, such as biology, chemistry, and physics, are necessary, as are math courses. These classes will not only provide you with an introduction to basic science and math concepts, but also allow you to determine your own aptitude in these areas. Since college will be your next educational step, it is also important to take English courses to develop your research and writing skills. Foreign language, social science, and computer classes will also help make you an appealing candidate for college admission as well as prepare you for your future undergraduate and graduate education. As a high school senior you may want to consider applying to colleges or universities that are also associated with a medical school. High school guidance counselors should also be able to provide you with information about such schools.

Postsecondary Training

Following high school, the next step to becoming an orthopaedic surgeon is to receive a bachelor's degree from an accredited four-year college or university. Typical college courses that may help you prepare for medical school include biology, chemistry, anatomy, psychology, and physics. English courses will help you to hone communication skills; other humanities classes, social sciences, and ethics will help prepare you for a people-oriented career.

If you choose to attend a college or university associated with a medical school that offers the accelerated medical program, your undergraduate education will be different from that of other undergrads. An accelerated program typically reduces or consolidates the number of years you spend as an undergraduate, thereby speeding up the your entrance into medical school. A six- or seven-year med student is actually enrolled for two or three years, respectively, of undergraduate school, plus the requisite four years of medical school.

After receiving an undergraduate degree, you must then apply to and be accepted by medical school. Most students apply to several schools early in their senior year of college. Admission is competitive; only about one-third of the applicants are accepted. Applicants must undergo a fairly extensive and difficult admissions process that takes into consideration grade point averages, scores on the Medical College Admission Test (MCAT), and recommendations from professors. Many medical schools also interview applicants.

A student who is not accepted on his or her first attempt to get into medical school should not despair. Many talented and highly regarded physicians were not accepted on their first try. Others have attended and graduated from foreign medical school programs. Dr. Toriello is one such example.

"I was planning to be a priest," Dr. Toriello says. "I went to seminary for two years. Having gone to a seminary, I didn't have the grades or the background to get into an American medical school. I didn't want to go to Mexico, so I decided to go abroad to study medicine in Italy." He acknowledges this was a difficult choice to make, since he would have to learn a new language while trying to learn medicine too. "It was a lot of work. All of the courses were in Italian. I went over three months early to go to an intensive language school, so that I would learn enough Italian to take the med classes," he explains. "The oral exams were intimidating, I'll tell you that much. It was tough, but I loved every minute of it." The University of Padova's medical school was a six-year program. At the end of five years, Dr. Toriello transferred to S.U.N.Y. at Buffalo's School of Medicine, where he studied for another two years.

In order to earn the degree doctor of medicine (M.D.), a student must complete four years of medical school study and training. For the first two years of medical school, students attend lectures and classes and spend time in laboratories. Courses include anatomy, biochemistry, physiology, pharmacology, psychology, microbiology, pathology, medical ethics, and laws governing medicine. Students learn to take patient histories, perform routine physical examinations, and recognize symptoms. "Anatomy was just pure rote memorization—no finesse, at all," says Dr. Toriello. "But I loved physiology. Physiology tells you how it all works. That's what put it all together for me."

In their third and fourth years, students are involved in more practical studies. They work in clinics and hospitals and are supervised by residents and physicians. They learn acute, chronic, preventive, and rehabilitative care. They go through what are known as rotations (brief periods of study) in a particular area, such as internal medicine, obstetrics and gynecology, pediatrics, dermatology, psychiatry, and surgery. Rotations allow students to gain exposure to the many different fields within medicine and to learn the skills of diagnosing and treating patients.

Upon graduating from an accredited medical school, physicians must pass a standard examination given by the National Board of Medical Examiners. Most physicians complete an internship, also referred to as a transition year. The internship is usually one year in length, and helps graduates to decide what their area of specialization will be.

Following the internship, the physicians begin what is known as a residency. Orthopaedics requires a minimum of five years of postgraduate study. There are 168 residency programs in the United States that offer approximately 2,000 residency positions to prospective orthopaedic surgeons. Competition for these positions is keen.

"I knew I liked surgery, so I began in general surgery," explains Dr. Toriello. "I saw how hard everybody worked throughout the residency, but I got discouraged when I saw that general surgery residents who were ahead of me in school were doing more run-of-the-mill surgeries afterwards. It was nothing like what they'd done while in their residencies. The coolest guys were in orthopaedics. I liked that it was positive surgery—no amputations," he adds. "And, unlike the general surgeons, the orthopaedic surgeons I rotated with were still doing challenging, interesting surgeries once they left their residencies."

Throughout the surgical residency, residents are supervised at all levels of training, with the attending surgeon ultimately responsible for the patient's care. Residents begin their training by assisting on and then performing basic operations. As the residency years continue, residents gain responsibility through teaching and supervisory duties. Eventually the residents are allowed to perform complex operations independently.

The residency years are as filled with stress, pressure, and physical rigor as the previous four years of medical school, perhaps even more so since residents are given greater responsibilities than medical students. Residents often work twenty-four-hour shifts, easily putting in eighty hours or more per week.

certification or licensing

Licensing is a mandatory procedure in the United States. It is required in all states before any doctor can practice medicine. In order to be licensed, doctors must have graduated from medical school, passed the licensing test of the state in which they will practice, and completed their residency.

Certification by the American Academy of Orthopaedic Surgeons, although voluntary, is highly recommended. Hospitals, for example, often refuse to extend privileges to noncertified physicians. Orthopaedic surgeons seeking certification must undergo a two-step process. After completing postgraduate training, the candidate must successfully complete the written examination. Then, after two years in practice, the candidate must successfully complete the oral examinations. The orthopaedic surgeon who passes both examinations is now eligible for membership in the American Academy of Orthopaedic Surgeons. The candidate must complete an application and interview, and be sponsored by two fellows in the Academy.

scholarships and grants

Scholarships and grants are often available from individual institutions, state agencies, and special-interest organizations. The book *Dollars for College: Medicine, Dentistry, and Related Fields* by Ferguson Publishing Company is an excellent source for this information. Many students finance their medical education through the Armed Forces Health Professions Scholarship Program. Each branch of the military participates in this program, paying students' tuitions in exchange for military service. Contact your local recruiting office for more information. The National Health Service Corps Scholarship Program also provides money for students in return for service. Another source for financial aid, scholarship, and grant information is the Association of American Medical Colleges. The Ruth Jackson Orthopaedic Society (named for the first woman to become an orthopaedic surgeon in the United States) was organized for women orthopaedists. The society offers scholarships and information helpful to women interested in orthopaedics. Remember to request information early for eligibility, application requirements, and deadlines.

Association of American Medical Colleges
2450 N Street, NW
Washington, DC 20037
TEL: 202-828-0400
WEBSITE: http://www.aamc.org
Specific information on financial aid programs can be found at:
WEBSITE: http://www.aamc.org/stuapps/finaid

Ferguson Publishing Company
200 West Madison, Suite 300
Chicago, IL 60606
TEL: 312-580-5480

National Health Services Corps Scholarship Program
U.S. Public Health Service
1010 Wayne Avenue, Suite 240
Silver Spring, MD 20910
TEL: 800-638-0824

Ruth Jackson Orthopaedic Society
6300 North River Road, Suite 727
Rosemont, IL 60018
TEL: 847-698-1693

who will hire me?

Orthopaedic surgeons typically practice in one of three settings. One option is to work as a solo practitioner. Solo practitioners work for themselves, although they may share office space with other orthopaedic surgeons or physicians. A second option is to work in an orthopaedic group practice. Typically in this setting, two to six orthopaedists work together, sharing costs for the office, seeing each other's patients, and providing continual coverage in hospital rounds. The third typical practice setting is in multi-specialty groups. In these groups a number of orthopaedists work together with other specialists, such as cardiologists or general practitioners.

Many orthopaedic surgeons are also involved in education, either as full- or part-time teachers. There are also orthopaedists who work for the military or in administrative positions for health care providers.

where can I go from here?

Orthopaedic surgeons usually advance their careers by increasing the size of their private practice, increasing their specialty knowledge by returning to school, or assuming additional responsibilities of administrative or supervisory positions. Prominence in the profession may also be gained by having papers or research results published in respected medical journals. Many physicians also give lectures at specialty conferences.

what are the salary ranges?

The national average salary for first-year residents in the mid-1990's was approximately $31,000. That average increased to $41,800 by the final residency year. Salaries will vary depending on the kind of residency, the hospital, and the geographic area.

According to surveys by the American Medical Association, annual income for surgeons in the mid-1990's ranged from approximately $140,000 to $300,000, with the median income at about $200,000. These figures are for all surgeons, and incomes may vary from specialty to specialty. Other factors influencing individual incomes include type and size of practice, hours worked per week, geographic area, and professional reputation.

what is the job outlook?

Orthopaedics is an expanding specialty, and the need for orthopaedic surgeons will increase markedly into the next century. Future opportunities in orthopaedics will be influenced by major trends in population aging (with its increasing numbers of fractures and reconstructive surgery), by trauma and injuries in sports and the workplace, and by continuing technological advancement.

how do I learn more?

professional organizations

Following are organizations that provide information on the profession and certifying process of orthopaedic surgeon.

American Academy of Orthopaedic Surgeons
6300 North River Road
Rosemont, IL 60018
TEL: 847-823-7186
WEBSITE: http://www.aaos.org

Ruth Jackson Orthopaedic Society
6300 North River Road, Suite 727
Rosemont, IL 60018
TEL: 847-698-1693

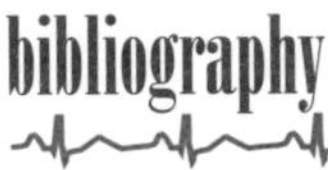

Following is a sampling of books and periodicals relating to the professional concerns and development of orthopaedic surgeons.

Books

Redford, John B., John V. Basmajian, and Paul Trautman, editors. *Orthotics: Clinical Practice and Rehabilitation Technology.* New York, NY: Churchill Livingstone, 1995.

Shankman, Albert L. *Fundamental Orthopedic Management for the Physical Therapist Assistant.* St. Louis, MO: Mosby, 1996.

Shurr, Donald G. *Prosthetics and Orthotics.* New York, NY: Appleton & Lange, 1990.

Periodicals

Journal of Prosthetics and Orthotics. Quarterly. Presents articles and reports from professionals on current topics in orthotics and prosthetics. American Academy of Orthotists and Prosthetists, 1650 King Street, Suite 500, Alexandria, VA 22314, 703-836-7116.

O & P Almanac. Monthly. Contains articles covering the professional, business, association, and government activities affecting the field. American Orthotic and Prosthetic Association, 1650 King Street, Suite 500, Alexandria, VA 22314, 703-836-7114.

orthotic and prosthetic technicians

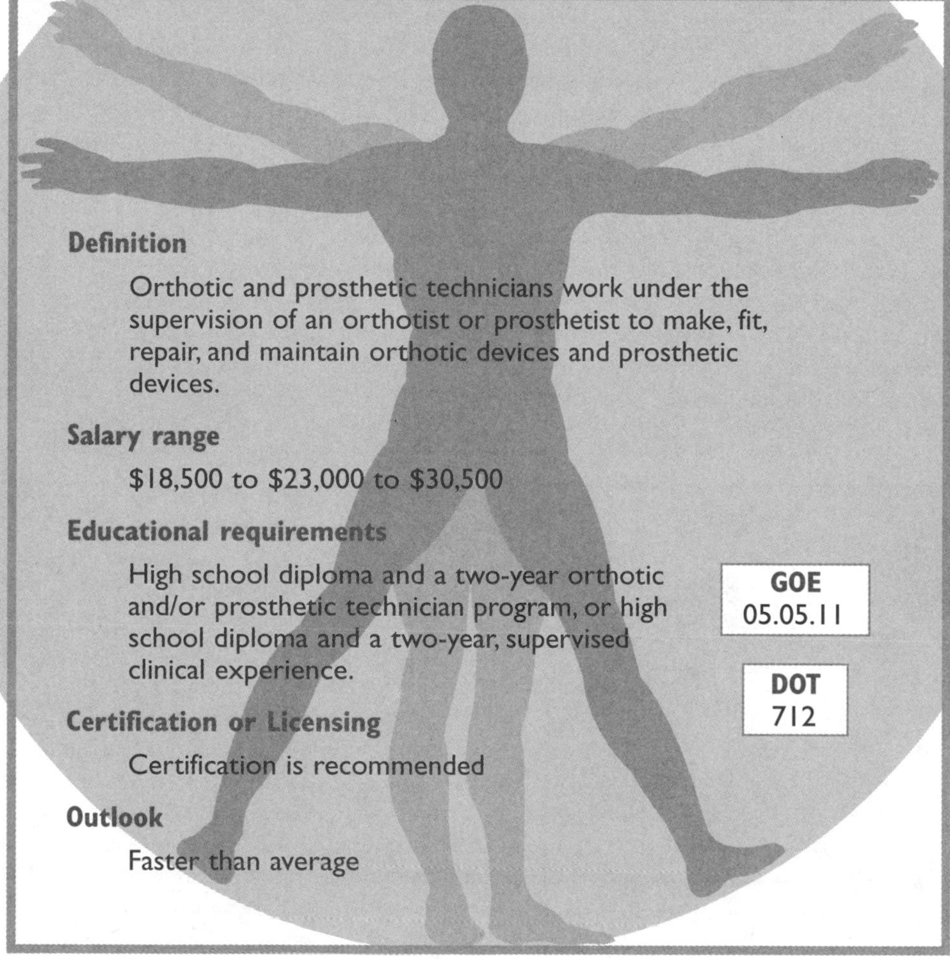

Definition

Orthotic and prosthetic technicians work under the supervision of an orthotist or prosthetist to make, fit, repair, and maintain orthotic devices and prosthetic devices.

Salary range

$18,500 to $23,000 to $30,500

Educational requirements

High school diploma and a two-year orthotic and/or prosthetic technician program, or high school diploma and a two-year, supervised clinical experience.

Certification or Licensing

Certification is recommended

Outlook

Faster than average

GOE
05.05.11

DOT
712

High School Subjects

Computer science
English
Mathematics
Metal shop
Plastic shop
Wood shop

Personal Interests

Creating and repairing things
Doing detailed, exact work
Helping people
Working with your hands

Walking down the hall, Jeff Borgman hears a shout from behind him. "Jeff!" the voice calls out. Turning around, he is met by a blur of pigtails and striped jersey. Jumping into his arms to give him a warm hug, the little girl says the unnecessary. "Thanks, Jeff," she whispers into his ear, and then as she bounces back down on the ground, she holds up a brightly striped prosthetic arm that matches the stripes of her jersey. "Check this out!" she says with a grin. She pauses for an instant and then dives into a cartwheel. Jeff almost forgets that the little girl is also using a prosthetic leg. He applauds loudly and beams at her, full of pride.

"Awesome!" he smiles and offers his arm to her. "Walk me back to the O & P department?" he asks her. She nods, and as they walk, tells him all about the upcoming gymnastics class she has that Saturday.

what does an orthotic or a prosthetic technician do?

Millions of people throughout the world require the use of special devices to help them perform the basic functions of daily living. Most of us take for granted activities like walking, eating an apple, running or skiing in a competition, or typing on a computer keyboard. The artificial leg (a prosthesis) that enables a person who is missing a leg to walk down the street or the back brace (an orthosis) that allows a person with a severely curved spine to stand tall while in line at the grocery store are made by skilled orthotic and prosthetic technicians. Orthotic devices support the spine or limbs weakened by disease, injury, or illness. Prosthetic devices, often referred to as artificial limbs, are used to assist patients with total or partial limb loss resulting from disease, injury, or illness. Although orthotists and prosthetists also know how to fabricate these devices, it is usually the *orthotic or prosthetic technician* who makes the orthosis or prosthesis.

Typically, a physician sends a prescription to the orthotist or prosthetist for a patient who needs either device. The prescription describes the specific device the physician believes the patient requires. The orthotist or prosthetist then sees the patient, conducts a diagnostic exam, and takes measurements. Sometimes the orthotist or prosthetist might suggest another type of device or make some modification to the device proposed by the physician. Finally, the orthotist or prosthetist takes the prescription, along with any notes and measurements he or she has made, back to the laboratory facility where the device will be constructed. After a consultation with the orthotist or prosthetist, the orthotic and prosthetic technician works from the prescription, notes, and measurements to create the desired orthosis or prosthesis.

At one time, the role of the technician would have been described as that of a skilled craft worker. Today, however, the technician's work is rapidly changing from a craft to a science. Many time-honored craft techniques are still utilized in the fabrication of these devices, but they are being blended with advanced technology.

Orthotic braces are often made of metal, plastic, or a combination of the two. Orthotic technicians must shape the materials into the proper forms. To be certain that the brace will fit the patient, they may use a cast model of the appropriate body part. In many cases, they have the responsibility of making this plaster or melted plastic model.

In order to shape the brace, the orthotic technician uses saws, welding equipment, and hammers. They also often use drills, to drill holes in the brace components, and then rivet the components together to form the device. When the brace is completely formed, the orthotic technician covers and pads it, using layers of rubber, felt, plastic, and leather. Often, fastening devices such as velcro straps or plastic hooks are attached.

Prosthetic devices are made of wood, plastic, metal, and fabric. Following the instructions of the prosthetist, the prosthetic technician uses rotary saws, cutting machines, and hand cutting tools to carve and grind materials to the correct dimensions. To assemble the prosthesis, the technician drills or taps holes

lingo to learn

AFO A brace supporting the ankle and foot area. The acronym stands for ankle-foot orthosis.

Grinding wheel A wheel or disk covered with abrasive material that is used to sand and finish metal, plastic, or other material.

KAFO A brace supporting the knee-ankle-foot area. The acronym stands for knee-ankle-foot orthosis.

Kinesiology The study of human movement.

Manual dexterity Skill in using the hands, requiring both small and large muscle coordination.

Plaster of Paris A white powder that can be mixed with water to form a paste. This paste can then be used to form a cast that will set into a hardened solid.

Physiology A type of biology that deals with the study of essential life functions, processes, and activities.

for rivets or screws, and then rivets, glues, sews, bolts, or welds the components together. Then, the prosthetic technician pads the prosthesis with layers of fiberglass, plastic, or leather and, finally, using sewing machines, riveting guns, and hand tools, fits the prosthesis with an outer covering. If it is necessary, coloring might be applied to the outer covering of the prosthesis so that it more closely matches the patient's skin tone. New techniques now allow technicians to use an almost limitless selection of colors, patterns, and designs for the outer covering.

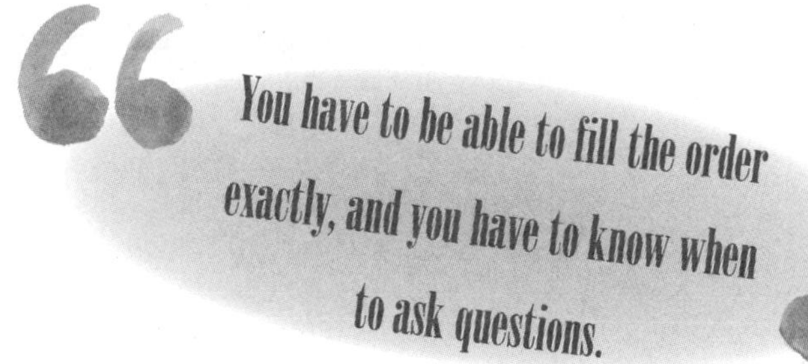

Prosthetic technicians, like orthotic technicians, may also build cast models of their patients, especially when making plastic cosmetic replacements, such as ears or hands. Of course, this is only possible if the patient has a remaining limb (also known as a residual limb). When making a cosmetic replacement for a nose, the prosthetic technician usually follows a standard model of a nose and then tailors or modifies it according to the appearance of the patient's face.

After the orthosis or prosthesis has been fabricated, it must be tested by the technicians for stability, the proper alignment of parts, and freedom of movement. Technicians are also responsible for maintaining the orthotic or prosthetic device, as directed by the orthotist or prosthetist. Sometimes an orthosis or prosthesis requires modifications or adjustments in order to remain comfortable and functional for the patient. In cases where orthotic or prosthetic devices have been designed for children, regular fittings and modifications are necessary in order to maintain a proper fit as the child grows. Repairs to orthotic and prosthetic devices are also the responsibility of technicians.

what is it like to be an orthotic or a prosthetic technician?

Jeff Borgman, a registered prosthetic technician at the Shriner's Hospital for Children in Minneapolis, Minnesota, specializes in custom pediatric prostheses. He has worked as a technician for fourteen years and still loves his job. "These are happy kids. We've really given them something to enhance their lives. Our kids play baseball, hockey, the violin—you name it and they do it," he says. "Where I work is a little different from the typical fabrication facility. In private facilities you tend to see the same, standard prostheses—above- and below-the-knee, above- and below-the elbow prostheses. At Shriner's, I see strange cases, special models. I do mostly custom work from scratch." He describes a piece that he is currently working on. "I'm making a knee-bearing prosthesis with outside joints. I'll make a skin from scratch, using traditional, old-world craft techniques, as well as cutting edge technology," says Jeff. "The bottom half is a custom-made wooden leg, labor-intensive and expensive," he says. "I asked the prosthetist how much this particular prosthesis would be in the regular market, and he guessed around $5,000." Jeff's employer, the Shriner's Hospital for Children, provides free medical care for the children accepted into the hospital, who range in age from roughly six months to twenty-one years. Everything, from diagnostic testing to medications to surgical procedures to rehabilitation to orthotics and prosthetics, is free. "There are screening clinics every week that kids and their parents attend to see if they qualify. And it's not always based solely on financial need."

Prior to working at Shriner's Hospital, Jeff worked in a private lab and a central fabrication facility. He enjoys the diversity of his present job and the increased contact with patients. "The amount of contact you have with patients really depends on the size of the facility," he explains. "In a large place, the orthotist or prosthetist is going to be the one going back to the patient and, as a tech, you're not going to have much contact with patients." At Shriner's, Jeff has a lot of contact with the patients, especially when fitting and making modifications to a prosthesis. "Patient contact is rewarding, but it also has a very practical side. The more information you have, the smoother the job will go."

Technology has advanced the technical details of the devices that Jeff and other prosthetic technicians create, and it has also done much in the way of improving the aesthetics of each piece—an important factor for patients of any age. "It really helps when you can make them feel better about the piece. For example, instead of white polypropylene, polyester fabric can be placed on the plastic while it's hot, and the heat, basically, pulls the inks through onto the prosthesis. Using this technique, we now do a lot of customized finishes, from camouflaged arms to writing their names on it in a fancy script. The patient is only limited by the fabric selection. And the kids feel like they have input," he says. "One little girl wouldn't wear an arm unless she could have it any color she wanted. So, she picked out a pretty floral pattern she liked, we heated it into the prosthesis, and her grandmother made her a couple different outfits that matched it. She was so excited, wearing it isn't a problem, now."

In addition to his own responsibilities as a prosthetic technician at Shriner's Hospital, Jeff teaches technicians-in-training. "When you teach, it really helps reinforce what you already know," he says. "You sometimes end up seeing things in a new or different light. Things you do every day, almost by instinct, you suddenly have to explain how to do them." Jeff truly enjoys this aspect of his work, realizing the need to pass along information to others. "In the 1950s and 60s," Jeff says, "specialists wouldn't share their knowledge. It was a form of job security. If no one else knew how to do what they did, they would always have work. I have a different perspective on it. My philosophy is that I'm there for the patient, so anything that helps the patient is good. I'm always more than happy to share what I know with others. After all, that's how you learn in the first place."

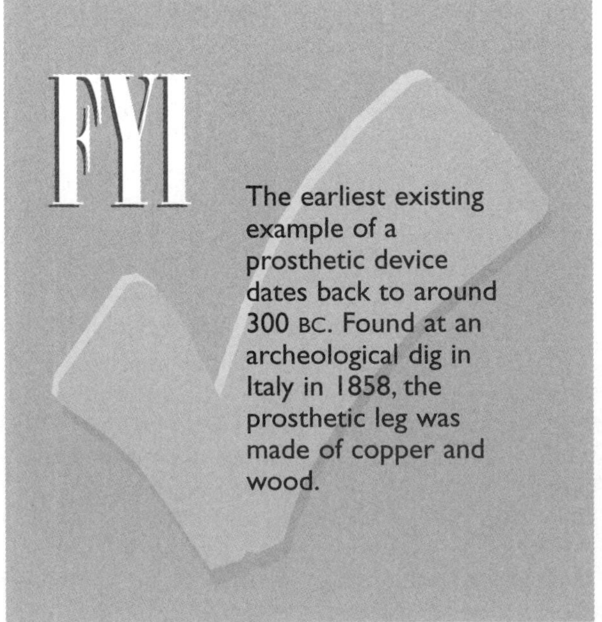

The earliest existing example of a prosthetic device dates back to around 300 BC. Found at an archeological dig in Italy in 1858, the prosthetic leg was made of copper and wood.

John Hebble works as an orthotic technician at Riley Children's Hospital in Indianapolis, Indiana. Presently, he is the only technician on staff, although the department employs three orthotic assistants who have many of the same responsibilities that he does.

John's regular work week, Monday through Friday, 8:00 AM to 4:30 PM, is spent in an area very different from the rest of the hospital. The brace shop, as it is commonly called, is a series of work rooms filled with machines, workbenches, and tools. John typically wears a lab coat to protect his clothes from the plaster dust. His day at work begins in the casting room, where he begins the process of creating cast models that will be used to form the braces he makes. He occasionally makes braces to fit around the patient's torso, but most often John is involved in forming leg braces. To make the cast, he uses an empty impression, or negative, of a leg which an orthotist has made. Wedging it in a box of sand to keep it upright, John mixes a batch of plaster of Paris, and carefully fills the empty cast. If there are more casts to be poured, he completes the process for each one and leaves them to harden.

Once the cast model is formed and broken out of its mold, there is still quite a lot of work to be done before it is finished. "This is what I think is the hardest part of the job," John says. "After you get the model, you have to sand it down or build it up to make sure the proportions match the measurement sheet exactly." According to John, the original model is almost never precisely right. "By the time the orthotist puts the cast on, then cuts it off, and puts it back together, there's always some distortion," he says. In order to work the cast into the exact dimensions required, John must sand and carve the plaster in the necessary places. Sometimes he must also use additional plaster to build up areas of the cast. It is painstaking work.

After the cast is finished to specification, John begins to form the actual brace, using the cast as a model. Most of the braces he creates are made out of plastic. "Plastic and plaster are what I mainly work with," he says. "But, now I'm starting to learn how to bend metal. That's pretty hard." A plastic brace is formed by heating a sheet of plastic in an infrared oven until it is pliable. In the oven room, John puts a milky-white plastic sheet in the oven and clamps the cast model onto the work table. He then begins to make the pads that will be used in the brace. Working from the measurement sheet, he selects the proper material, and cuts it into the right shape. "We use different thicknesses of padding for different areas," John says. After the pad is cut, its edges must be beveled, using a grinding wheel. When the edges are smooth, John covers one side of the pad with glue, and heats it in the oven. He then attaches it to the model, which has been covered with a stocking to allow the plastic to pull away easily from the plaster.

When all the pads have been formed and placed, John must then mold the heated plastic around the cast to make the actual brace. When the plastic has changed from milky-white to clear, he puts on work gloves, pulls the pliable sheet from the oven, and wraps it around the model, making it conform to the shape beneath. "You have to be careful not to get any bubbles or folds," he says. A vacuum hose attached to the bottom of the cast helps draw out the air, and mold the plastic more tightly to the form of the cast. After the plastic-covered cast has cooled, it is given back to the orthotist. He or she then diagrams the areas that will be cut out of the device to form the brace. John then makes the prescribed cuts with a cast saw and then pulls the plastic brace off of the cast, or model. Now, he begins the process of smoothing and beveling the edges, again using various grinding wheels with different grades of coarseness. When the brace has finally been formed and sanded smooth, it is given to an assistant who specializes in attaching the fastening mechanisms.

Although the great majority of John's day is spent in actual preparation of various braces, he does spend a small amount of time performing other duties, such as storing materials, cleaning the work area and equipment, repairing damaged braces, and attending departmental meetings.

To be a successful orthotic and prosthetic technician, you should

- Enjoy working with your hands
- Have good hand-eye coordination and manual dexterity
- Be able to follow written and oral instructions
- Be able to listen and communicate well
- Have mechanical aptitude
- Possess strong problem-solving skills

have I got what it takes to be an orthotic or a prosthetic technician?

"There's nothing like it when you get a handshake or a hug from a grateful kid," says Jeff of his work at Shriner's Hospital. Helping children to walk, to run, even to perform gymnastics is very gratifying. "It's a humbling job, knowing that your problems aren't big by comparison to the ones these kids face. You're really helping them. In turn, they help you remember why you're there," says Jeff.

In spite of the wonderful rapport a technician can develop with patients, there are times when egos can cause problems. "I see a lot of arrogance in this field," Jeff says, "where there should be none at all. Personally, I'd rather let my work speak for me." Having a positive, self-confident, but not arrogant, outlook will help the technician work with the wide variety of personalities that are present among both patients and other allied health professionals.

Speaking of his work at Riley Children's Hospital, John notes that following directions is extremely important. Technicians are given a sheet with the patient's measurements and instructions on what type of orthosis or prosthesis to form. It is important that they be able to comprehend and follow those instructions to the letter. "You have to be able to fill the order exactly," John says, "and you have to know when to ask questions. If you make assumptions, it can really backfire."

Jeff agrees that communication is definitely a crucial part of the job. During the course of creating a device for a patient, an orthotic and prosthetic technician works with other technicians and an orthotist or prosthetist, as well as possibly having some contact with other members of the patient's rehabilitative team, such as the orthopaedist or physical therapist. Orthotic and prosthetic technicians need to be able to communicate their thoughts and opinions clearly at all times. "It shouldn't be intimidating," Jeff says. "You're there to help someone, you have to remember that. Don't let people intimidate you." Also, patients are sometimes more comfortable with a technician than with a physician, or even the orthotist and prosthetist. A patient may feel uncertain about voicing a complain in front of them, but feel perfectly at ease in sharing it with the technician. In such a case, it would be essential for the technician to share this information with the orthotist or prosthetist.

Part of the technician's job, like any other medical professional, is learning from experience. Mistakes are sometimes made. Jeff counsels prospective technicians to take it all in stride. "You have to learn not to take criticism personally. Just learn from your mistakes," he advises. "I like to think of myself this way: I'm not good, I just don't make that many mistakes." Taking criticism well is also extremely important when that criticism comes from the patient. "Listen," Jeff advises others. "The patient is telling you what needs to happen to that piece. He's actually making your work easier."

Orthotic and prosthetic technicians must be skillful with their hands. Technicians spend the majority of their day sanding, carving, grinding, and shaping the base materials to meet very exact specifications. "It's a craft," John says. "You definitely have to be able to work well with your hands and with machinery. That's what it's all about." Being able to create with his hands is also what John likes best about his job. "You take pride in what you do, and do it as well as you can. Then you can say, 'I built that.' It's like a carpenter saying he built a house." He also finds it rewarding to see the entire process through, from beginning to end. "It's not like working in a factory," he says, "where you just do one thing over and over and never get to see the finished product."

Jeff agrees. "A technician needs good hand-eye coordination, should be mechanically-inclined, and must be somewhat artistic in order to shape an aesthetically pleasing prosthesis."

Finally, it is important that the technician be able to focus on what he or she is doing, even while working in a very distracting environment. "This shop is really dusty," John says. "Really cluttered, and really noisy. There are machines running all the time. You have to get used to that." Technicians may also be working from time to time in uncomfortably hot conditions. "In the oven room, it can get pretty miserable, especially in the summer," admits John. He also stresses the need for caution when working with both the machines and the oven. "It's easy to get little nicks and burns," he says, "but if you're careful, you'll be okay."

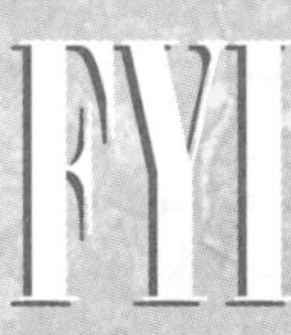

Did you know that there are a number of jobs related to those of the orthotic and prosthetic technicians?

Similar positions include those who make dental devices, glass eyes, medical instruments, and light or heat instruments. Among the related jobs are:

artificial-glass-eye makers
biomedical equipment technicians
dental ceramists
dental laboratory technicians
lens mounters
optician apprentices

how do I become an orthotic or a prosthetic technician?

Jeff Borgman was working for a gas station as a tow truck operator and restoring Oldsmobile Cutlasses with his father and brothers, when his mother, a nurse's assistant, suggested he go next door to the orthotic-prosthetic laboratory in search of a job. "While trying to reupholster a the back seat of a '63 Plymouth, I took an upholstery class, where I learned how to sew leather and fabric. But it wasn't for me," says Jeff. "Mom worked next door to this orthotic-prosthetic lab, and she said I should look into that. The rest is history."

Before beginning his job in orthotics, John Hebble had done various jobs that involved using his hands, such as factory-line work. He remembers always tinkering around, making and repairing things with his hands. He especially enjoyed shop classes in high school.

Advancement Possibilities

Orthotists design and fit orthotic braces, under direction of a doctor, to treat patients with disabilities of the spine and limbs; evaluate the effectiveness of braces on a patient; prescribe adjustments; and may supervise orthotic technicians.

Prosthetists plan and write specifications, under direction of a doctor, for prosthetic devices to assist patients with partial or total limb loss; formulate prosthesis design; select materials; fit and evaluate the effectiveness of the device on the patient; and may supervise prosthetic technicians.

Prosthetist/Orthotist is a position combining the responsibilities of both the prosthetist and the orthotist.

education

High School

A high school diploma, or its equivalent, is the minimum educational requirement for becoming an orthotic and prosthetic technician. The prospective technician should be sure to take as many shop classes as possible, including metal, plastic, and wood shop classes. An exposure to working with several different kinds of materials and machines will build a good foundation for later work as an orthotic or prosthetic technician. Also, the shop classes will provide students with both experience and practice working with their hands, as well as improving manual dexterity and hand-eye coordination.

In addition, skills learned in English class are very important. Technicians must be able to communicate and work well with both practitioners and patients. Comprehension of written and oral instruction is also vital. Any classes that build solid communication and comprehension skills are good choices.

Finally, math courses will benefit the prospective orthotic or prosthetic technician. The ability to measure in exact increments, work with fractions, and use angles and degrees are all part of the technician's work. Geometry and algebra are good courses to take, as well as physics and computer science.

Many orthotic and prosthetic technicians eventually become practitioners. If you are interested in becoming an orthotist or prosthetist, the educational requirements include a college or university degree, practical experience in the field of orthotics and prosthetics, and completion of a residency program or one-year supervised work. Many more math, science, and computer courses are needed, so prospective technicians thinking of advancing to the practitioner level, should keep that in mind. For more information on the career of a practitioner, see the chapter "Orthotist and Prosthetist."

High school students interested in the prosthetics and orthotics field might also want to work with a high school teacher or guidance counselor to arrange a visit to an orthotic and prosthetic fabrication facility or the orthotics and prosthetics department at a local hospital. This would allow the student to watch technicians at work and to talk with them about their jobs.

Postsecondary Training

There are two paths to becoming an orthotic and prosthetic technician. The first, and most common, is to begin a two-year program of supervised clinical experience. Basically, this amounts to on-the-job training during which the trainee learns the methods of fabricating an orthosis or prosthesis. During the training, he or she must work under the supervision of a certified orthotist, certified prosthetist, or certified orthotist-prosthetist. Depending on the department and the supervisor, the technician-in-training may work in both orthotics and prosthetics or in just one of the two disciplines. The two-year training program ends with the trainee achieving technician status.

The second method of becoming a technician is far less common. In this method, interested students enroll in a one- or two-year training program of formal instruction and practical clinical experience. This program leads to the technician-in-training earning a certificate, or associate's degree, in orthotics-prosthetics technology. These programs usually offer courses in anatomy, physiology, material science, and fabrication, as well as supervised clinical experience.

Currently there are only two such technician-level programs in the United States that are accredited by the National Commission on Orthotic and Prosthetic Education (NCOPE). These programs are Spokane Falls Community College, in Spokane, Washington, and Northeast Metro Technical College, in White Bear Lake, Minnesota. Jeff is a graduate of the program at Northeast Metro Technical College. This method of learning to be an orthotic or prosthetic technician is less common mainly because of the scarcity of programs available.

certification or licensing

Currently licensing is not required for orthotic and prosthetic technicians. Certification, while not required, is recommended. Certification takes place through a registration program conducted by the American Board for Certification in Orthotics and Prosthetics, Inc. (ABC).

In order to qualify for registration, the technician must first meet the educational and work experience requirements discussed in the previous section. In addition, all candidates must take and pass a certifying examination administered by the board. The exam is given three times each year and consists of two parts. The first part is a one-hour multiple choice written test, and the second part is a seven-hour practical exam designed to assess the technician's skills and knowledge. Depending on their area of concentration, technicians who pass the exam are designated registered technician (orthotics), registered technician (prosthetics), or registered technician (orthotics-prosthetics).

> There's nothing like it when you get a handshake or a hug from a grateful kid.

When Jeff suggested that a registered technician should be involved in administering and scoring the practical exam for the orthotic-prosthetic technicians, the testing administrators agreed. They asked him to do just that on the fall and spring examinations. "It was nice to give something back to the field," he says of the experience.

Technicians may retain their registered status by paying an annual renewal fee. There is, however, no continuing education requirement. Registered technicians receive a subscription to both the monthly *O & P Almanac* and the newsletter *O & P Now.* More significantly, perhaps, registered technicians tend to receive a higher rate of pay than those technicians without certification. The probability of higher pay makes the certification process well worth considering.

who will hire me?

Hospitals and other medical institutions are a major source of jobs for orthotic and prosthetic technicians. Often, these facilities have their own orthotics and prosthetics departments, complete with machine shop. Another large employer of orthotic and prosthetic technicians is the private orthotic-prosthetic fabrication facility. Private facilities work under contract with HMOs and hospitals that do not have their own orthotic-prosthetic departments. Finally, orthotic and prosthetic technicians may work in rehabilitation centers, especially those that specialize in orthopaedic surgery and orthotic and prosthetic work.

Many hospitals, private fabrication facilities, and rehabilitation centers sponsor in-house training programs like those discussed in the section on education. One of the best ways to find out which institutions and companies offer these programs is to contact their personnel departments.

Graduates of the one- or two-year training programs in orthotics and prosthetics may find their job search somewhat easier for several reasons. First, the technicians in these programs are taught by certified practitioners in orthotics and prosthetics who are familiar with, and work in, the orthotics and prosthetics industry. These contacts can be very helpful to the new technician looking for a job. Second, because of the school's status as a training center for orthotic and prosthetic technicians, hospitals, rehab centers, and private companies are more likely to go directly to one of these schools when searching for new technicians. Finally, the placement offices at these institutions work hard to find jobs for their newly graduating technicians.

Prospective orthotic and prosthetic technicians might consider subscribing to publications geared toward the orthotics and prosthetics industry. Many of these publications feature classified advertisement sections in which employers advertise job openings for technicians and practitioners.

where can I go from here?

Depending on the size of the facility, an orthotic or prosthetic technician may advance quickly to a supervisory position. In larger facilities, technicians advance relatively more slowly, because they have more positions to advance through.

In the orthotics department where John works, for example, there is a specified advancement ladder. John has already advanced twice, first from junior plastics technician trainee to plastics technician, and then a second time from plastics technician to orthotic technician. The next level of advancement for him is to move up to senior orthotic technician. Eventually, he will gain the title of orthotic assistant. At that time, he can decide whether or not he is interested in going back to school to become an orthotist or prosthetist.

Short of enrolling in an NCOPE-accredited residency program for practitioners of orthotics and/or prosthetics, an orthotic and prosthetic technician can advance by specializing in a particular type of orthoses or prostheses, such as leg braces or prosthetic hands.

Jeff is happy where he is. "I put myself through school," he says. "And I just didn't have the time, money, or interest to go on and train to become a prosthetist," he explains. "Personally, I'm comfortable making the piece."

what are the salary ranges?

Although earnings depend on many factors, including expertise, experience, and geographic location, a technician in an entry-level position can expect to earn approximately $8 to $9 per hour. A technician with five to ten years experience could expect to earn roughly $11 to $13 per hour. A technician with ten or more years experience and a good record of employment showing his or her advancements can expect to earn between $15 and $20 per hour. Put in terms of an annual salary, an average technician with five years experience working a forty-hour week will earn approximately $23,000.

Technicians in the New England area are among the highest paid, with those in the western third of the country earning the second highest salaries. The most significant factor in salary levels among orthotic and prosthetic technicians, however, is certification. Technicians with certification earn, on the average, $3 more per hour than do those technicians without certification—which translates into a difference of $6,000 per year. Sometimes, however, hospitals or other medical institutions do not honor or recognize the distinctions of certification.

what is the job outlook?

The health care industry is thriving, and the employment of physicians and technicians in almost all fields is expected to grow much faster than the average for all occupations through the year 2005.

Specifically, the future looks good for orthotic and prosthetic technicians. An increasing number of people are now receiving access to medical and rehabilitative care through private and public insurance programs, and more will do so in the coming years as baby boomers age and develop injuries, illnesses, and diseases that make them candidates for orthoses and prostheses. For example, in the United States 1.5 million people have amputations each year, and that number is expected to increase as the population ages.

In addition, as medical technology advances to create life- and limb-saving techniques, patients with new and different disabilities will need new and different orthoses and prostheses to help them regain an active life. This need translates into more technician-level jobs in the orthotic-prosthetic industry.

how do I learn more?

professional organizations

Following are organizations that provide information on the professions of orthotic and prosthetic technicians.

American Academy of Orthotists and Prosthetists
1650 King Street, Suite 500
Alexandria, VA 22314
TEL: 703-836-7118
WEBSITE: http://www.oandp.com/academy

American Orthotic and Prosthetic Association
1650 King Street, Suite 500
Alexandria, VA 22314
TEL: 703-836-7116

American Board for Certification in Orthotics and Prosthetics
1650 King Street, Suite 500
Alexandria, VA 22314
TEL: 703-836-7114

bibliography

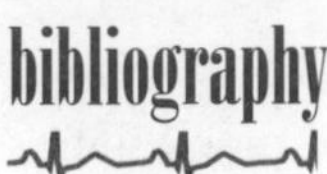

Following is a sampling of books and periodicals relating to the professional concerns and development of orthotic technicians and prosthetic technicians.

Books

Redford, John B., John V. Basmajian, and Paul Trautman, editors. *Orthotics: Clinical Practice and Rehabilitation Technology.* New York, NY: Churchill Livingstone, 1995.

Shankman, Albert L. *Fundamental Orthopedic Management for the Physical Therapist Assistant.* St. Louis, MO: Mosby, 1996.

Shurr, Donald G. *Prosthetics and Orthotics.* New York, NY: Appleton & Lange, 1990.

Periodicals

Journal of Prosthetics and Orthotics. Quarterly. Contains articles and reports from professionals on current topics in orthotics and prosthetics. American Academy of Orthotists and Prosthetists, 1650 King Street, Suite 500, Alexandria, VA 22314, 703-836-7116.

O & P Almanac. Monthly. Covers the professional, business, association, and government activities affecting the field. American Orthotic and Prosthetic Association, 1650 King Street, Suite 500, Alexandria, VA 22314, 703-836-7114.

orthotist and prosthetist

Definition

Orthotists design, make, and fit braces to support the spine or limbs weakened by illness. Prosthetists design, make, and fit artificial limbs for persons missing an arm, leg, or other body part as a result of injury or illness.

Salary range

$30,000 to $60,000 to $120,000

Educational requirements

Bachelor's degree, one year in a certified Orthotics and/or Prosthetics residency program or one year clinical experience under an ABC-certified practitioner

GOE
05.05.11

DOT
078

Certification or Licensing

Certification highly recommended; licensing mandatory in some states

Outlook

Much faster than average

High School Subjects

Biology
Chemistry
English
Mathematics
Shop classes

Personal Interests

Designing and problem solving
Helping people
Working with your hands
Working with technology

Waiting anxiously while his orthopaedic surgeon conferred with the prosthetist in the hallway just outside of his hospital room, Randall thought of all the things he would be able to do with his new prosthetic leg. He had had surgery seven times and had spent months recovering. Now he was about to be measured for the leg that would allow him to run, jump, dance, and drive a car again. A moment later, the prosthetist entered his room and introduced herself. Randall barely heard her. She smiled and took a seat next to the bed. For the next several minutes, Randall tried to suppress his excitement while keeping his mind focused on the questions she was asking during the exam and watching how she measured his thigh with calipers. Then she looked up at him. "Please," she said, "If you have any questions, ask them."

"How soon before I get to try it out?" Randall asked.

She smiled, "Is tomorrow afternoon too soon?"

Orthotists and prosthetists can help patients regain the ability to participate in almost any activity—from walking to rock climbing to golfing to playing tennis. Some orthotists and prosthetists also work to develop specialized devices made from sturdy, ultralight materials. These orthoses or prostheses can help athletes with disabilities achieve world-class performances. The Paralympic Games is known for attracting, from all over the world, elite athletes with disabilities. These athletes qualify and compete using guidelines similar to those of the Olympic Games, and their athletic abilities rival those of Olympic star athletes. Some lower-limb amputees, for example, run the 100-meter race only a split second slower than non-amputee sprinters.

what does an orthotist or a prosthetist do?

Every year in the United States, more than 125,000 people lose a limb to an accident or disease, and many others require special, corrective devices to help them perform activities ranging from eating and walking to playing a sport to pursuing a career. *Orthotists* evaluate and design braces and strengthening devices (known as an orthosis, plural orthoses) for those needing protective support or correction due to muscle/bone impairment, disease, or deformity. Prosthetists evaluate, design, and fabricate artificial limbs (a prosthesis, plural prostheses) for persons who have amputations due to accidents, birth abnormalities, or disabling diseases. Both practitioners work with their patients to make certain that the specific devices fit and are as comfortable as possible. Both practitioners are also members of a rehabilitation team that is dedicated to helping the patient regain his or her mobility, strength, and independence.

lingo to learn

AFO A brace supporting the ankle and foot area. The acronym stands for ankle-foot orthosis.

Anatomy A science dealing with the structure of organisms.

CAD/CAM computer programming that can be used to design and produce orthoses or prostheses.

Calipers A two hinged, adjustable instrument with curved legs that are used to measure thicknesses.

KAFO A brace supporting the knee-ankle-foot area. The acronym stands for knee-ankle-foot orthosis.

Kinesiology The study of human movement.

Orthotists work with patients of all ages who have a wide range of problems. Their patients may include an elderly woman who has suffered a stroke, a child with muscular dystrophy, and an accident victim with a damaged back. In each case, the orthotist needs to create a custom brace to match the precise specifications of the individual patient. A patient may come to the orthotist's office with a prescription from a physician for a particular orthosis, or the physician may send the prescription to the orthotist and ask that he or she visit the patient in the hospital or at the nursing home or at the patient's home. The prescription only tells the orthotist the specifics of the patient's problem and which orthosis the physician would like created for the patient. For example, the prescription might only say, "Fit Patient X with an AFO." The orthotist knows that an AFO is an ankle/foot orthosis and so has an idea of what type of device is needed. The orthotist then meets with the patient to evaluate the problem firsthand, take measurements for the orthoses, and may then make revisions to the original prescription based on the evaluation of the patient. The orthotist discusses any revisions he or she has made with the physician.

Prosthetists work in a similar fashion, although their patients are amputees who have lost, for example, a hand or an arm or a foot. These patients may be diabetic (or suffering from some other type of vascular disease which results in poor circulation and, subsequently, amputation of a limb), or they may be trauma victims who have lost a limb in an accident. Like orthotists, prosthetists work from prescriptions written by a patient's physician. Prosthetists may suggest changes to the prescription based upon their evaluation of the patient and his or her situation.

The orthotist's evaluation includes several steps. First the orthotist reads the patient's chart to see if other problems might complicate, or be affected by, the use of an orthosis. The orthotist conducts manual muscle testing, which is a testing of the strength of different muscle groups (hamstrings, biceps, etc.). The orthotist also checks the patient's range of motion and assesses any gait problems. Based on such tests, the orthotist determines if an orthosis can remedy whatever problem exists. Other decisions, such as the type of orthosis to use and if the bracing system should be rigid or allow for movement, are also made at this time.

The prosthetist's evaluation is done in a similar manner. The prosthetist takes the patient's past medical history, notes any medical complications, and performs physical testing of the patient to determine the best type of prosthesis.

During the evaluation, both orthotists and prosthetists use tape measures, calipers, and other precision measurement tools to measure the area of the patient's body for which an orthosis or prosthesis will be made. The orthotist takes these measurements back to the laboratory to make an impression in plaster. Sometimes the orthotist uses the patient's ankle, leg, or arm to make the cast, wrapping the patient's limb with plaster and material just as if applying a cast to a broken limb. If the brace is unusual or complex, the orthotist might make drawings or blueprints of the proposed orthosis. In either case, the orthotist then fabricates the orthosis or supervises a technician in fabricating it.

Sometimes the measurements alone are used to create the orthosis. For example, the physician of an accident victim with an injured spine will write a prescription for a back brace. If the patient has just had surgery, the physician will want that brace on the patient as soon as possible. The orthotist would immediately take the patient's measurements and create the brace. On the other hand, if an ankle-foot orthosis were prescribed, the orthotist would actually wrap the patient's foot in a plaster cast, allow it to dry to form a negative mold of the patient's foot and ankle, and remove the mold. The orthotist would then take the mold back to the lab and have a technician fill the mold with plaster in order to create a positive mold of the patient's foot and ankle. Only after that would the ankle-foot brace be fabricated.

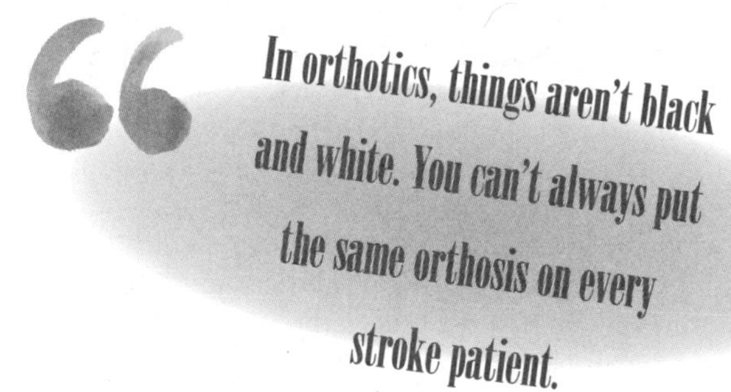

The prosthetist, however, must take measurements of the remaining limb (also known as the residual limb) from which he or she will create a plastic impression of that limb. The prosthetist takes these measurements back to the laboratory, where a technician fills the cast with a thermoplastic material that is somewhat malleable and can be adjusted. The prosthetist then returns to the patient with this transparent cast and places it on the patient's residual limb. Through the transparent plastic, the prosthetist can see how well it fits. High and low pressure points (that is, where the skin presses into the plastic, where a large gap exists between the cast and the skin) are clearly visible to the prosthetist, and he or she marks these points on the cast with a pencil. Later, these marks will help the technician to craft a better fitting prosthesis.

After the cast is modified with any corrections, the prosthesis is made from it. As the patient uses the prosthetic limb, the prosthetist assesses the patient's movement and makes any further alterations necessary for a good fit. If all goes well, the patient goes to physical therapy with the new limb to learn how to use it.

Orthotists and prosthetists also use computer programming, called Computer-Aided Design/Computer-Aided Manufacture (more commonly referred to as CAD/CAM), to design and fabricate orthoses or prostheses. They can either keyboard the patient's measurements into a computer or scan the patient's limb with an optical scanner to input the measurements directly into the computer. The computer produces a detailed, three-dimensional blueprint of the orthosis or prosthesis needed. The blueprint is then fed into a machine that shapes the device.

Orthotists and prosthetists select materials for each orthosis or prosthesis to match the needs of the patient. Considerations range from the patient's height and weight to the patient's activities. Materials used in the construction of orthoses and prostheses include wood, foam, plastics, fabric, steel, aluminum, fiberglass, and leather, as well as newer, composite materials, such as carbon-graphite. Orthotists and prosthetists use hand and power tools, such as saws, drills, and sewing machines, to skillfully manipulate these materials into the desired designs. They may glue, bolt, weld, sew, and rivet parts together or take advantage of advanced thermoforming techniques (techniques using heat) to mold and form parts. Straps or velcro may be added to help customize the fit.

The patient has several fitting sessions with the orthotist or prosthetist to ensure the best fit and maximum comfort of the finished orthosis or prosthesis. The orthotist or prosthetist may work alone or with the patient's entire rehabilitation team. This team may include the the patient's physician, a physical therapist, an occupational therapist, an orthopaedic surgeon, and a physical medicine and rehabilitation doctor, also known as a PMR. The orthotist and prosthetist evaluate the fit, alignment, and stability of the orthosis or prosthesis, and check to see that it functions as intended, making adjustments as needed. They teach the patient how to put on and use the orthosis or prosthesis, and how to adjust the velcro straps or buckles that enhance the custom fit of the device. In addition, the orthotist and prosthetist make certain that the patient finds the device usable, comfortable, and aesthetically acceptable. Finally, the finished orthosis or prosthesis must be approved by the physician who prescribed it.

Prosthetists are also involved in the development and creation of myoelectric and externally-powered prostheses. A patient with a myoelectric prosthesis can utilize the electrical impulses of his or her muscles to power a prosthetic limb. To accomplish this, an electrode is placed on the skin over a muscle. When the patient contracts that muscle, the electrode picks up and amplifies the electrical activity from the muscle. This electrical signal then activates a battery-powered motor in the prosthetic that causes the device to move.

At present, myoelectric prostheses are used exclusively on the upper-body, primarily because the fine motor skills of the hand lend themselves more easily to myoelectrics. Because of the many tasks that we accomplish with our hands and fingers, the muscles here are more finely developed. Also, the myoelectric systems are not very durable. Used on the hand and upper-body, they do not experience as much wear and tear as they would if they were trying to power a prosthetic leg. Externally-powered prostheses use motors, not electrodes, and these prostheses are generally used on higher-level amputations, such as the shoulder or upper-arm.

Myoelectric and externally-powered prostheses are made the same way as regular prostheses. After fitting the patient with the prosthetic, the prosthetist also fits the patient with electrodes. Then the prosthetist analyzes the function of the prosthetic, a hand-elbow for example, and adjusts the electrodes until the device works smoothly. After this, the patient just needs time and practice with the prosthetic limb.

Patients usually return to the same orthotist or prosthetist for replacement braces or limbs or for future adjustments. In particular, the orthoses or prostheses made for children need to be adjusted as the child grows. Eventually these devices are replaced by new ones.

more lingo to learn

Myoelectrics Technology using electrical impulses from muscles to trigger a motorized component in a prosthesis which, in turn, causes the prosthesis to move.

Rivet A small bolt of metal with a head on one end. It is used to join two or more pieces of material (such as leather or metal) together. The rivet is passed through a hole in each piece of material. The plain end of the bolt is then beaten down to make a second head, which secures the materials.

Thermoforming Using heat and sometimes pressure to shape a substance such as plastic.

what is it like to be an orthotist or a prosthetist?

"There's a tangible end result," says Mark Edwards of his work as a certified prosthetist. "The person ends up walking or using the prosthesis." All day long, prosthetists see patients who have lost a limb. A majority of these patients are diabetic and have poor circulation. Others smoke or are obese and, as a result, also have poor circulation in their extremities. In any of these cases the poor circulation can lead to amputation of a hand or foot. Still other patients have been in accidents that claimed a limb. "The patients aren't usually in acute-care when we visit them for an evaluation," Mark says. "But you may talk to them about a pre-prosthesis." A pre-prosthesis, or temporary prosthesis, is a device that is worn at first for short periods of time to accustom the residual limb to it. When the tissues of the residual limb have healed completely, the permanent prosthesis can be developed.

To be a successful orthotist or prosthetist, you should

- Enjoy helping people
- Have good hand-eye coordination and manual dexterity
- Be able to listen and communicate well
- Be able to demonstrate compassion
- Be able to collaborate with others

Following the evaluation, the prosthetist does a casting of the patient's residual limb. "By taking a plastic impression of the residual limb, you can identify those areas that might be pressure sensitive, like bony areas," explains Mark. "The plastic impression is like a cast, but thinner, with no padding."

Back in the laboratory, a technician fills the cast and modifications are made based on the prosthetist's notes. "If it fits, we set it up on an adjustable leg or an alignment fixture and the patient tries it out while we assess his gait pattern. By working with the prosthetist and physical therapist, the patient learns how to walk easily and naturally." Mark adds, "The greatest innovations have occurred in technology and cosmetics."

A typical day for Mark is spent supervising and administering the certificate program in prosthetics at Northwestern University Medical School, Prosthetic-Orthotic Center, in Chicago, Illinois. As the Director of Prosthetic Education, it is his duty to see to it that students enrolled in the program are learning the required coursework. From 8 AM until 4 PM most days, Mark is somewhere on campus. He might be delivering a lecture, supervising fabrication in the prosthetic laboratory, or in the middle of clinical work with patients and students. On some days, he also sees patients at the Rehabilitation Institute of Chicago.

Bryan Malas, a certified orthotist, loves his work. "The best thing about this work, besides helping patients, is the versatility of the job. You're always doing something different. Either you're in the lab, you're with patients, you're giving lectures, and on and on. There's no monotony." He currently spends 20 percent of his time with patients and 80 percent of his time teaching or occupied with administrative tasks. Bryan is Director of Orthotic Education at Northwestern University Medical School and his days are similar to Mark Edwards'. Administrative duties take up a good portion of his time, duties which he describes as, "putting out fires, answering calls, and helping students." Often, he says, he either stays late to finish writing his lectures, or he works on them at home. In addition to teaching, he is responsible for creating and coordinating class schedules, devising the curriculum, and monitoring the students' interaction with patients in clinics.

For these clinics, the school hires professional patients to work with the students. These people are called "professional patients" because, due their experience living with orthoses, they know almost more about the devices than the students do. The school asks them to come back every semester to help the students learn. In return, they are paid a small stipend for their time. The professional patients have real case histories that the students evaluate. Students then come up with recommendations for new orthotic devices. Eventually, the students fabricate the orthoses they believe the patients should have. They then fit the patients with the devices they have created. "The presentation of the orthosis is very stressful," Bryan says. "The students present their orthoses in front of everyone, but they learn so much. They're critiqued by everyone, including the patient."

Learning from the patients is a powerful example, according to Bryan. In addition to practical technical knowledge, students learn how to listen to the patient's input. "Most kids out of a four-year college are used to right and wrong answers. In orthotics, things aren't black and white. You can't always put the same orthosis on every stroke patient," explains Bryan. "The textbook is usually the ideal situation, which is a good starting point. But it's not always the way to get the best results." One of the most important aspects of school is the interaction students have with real patients during the clinics. According to Bryan, "It's challenging. The student sees patients with deficits, learns all the information about them, and then chooses the best orthoses to improve the patients' problems."

Most practitioners of orthotics and prosthetics, however, do not teach. Bryan describes what a typical day might include for a certified orthotist (CO) or certified prosthetist (CP) working at an orthotic-prosthetic facility. "He might respond to phone calls or focus on getting contracts with HMOs. He would undoubtedly see patients, making hospital visits or house calls, as necessary." Depending on the size of the facility, the CO or CP might be helped with the fabrication of orthoses or prostheses by assistants or technicians.

have I got what it takes to be an orthotist or a prosthetist?

"You need to be able to collaborate with others," says Bryan. "It's best when the whole medical team is involved and everyone sits down to come together for a common goal—to help the patient. When everyone's involved, all facets of the picture are represented." Orthotists and prosthetists work closely with members of the rehabilitation team. They should be able to function equally well by themselves and in small to large groups. The orthotist and prosthetist must not be intimidated by physicians or surgeons but must be able to speak his or her mind clearly and firmly, if necessary.

Although many patients justly view an orthosis or prosthesis as a means of regaining normal lives, many new patients, as well as familiar patients, may understandably voice fear, concern, or even embarrassment or anger at the prospect of using an orthosis or prosthesis. Orthotists and prosthetists need to develop and demonstrate compassion and sensitivity when dealing with patients. "You have to have empathy and enjoy working with people," says Mark. "It's not enough to have the necessary knowledge. You need to be a good communicator, too." Orthotists and prosthetists need to be able to explain technical issues to the patient, so that the patient, in turn, can communicate whether or not a device is working as it should.

Patience is also necessary when dealing with patients who are trying to adjust to a new device. Practitioners need to remind themselves that although they, themselves, may have conducted a thousand evaluations or fittings, this is the first time for the patient. He or she may need time to emotionally adjust and to practice with the device.

"You're always doing something different....There's no monotony."

how do I become an orthotist or a prosthetist?

education

High School

Anyone interested in becoming an orthotist or a prosthetist should take high school courses that are college preparatory. Mathematics classes such as algebra and geometry will be useful. Also of importance are biology, physics, and chemistry classes. These classes will familiarize you with basic anatomy and the properties of various materials. Computer science courses will prepare you for a future career in which you will make use of technology. Shop classes in metal, plastic, or wood may also offer the opportunity to work with many materials the orthotist or prosthetist uses in creating braces or artificial limbs. In addition, English classes that teach communication, research, and writing skills are essential to take. These skills will help you in your college years and, later, when you begin to work with patients and other health professionals.

Postsecondary Training

Your next step to becoming an orthotist or a prosthetist is to receive a college degree. You may choose to get a bachelor of science (B.S.) degree in orthotics and prosthetics from an NCOPE-accredited school. (NCOPE is the National Commission on Orthotic and Prosthetic Education.) Or you may get a bachelor of art (B.A.) or B.S. degree in any field. If you take your B.A. or B.S. degree in a field other than orthotics and prosthetics, you will then need to complete a one year certificate program following college. In either case, your college course work should include classes in anatomy, biology, chemistry, computer science, physics, math, and English.

After receiving a college degree, and completing the one year certificate program if necessary, the next step taken by most practitioners is to enter a one year clinical residency program. These programs are also NCOPE accredited and a listing of them can be requested from this organization (see Professional Organizations for the address).

Another option for someone pursuing an orthotist or prosthetist career is to do what is commonly called a 1900 hour program. The 1900 hour program is a one-year clinical experience under the supervision of an ABC-certified practitioner. (ABC stands for American Board for Certification in Orthotics and Prosthetics, Inc.)

Residency programs are much more commonly done, however, due to their excellent structure and organization. Currently there are nineteen NCOPE-accredited residency programs in both orthotics and prosthetics; eleven in orthotics only; and six in prosthetics only.

In addition to a college degree, students should be aware that most orthotic and prosthetic residency programs usually do not accept candidates who lack prior experience in either field. Bryan suggests that students work for an orthotic or prosthetic facility. "Following a tech or practitioner around is a great way to learn. The more interaction with the orthotist or prosthetist, the better."

Both Mark and Bryan worked with prostheses and orthoses early in their careers. Mark first started working with amputees as a physical therapist at the Veterans Administration Hospital. Bryan's mother was a physical therapist who knew the local orthotist and managed to get him a job there after school at age thirteen. He worked in the facility, filling impressions and cleaning up the laboratory. While working there, he became interested in pursuing the field as a career.

"We look for the best combination of education and practical experience," Mark says of the candidates who apply for admission to the residency program at Northwestern University Medical School, Prosthetic-Orthotic Center. "Good advice for prospective students," he says, "is to start out at a facility and train to be a technician."

After a residency or clinical supervision program, ABC certification is the final step to becoming a certified professional. Although ABC certification is not mandatory, it is highly recommended.One benefit of certification is that it will increase the number of employers willing to hire you. In fact, some employers, such as the Department of Veterans Affairs, require certification for employment.

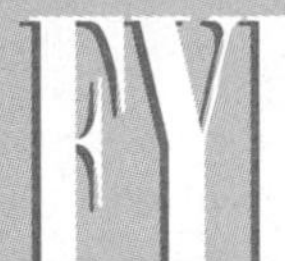

Cost of Amputations

Studies have shown that every dollar spent on rehabilitation, including orthotic and prosthetic care, saves more than $11 in long-term care health-costs. Rehabilitation enables patients to resume active daily lives, which can include returning home and to work or school. It is estimated that the 49 million people in the United States who have disabilities represent $700 billion in income, from which they return huge funds to society through taxes and economic activity.

Conversely, if long-term care is required, institutionalization can cost $25,000 to $50,000 per patient per year; adult day care can be $10,000 per patient per year; and custodial care at home can cost more than $7,000 per patient per year.

All statistics are from the Orthotists and Prosthetists National Office, 1650 King Street, Suite 500, Alexandria, VA 22314

certification or licensing

Depending on the state, licensing may be required for an orthotist or a prosthetist. Practitioners will need to check with the laws of the state in which they intend to practice for licensing requirements.

Certification, as mentioned in the previous section, is highly recommended. The American Board for Certification in Orthotics and Prosthetics, Inc. grants three credentials. These credentials are certified orthotist (CO), certified prosthetist (CP), and certified prosthetist-orthotist (CPO).

To earn certification in either or both fields, practitioners must hold a degree from an accredited four-year college or university, have successfully completed an accredited residency or clinical supervision program, and have at least one year of patient management experience. In addition, candidates for certification must pass a written examination, a written simulation, and a three-day clinical examination that tests their abilities to design, fabricate, and fit a variety of orthoses and prostheses.

Every five years, certified practitioners renew their credentials by demonstrating their knowledge of the latest developments in technology and patient management by meeting continuing education requirements.

scholarships and grants

Students interested in learning about scholarships and grants for study in orthotics and/or prosthetics, should contact the following organizations.

NCOPE
1650 King Street, Suite 500
Alexandria, VA 22314
TEL: 703-836-7114

Orthotic and Prosthetic Educational and Development Fund, Inc.
1650 King Street, Suite 500
Alexandria, VA 22314
TEL: 703-836-7114

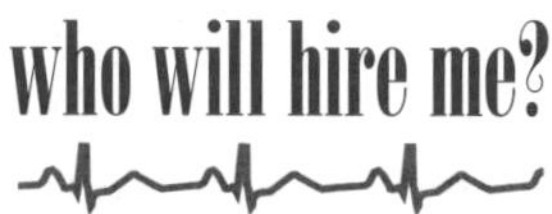

Orthotists and prosthetists work in several different practice settings. Many are self-employed in private practice. Others work in privately-owned laboratories, at hospitals, in rehabilitation clinics, or for government agencies. In a small facility, the orthotist or prosthetist alone might evaluate, design, and custom-fit a patient's device. At a larger facility that has numerous staff members, the orthotist or prosthetist might be assisted by an orthotic or prosthetic technician who would help with the fabrication and production of each device. In such cases the orthotist or prosthetist has more time to see and work with patients.

A small number of orthotists and prosthetists also teach. In addition to teaching, administration is another area where orthotists and prosthetists can work. After accumulating experience, orthotists or prosthetists may go into administration, directing or supervising the training programs.

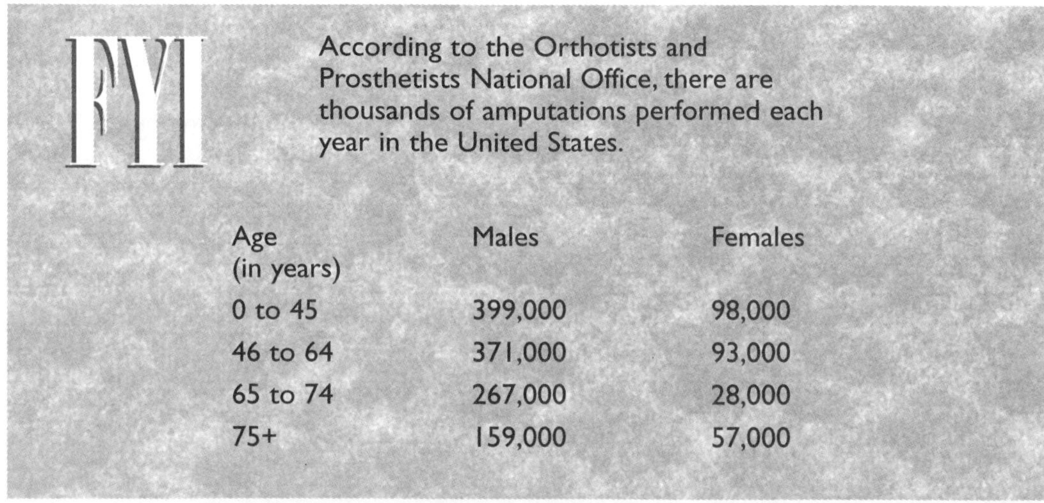

FYI

According to the Orthotists and Prosthetists National Office, there are thousands of amputations performed each year in the United States.

Age (in years)	Males	Females
0 to 45	399,000	98,000
46 to 64	371,000	93,000
65 to 74	267,000	28,000
75+	159,000	57,000

where can I go from here?

Orthotists and prosthetists who work for themselves can work to increase the size of their companies and facilities by expanding the number of clients for whom they work. If the practitioners are employed by private or government agencies, they can advance to supervisory positions. The same is true for those practitioners who teach in residency programs. Most practitioners like to do a combination of these activities, especially by maintaining at least a small practice to keep their diagnostic skills up to date.

what are the salary ranges?

Salaries for both types of practitioners will vary according to the size and type of facility, as well as the geographic location. On the average, practitioners who work for hospitals or an orthotic-prosthetic facility earn between $30,000 and $70,000, depending on their expertise and the number of years they have been in the field.

Those practitioners who work on their own earn substantially more than those who work for others. These practices can be extremely lucrative, but success does hinge on the practitioner's ability to draw new clients to his or her business. Salaries for independent practitioners usually range between $60,000 and $120,000 per year.

what is the job outlook?

In general, the health care industry is thriving and the employment of practitioners, technologists, and technicians, in almost all fields, is expected to grow faster than the average for all occupations through the year 2005.

In March of 1996, there were approximately 3,000 ABC-certified practitioners of orthotics and prosthetics in the United States. According to a 1991 National Health Interview study, approximately 1.5 million patients require orthotic and/or prosthetic care and management. Mark reports that the future of the field looks good for two reasons. "One, the number of individuals with amputations will only increase as the baby boomer generation ages. And two, the current number of graduates won't keep up with the increase in amputee patients."

Advancements in technology and new, lightweight materials will only increase the value of those individuals who can design and fabricate attractive orthoses and prostheses. "CAD/CAM is definitely pushing the profession in a new direction," Mark says of prosthetics. "It's changing from a craft to a science."

how do I learn more?

professional organizations

Following are organizations that provide information on the profession of orthotist and prosthetist and accredited schools.

American Academy of Orthotists and Prosthetists
1650 King Street, Suite 500
Alexandria, VA 22314
TEL: 703-836-7118
WEBSITE: http://www.oandp.com/academy

American Board for Certification in Orthotics and Prosthetics, Inc.
1650 King Street, Suite 500
Alexandria, VA 22314
TEL: 703-836-7114

NCOPE
1650 King Street, Suite 500
Alexandria, VA 22314
TEL: 703-836-7114

bibliography

Following is a sampling of materials relating to the professional concerns and development of orthotist and prosthetists.

Books

American Academy of Orthopaedic Surgeons Staff. *Atlas of Orthotics Assistive Devices*, 3rd edition. St. Louis, MO: Mosby, 1996.

Geering, Alfred H., Martin Kundert, and Charles Kelsey, editors. *Complete Denture and Overdenture Prosthetics.* New York, NY: Thieme Medical Publishers, 1993.

Lucas, Michael S., and Paul Martin. *Attachments for Prosthetic Dentistry: Introduction and Application.* Carol Stream, IL: Quintessence Publishing Co., 1995.

MacGregor, A. Roy. *Clinical Dental Prosthetics,* 3rd edition. Newton, MA: Butterworth-Heinemann, 1989.

Nawoczenski, Deborah A., and Marcia E. Epler. *Orthotics in Functional Rehabilitation of the Lower Limb.* Philadelphia, PA: W.B. Saunders, 1997.

Redford, John B., John V. Basmajian, and Paul Trautman, editors. *Orthotics: Clinical Practice and Rehabilitation Technology.* New York, NY: Churchill Livingstone, 1995.

Shurr, Donald G. *Prosthetics and Orthotics.* New York, NY: Appleton & Lange, 1990.

Thomas, Keith F. *Prosthetic Rehabilitation.* Carol Stream, IL: Quintessence Publishing Co., 1994.

Periodicals

Journal of Prosthetic Dentistry. Monthly. New techniques, evaluation of dental materials, and patient psychology. Academy of Prosthodontics, Mosby, 11830 Westline Industrial Drive, St. Louis, MO 63146, 314-872-8370. 800-324-4177.

Journal of Prosthetics and Orthotics. Quarterly. Presents articles and reports from professionals on current topics in orthotics and prosthetics. American Academy of Orthotists and Prosthetists, 1650 King Street, Suite 500, Alexandria, VA 22314, 703-836-7116.

Journal of Prosthodontics. Quarterly. Contains original articles, reviews of new techniques and instrumentation, and instructive case reports. American College of Prosthodontists, W.B. Saunders Co., Curtis Center, 3rd Floor, Independence Square West, Philadelphia, PA 19106, 215-238-7800.

O & P Almanac. Monthly. Covers professional, business, association, and government activities affecting the field. American Orthotic and Prosthetic Association, 1650 King Street, Suite 500, Alexandria, VA 22314, 703-836-7114.

osteopathic physician

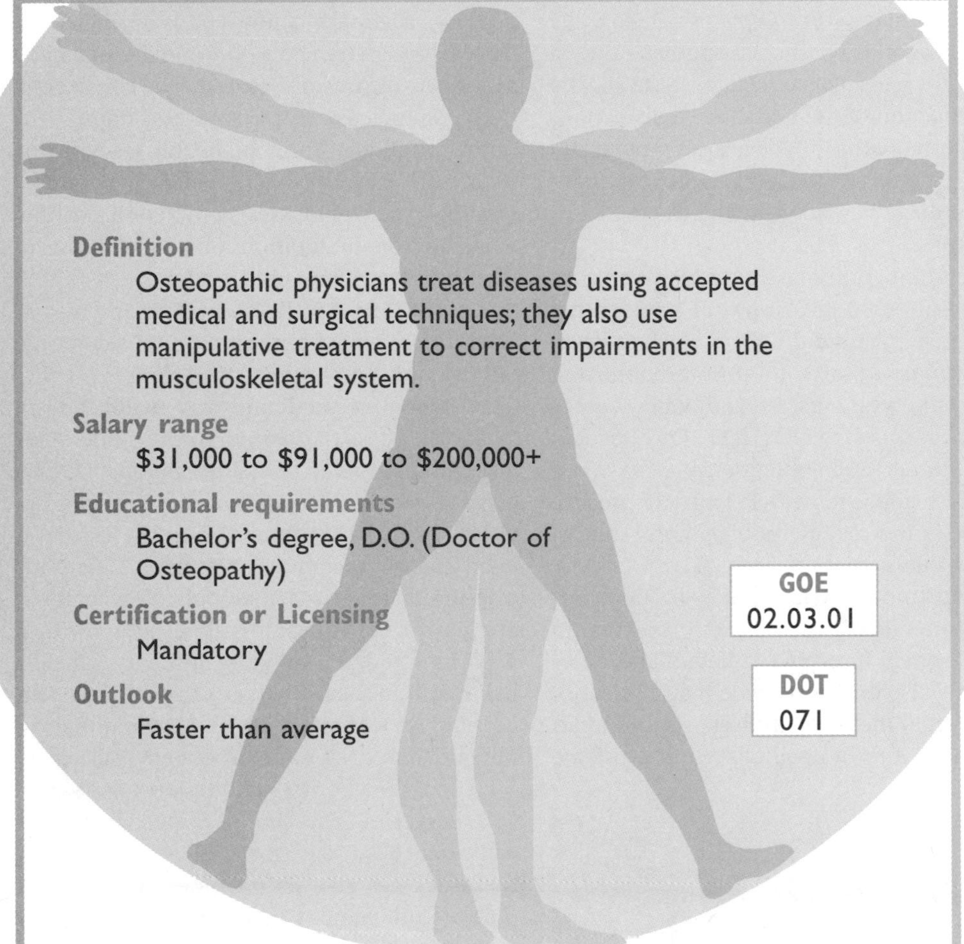

Definition

Osteopathic physicians treat diseases using accepted medical and surgical techniques; they also use manipulative treatment to correct impairments in the musculoskeletal system.

Salary range

$31,000 to $91,000 to $200,000+

Educational requirements

Bachelor's degree, D.O. (Doctor of Osteopathy)

Certification or Licensing

Mandatory

Outlook

Faster than average

GOE
02.03.01

DOT
071

High School Subjects

Biology
Chemistry
Mathematics
Physics

Personal Interests

Science
Health and fitness
Helping people

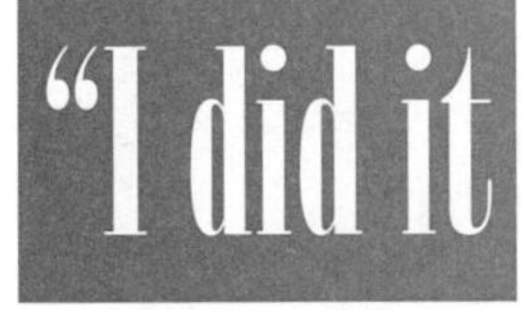

"I did it while stepping down off a forklift," said Bill, as he gingerly made his way to the examining table. Dr Pappas helps Bill ease down and carefully inspects the ankle. "You sure did, Bill. Looks like a nasty sprain. Let's begin with some ice for the swelling and then we'll progress with further treatments. Say, how's that shoulder of yours doing?"

Bill, a warehouse worker at a local food processing plant, has sought out the services of his trusted doctor. Dr George Pappas, however, is not your typical physician. The initials after the name on his license are D.O., not M.D., yet he has all the professional responsibilities and privileges of a medical doctor. Dr. Pappas is an osteopathic physician and part of the growing field of osteopathic medicinc.

what does an osteopathic physician do?

Many people think osteopathic medicine is a medical specialty or a type of "alternative" medicine. It is neither. *Osteopathic physicians*, like chiropractors, place particular emphasis on the role of the musculoskeletal system in the healthy function of the body. But, unlike chiropractors, osteopathic physicians are trained and licensed to perform all aspects of medical care—including diagnosis, surgery, and the prescription of drugs.

For certain conditions, osteopathic physicians use a technique known as osteopathic manipulative treatment (OMT), which involves applying manual force to an interconnected network of nerves, muscles, and bones. Osteopathic doctors use their hands to apply traction, pressure, thrust, and counterforce to body systems. These applications relax muscles, relieve tenderness, and restore mobility and range of motion to joints and muscles.

Osteopathic physicians can be found in virtually all medical specialties, but most are in family practice, internal medicine, and pediatrics. They use the most modern and scientifically accepted methods of diagnosis and treatment. They work in hospitals, clinics, private offices, nursing homes, and other health care settings.

Osteopathic physicians treat a wide range of patients and ailments. They treat children with colds, elderly people with arthritis, athletes with sports-related injuries, new mothers and infants, or workers with occupational injuries.

It is the osteopathic philosophy that distinguishes osteopathic physicians from M.D.s. Osteopaths are trained to view the human body as a single organism. Because they consider all body systems as interrelated and dependent upon one another for good health. Osteopathic physicians have a holistic view of medicine, treating specific illnesses in the context of the whole person. In addition to using all forms of medical treatment, osteopaths use OMT to diagnose illness. Reflecting their interest in treating the whole patient, many osteopathic physicians become family practitioners.

Osteopathic medicine was established in 1892 by a physician named Andrew Still. After losing three sons to spinal meningitis, Dr. Still came to believe that some current medical practices were inadequate or even harmful. He developed his own method of treatment, which was comprised primarily of manipulative techniques applied to the musculoskeletal system. In a departure from the thinking of the day, Dr. Still believed that the body has a capacity for self-healing. He was one of the first proponents of physical fitness as a route to better overall health.

There are about 35,000 practitioners with D.O. degrees in the United States, compared with about 600,000 with an M.D. degree. Both of these degrees give their holders the right to practice medicine. However, there is a widespread ignorance of the osteopathic medical profession, not only of how it compares to traditional medical practice, but that it exists at all.

lingo to learn

Chiropractic a system of health care that emphasizes the relationship between the structure and the function of the body.

Holistic emphasizing the importance of the whole body and the interdependence of its parts.

Osteopathic manipulative treatment applying manual force to an interconnected network of nerves, muscles, and bones.

Palpation examining by touching to detect soft tissue changes or structural defects in the body.

Strain-counterstrain therapy an osteopathic treatment technique used to identify trigger points in the body and the use of manipulative techniques to relieve pain caused by these trigger points.

what is it like to be an osteopathic physician?

Dr. George Pappas is the medical director and co-owner of Tyler Medical Services, in St. Charles, Illinois. He is an osteopathic physician specializing in occupational medicine, or treating and preventing work-related illnesses and injuries. He views his specialty as being similar to that of a sports physician. "Treating injured workers is not unlike the way a team physician would treat an injured athlete . . . it's just that you have an industrial athlete . . . the challenges are the same, getting them back in the game as quickly as possible."

Tyler Medical Services is a comprehensive medical facility. On-site are two other osteopathic physicians, and a massage therapist, a physical therapist, and an occupational therapist. In addition, Dr. Pappas contracts out with three additional physicians: a neurologist, a neurosurgeon, and an orthopedic specialist. According to him, he does this to "provide a greater ability to treat people in a broader spectrum of care."

Dr. Pappas spends about 80 percent of his day with patients and about 20 percent attending to administrative work. He generally works fifty hours a week, with some Saturdays. In the course of a day he sees about thirty patients, half of which have musculoskeletal problems where he can apply osteopathic manipulative treatments, or what he calls, "hands-on medicine." He feels that this is the core of his practice—"the actual laying on of the hands, where you are touching a patient and providing them with hands-on medicine is very therapeutic. . . . You develop a link with the patient."

Like most osteopathic physicians, Dr. Pappas does not forsake traditional medical treatments when needed. He views these treatments as a part of his arsenal, an adjunct to osteopathic treatments. He will prescribe drugs and when faced with a severe condition, such as a herniated disk, will recommend a specialist, who may oftentimes be an M.D.

Most of the patients who have come in to his office are there because they feel like he actively involves them in decisions. According to Dr. Pappas, "they [patients] are seeking out osteopathic physicians because of their ability to include them in their decisions with health care."

Dr. Pappas quickly responds when you ask him what he likes most about being an osteopathic physician—it's "the reward of the satisfaction of a patient saying 'you made me feel better' . . . it's a high."

have I got what it takes to be an osteopathic physician?

The practice of osteopathy usually involves a lot of personal interaction and touch, which can make some patients feel uncomfortable. Osteopathic physicians need excellent communication skills to let patients know what is going on.

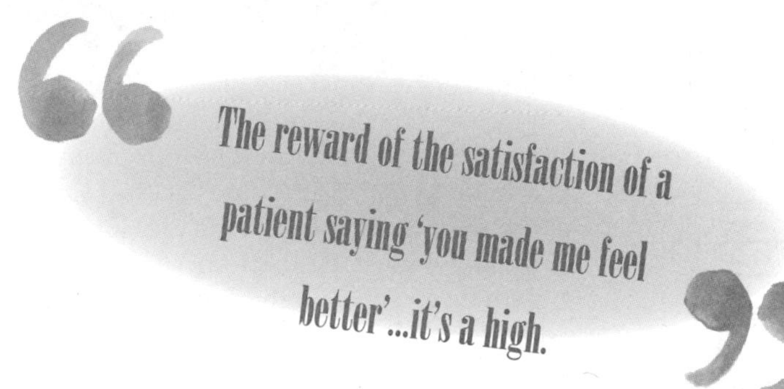

Good communication skills are also necessary to treat patients well. "You have to be able to communicate what your thoughts are," says Dr. Pappas, "if the patient does not understand what you're telling them, chances are they're not going to do what you tell them to do." Dr. Pappas also stresses the need to be a perceptive listener.

Since most osteopathic physicians work in private practices, business and management skills are very useful. You also need to work well with others. Having good manual dexterity is necessary to use osteopathic manipulative techniques effectively.

Most importantly, you need to have a true commitment to caring for people. Lesser goals may not provide sufficient motivation for the completion of difficult medical training.

how do I become an osteopathic physician?

After college graduation, Dr. Pappas worked at a YMCA health care facility. It was here that he was introduced to osteopathic medicine and became intrigued. He took the Medical College Admission Test (MCAT) and later got accepted into programs at an osteopathic as well as a traditional medical school. According to Dr. Pappas, he chose the Chicago College of Osteopathic Medicine because the "philosophies and principals [of osteopathy] fit with who I am."

education

High School

Students who plan to become doctors should take a college preparatory program in high school. You should have a good foundation in the sciences, especially biology, chemistry, and physics. You should also take English, foreign languages, and history. If possible, volunteer at a hospital or health care facility. This is an excellent way to observe the workings of a hospital and its staff, and to become acquainted with the health care community and its goals.

Postsecondary Training

It generally takes about eleven years to become a physician. Four years of premedical undergraduate courses include physics, biology, mathematics, organic and inorganic chemistry, and English. Premed students who wish to become osteopaths are strongly urged to take psychology, sociology, communications, and history. It is possible to enter an osteopathic school with only three years of undergraduate study, but most applicants have a bachelor's degree. Most schools recommend science majors for premed students.

After completion of the Medical College Admissions Test, the student studies another four years at an accredited osteopathic college. Currently, there are seventeen colleges of osteopathic medicine in the United States, compared to some 125 medical schools. Most of these schools are in the Midwest and Northeast, though there are some in Florida, Missouri, Texas, and California. Classes include biochemistry, anatomy, physiology, pharmacology, psychology, microbiology, pathology, and medical ethics. Students also learn the principles of osteopathic manipulation and palpatory diagnosis.

According the American Association of Colleges of Osteopathic Medicine, "The curriculum reflects the osteopathic philosophy, with an underlying emphasis on preventative, family, and community medicine. Clinical instruction emphasizes looking at all patient characteristics (including behavioral, environmental, etc.) and how various body systems interrelate." The philosophical basis of osteopathy is woven into the fabric of the curriculum, giving osteopathic students a holistic approach to health care.

After graduation from medical school, osteopathic students are expected to complete one year of rotating internship in such areas as internal medicine, obstetrics/gynecology, and surgery. Each year Dr. Pappas has several students rotate through his practice. Following rotations, students spend two to six years in residency training if a specialty is desired.

One of the difficulties facing the profession of osteopathy is that its schools produce more students than there are available spaces for residents in osteopathic hospitals. Graduates of osteopathic programs must increasingly find residencies in traditional medical facilities. Though increasing the awareness of osteopathy as a profession, some osteopathic physicians feel that residencies in traditional hospitals make it difficult to adhere to the osteopathic philosophy that is central to their training.

FYI

The single largest group (nearly 32 percent) of all practicing osteopathic physicians in the United States are in solo private practice.

certification or licensing

At an early point in the residency period, all physicians must pass a state medical board examination in order to obtain a license and enter practice. Each state sets its own requirements and issues its own licenses, though some states will accept licensing from certain other states.

Many osteopathic physicians belong to the American Osteopathic Association (AOA). To retain membership, physicians must complete 150 hours of continuing education every three years. Continuing education can be acquired in a variety of ways, including attending professional conferences, completing education programs sponsored by the AOA, osteopathic medical teaching, and publishing articles in professional journals. Dr. Pappas acquires many of his hours through teaching osteopathic medical students. He finds that teaching is the best way to stay current because "students are going to ask the best questions, they're going to challenge you, [and] they're going to make you stay in touch."

The AOA offers board certification. Certification has many requirements, including passing a comprehensive exam as well as a practical test where you must demonstrate osteopathic manipulative techniques. The AOA offers specialty certification in more than 100 specialties. Some osteopathic physicians are certified by both the AOA and the American Medical Association.

scholarships and grants

Scholarships and grants are often available from individual institutions, state agencies, and special-interest organizations. The book *Dollars for College: Medicine, Dentistry, and Related Fields* by Ferguson Publishing is an excellent source for this information. Many students finance their medical education through the Armed Forces Health Professions Scholarship Program. Each branch of the military participates in this program, paying students' tuitions in exchange for military service. Contact your local recruiting office for more information on this program. The National Health Service Corps Scholarship Program also provides money for students in return for service.

Ferguson Publishing Company
200 West Madison, Suite 300
Chicago, IL 60606
TEL: 312-580-5480

National Health Services Corps Scholarship Program
U.S. Public Health Service
1010 Wayne Avenue, Suite 240
Silver Spring, MD 20910
TEL: 800-638-0824

who will hire me?

Osteopathic physicians may begin their career in one of several ways. They may set up a private practice. This route is relatively rare because of the high cost and the need to establish a client base. Many osteopathic physicians begin by taking salaried jobs in group medical practices, clinics, or in health management organizations. These positions offer regular hours, a regular salary, and the opportunity for consultation with peers. After completing his residency, Dr. Pappas joined a private group medical practice as an associate.

To be a successful osteopathic physician you should

- Have excellent communication skills
- Be dedicated to helping others
- Be a very good listener
- Enjoy working with a variety of people
- Have good manual dexterity
- Be committed to completing an arduous training regimen, including osteopathic medical school, internship, and residency

Osteopathic physicians advance in earnings and stature as they build up a practice. Income usually rises substantially as the practice becomes established. Some osteopathic physicians continue their studies to quality for a specialty. These fields offer a higher income. Currently, Dr. Pappas is working on specialty certification in occupational medicine.

About 60 percent of all practicing osteopathic physicians are currently involved in direct patient care—in a hospital, clinic, or private practice. At present, only a handful of osteopaths are employed as consultants, but this may change as patients become aware of osteopathic options and demand access to osteopathic treatment.

Osteopathic physicians, who represent 5.5 percent of the total physician population in the U.S., comprise 10 percent of all U.S. military physicians. The federal government also employs osteopathic physicians as public health physicians. Government job listings are available in most state and federal institutions.

Sports medicine is a natural outgrowth of osteopathic practice, because of its focus on the musculoskeletal system, manipulative treatment, diet, exercise, and fitness. Many professional sports team physicians, Olympic physicians, and personal sports medicine physicians are osteopathic physicians.

where can I go from here?

Osteopathic physicians may work toward earning a specialty degree—in obstetrics or gynecology, for example—to better serve a general practice clientele. Some choose to go into administration so that they can influence hospital- and public-policy making. There is a also need for research on osteopathic medicine and techniques, and some osteopaths may find this path to be a rewarding alternative to patient care.

About a year after being hired as an associate, Dr. Pappas opened Tyler Medical Services. He offers a word of advice concerning hiring associates—"you have to realize that it is much more than just a business. You have to choose associates who have similar philosophies to you, because you are going to be judged on your group as a whole." Dr. Pappas has seen his practice grow tremendously and hopes to open another facility in the near future.

what are the salary ranges?

The national average salary for first-year residents in the mid-1990's was approximately $31,000. That average increased to $41,800 by the final residency year. Salaries will vary depending on the kind of residency, the hospital, and the geographic area.

According to surveys by the American Medical Association, practitioners of internal medicine in the mid-1990's had a salary range of approximately $95,000 to $200,000. The median income was about $130,000. These figures are for all doctors of internal medicine, and income for osteopathic physicians may vary from these numbers. Other factors that influence annual income include size and type of practice, hours worked per week, professional reputation of the individual, and the geographic location.

what is the job outlook?

The outlook for osteopathic physicians is bright. Population growth, longer life spans, and an increase in the number of people covered by medical insurance has contributed to the growing demand for osteopathic physicians. The greatest need is for primary care doctors—family practitioners, internists, pediatricians, and obstetricians. Since most osteopathic practitioners fall into these categories, the outlook for a continued demand for their services is good. Opportunities for new osteopathic physicians are opening up in rural regions, small towns, and the suburban areas.

The American Osteopathic Association estimates that there will be 45,000 osteopathic physicians practicing in the U.S. by the year 2000, up 10,000 from its current figure

how do I learn more?

For additional information on becoming an osteopathic physician, contact the following:

professional organizations

American Association of Colleges of Osteopathic Medicine
6110 Executive Blvd., Suite 405
Rockville, MD 20852
TEL: 301-468-0990
WEBSITE: http://www.aacom.org

American Osteopathic Association
142 E. Ontario Street
Chicago, IL 60611
TEL: 312-280-5800
WEBSITE: http://www. am-osteo-assn.org

bibliography

Following is a sampling of materials relating to the professional concerns and development of osteopathic physicians.

Books

Belshaw, Chris. *Osteopathy: Is It for You?* Rockport, MA: Element Books, 1993.

Ward, Robert C., and others, editors. *Foundations for Osteopathic Medicine.* Baltimore, MD: Williams & Wilkins, 1996.

Periodicals

Journal of Bone and Joint Surgery. Monthly. Journal of Bone and Joint Surgery, Inc., 20 Pickering Street, Needham, MA 02192-3157, 617-449-9738.

Journal of Musculoskeletal Medicine. Monthly. Provides practical information on diagnosis and management of a wide variety of common disorders. Cliggott Publishing Co., 55 Holly Hill Lane, Box 4010, Greenwich, CT 06830, 203-661-0600.

pathologist

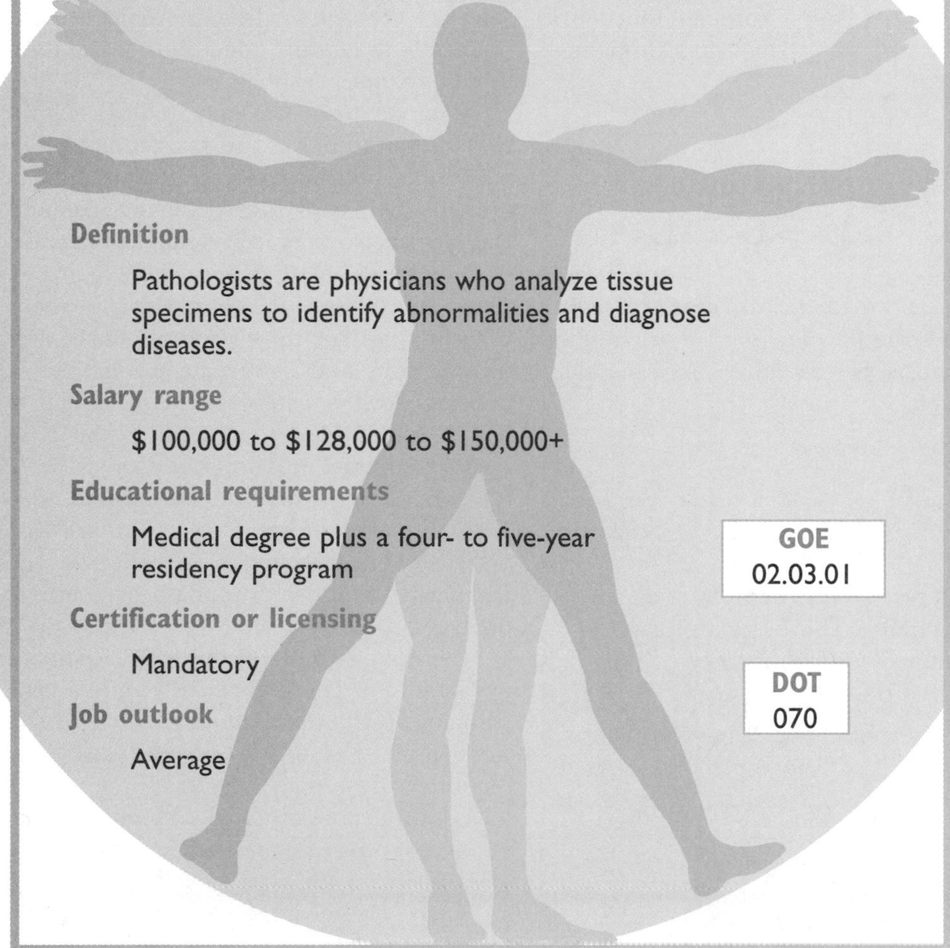

Definition

Pathologists are physicians who analyze tissue specimens to identify abnormalities and diagnose diseases.

Salary range

$100,000 to $128,000 to $150,000+

Educational requirements

Medical degree plus a four- to five-year residency program

Certification or licensing

Mandatory

Job outlook

Average

GOE
02.03.01

DOT
070

High School Subjects

Biology
Chemistry
English
Physics
Psychology

Personal Interests

Art
Health
Helping people

The surgeon reached for his saw to amputate the patient's leg. The pathology resident had just informed him that her analysis of tissue from a tumor on the leg showed that the tumor was malignant, or cancerous. The leg would have to be amputated to prevent the cancer from spreading to other parts of the body.

The resident, meanwhile, returned to the lab, where she saw the hospital's attending pathologist bent over a microscope, examining the slide of the tumor.

The pathologist said, "That's a nice slide of a fibrous histiocytoma you've got there."

The resident looked confused. "Excuse me, sir?"

"You know, the tissue you left in the microscope. It's a nice fibrous histiocytoma."

The resident turned pale. "But a fibrous histiocytoma is benign; it's noncancerous! I just told the surgeon the tumor is malignant! He's about to amputate the patient's leg!"

They ran to the operating room. The surgeon held the saw in the air above the patient's leg.

The resident burst through the doors. "Stop!" she shouted. "It's benign! Don't amputate that leg!"

what does a pathologist do?

Pathologists provide information that helps physicians care for patients; because of this, the pathologist is sometimes called the "doctor's doctor." When a patient has a tumor, an infection, or symptoms of a disease, a pathologist examines tissues from the patient to determine the nature of the patient's condition. Without this knowledge, a physician would not be able to make an accurate diagnosis and design the appropriate treatment. Because many health conditions first manifest themselves at the cellular level, pathologists are often able to identify conditions before they turn into serious health problems.

Many people associate pathologists only with the performing of autopsies. In fact, while pathologists do perform autopsies, much more of their work involves living patients. Pathologists working in hospital laboratories examine the blood, urine, bone marrow, stools, and tumors of patients. Using a variety of techniques, pathologists locate the causes of infections and determine the nature of unusual growths. Pathologists consult with a patient's physician to determine the best course of treatment. They may also talk with the patient about his or her condition. In a sense, the work of pathologists is much like detective work. It is often through the efforts of pathologists that health conditions are recognized and properly treated.

There are two main divisions of pathology—anatomic pathology (AP) and clinical pathology (CP). A pathologist may choose to work either in AP or CP, or in both divisions. Anatomic pathology covers three major areas—surgical pathology, cytology, and autopsies. Clinical pathology covers several areas, including toxicology and immunology.

Surgery pathology is concerned with biopsies, the examination of tissues removed from patients. Pathologists examine tumors, for example, to determine if they are malignant (cancerous) or benign (noncancerous). After a surgeon removes a malignant tumor, a pathologist examines it to make sure that the surgeon has not left any of the tumor in the patient's body, where it can continue to grow. Pathologists are often called upon to examine samples of patients' tissues while the patients are undergoing surgery. The tissue samples pathologists look at are called frozen sections; they are prepared for analysis by freezing them with liquid nitrogen. After examining a frozen section, a pathologist immediately recommends to the surgical team the proper course of action for treating the patient, such as the removal of an organ or other body part. For example, after examining tissue from a lump in a patient's breast, a pathologist directs the surgical team to perform either a lumpectomy (removal of

lingo to learn

Autopsy, or **post-mortem examination** The inspection and dissection of a dead body to determine the cause of death.

Benign Noncancerous; used in reference to tumors.

Cytology The study of the structure, function, and formation of cells.

Fine needle aspiration A technique in which a thin needle is used to collect cells from a patient; the cells are then examined under a microscope.

Forensic A term denoting a relationship to legal matters and courts of law. Forensic medicine and forensic pathology apply medical knowledge to civil and criminal law.

Frozen section A technique, involving liquid nitrogen, for rapidly preparing tissue specimens for microscopic examination. The term is also used to refer to the specimens themselves.

Lesion Any abnormal change in the structure of a body part.

Malignant Cancerous; used in reference to tumors.

Tumor, or **neoplasm** An abnormal growth or swelling in any part of the body.

the lump) or a mastectomy (removal of the entire breast).

Cytology is concerned with individual cells rather than with larger sections of body tissue. Pathologists working in this area commonly use a technique called fine needle aspiration (FNA) to collect cells from patients. Using this technique, a pathologist aspirates, or collects, a sample of tissue with a thin needle; the cells of the tissue are then analyzed under a microscope. Fine needle aspiration makes it possible to identify the nature of a condition without a surgical procedure.

Autopsies are concerned with the cause of death. Many people associate autopsies with forensic science, in which pathologists work with law enforcement officials to help solve homicide cases. But a primary purpose of autopsies is to provide greater understanding of diseases so that physicians will be better able to identify them while patients are still alive. Performing an autopsy enables a pathologist to determine if a physician's diagnosis was correct. During an autopsy, a pathologist may discover new information that can aid in diagnosing and treating other patients.

Clinical pathology is primarily concerned with the analysis of body fluids, such as blood and urine. Clinical pathologists analyze these fluids using various laboratory tests. There are a number of different areas a pathologist can work in within clinical pathology. Toxicology is concerned with the levels of drugs and toxic chemicals in the body. Clinical chemistry is concerned with the levels of such necessary substances as sodium and potassium in the blood and other body fluids. Clinical microbiology is concerned with bacteria, fungi, and viruses that cause illnesses. One of the main duties of clinical pathologists in this area is to make sure that hospitals maintain blood supplies that are free of harmful microorganisms. Clinical immunology is concerned with the patient's immune system and such diseases as AIDS. Hematopathology is concerned with diseases of the blood, such as hemophilia, anemia, and leukemia.

what is it like to be a pathologist?

David Cheng is a third-year resident in the University of Chicago Hospitals Pathology Program. Although he will not formerly qualify as a pathology specialist for two more years, David is already actively involved in many of the duties that a hospital's pathologist performs. "I'm following a five-year combined AP/CP program," David says. "The AP part involves actually working as a pathologist in the hospital's pathology laboratory. The CP part is more straight education—attending lectures and doing a lot of reading about pathology."

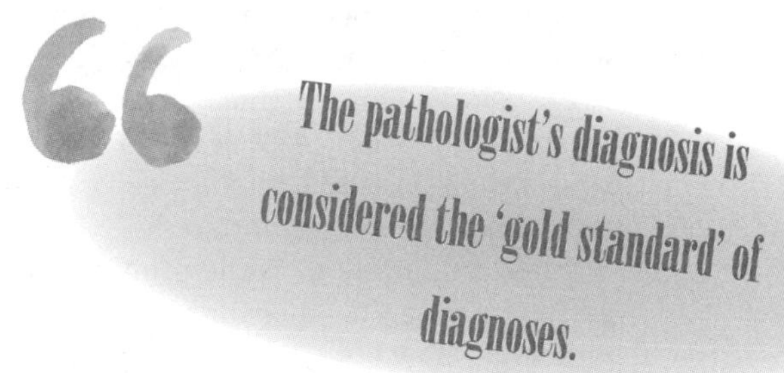

David's work in the laboratory is supervised by the hospital's attending pathologist. "That story about the resident and the patient's leg (at the beginning of this article) actually happened, and it shows how important it is for us to get a diagnosis right," David says. "There's a lot of training involved in becoming a pathologist. And experience is important, too. I like it that the attending pathologist was able to look at the resident's slide and see right away that that tumor was benign. That patient could have lost his leg if not for the attending pathologist!"

Pathology, which means the study of disease, is the only medical specialty that is also a basic science. "I honestly didn't know about pathology before I went to medical school," David admits. "My introduction came in my first year. All medical students take pathology courses in their first and second years. And I was impressed by the breadth and depth of knowledge that a pathologist has to have."

As a resident, David is involved in the main areas of pathology. "I do some autopsies. Autopsies are very hands on. First I'll do a gross analysis, that is, an examination of the organs and systems. Then I'll do a microscopic analysis of the tissues. An autopsy requires great attention to detail. What we try to do with an autopsy is to fit the cause of death with the patient's medical history." David's work also involves the area of cytology. "That's when we look at individual cells. To do this, we take smears, like PAP smears or throat cultures; or we draw cells from patients with fine needles. Sometimes we examine cells in body fluids. Cytopathology is becoming more and more important. It's non-invasive, for one thing, which means there's less risk to the patient. And it's also much less expensive to do. And with managed care, that's become increasingly important."

Surgical pathology is the primary focus of David's training. "I'm most interested in surgical pathology," David says. "There's a strong sense that what I'm doing is very important, because it's still relevant—the patient is still alive." When David is assigned to a surgical pathology rotation, he typically begins his work day at 7:00 AM "As a resident, my schedule parallels the hours that the pathology lab is open. And unlike most medical specialties, pathologists' hours are pretty normal. I'll generally work fifty hours a week. Depending on the rotation, I'll work from 7:00 AM to 6:00 PM or from 9:00 AM to 5:00 PM." A pathologist must be able to respond in an emergency, however. "Surgical pathology is very services oriented," David says. "A hospital cannot run without pathologists."

David's day begins in the pathology lab. "I spend the first part of the day grossing-in specimens. That means I'll examine them as larger samples first. Then I'll cut into the specimens and select portions to be processed into slides, which usually is done overnight, so they can be examined more closely under a microscope." A primary duty for any pathologist is recording his or her observations. "While I'm working, I'm also dictating what I see. You can use a dictaphone or some other recording device for that. But it's important that our observations are precisely documented." David is very aware of the need for detail when examining specimens. "I know that I'm dealing with live patients. The patient's physician has already made a diagnosis. It's my responsibility to either confirm that diagnosis or to come up with a corrected diagnosis."

Depending on the work load, David may spend the entire day grossing-in specimens. On other days, he may only spend half the day doing that. "Then in the afternoon, I'll look at slides from the day before. That's when I work closely with the attending pathologist. He'll go over my diagnoses, make changes where necessary, and do a lot of teaching."

When a patient is on the operating table, David must be prepared to assist the surgical team. "When a frozen section comes in, I'll do an immediate analysis of it. I have to make an analysis within minutes. The surgeon needs to know right then and there, while the patient is on the table. For example, the surgeon might remove a tumor and send that to me. I have to examine the tumor and make a diagnosis. And if it's a malignant tumor, I have to look closely at the margins and make sure they're clear. That means I make sure that none of the tumor is left in the patient."

David likes the fact that pathologists don't have to get involved in guesswork; their diagnoses are all based on scientific tests. "What impressed me when I first began to consider a pathology specialty," David says, "was that what pathologists do is more concrete than other medical specialties. You're not dealing with something vague, like a patient's symptoms. You get to look at the tissues themselves and give a more concrete, more substantive diagnosis. The pathologist's diagnosis is considered the 'gold standard' of diagnoses. You really have an impact on a patient's care."

FYI

Among the major causes of disease are the tiny organic particles called viruses. Though viruses have DNA and RNA, as living organisms do, most biologists do not consider viruses to be living organisms. This is because viruses cannot make proteins or obtain energy from food.

have I got what it takes to be a pathologist?

"I think the most frustrating part about being a pathologist is not the work itself, but the public's perception of what we do," David Cheng says. "I think people still perceive pathology as odd. They don't look at you the same way they look at other doctors. A lot of people think that all we do are autopsies. And it's frustrating because most of the time we're working with living patients." Because pathologists generally work behind the scenes, they are not as visible as other physicians and are not always recognized as vital members of the health care team. "Other physicians don't seem to speak to us as equals," David says. "There's a bit of a prejudice against people who are not predominantly involved in direct patient care. People, even other physicians, don't always see that what we do is important. A physician cannot make decisions without us. So it's frustrating that we don't always get the credit we deserve."

Part of the image problem pathologists face stems from the specialty's history. Pathology is a fairly young medical specialty, and until about twenty years ago, a pathologist was likely to be chiefly involved in performing autopsies. But the growth in medical testing and diagnostic techniques has greatly expanded a pathologist's potential to have an impact on patient care. Pathologists now have the ability to perform a broad range of tests and to diagnose health conditions affecting virtually every function and part of the human body. This ability has brought pathologists into the front lines of patient care and made them an integral part of the health care team. "That's why I'm most interested in surgical pathology. I'm communicating constantly with surgeons, and I find that really rewarding," David says. "When things are clicking, and when you have a good mesh with the surgical team, it feels really good."

Anyone interested in pathology as a specialty will be confronted with working with body fluids, tissues, and other potentially unpleasant aspects of health care. Most pathologists in general practice will be called upon to perform autopsies. "I'm not different from anyone else," David admits. "I have no affection for dead bodies. But autopsies are important as a quality control for the health care process. Often during an autopsy, you'll find lesions or tumors that were missed."

Pathologists generally work more regular hours than other physicians. "The hours are definitely more reasonable. You're not on call twenty-four hours a day like other physicians. So I'd say the lifestyle is more attractive than for other specialties."

To be a successful pathologist, you should

- Have an eye for detail
- Be able to concentrate intently on your work
- Be able to work well with others
- Have strong communication skills
- Be able to accept a great deal of responsibility and perform well under pressure
- Be patient, thorough, and confident in your decisions

how do I become a pathologist?

Like any medical specialist, a pathologist must complete a medical school program before attending a residency program. A pathology resident may choose to specialize in anatomical pathology or clinical pathology, each of which generally requires a four-year residency program. Many pathologists, however, prefer to specialize in both anatomical and clinical pathology; licensing as an AP/CP pathologist requires a five-year residency.

Admission to premedical and medical school programs is highly competitive. Prospective pathologists should begin preparing for this career while still in high school.

education

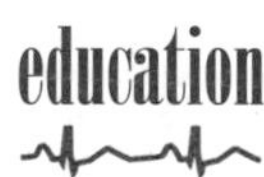

High School

While in high school, all students interested in medical careers should follow course programs that will enable them to compete for placement in college-level premed programs. Courses should include mathematics and such basic sciences as biology, chemistry, and physics. Especially important are any courses emphasizing laboratory work. Students should also develop strong communication skills, including writing, reading, and speaking, since these are essential for a successful career. Outside of school, students can volunteer or work part-time at local hospitals. This experience will help a student determine if a career in health care is right for him or her.

Postsecondary Training

Most colleges offer premedical degree programs that prepare students for entry into medical school. Majoring as a premed is not mandatory, however. Students pursuing other majors can enter medical school if they fulfill certain basic requirements. "In fact, I was an anthropology major as an undergraduate," David Cheng says. "I knew I'd be going to medical school, so I took the opportunity to pursue my interest in anthropology. I think it helps to have a well-rounded education. Knowing that I would go for a medical career gave me the safety net to study something like anthropology, which doesn't offer the same kind of job security."

David recommends that undergraduate students try to gain as much laboratory experience as possible. "You could work as a laboratory technician, for example. That way you'll get experience while earning money too. A lot of what pathologists do is in the laboratory, and it's good to build those skills and gain familiarity with the fastidiousness that lab work requires. Working in a lab teaches you to be neat and focused. We have to go through elaborate procedures to avoid contamination."

David also suggests that students pursue activities that will help them develop other skills important for their careers. "I'd recommend that they take art and art history classes," David says. "The bulk of pathology is the analysis of tissues. Developing a good eye for detail and the ability to pick out things will be very helpful. I think art history classes would be good for that, but I recommend anything that will help train your eyes to see detail."

certification or licensing

After completing a medical degree, a pathologist must be accepted into a four- to five-year residency program. As stated earlier, a pathologist can pursue certification along three primary paths—an anatomic pathology program, a clinical pathology program, or a combined anatomic and clinical pathology program. Once a pathologist has completed certification, he or she can choose to specialize in a particular area of pathology. Gaining certification in a specialty generally requires an additional one to two years of training, although there is a potential for combining this training with the standard pathology residency program.

who will hire me?

About 75 percent of pathologists work in community hospitals, directing the activities of pathology laboratories. Most pathologists working in hospitals are responsible for the blood bank supplies. Many also perform laboratory services for physicians and medical clinics affiliated with the hospitals. In most hospitals, pathologists work in a group, sharing various duties. They may, for example, each specialize in a different area of clinical pathology.

Medical schools and university hospitals offer pathologists the best opportunities for specialization. Pathologists in these settings will also have opportunities to become actively involved in teaching pathology to medical students.

As health care moves toward more outpatient and ambulatory care services, there will be increasing opportunities for pathologists to work in clinics, group practices, and their own private practices. There are many independent laboratories that require pathologists. A relatively small number of pathologists work for local, state, and federal governments as forensic pathologists assisting law enforcement agencies. The military services and such government agencies such as the National Institutes of Health and the Food and Drug Administration also employ pathologists.

where can I go from here?

"I definitely see myself working in a community hospital setting," David Cheng says, "because I'm most interested in surgical pathology. But I may decide to try to win a fellowship and train in a specialty before going into community practice. And if you're interested in academic work, you'll definitely want to continue training. A fellowship will help open doors to an academic position."

After gaining enough experience, a pathologist may become director of a hospital pathology laboratory. With even more experience, a pathologist may advance to serving in a hospital's administration. A pathologist working in an academic capacity may advance to direct a medical school's pathology program. Some pathologists open independent pathology laboratories, or join with other physicians to form private group practices.

what are the salary ranges?

Beginning pathologists are likely to earn around $100,000 per year, while experienced

in-depth

Pathology Specializations

Many pathologists, especially those working in university or medical school hospitals, choose to specialize in specific areas of pathology. Specialties (and the areas of their concern) include the following.

Cardiovascular pathology Heart and blood vessels

Cytopathology Cells

Dermatopathology Skin

Environmental pathology Disease caused by environmental factors

Gastrointestinal pathology Stomach and digestive tract

Gynecologic/obstetrical pathology Female reproductive system and childbirth

Hematopathology Blood

Immunopathology Immune system

Neuropathology Nervous system

Ophthalmic pathology Eyes

Pediatric pathology Children

Pulmonary pathology Lungs

Renal pathology Kidneys

pathologists may earn $150,000 per year or more. The average earnings of all pathologists is about $128,000 per year. Forensic pathologists and other pathologists working for government agencies generally earn lower salaries than those involved in community practice.

what is the job outlook?

The outlook for careers in pathology is very good. New medical tests are constantly being developed and refined, making it possible to detect an increasing number of diseases in their early stages. The medical community depends on pathologists to analyze results from these tests. Another factor favorably affecting the demand for pathologists is the shifting of health care to cost-conscious managed care services. Testing for, diagnosing, and treating a disease or other health condition in its early stages is much less expensive than treating a health condition in its advanced stages.

how do I learn more?

professional organizations

Following are organizations that provide information on pathology careers, accredited schools, and employers.

American Board of Pathology
P.O. Box 25915
Tampa, FL 33622
TEL: 813-286-2444

College of American Pathologists
325 Waukegan Road
Northfield, IL 60093
TEL: 847-832-7000
WEBSITE: http://www.cap.org

Intersociety Committee on Pathology Information
4733 Bethesda Avenue, Suite 700
Bethesda, MD 20814
TEL: 301-656-2944

United States and Canadian Academy of Pathology
3643 Walton Way Extension
Augusta, GA 30909
TEL: 706-733-7550

bibliography

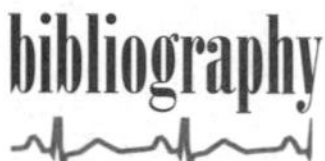

Following is a sampling of materials relating to the professional concerns and development of pathologists.

Books

Burke, Shirley R. *Human Anatomy and Physiology*, 3rd edition. Albany, NY: Delmar, 1993.

Chandarasoma, Parakrams. *Pathology*, 2nd edition. New York, NY: Appleton & Lange, 1994.

Govan, Alasdair, D.T., and others. *Pathology Illustrated*, 4th edition. New York, NY: Appleton & Lange, 1994.

Harruff, Richard C., and Ruth Viste. *Pathology Facts*. Philadelphia, PA: Lippincott-Raven, 1993.

Kumar. *Basic Pathology*, 6th edition. Philadelphia, PA: W.B. Saunders Co., 1997.

Mitchinson, Malcolm J., and others, editors. *Essentials of Pathology*. Cambridge, MA: Blackwell Science, 1995.

Pathology as a Career in Medicine. Bethesda, MD: Intersociety Committee on Pathology Information, n.d.

Sinard, John H. *Outlines in Pathology*. Philadelphia, PA: W.B. Saunders Co., 1996.

Standler, Nancy. A *Short Course in Pathology*. New York, NY: Churchill Livingstone, 1994.

Periodicals

American Board of Family Practice Journal. Bimonthly. Covers clinical studies that have relevance for improved patient care in family medicine. American Board of Family Practice, 2228 Young Drive, Lexington, KY 40505, 606-269-5626.

American Family Physician. 16 per year. Provides continuing medical education for doctors involved with primary care. American Academy of Family Physicians, 8880 Ward Parkway, Kansas City, MO 64114, 816-333-9700.

American Journal of Clinical Pathology. Monthly. Helps pathologists and other clinical laboratory scientists keep their professional knowledge current. Publishes original investigations and observations in clinical pathology. Articles cover a broad spectrum of subspecialty topics. American Society of Clinical Pathologists, Lippincott-Raven Publishers, 227 E. Washington Square, Philadelphia, PA 19106, 215-238-4200.

American Journal of Pathology. Monthly. Publishes research papers on the cellular and molecular mechanisms of disease, without preference for specific methods of analysis. American Society for Investigative Pathology, 9650 Rockville Pike, Bethesda, MD 20814, 310-530-7130.

Modern Pathology. 9 per year. Provides a forum for the presentation of advances in the understanding of pathological processes. It is practice-oriented and concentrates on diagnostic human pathology. United States and Canadian Academy of Pathology, Williams & Wilkins, 428 E. Preston Street, Baltimore, MD 21202, 410-528-4000, 800-638-6423.

Pathology Annual. Semiannual. Original articles written by an international contingent of scientists for practicing pathologists. Appleton & Lange, 25 Van Zant Street, Box 5630, Norwalk, CT 06856, 203-838-4400.

pediatrician

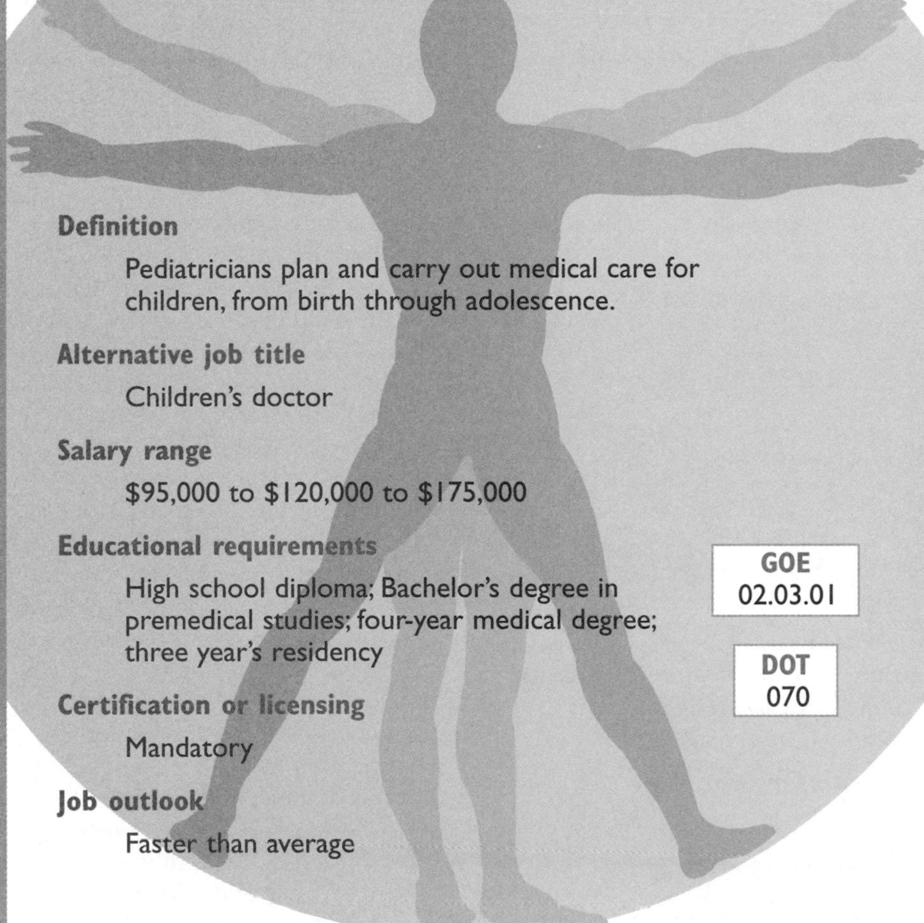

Definition

Pediatricians plan and carry out medical care for children, from birth through adolescence.

Alternative job title

Children's doctor

Salary range

$95,000 to $120,000 to $175,000

Educational requirements

High school diploma; Bachelor's degree in premedical studies; four-year medical degree; three year's residency

Certification or licensing

Mandatory

Job outlook

Faster than average

GOE 02.03.01

DOT 070

High School Subjects

Biology
Chemistry
Mathematics
Physics
Physiology

Personal Interests

Children
Health
Helping people
Medicine

Watery-eyed and flushed, five-year-old Benjamin is sitting on his mother's lap as Dr. David Esary walks into the examining room.

"How are you, Ben?" Dr. Esary asks, sitting down and opening his file. "Are you a sickie today?"

Ben stirs slightly on his mother's lap. "I don't feel good," he says. "My brain hurts."

Dr. Esary smiles and rolls his stool closer. "How long has he been running a fever?" he asks the little boy's mother.

"The fever just started last night," she responds, "but he's had a cough and a runny nose for about three days."

"He may have an infection," Dr. Esary says, making a quick note on the chart. Holding out a hand to Ben, he asks, "Can you stand up for me just a minute, guy? I want to take a peep in your ears and see if any birds have nested in there."

what does a pediatrician do?

Infancy and childhood are the most critical periods of life in a person's development; the body is growing rapidly, and motor, speech, and cognitive skills are evolving. Thorough health care during this time of growth and development is extremely important. An infant or child who doesn't get proper nourishment or medical treatment may face a lifetime of health problems. Likewise, a child who doesn't receive all the necessary immunizations against childhood diseases risks permanent damage, or even death.

Pediatricians are physicians who provide health care to infants, children, and adolescents. Typically, a pediatrician meets a new patient soon after birth, and takes care of that patient through his or her teenage years.

A significant part of a pediatrician's job is preventive medicine—what is sometimes called "well care." This involves periodically seeing a patient for routine health checkups. During these checkups, the doctor physically examines the child to make sure he or she is growing at a normal rate and to look for symptoms of illness. The physical examination includes testing reflexes, listening to the heart and lungs, checking eyes and ears, and measuring height and weight.

During the checkup, the pediatrician also assesses the child's mental and behavioral development. This is done both by observing the patient's behavior and by asking the parents questions about their child's abilities.

Immunizing children against certain childhood diseases is another important part of preventive medicine. Pediatricians administer routine immunizations for such diseases as rubella, polio, and smallpox as children reach certain ages. Yet another part of preventive medicine is family education. Pediatricians counsel and advise parents on the care and treatment of their children. They provide information on such parental concerns as safety, diet, and hygiene.

In addition to practicing preventive medicine, pediatricians also treat sick infants and children. When a sick or injured patient is brought into the office, the doctor examines him or her, makes a diagnosis, and orders treatment. Common ailments include ear infections, allergies, feeding difficulties, viral illnesses, respiratory illnesses, and gastrointestinal upsets. For these and other illnesses, pediatricians prescribe and administer treatments and medications.

If a patient is seriously ill or hurt, a pediatrician arranges for hospital admission and follows up on the patient's progress during the hospitalization. In some cases, a child may have a serious condition, such as cancer,

lingo to learn

Acute Having a sudden onset, sharp rise, and short course.

Chronic Marked by long duration or frequent recurrence. A chronic illness may become more serious over time.

Managed Care A system of providing health care through a program that is designed to control costs. HMO's and PPO's provide managed care.

Health Maintenance Organization (HMO) A health care organization that is financed by fixed periodic payments. An HMO has member physicians that sometimes refer patients to outside specialists.

Preferred Provider Organization (PPO) A health care organization that provides economic incentives for people to use certain physicians and hospitals. These physicians and hospitals agree to supervision and reduced fees.

Preventive medicine A branch of medical science emphasizing methods of preventing disease. It is sometimes called "well care."

Vaccine A preparation of killed or disabled microorganisms that is administered to produce or increase immunity to a particular disease.

cystic fibrosis, or hemophilia, that requires the attention of a specialist. In these cases, the pediatrician, as the primary care physician, will refer the child to the appropriate specialist.

Some pediatric patients may be suffering from emotional or behavioral disorders or from substance abuse. Other patients may be affected by problems within their families, such as unemployment, alcoholism, or physical abuse. In these cases, pediatricians may make referrals to such health professionals as psychiatrists, psychologists, and social workers.

Pediatricians that are in general practice usually work alone or in partnership with other physicians. Their average workweek is fifty to sixty hours, most of which is spent seeing patients in their offices. They also make hospital rounds to visit any of their patients who have been admitted for treatment or to check on newborn patients and their mothers. Pediatricians spend some time on-call, taking care of patients who have emergencies. A pediatrician might be called to attend the delivery of a baby, to meet an injured patient in the emergency room, or simply to answer a parent's question about a sick child.

Some pediatricians choose to pursue pediatric subspecialties, such as the treatment of children who have heart disorders, kidney disorders, or cancer. Subspecialization requires a longer residency training than does general practice. A pediatrician practicing a subspecialty typically spends a much greater proportion of his or her time in a hospital or medical center than does a general practice pediatrician. Subspecialization permits pediatricians to be involved in research activities.

what is it like to be a pediatrician?

A fish tank covers most of one wall. Toys are scattered on the floor and chairs. At a low table in the corner, two toddlers are playing with busy beads, while a five-year-old painstaking sounds out words in a Dr. Seuss book. It may sound like a preschool, but it's actually Dr. David Esary's waiting room. The examination rooms, where Dr. Esary takes care of his young patients, are through a set of double doors and down a short hallway.

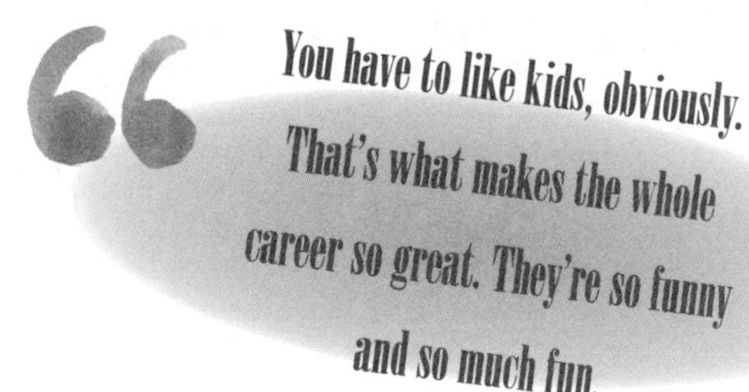

Although he spends the great majority of his time in the office, Dr. Esary's day always begins with a visit to the hospital. "I usually start out at 7:30 at the hospital, making rounds," he says. "I usually have a few newborns to see, and maybe some sick kids in the pediatric ward."

Around 8:30, he returns to his office to see the morning's scheduled patients. On a typical day, he sees anywhere from fifteen to twenty-five patients in the morning, and another fifteen to twenty-five in the afternoon. "I try to have eight to ten appointments each half day be checkups, and the rest be sick visits," he says. "Sick visits take much less time, because you can just concentrate on what the problem is."

The problem may be anything from recurring difficulties with asthma to an ear infection to a small hole in the heart. Dr. Esary treats anything that falls under the category of general pediatric care. He refers more severe disorders to specialists.

Checkups take up a large part of Dr. Esary's time. These are routine physical examinations that are usually scheduled for certain ages in a child's life. Newborns, for example, are typically scheduled for a visit to Dr. Esary every three months. After a child's first year, checkups are generally less frequent.

A total checkup is a head-to-toe examination. Dr. Esary says, "I check the eyes, ears, nose, and throat, check movement of the extremities, palpate the abdomen, check for hernias, check genitals, and make sure that everything is generally okay neurologically. Plus, I take a little time to play. I also take a developmental history and talk with the parents about habits, appetite, diet, elimination, and any concerns they might have."

Family education is an important element of checkups. "During checkups, I spend a lot of time talking with the parents about things to avoid, proper diet, the importance of immunizations, the risk of poisoning and accidents—that sort of thing," Dr. Esary says.

In addition to treating his existing patient base, Dr. Esary is sometimes called upon to attend the delivery of a new patient—particularly if the baby may be at risk. "If there's a chance that the baby will need immediate care, I'll get called into the delivery," he says. "If, for example, the baby's heart rate drops during labor, or if there are other complications." He shares the responsibility of being on-call for such emergencies with six other pediatricians, which means that he does a twenty-four hour on-call shift about four times each month.

While on-call, he may be summoned to the emergency room to help attend a sick or injured child. He may take phone calls and answer questions from parents who need to know what to do with a child who is ill or hurt.

Because Dr. Esary practices alone rather than in a physician's group, clinic, or hospital, he serves as his own business manager. This involves overseeing the office finances and supervising his six-person staff. Billing, insurance, and inventory are handled by staff members, as is patient check-in and check-out.

have I got what it takes to be a pediatrician?

What personal quality is most important for pediatricians? "You have to like kids, obviously," Dr. Esary says, laughing. "That's what makes the whole career so great. They're so funny and so much fun."

Treating children can be much different than treating adults. Children, especially very young ones, can't verbalize what is wrong with them. They can't control emotions, such as fear and anger, as well as most adults can. Therefore, it takes much patience and understanding to work effectively with them.

"Most kids don't want you to do whatever it is you're trying to do to them, so you can't be too easily frustrated," Dr. Esary says. "You also have to be fairly calm. Someone who's loud and aggressive might do well in another field, but that person would probably scare a child."

It is also important that pediatricians be willing to keep up with newly-emerging technologies and medical advances. "I think you have to be a little bit obsessive-compulsive," says Dr. Esary. "You have to keep up on the latest information by attending conferences and reading the literature as much as you can."

Pediatricians need a great deal of commitment in order to cope with the negative aspects of the job. For example, they may be under considerable stress, both during their years of training and in their careers. They work long, irregular hours, and often face interruptions to their personal lives. In addition, they must be able to handle very depressing situations. "The downside is the occasional sick child that you lose," says Dr. Esary. "Even though some of the cancers are very curable now, telling a family that a child has leukemia is very hard."

Despite the long hours, the stress, and the occasional loss, pediatrics is a very rewarding career. It is gratifying for a physician to know that he or she has helped a child get well, and it is enjoyable to watch patients grow and develop. Pediatricians have the pleasure of knowing that they are helping protect and care for an important human resource.

FYI

Pediatrics became a separate medical specialty during the 19th century. The first pediatric clinic in the United States opened in New York City in 1862. About that same time, several children's hospitals opened in Europe.

how do I become a pediatrician?

Dr. Esary knew he wanted to be a doctor when he was in the seventh grade. He didn't, however, plan to be a pediatrician. "I went from the seventh grade all the way through high school and college, and then through my first two years of med school planning to be an ophthalmologist," he says. He changed his mind in his junior year of medical school when he started doing rotations, specified periods of time in various hospital departments. "Just by coincidence, all the rotations I took were oriented towards kids," Dr. Esary says. "I enjoyed it too much. So, I decided to pursue pediatrics instead of ophthalmology."

To be a successful pediatrician, you should

- Like children and adolescents
- Have patience, compassion, and a good sense of humor
- Be willing to continually learn
- Have a desire to help others
- Be able to withstand stress and make sound decisions

education

High School

While in high school, prospective pediatricians should take college prep classes, with a heavy emphasis on science and math. Biology, chemistry, physics, and physiology are important science classes. Any advanced math courses are also excellent choices.

Classes in English, foreign languages, and speech will enhance communication skills, which are vital to being a successful physician. Such social sciences as psychology and sociology, which increase one's understanding of others, are also beneficial to the prospective pediatrician.

In addition to carefully selecting curriculums, there are other ways high school students can prepare for medical school and careers in pediatrics. Participation in science clubs, for example, will allow for in-depth explorations of some areas of science. Volunteer work at hospitals or other health care institutions will allow students to see many aspects of medical care. Such volunteer work can also provide a taste of what a physician's career entails, and help a student decide if he or she is suited for it.

Postsecondary Training

After high school, prospective pediatricians must attend a four-year college and complete a bachelor's degree in premedical studies. Required undergraduate courses include physics, biology, and organic and inorganic chemistry. Some classes in English, mathematics, social sciences, and the humanities are also required. Medical schools are very selective, so a good grade point average is a must.

In the final year of college, prospective physicians should apply to medical schools. Applicants must submit transcripts of their premedical studies, letters of recommendation, and scores from the Medical College Admission Test (MCAT). In addition, an applicant is typically interviewed by an admissions officer, who evaluates the applicant for character, personality, and leadership qualities.

A student's first two years of medical school are spent in classrooms and laboratories. Such courses as anatomy, biochemistry, histology (the study of tissues) pathology, physiology, pharmacology, psychology, medical ethics, and medical law make up the standard curriculum. Students are also taught to take medical histories of patients and to examine patients for symptoms of various diseases.

During the third and fourth years of medical school, students work in hospitals and clinics, under the supervision of experienced physicians. They do rotations in different departments to learn various aspects of medicine. Rotations may include family practice, obstetrics and gynecology, pediatrics, internal medicine, psychiatry, and surgery.

Once the medical student has successfully completed four years of medical school, the student takes the medical boards. Upon passing the boards, the student is granted a medical degree.

In order to become a pediatrician, the new graduate must complete a three-year residency program in a hospital. The pediatric residency provides extensive experience in ambulatory pediatrics, the care of infants and children who are not bedridden. Residents also spend time working in various specialized pediatric units, including neonatology, adolescent medicine, child development, psychology, special care, intensive care, and outpatients.

certification or licensing

All physicians must be licensed by their state in order to practice medicine legally. Certification by the American Board of Pediatrics (ABP) is recommended. A certificate in General Pediatrics is awarded after three years of residency training and the successful completion of a two-day comprehensive written examination. A pediatrician who specializes in cardiology, infectious diseases, or other area must complete an additional three-year residency in the subspeciality before taking the certification examination. To remain board-certified, pediatricians must pass an examination every seven years.

scholarships and grants

Most medical schools offer scholarships to qualified students. Students should check with the financial aid offices of the schools they are considering to learn what assistance might be available.

There are several organizations offering scholarships and loans to medical students. A good place to look for information on these organizations is a local library, where reference librarians may be able to provide a list of available assistance programs. For those students who have access to the Internet, simply performing a keyword search on "scholarships" or "financial aid" should produce a multitude of resources to explore.

Another option is to contact the National Association of Student Financial Aid Administrators (NASFAA) for a list of possibilities. They can be reached at the following address and Website.

NASFAA
1920 L Street NW, Suite 200
Washington, DC 20036
WEBSITE: http://www.finaid.org/nasfaa/

Finally, there are some not-for-profit lenders who offer loans targeted at medical students. The following is a list of some of the most popular programs. They may be contacted directly for information.

MEDFUNDS
10515 Carnegie Avenue
Cleveland, OH 44160

Nellie Mae-MedDent
EXCEL Program
50 Braintree Hill Park
Suite 300
Braintree, MA 02184
TEL: 800-9-TUITION
WEBSITE: http://www.nelliemae.org/

The Education Resource Institute,
Professional Education Program
330 Stuart Street,
Suite 500
Boston, MA 02116
TEL: 800-255-TERI
WEBSITE: http://www.teri.org/pep.html

who will hire me?

Dr. Esary found a job during the second year of his residency. "A friend mentioned that she'd seen a letter from a multispecialty clinic saying it needed a pediatrician," he says. "So I contacted them, and we agreed that I would start as soon as I wrapped up my residency." While it's uncommon to win a position so early in one's residency, most pediatricians do not have trouble finding work.

The majority of pediatricians are involved in direct patient care. Of these, about one-third have private practices. The others work in group practices, community clinics, hospitals, university-affiliated medical centers, and health maintenance organizations. Only about 10 percent of pediatricians work in administration, teaching, or research.

For the pediatrician who plans to set up a private practice, it is wise to consult with his or her medical school placement office to find a suitable geographic location in which to do so. Certain locations, such as rural areas and small towns, offer less competition for patients and, therefore, better chances of success.

Many newly-licensed pediatricians take salaried jobs until they can pay off some of their medical school debt, which is likely to total more than $50,000. Medical school placement offices should be able to recommend hospitals, clinics, HMOs, and group practices that are hiring pediatricians.

There are some professional organizations of pediatricians that offer job placement and recruitment services for their members. Both the American Academy of Pediatrics and the Ambulatory Pediatric Association offer such services. These and other professional organizations are listed later in this article, under the heading, "how do I learn more?"

If a pediatrician has a specific location in mind, such as his or her home town, it might be wise to approach potential employers directly.

where can I go from here?

The most common method of advancement for pediatricians is subspecialization. There are several subspecialties open to the pediatrician who is willing to spend the additional time training for one. A subspecialty requires three to four more years of residency training.

For awhile, Dr. Esary considered entering the subspecialization of neonatology, the care of sick newborns. But he ultimately decided against it. "The problem with neonatology is that once you cure the babies and get them healthy, they go home and you never see them again," he says. "I like general practice because you get to watch the kids grow up."

Some of the other subspecialties a pediatrician might acquire training for include adolescent medicine, pediatric cardiology (care of children with heart disease), pediatric critical care (care of children requiring advanced life support), pediatric endocrinology (care of children with diabetes and other glandular disorders), pediatric neurology (care of children with nervous system disorders), and pediatric hematology/oncology (care of children with blood disorders and cancer).

> "Even though some of the cancers are very curable now, telling a family that a child has leukemia is very hard."

Some pediatricians pursue careers in research. Possible research activities include developing new vaccines for infections, developing treatments for children with heart disease, and developing treatments for infants born with severe abnormalities.

Another way for pediatricians to advance is to move into the field of education, where they can teach medical students and resident physicians about particular areas of pediatrics.

what are the salary ranges?

Pediatricians, while at the low end of the earning scale for physicians, still have among the highest earnings of any occupation in the United States.

During their residencies, pediatricians commonly earn between $30,000 and $42,000. For pediatricians who have completed their residency, the median net income is about $120,000, according to a 1995 American Medical Association survey. After several years in practice, it is possible to make between $150,000 and $200,000 yearly.

The earnings of pediatricians are partly dependent upon the types of practices they choose. Those who are self-employed tend to earn more than those who are salaried. Geographic region, hours worked, number of years in practice, professional reputation, and personality are other factors which can impact a pediatrician's income.

in-depth

An ounce of prevention...

Some of the most significant breakthroughs in children's health care have been in disease prevention. Perhaps the most well-known method of prevention is the use of vaccines.

The first vaccine was developed in 1796 by Edward Jenner, an English physician. At that time, the viral disease smallpox disfigured and killed thousands of people each year. Jenner noticed that people who had developed a similar but less severe disease, called cowpox, never developed smallpox, even when exposed to it.

Curious about this, Jenner took material from a cowpox sore and scratched it into the arm of a healthy eight-year-old boy. The boy, as expected, developed cowpox. Jenner then scratched material from a smallpox sore into the boy's arm, but the boy did not develop smallpox.

Jenner named the material from the cowpox sore "vaccine," and the process in which he used it "vaccination." Both words are from the Latin "vaccinus," meaning "of or from cows." The use of the vaccine spread quickly, and within 200 years, smallpox had been eliminated from the world.

Vaccines are now available for a wide variety of diseases. Thanks to Jenner's pioneering work, many childhood diseases that once posed serious threats are virtually unheard of.

Yet another factor impacting earnings is how much of a pediatrician's revenue comes from patients who are enrolled in managed care plans. Under these plans, insurance companies sometimes reimburse physicians at a relatively low rate.

what is the job outlook?

According to the United States Department of Labor, employment of all physicians is expected to grow faster than the average for all occupations through 2005. The employment prospects for pediatricians—along with other general practitioners, such as family physicians—are especially good. This is because of the increasing use of managed care plans.

In a managed care plan, an insurance company controls which physicians the plan members see. In a typical plan, the insurance company contracts with several physicians to provide service. Each plan member is then given a "menu" of physicians to choose from. A patient selects a primary-care doctor, who oversees the patient's medical care and refers the patient to specialists as needed. Pediatricians, under these plans, are considered to be primary-care providers rather than specialists. Most managed care plans have several pediatricians for patients to select.

Because managed care plans rely so heavily on primary-care physicians, there is a growing need for such doctors, including pediatricians. Since the use of specialists is limited under these plans, however, there may be a decreased need for those pediatricians who choose to pursue subspecialties.

The move toward primary care is reflected in the increasing number of medical school graduates entering residency programs in pediatrics, family practice, and internal medicine. In 1996, according to the National Resident Matching Program, a record number of graduates (1,593) entered residencies in pediatrics. This is a 6.1 percent increase over 1995.

Another factor which may influence a pediatrician's employment prospects is location. Employment possibilities will probably be the best in rural regions and small towns.

Some of the larger metropolitan areas, are already well-supplied with pediatricians, thus they may offer fewer chances for establishing practices.

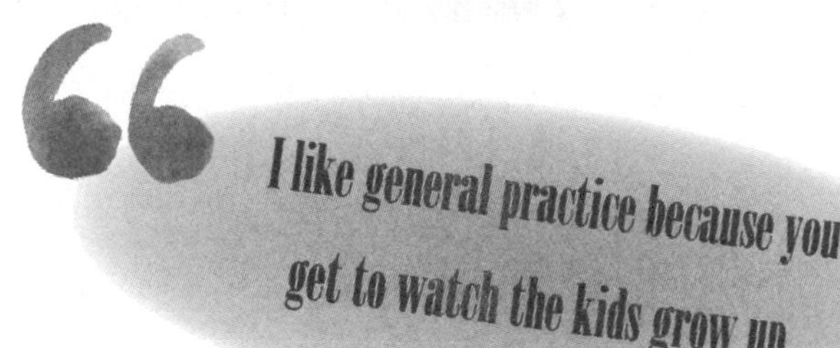

how do I learn more?

professional organizations

Following are organizations that provide information on pediatric careers, accredited schools, and employers.

American Academy of Pediatrics
141 Northwest Point Blvd.
P.O. Box 927
Elk Grove, IL 60007
TEL: 847-228-5005
WEBSITE: http://www.aap.org

American Medical Association
515 North State Street
Chicago, IL 60610
TEL: 312-464-5000
WEBSITE: http://www.ama-assn.org

American Pediatric Society
TEL: 281-296-0244

Ambulatory Pediatric Association
6728 Old McLean Drive
McLean, VA 22101
TEL: 703-556-9222
WEBSITE: http://www.ambpeds.org

bibliography

Following is a sampling of materials relating to the professional concerns and development of pediatricians.

Books

Avery, Mary E., and Lewis R. Frost. *Pediatric Medicine,* 2nd edition. Baltimore, MD: Williams & Wilkins, 1993.

Behrman, Nelson. *Textbook of Pediatrics,* 15th edition. Philadelphia, PA: W.B. Saunders Co., 1996.

Burns, Catherine E., and others. *Pediatric Primary Care: a Handbook for Nurse Practitioners.* Philadelphia, PA: W.B. Saunders Co., 1996.

Grossman, Elmer. *Everyday Pediatrics.* Philadelphia, PA: W.B. Saunders Co., 1993.

Hull, David, and Derek I. Johnston, editors. *Essential Pediatrics,* 3rd edition. New York, NY: Churchill Livingstone, 1993.

Kaye, Robert, and others. *Core Textbook of Pediatrics,* 3rd edition. Philadelphia, PA: Lippincott-Raven, 1988.

McCarthy, Claire. *Learning How the Heart Beats: the Making of a Pediatrician.* New York, NY: Viking Penguin, 1995.

Periodicals

Archives of Pediatrics and Adolescent Medicine. Monthly. Publishes original clinical studies, practice commentaries, updates on clinical science, and practice management articles. Provides a forum for dialogue on clinical, scientific, advocacy, and humanistic issues relevant to the care of pediatric patients from infancy through young adulthood. American Medical Association, 515 N. State Street, Chicago, IL 60610, 312-464-5000, 800-262-2350.

Clinical Pediatrics. Monthly. For practitioners in all areas of child care. Contains articles on pediatric practice, clinical research, behavioral and educational problems, community health, and subspecialty or affiliated specialty applications.

Cortlandt Group, Inc., 500 Executive Boulevard, Suite 302, Ossining, NY 10562, 914-672-0647.

Journal of Pediatric Health Care. Bimonthly. Provides information on examination and developmental assessments, treatment, and coordination of care for various childhood illnesses. National Association of Pediatric Nurse Associates and Practitioners. Mosby, 11830 Westline Industrial Drive, St. Louis, MO 63146, 314-872-8370, 800-325-4177.

Journal of Pediatrics. Monthly. Offers practical guidance for physicians who diagnose and treat disorders in infants and children. Mosby, 11830 Westline Industrial Drive, St. Louis, MO 63146, 314-872-8370, 800-325-4177.

Pediatrician. Quarterly. For pediatricians and their patient families with pre-school children. Covers advances in neonatal and pediatric medicine, psychology, and dentistry, plus relevant consumer product information. E P I, Inc., 8003 Old York Road, Elkins Park, PA 19117, 215-635-1700.

Pediatrics. Monthly. Includes employment listings. American Academy of Pediatrics, 141 Northwest Point Boulevard, Box 927, Elk Grove Village, IL 60009, 847-228-5005, 800-433-9016.

pedorthist

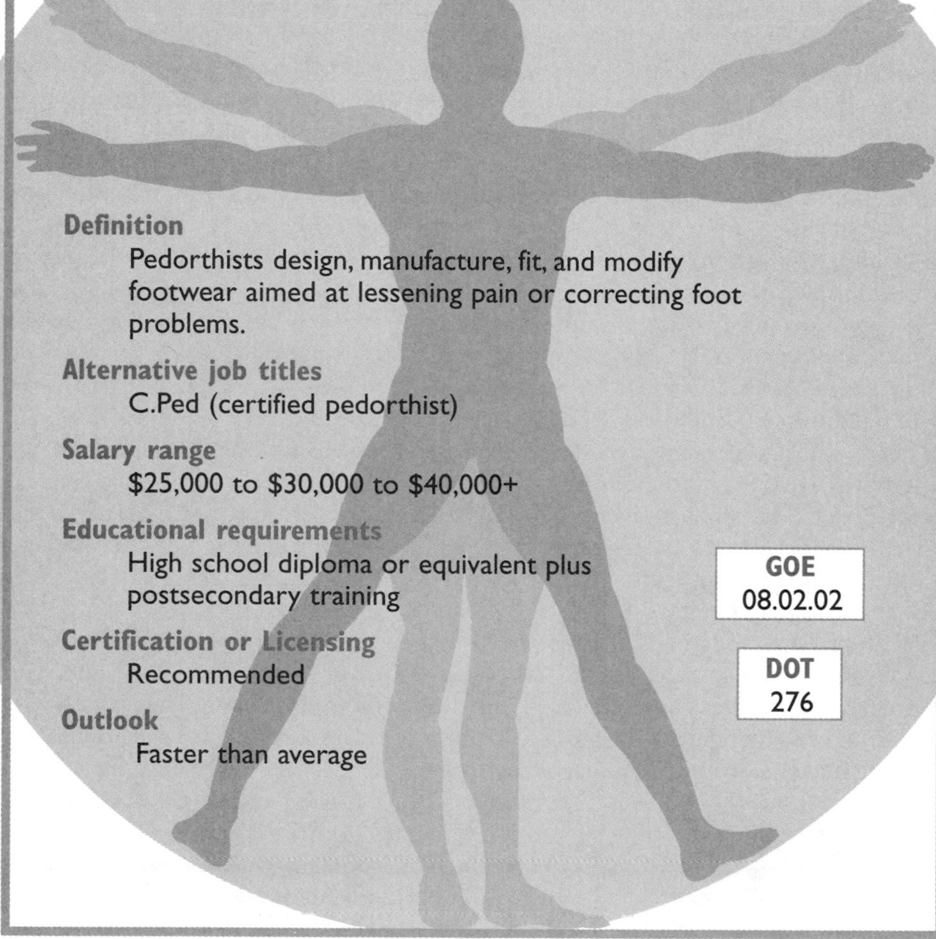

Definition

Pedorthists design, manufacture, fit, and modify footwear aimed at lessening pain or correcting foot problems.

Alternative job titles

C.Ped (certified pedorthist)

Salary range

$25,000 to $30,000 to $40,000+

Educational requirements

High school diploma or equivalent plus postsecondary training

Certification or Licensing

Recommended

Outlook

Faster than average

GOE
08.02.02

DOT
276

High School Subjects

Biology
English
Shop (Trade/Vo-tech)
Speech

Personal Interests

Health
Helping others
Science
Shoes
Sports

A deafening roar pours through the stadium. Nearly seven feet tall, the pro basketball player lopes down the court and moves into position. It's a routine setup. But suddenly he's on the floor, his long body jackknifed in pain, his hands reaching down to grasp one foot. "I think I pulled something," he gasps as a trainer quickly appears at his side. "My arch. . . ." His teammates hover close by and exchange worried glances. Will he be able to get up and play? Will this put him out of commission? For how long?

Watching the game is Ron, a certified pedorthist who works in a nearby sports medical facility. He can't tell how serious the problem is, but he bets this player is on the way to see a doctor. Maybe surgery will be needed. Maybe rehab after that. If footwear can help in any part of the player's recovery, Ron hopes the player comes to see him.

what does a pedorthist do?

A lot of things can go wrong with feet. Some common problems include bunions, claw toes or hammertoes, fallen arches, swelling from arthritis, and ulcers from diabetes. When a doctor examines your feet and decides special shoes or footwear could help, you could be on your way to see a *pedorthist.*

Pedorthists design, manufacture, fit, and modify shoes or therapeutic devices (such as braces) aimed at lessening pain or correcting foot problems. Trained in anatomy and shoe construction, pedorthists understand what has physically gone wrong with the foot and what shoe, insert, brace, pad, or other device will help. Whether designing a new shoe or just adding a modification, pedorthists play a key role in putting people back on their feet.

A certified pedorthist (C.Ped) works as part of a team of health care professionals treating a patient. Pedorthists never diagnose problems; that is done by a doctor, surgeon, or podiatrist. These physicians write out a prescription explaining what should be done and send the person to see a pedorthist. Pedorthists also may confer with physical therapists, nurses, orthotists, and other health care professionals.

Patient evaluation is the first step for pedorthists. They gain an understanding of the problem and what the doctor wants to accomplish. During an evaluation, pedorthists may observe the patient's gait (walk) and range of motion. They also may check back with the doctor if there are any questions.

Generally, a "corrective" or "accommodative" shoe or device is needed. Corrective footwear fixes a problem—bringing pigeon toes into alignment, for example. Accommodative footwear eases but does not fix a problem. It mainly makes the patient more comfortable. For example, feet that are greatly swollen may need shoes that are deeper than normal or that have a wider toe-box.

After determining the patient's needs, a pedorthist takes foot impressions. In a floor reaction imprint, the patient walks on a kind of slanted inked mat. The resulting footprints clearly show the foot's shape, pressure points, stride, and other characteristics. The patient also may step barefoot into plaster, wax, or other material. A plaster model of a person's feet can be made from this impression and used in making the patient's shoe or device.

Sometimes, the pedorthist can adapt an off-the-shelf product (like a shoe or insert) for the patient. Perhaps the shoe can be stretched, or the insert cut. Other times, a new shoe or a therapeutic device needs to be made.

To help them get the proper design, pedorthists may use computer-aided design (CAD) and 3D computer modeling. They then make the shoe or device or send the specifications to a manufacturing facility. Pedorthists are trained to know the right materials to use, such as plastic or leather. Some pedorthists have equipment in their office for making shoes or devices.

Fitting and follow up are the last steps. Pedorthists put the shoe or device on the patient and check the fit. Any necessary adjustments are made. (Sometimes this requires more than one visit.) Pedorthists make sure the patient understands how to use and maintain the footwear. In some cases the patient will start out using the new footwear for only an hour or so a day, building up gradually to a full day.

In follow up visits, pedorthists check to see if the desired results are being achieved. They will keep careful records and check back with the physician if something else needs to be done.

Pedorthists may work with anyone from babies to elderly people. That's because foot problems can happen at any age. Areas of specialization in pedorthics include adult foot deformities, amputations, arthritis, congenital deformities, diabetes, geriatrics, overuse injuries, pediatrics/rotational disorders, post-polio symptoms or late effects of polio, sports-related injuries, and trauma.

lingo to learn

Accommodative shoe or device It eases but does not fix a foot pain or problem. It mainly makes the patient more comfortable. Also may be called functional shoe or device.

Corrective shoe or device It fixes a problem—bringing pigeon toes into alignment, for example.

Custom A device or shoe that is made specifically for the patient.

Floor reaction imprint An impression of the bottom of the patient's foot showing foot shape, pressure points, stride, and other characteristics.

Prosthesis A device that replaces a missing body part or improves body function.

what is it like to be a pedorthist?

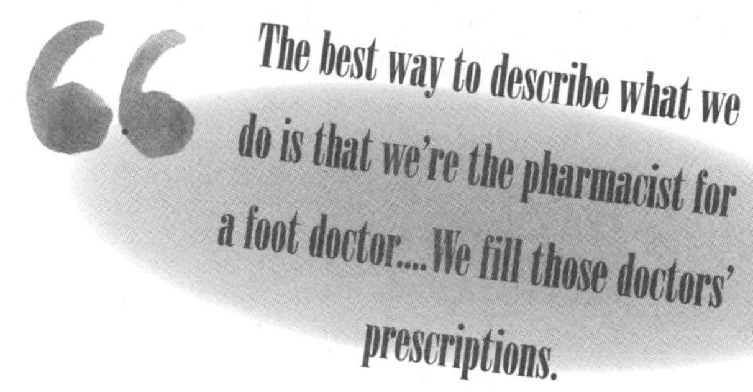

Rhona Chick, C.Ped, works for Ballert Orthopedic of Chicago, a health care facility specializing in orthotics and prosthetics (artificial limbs). People come here for everything from braces to prosthetics for amputees. Ballert staff also travel to nearby hospitals, clinics, nursing homes, and other health care facilities to see patients. Rhona has been working in the field for twelve years, and she definitely likes her job.

Rhona's cases fall into two major categories: children and adults. "We see a lot of kids from about age one or two to age seven for malalignment of feet," she says. Feet generally should be in a straight line but sometimes a child's foot has not developed properly. For example, a heel may be splayed or tilted to the outside. "These problems often happen in utero [in the womb]," Rhona notes.

Since a child's body is not fully formed yet, the right footwear can encourage the feet to grow in proper alignment. "The body will respond, especially with younger children," says Rhona.

A cast is made of the child's feet and footwear is designed that will hold the foot in the proper anatomical alignment. Ballert has its own on-site facilities for manufacturing the needed shoes or devices. (Although Rhona knows how to fabricate shoes, at Ballert, technicians handle this part.)

The child is fitted with the shoes and wears them for about a year until the problem is fixed. During that time, Rhona will see the patient periodically to check on his or her progress.

By contrast, adults are "skeletally mature" — their bones are fully formed—so it's less likely that footwear will correct alignment problems. Instead, accommodative shoes or devices are prescribed. Rhona's adult patients may also have foot problems caused by diabetes, arthritis, heart disease, or other medical conditions, as well as overuse or years of wearing the wrong shoes.

Each adult case is unique and Rhona has to be careful to think about all aspects of the problem. A patient may need better balance to avoid falls that could cause injury. Ulcers on the feet can become infected and the patient could lose a limb.

For her adult patients, Rhona may adapt an off-the-shelf shoe or device. For example, she may stretch a shoe or trim an insert to accommodate a problem. She may also create a special insert. "All of our footwear is extra-depth to accommodate an insert," says Rhona. Or, she may create a shoe or device from scratch.

Rhona learned in school that about 85 percent of the population needs orthotics, but most people don't know it. "Women generally have more problems than men because of high heels and other fashionable shoes," she adds. "Before I was a pedorthist, I always wondered why I'd see women walking to work downtown in bobby socks and gym shoes. But I know now. High heels are the worst thing for feet."

Rhona sees fewer sports-related injuries than high-heel injuries. This is partly because athletes protect themselves with good shoes. "Gym shoes today are made with lots of shock absorption," she points out. Still, sports-related injuries do occur—like plantar fasciitis or heel pain, such as what Toni Kukoc of the Chicago Bulls suffered during the 1996-97 season. "Maybe he landed weird on it, maybe it was a weakness that came to climax," Rhona speculates. Heel cups or arch supports might help in his case. However, Kukoc may eventually require surgery, which a pedorthist doesn't do.

Because Rhona is also a prosthetist, part of her job includes working with amputees to ensure proper design, fit, and wear of their artificial feet. Is that difficult? "To someone in the field, no," says Rhona. "You're glad to be able to help." This is true for all the problems she sees. "Someone might come in with an open oozing ulcer, and to me that's interesting. I can help them," she says.

Pedorthists are unusual in that they may also work in retail. For example, Lyle Rosen, C.Ped. spends most of his time working in a shoe store called Corrective Measures Plus. Like Rhona, he also sometimes visits patients in various hospitals, clinics, or nursing homes in the area, particularly elderly people, if a doctor calls and asks him to.

"The best way to describe what we do is that we're the pharmacist for a foot doctor," says Lyle. "We fill those doctors' prescriptions." Lyle's workplace looks like a typical shoe store from the outside, with nice-looking shoes on display in the windows.

As a certified pedorthist, Lyle does the same types of things that Rhona does, including evaluations, foot impressions, fittings, and follow-up checks. He does, however, send the fabricating work out to a local manufacturer.

Lyle says he's seeing a lot of foot problems these days from arthritis and diabetes. "Both are going up in numbers," he says. He also sees many stroke and heart disease patients. Many of these people are definitely hurting. For example, heart disease patients can suffer severe edema (swelling). "Their feet become very sensitive," says Lyle.

have I got what it takes to be a pedorthist?

A pedorthist needs to be able to talk to patients, ease their fears, teach them about the device or shoe, and make sure the patient complies with the treatment. Some people may resist wearing a corrective or accommodative shoe or device because they think it's not fashionable. Pedorthists should make sure the shoe or device is as appealing as possible. They should also explain how the shoe or device will help the patient and encourage the patient to comply with treatment in order to correct a problem or prevent further damage.

Usually a patient visits a pedorthist several times—for evaluation, fitting, and follow up. It's important to be able to develop rapport with patients to make sure you're giving them the best possible care and that they're following your instructions carefully.

"It's definitely a people job," says Rhona. manual dexterity is also important, she says, for the fabrication parts of the job. Patience, problem-solving skills, and conscientiousness are other desirable traits she adds. Besides dealing with the public, pedorthists need to be able to work cooperatively with physicians, physical therapists, nurses, and others on the patient's health care team.

how do I become a pedorthist?

"I was premed in college at the University of Illinois-Champaign," recalls Rhona. By junior year, however, she knew she wasn't going to be going on to medical school. She discovered pedorthics through a career guide in the library and decided it was for her.

Lyle had already been in the shoe business for many years when he decided to become certified in pedorthics.

education

High School

A high school diploma or equivalent is a requirement to be a certified pedorthist. You do not need to take any special classes in high school but you should take plenty of science courses. Biology would be an especially useful class. Because effective communication is always important, classes in English or speech would also be useful. Finally, since some pedorthists manufacture footwear or therapeutic devices, classes that teach you how to use various machines would be very beneficial.

Postsecondary Training

Many jobs in the field of pedorthics require at least some college-level coursework. Appropriate fields of study include courses in medicine, engineering, biomechanics, anatomy, and physical therapy.

certification or licensing

The Pedorthic Footwear Association (PFA), which certifies people in this field, requires at least a high school diploma or equivalent to start training in pedorthics. Beyond the high school requirement, you can take one of three paths to gain admission to the PFA certification program:

The first way is to get your associate's degree from an accredited college or university. The degree should be in a health or science-related field.

A second way is to get a bachelor's degree or higher from an accredited college or university. (This is what Rhona did.)

The third way is to earn 300 "points" from PFA by doing one or more of the following (PFA assigns the point totals): Complete science courses at an accredited college or university; do an internship in pedorthics, working under a C.Ped; or complete PFA-approved courses and seminars.

Once you've fulfilled one of the three options, you qualify to take PFA's certification exam. You must pass this exam to earn your certification.

Training doesn't stop after you've earned certification. "There's always continuing education requirements that you must meet," says Rhona. To keep your certification, you need to earn 150 continuing education "points" every three years as long as you're working in the field. Points are earned by going to approved classes, seminars, and workshops; retaking and passing the certification exam; providing in-service training; studying videos and books; and taking various other steps spelled out by PFA. For each activity, certain documentation must be submitted to and approved by PFA.

To be a successful pedorthist you should

- Have manual dexterity
- Be good at solving problems
- Be conscientious
- Enjoy working with people
- Have good communication skills

internships and volunteerships

"An internship is definitely a plus," says Rhona. "It's to one's interest and benefit." Rhona interned at a prosthetics and orthotics facility in Champaign, Illinois, where she mainly did observation. "Hands-on work is the best, though," she says. She recommends that you look in the Yellow Pages for such facilities and call them to ask about internship opportunities. "For example, there are 56 prosthetic and orthotic facilities or labs listed in the Yellow Pages" for the Chicago area, says Rhona.

who will hire me?

Pedorthists are employed in three major areas, manufacturing, retail, and clinical. Rhona is an example of someone from the clinical area. Lyle works in both the retail and clinical areas.

In clinical environments, pedorthists work in hospitals, clinics, nursing homes, or other health care facilities. Some pedorthists own their own companies, specializing in providing pedorthic services to others. A facility can become PFA-certified by meeting certain requirements. Like Rhona, you may work out of one clinical facility but routinely visit others because the patients can't come to you.

In manufacturing environments, pedorthists work for shoe and device manufacturers. These companies focus on fabricating pedorthic shoes and devices to supply to other pedorthists. For example, Lyle uses these types of companies because he doesn't have the facilities at his store to make the shoes and devices himself. Having pedorthists on staff can help manufacturers ensure they are properly filling orders for shoes or devices.

In retail environments, pedorthists work in specialty shoe stores. Most of the customers that go to these stores will have been sent by a doctor. But sometimes you will also get people off the street who like the idea of buying extra-care shoes.

Education, government affairs, research, and association work are other possible areas of employment. A source of potential employers is PFA's Directory of Pedorthics, which lists all PFA members. You may also wish to contact this association directly for information about employment opportunities in the field.

Rhona was hired by Ballert out of college. Lyle already had a job in retail shoes before he became a certified pedorthist. Good bets for finding your first employer start with your internship. If the pedorthist you intern for can't hire you, ask if he or she can recommend you to someone who can. Also check with the placement department of your school. Beyond that, develop your resume, turn to your PFA directory and your Yellow Pages, and start sending out letters to prospective employers.

where can I go from here?

Bill Boettge, Executive Director of PFA, says ownership and additional duties are two keys to advancement. "The C.Ped may branch out and open his or her own facility," he says. " Or he or she may take on additional responsibilities besides patient care, such as managing inventory, supervising others in the office, or marketing pedorthic services to doctors or managed care firms," he adds. Each of these things would constitute advancement and command a higher salary.

what are the salary ranges?

Salaries differ by geographic area and by level of education, says Bill Boettge of the PFA. Salaries in heavily populated metropolitan areas tend to be higher than those in less populated areas. In general, entry-level salary is about $25,000, according to Bill—less if the person is just out of high school and working towards certification, more if the person has a year or two of experience and is certified. A mid-level salary is about $30,000, with the C.Ped primarily focusing on patient care. A high-level salary is about $40,000 and up, with the highest pay going to those who own their own practice or have responsibilities beyond patient care.

what is the job outlook?

Pedorthics is still a fairly small field. According to Bill, there are about 1,400 people currently certified through PFA. The outlook for growth, however, is excellent. Pedorthic care is no exception. As Lyle noted, professionals already are seeing growing numbers of cases where arthritis, diabetes, heart disease, and strokes are involved with foot problems. Pedorthists can often help ease the pain associated with these foot problems. Everyday wear-and-tear problems associated with feet, including overuse and sports injuries will also keep tomorrow's pedorthists busy.

Also key to the growth of the industry will be awareness. "Pedorthist" is not exactly a household world, and even some health care professionals are not familiar with the specialty. Pedorthists actively network with physicians. Associations like PFA have public education initiatives to teach the general public and health professions about pedorthics and its benefits.

PFA also has professional liaisons with medical and allied health organizations such as the American Diabetes Association, American Orthopaedic Foot & Ankle Society, American Orthotic and Prosthetic Association, American Podiatric Foundation, National Association of Athletic Trainers, and the like.

how do I learn more?

professional organizations

To find out more about becoming a pedorthist and to receive free brochures, please contact:

Pedorthic Footwear Association (PFA)
9861 Broken Land Parkway, Suite 255
Columbia, MD 21046
TEL: 410-381-7278 or 800-673-8447
WEBSITE:
http://www.cloudnet.com/~oandpnet/PFAPFA.html

For information on certification requirements and procedures, write to:

Board for Certification in Pedorthics (BCP)
9861 Broken Land Parkway, Suite 255
Columbia, MD 21046
TEL: 410-381-5729
WEBSITE:
http://www.cloudnet.com/~oandpnet/TBFCIP.html

bibliography

Following is a sampling of materials relating to the professional concerns and development of pedorthists.

Books

Awad, Elias M., and M. David Tremaine. *The Foot and Ankle Source Book: Everything You Need to Know.* Los Angeles, CA: Lowell House, 1996.

Cailliet, Rene. *Foot and Ankle Pain,* 3rd edition. Philadelphia, PA: F.A. Davis Co., 1996.

Hurwitz, Shepard R., Panos A. Labropoulos, Henry L. Feffer, and Sam W. Wiesel. *Foot and Ankle Pain.* Charlottesville, VA: MICHIE, 1988.

Michaud, Thomas C. *Foot Orthoses and Other Forms of Conservative Foot Care.* Baltimore, MD: Williams & Wilkins, 1993.

Periodicals

Pedoscope. Bimonthly. Newsletter. Pedorthic Footwear Association, 9861 Broken Land Parkway, Suite 255, Columbia, MD 21046, 410-381-7278.

perfusionist

Definition

Perfusionists operate and monitor extracorporeal circulation equipment, such as heart-lung machines and artificial hearts, during any medical situation where it is necessary to support or temporarily replace the patient's cardiopulmonary-circulatory function.

Alternative job titles

Cardiovascular perfusionists
Extracorporeal technologists
Perfusion technicians

Salary range

$50,000 to $70,000 to $120,000

Educational requirements

High school diploma; bachelor of science degree; twelve to forty-eight months of specialized training

Certification or licensing

Highly recommended

Outlook

Faster than average

GOE
10.03.02

DOT
078

High School Subjects

Biology
Chemistry
Mathematics
Physics

Personal Interests

Helping people
Human anatomy
Working as part of a team

Carol Zografas shuts the door behind her and glances around the sterile cardiac operating room. It is only 7:00 AM and she has already read her patient's chart and knows what to expect. It is the first procedure of the day, a neonatal case involving two-month-old Kristen. Carol will be working with Maxine, the anesthesiologist, and Dr. Cardwell, the heart surgeon, as well as with the other operating room staff, to repair complex defects in Kristen's heart.

Carol turns on the heart-lung machine and goes through her preoperative checklist. Is the tubing the right size for the infant? Are all the parts of the machine working properly? She checks off one item after another on her list. Once the operation begins, Kristen's life could depend on Carol's skills and the heart-lung machine.

Finally, she puts the list down, satisfied that she is as prepared as she can be to begin the operation. She looks across the room at Maxine. "I'm all set, Max. Are you ready?" she asks.

what does a perfusionist do?

The heart is an amazing and compelling organ of the human body. It is the main tool of the circulatory system, beating about seventy times a minute to circulate the oxygen and nutrients that provide energy for human action and thought. This tool, basically a life-giving pump, must move the equivalent of two thousand gallons of blood through the body every day without stopping.

lingo to learn

Blood salvaging Using as much of the patient's blood as possible so as not to depend on donated blood. Some patients donate their own blood supply prior to their surgery.

Cardiac Relating to the heart.

Cardiologist Heart surgeon.

Cardiopulmonary Relating to the heart and lungs.

Cell savers Machines that separate plasma, damaged platelets, and saline from blood that should not be returned to the patient's body.

Extracorporeal circulation Circulation of the patient's blood outside the body.

Heart-lung machine A machine used to take over the function of the patient's heart and lungs during surgery or respiratory failure. The machine draws blood from the patient's body, reoxygenates it, and pumps it back into the patient's body.

Induced hypothermia A condition that the perfusionist may inflict on the patient to reduce body temperature to 70 degrees or below; this slows the patient's metabolism and reduces stress on the heart.

Pulmonary circulation Blood flow to and from the lungs.

When one's heart is not functioning correctly, or when one has a heart disease, surgery is often performed to repair the damage or to control the illness. During an operation such as open heart surgery, coronary bypass, or any other procedure that involves the heart and lungs, the *perfusionist* is indispensable. Before the cardiologist can begin to operate on the heart, it is necessary to interrupt or replace the functioning of the heart by circulating the blood through machines outside of the patient's body. This process of circulating the blood outside the patient's body is called "extracorporeal circulation."

Perfusionists are experts in extracorporeal circulation. They perform complex, delicate procedures to transfer the functions of the heart to special machines while the cardiologist operates on the patient. These machines are called heart-lung machines; they take over the job of the heart and lungs. When the surgery is over, perfusionists also may help to start the heart pumping again if it doesn't start up by itself.

During heart surgery, the doctor will pierce the patient's breastbone and the membrane surrounding the heart (called the "pericardial sac"). Then the perfusionist will activate the heart-lung machine by inserting two tubes into the heart; one tube circulates blood from the heart to the machine, and the other tube circulates blood from the machine back into the heart. Using the heart-lung machine, the perfusionist maintains the functions of the patient's circulatory system and the appropriate levels of the patient's heart, including oxygen, carbon dioxide, and other nutrient levels.

Operating the heart-lung machine is the foundation of the perfusionist's job. During the medical procedure, perfusionists may also administer prescriptive drugs, anaesthetic agents, or blood products through the blood. They may also induce hypothermia, which means that the patient's body temperature is lowered to about 70 degrees (our average body temperature is about 98 degrees) so that the metabolism and stress levels are slowed down, allowing for less risk to the patient's body functions. Perfusionists use probes in other parts of the body to monitor the blood pressure and kidney activity during the surgical procedures. They also perform blood gas analysis and check for normal brain activity.

Perfusionists perform a technique called blood salvaging, which means that they try to save as much of the patient's blood as possible so they don't have to depend on donated blood. Blood salvaging is especially important these days because of the high rate of AIDS cases; the HIV virus, which causes AIDS, is transmitted through blood (as well as through other body fluids). Some patients donate their own blood supply prior to their surgery. Perfusionists also sometimes work with cell savers, which are machines that separate plasma, damaged platelets, and saline from blood that should not be returned to the patient's body.

When being operated on, a patient must have a precise and consistent amount of blood flowing through the body and to the brain. The perfusionist must make sure that the heart-lung machines are delivering the proper amount of blood back into the patient's body to prevent damage to the brain and other major organs. Before the patient is taken off the heart-lung machine, the perfusionist makes sure that the patient's temperature is back to normal; he or she also does a blood test (called a "hematocrit") on the patient to ensure that the red blood cell count is normal.

After surgery, the perfusionist slows down the blood flow to the patient and shuts off one of the lines to the heart-lung machine. When the patient's body takes over on its own, the machinery is shut off. If the patient's heart does not start on its own, the perfusionist may have to provide temporary cardiac support (with either the heart-lung machine or an artificial heart), until the patient's heart is ready to beat on its own.

Perfusionists are responsible for assembling, setting up, monitoring, and operating all the equipment that assists the circulation of blood during a medical procedure. They may also be responsible for ensuring that the equipment is maintained in accurate working order.

Specialized perfusionists assist at-risk patients such as premature babies and heart patients who have just had surgery (that is, "postoperative," or "post-op," patients). In these cases, the workers perform extracorporeal membrane oxygenation, using a machine that draws blood from the patient's body, reoxygenates it, and pumps it back into the patient through the arteries. For newborns and very young infants, this buys crucial time until the infant's respiratory and circulatory systems can work on their own; for heart patients, it may buy time until the heart is able to pump on its own or until a donor heart is found.

Perfusionists have also recently become important in the treatment of trauma. In such cases, they are called upon to rapidly infuse or replace lost blood or to lower the blood volume.

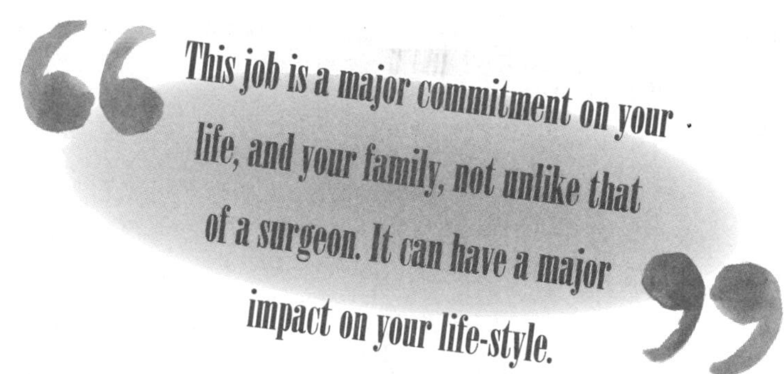

Perfusion is now being used in the treatment of patients undergoing cancer surgery, organ transplants, and orthopedic surgery. As medical technology evolves, new uses for perfusion will most likely continue to be developed.

what is it like to be a perfusionist?

Carol Zografas is the chief cardiovascular perfusionist at Maine Medical Center, in Portland, Maine. It is 6:30 in the morning when she arrives at the hospital. She checks the schedule to find out what procedure she will be doing today. She finds that she will be assisting the surgical team to repair extensive defects in the heart of a newborn baby.

Carol reads the patient's chart and looks for anything out of the ordinary that she may have to consult with the surgeon about. Does the baby have diabetes? Is the kidney function normal? It will be Carol's job to monitor and adjust the infant's kidney function, blood sugar, brain activity, and other body functions while the infant is in surgery.

After she is sure she knows all she needs to know, Carol gathers her equipment together and assembles it in the cardiac operating room. She needs some special equipment because the patient is an infant.

After assembling the equipment, Carol goes through her page-long preoperative checklist to be sure that all the equipment is running properly. She checks the contents of the prepackaged parts for sterility and integrity. Are the tubes for the artificial heart placed in the right areas to make sure the circuits are complete? Have the proper drugs been administered in the prime fluid? Are all the parts of the heart-lung machine working properly? Are all the alarms operational?

When Carol is satisfied that her checklist is complete, she is ready to begin her work with the rest of the surgical team. She will be in the operating room anywhere from four to six hours for a typical surgical procedure. Her machinery is next to the operating table, and she works closely with the surgeon, the anesthesiologist, and other operating room staff.

Carol and her staff will perform approximately 150 procedures each year. As chief of her department, Carol usually performs perfusions two days a week. The remaining hours in her work week are filled with administrative and managerial tasks and teaching. Maine Medical Center has one of the three largest heart programs in New England and is a clinical teaching site for Northeastern University in Boston.

Carol supervises seven full-time and one half-time staff members. For quality control reasons, she tries not to schedule her staff for more than one procedure per day; she fills in herself when someone gets sick. The rest of her time is spent monitoring quality standards, performing preventive maintenance on equipment, solving staffing problems, chairing department meetings, attending meetings with other departments, counseling staff, and keeping up with the accreditation requirements for hospitals.

Carol's day begins at 6:30 in the morning, and she is never sure when it will end. "All the perfusionists in my department average about five hours of overtime per week. Overtime has its peaks and valleys," she says. "We always have two staff members on call in case of an emergency, and we work every day of the week."

To be a successful perfusionist, you should

- Have the ability to concentrate for long periods of time
- Have good communication skills
- Have a strong sense of responsibility
- Work well as part of a team
- Know how to take and carry out orders
- Think independently
- Have the ability to respond to emergencies quickly and correctly
- Be able to use your common sense and good judgment
- Cope well under extreme stress
- Know how to cope with occasional failure

have I got what it takes to be a perfusionist?

Perfusionists perform some of the most delicate and vital services for patients during heart and lung surgery, yet most patients have never heard of perfusionists and aren't aware of the services they perform. Although their profession is not well known, perfusionists can take pride in the knowledge that the procedures they perform are crucial to their patients' lives.

Perfusionists make decisions that could affect the well-being of the patient for years to come. "It is so technical," Carol says. "There is always the possibility of us doing some permanent damage. This is why we have so many checklists and check things so often. We build our systems to be as safe as possible."

Carol tries not to schedule her staff for more than one procedure per day, because each procedure takes hours of total focused concentration. "This is not a job you should take because you want to make money," Carol says. "You have to be able to commit yourself to each and every patient, and that takes a lot of compassion. You have to be able to react quickly in emergency situations, keep a cool head. Suppose you've got a patient who comes in to the emergency room, and his heart isn't working. You've got to keep your head and get that patient on bypass as soon as possible." She concludes, "This job is a major commitment on your life, and your family, not unlike that of a surgeon. It can have a major impact on your life-style."

Occasionally, medical situations occur in which all the combined effort and talent of the surgical team is unable to help the patient. Perfusionists must have strength of character to accept the limitations of modern medicine, as well as its successes. "You need to know how to deal with death," Carol says, "and sometimes that only comes with age. It's really hard when you have children you're working with and you lose a patient. You have to learn some way to deal with it."

What Carol likes best about her job is the peace of mind she gets from knowing she's helped another human being. She especially likes working in the neonatal department. It gives her a sense of satisfaction to see a listless newborn with pale, clammy skin transformed through the surgery into a healthy, rosy-skinned infant. Carol's satisfaction comes from

in-depth

The Heart of the Matter

Considering the age of humankind and the evolution of the medical sciences, heart surgery is still in its infancy. The first bypass operation was performed in 1944 by Dr. John Blalock, whose patient was a newborn infant with oxygen-poor blood. The baby was born with a bluish tint because blood was not circulating correctly. Dr. Blalock operated on the baby, bypassing a blocked blood vessel.

The most significant breakthrough in open heart surgery occurred ten years later, when Dr. John Gibbon used a machine to pump blood and supply oxygen to an eighteen-year-old patient, giving the surgeon needed time for delicate heart surgery. The machine was the heart-lung machine, which is now a standard fixture in cardiac operating rooms.

knowing that the contributions she makes during any successful surgical procedure help the patient to live a normal life.

Carol likes working in a field where new developments and new technologies are always coming along. She never has time to be bored. She also enjoys teaching. Because Maine Medical Center is a clinical supervision site for Boston's Northeastern University, Carol is able to share her skills with students.

Carol says that it helps to have a great staff. "The surgeons here are wonderful," she says. However, she doesn't really enjoy the administrative work as much as working in the operating room. She also doesn't like what's happening in the health care industry itself. "It's so cost-driven these days," she says. "All you hear is cost, cost, cost; streamline your team. I'm concerned that there isn't much nonprocedural time left for my staff to keep educated about new developments. I'm also concerned that cutting the costs of medical services will adversely affect patient care, although this hospital has assured us over the years that would never happen here." Carol regularly reads various professional journals and annals to keep up with new developments in her field.

how do I become a perfusionist?

Carol Zografas was an operating room nurse at Maine Medical Center in 1967 when she entered an on-the-job training program for perfusionists. She characterizes her training as rigorous "baptism by fire." She became board-certified when that became standard, which was in 1972. She says that today you cannot learn perfusionism on the job alone. There is too much technical knowledge required, and too many technological developments have occurred for that to work.

When Carol began her studies, her nursing background was helpful to her, but she had to take a lot of extra classes and study a lot on her own to be successful.

education

High School

In preparation for any perfusion technology program, it is very important to take natural science classes such as biology and chemistry. Also essential are courses in higher mathematics and physics. You must have a high school diploma before you will be accepted in an accredited educational program.

Postsecondary Training

On-the-job training and apprenticeships are no longer available for positions in the perfusion field. To prepare for a career in perfusion, you must attend one of the twenty-eight nationally accredited schools in the United States. Some of these schools require you to have a bachelor's of science (B.S.) degree before you enter their program; others include coursework toward the B.S. as part of their training. Program length varies from one to four years, depending on the schooling required for acceptance.

Occasionally, an accrediting institution will accept applicants who have trained at nursing schools or other technical schools and who have had experience as nurses or health technicians.

The accredited school carefully examines the student's personal character, academic achievement record, and personal temperament before accepting new students. There is intense competition for admission to these programs. Only 10 to 20 percent of the applicants are accepted.

It takes a unique type of person to work successfully under the kind of stress and challenge required. Intense coursework is preparation for such a challenging job. Courses include physiology, cardiology, respiratory therapy, general surgical procedure, and pharmacology. Also covered are courses in heart-lung bypass for adult, young children, and infant patients undergoing heart surgery; extracorporeal circulation; monitoring of the patient; and special applications.

Students also receive clinical training for one and a half to two years. Most of the accredited perfusion programs try to begin their students' clinical training as soon as possible. The practice of perfusion requires extensive actual operating room experience. It is in the operating room that students observe and learn about extracorporeal circulation, respiratory therapy, general surgical procedures, and anaesthesia. In clinical practice, students begin to perform perfusion procedures and perfect their skills.

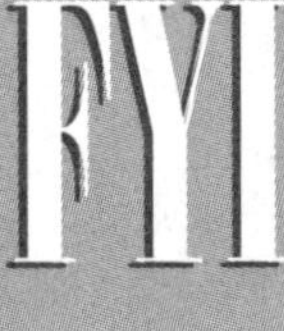

What is a Coronary Bypass?

A surgical procedure performed on patients with diseased or obstructed coronary arteries or veins. During surgery, a nonessential vein from another part of the patient's body is grafted onto the obstructed coronary artery, thus bypassing it and allowing essential blood flow to and from the heart.

certification or licensing

When students complete their study and training, they must then take written and oral tests given by the American Board of Cardiovascular Perfusion. The written test must be passed first. Each year, the examination location is different. There is a fee for taking the exam,and you must pay your travel expenses. Once certified, perfusionists pay an annual fee to maintain their certification.

After completing the tests, which can be taken only three times, the student receives certification and may legally perform perfusion. At one time, students who were trained on the job could take the certification tests without having to pass an exam. This is no longer the case. For liability reasons and quality control, most hospitals will not hire perfusionists who are not certified.

scholarships and grants

Scholarships for perfusion programs are available from the American Society of Extra-Corporeal Technology (AmSECT) and the American Board of Cardiovascular Perfusion (ABCP). Be sure to write well in advance of your planned study for application requirements and procedures. In addition, financial aid in the form of scholarships and grants is often available through the financial aid office where the student is applying for school.

who will hire me?

Carol Zografas's first job experience was at Maine Medical Center, the hospital where she continues to work today. Typically, the perfusionist works in the cardiac operating room in a hospital as part of the surgery team. The perfusionist might be employed by the hospital itself, by a medical services group, or even by an individual cardiologist.

Advancement Possibilities

Chief cardiovascular perfusionists are in charge of the perfusionists on staff at a hospital. The chief perfusionist supervises others' work, performs administrative tasks, counsels staff, and maintains and monitors quality standards. If the hospital where you work is part of a university or other educational setting, as chief perfusionist you would instruct students and others and perhaps do research on your work.

Many perfusionists are self-employed, meaning that they are independent contractors who offer their services to one or more hospitals. Those who are self-employed must take care of their own business affairs, including purchasing medical insurance, scheduling vacation time, and buying uniforms and other necessary materials.

A clinical perfusionist may find employment in any of the hospitals with open heart surgery facilities in the United States. Some perfusionists find work as clinical consultants for companies that develop and sell perfusion equipment to hospitals. Perfusionists with graduate school education may conduct research and write about their findings.

AmSECT, the professional society for perfusion technologists, recommends that students who have entered a program investigate the field first with professors and teachers, and then join the AmSECT student membership division. This group holds meetings and conferences where you can get information on job openings in the field.

where can I go from here?

Perfusionism is a highly specialized field. Carol Zografas has reached the pinnacle of success as chief perfusionist in her department at Maine Medical Center. Her position requires her to be responsible for managing a large staff as well as maintaining quality control. She is also responsible for supervising the purchase of supplies and equipment and for educating her staff about new techniques.

The typical career path involves learning more complex and specific procedures. Carol says that the foreseeable future in perfusionism will be increasingly technological and specialized. Neonatal perfusionism, one of Carol's most rewarding job responsibilities, is a good example of one specialization.

Perfusionists with graduate education and experience may conduct research and write about their work. Others choose to teach in colleges and accredited schools.

what are the salary ranges?

Beginning perfusionists may start their careers earning about $40,000 a year. Experienced perfusionists average about $55,000, and the top salary level is about $70,000 a year. Some perfusionists who are employed by a physician and those with successful private practices may earn as much as $120,000 or more a year.

There was until recently a great demand for trained individuals in this field, so salaries were quite high. However, salaries have "bottomed out" (meaning that they have reached a low point) because supply has caught up with demand.

Perfusionists employed by hospitals and medical services groups get benefits such as sick leave, vacation, and medical insurance. Self-employed and physician-employed perfusionists usually pay for their own insurance, as well as for such items as uniforms and other minor equipment needed on the job.

what is the job outlook?

The field of open-heart surgery has expanded considerably since the 1980s and it is expected to continue to expand, providing greater opportunities for perfusionists. Overall, job opportunities for perfusionists are expected to grow faster than the average for all occupations through 2005.

how do I learn more?

professional organizations

Following are organizations that provide information on perfusionist careers, accredited schools and scholarships, and employers.

American Society of Extra-Corporeal Technology (AmSECT)
11480 Sunset Hills Road
Suite 200E
Reston, VA 22090
TEL: 703-435-8556
WEBSITE: http://www.amsect.org

American Board of Cardiovascular Perfusion (ABCP)
207 North 25th Avenue
Hattiesburg, MS 39401
TEL: 601-582-3309

American Medical Association
515 North State Street
Chicago, IL 60610
TEL: 312-464-5000
WEBSITE: http://www.ama-assn.org

bibliography

Following is a sampling of materials relating to the professional concerns and development of perfusionists.

Books

Kamada, T., T. Shiga, and R. S. McCuskey. *Tissue Perfusion and Organ Function.* New York, NY: Elsevier Science, 1996.

Periodicals

Heart Direct. Quarterly. Newsletter discussing all aspects of cardiovascular health. McMurry Publishing, Inc., 8805 North 23rd Avenue, Suite 11, Phoenix, AZ 85021, 602-395-5850.

Heartbeat. Quarterly. Directed toward patients, this magazine covers cardiovascular health. Health Team Interactive Communications, 274 Madison Avenue, 19th Floor, New York, NY 10016, 212-689-1520.

Heartline. Monthly. Discusses all aspects of heart care. Coronary Club Bulletin, Coronary Club, Inc., 9500 Euclid Avenue, Suite E4-15, Cleveland, OH 44195, 216-444-3690.

Heart Disease and Stroke: a Journal for Primary Care Physicians. Bimonthly. Includes information on the diagnosis, treatment, and management of these two diseases. American Heart Association, 7272 Greenville Avenue, Dallas, TX 75231, 214-706-1426.

Perfusion Life. Monthly. Discusses news and events. American Society of Extra-Corporeal Technology, Inc., Golf Course Plaza, Suite 100E, 11480 Sunset Hills Road, Reston, VA 22090, 703-435-8556.

Perfusion Review. Quarterly. Trade publication. D M R Publishing, Box 85099, Los Angeles, CA 90072, 213-464-1959.

periodontist

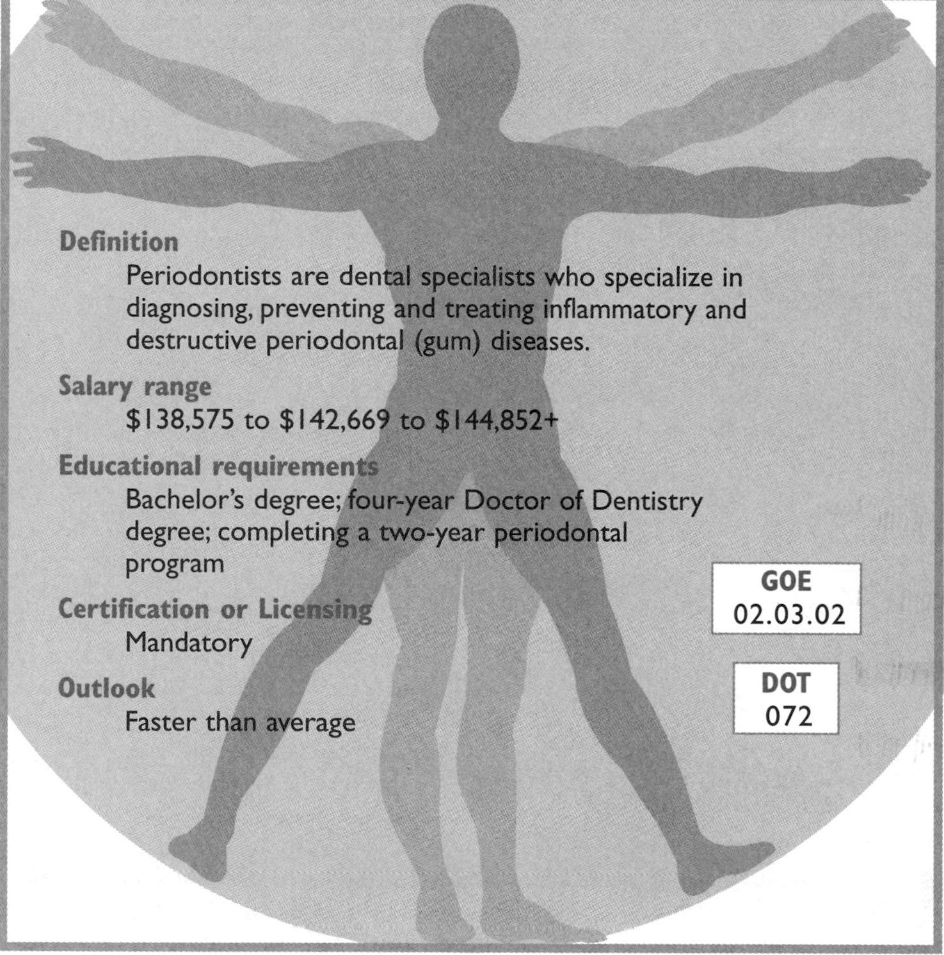

Definition
Periodontists are dental specialists who specialize in diagnosing, preventing and treating inflammatory and destructive periodontal (gum) diseases.

Salary range
$138,575 to $142,669 to $144,852+

Educational requirements
Bachelor's degree; four-year Doctor of Dentistry degree; completing a two-year periodontal program

Certification or Licensing
Mandatory

Outlook
Faster than average

GOE
02.03.02

DOT
072

High School Subjects

Accounting
Business
English
Math
Science

Personal Interests

Building models
Hobbies involving working with hands
Reading
Scientific and medical discoveries

Tom's gums had shrunk. At age twelve, Tom was nervous as he entered the periodontal office of Sara Whitener, D.D.S, M.S. What if she couldn't fix it? What if it got worse? He already felt self-conscious enough about wearing braces, and now this.

"Well, Tom, it looks like your orthodontist was right. The periodontal, or gum, tissue around your lower front teeth has receded a bit. I have reviewed your medical history, and you don't have any systemic diseases and don't take prescription drugs. So, the cause of this could be hereditary, a reaction to getting braces, or because you may not be effectively cleaning all the plaque off your teeth around your braces. Plaque and tartar irritate gums," Whitener said, "And sometimes they react."

"What's going to happen, doctor?" Tom asked, looking worried. Whitener sat down next to Tom. "Periodontal tissues are important Tom. They visually frame our teeth, almost like window shades. Some people have too much gum tissue and their teeth look too short. Other people, like you, have too little tissue in some places and those teeth look longer. Gum tissue not only helps our teeth to look attractive, they help support and stabilize our teeth. Teeth with insufficient periodontal tissue can shift and drift, becoming crooked or even loose."

"Can you treat my problem?" Tom asked."Luckily, your orthodontist sent you to a periodontist. We can do a tissue graft onto your existing periodontal tissue, which would effectively repair the damage done. It's an uncomplicated in-office procedure that I do every week," Whitener said.

"And it works?" Tom asked. "All the time," she said. "Let me talk with you and your mom about what's involved and then we'll make an appointment."

lingo to learn

Alveolar bone The bone that makes up the tooth socket onto which periodontal fibers attach the tooth.

Anesthesia Loss of feeling, also known as numbness, caused by an anesthetic agent applied, injected or inhaled, which permits diagnostic and treatment procedures to be performed comfortably.

Cementum Thin covering of calcified tissue on tooth.

Flap A surgically loosened section of gum or oral tissue that is separated from the tissue while still connected at its base.

Gingiva Gums.

Gingivitis Inflamed gums.

Infection Disease process involving inflammation and sometimes pain caused by microorganisms invading a particular site.

Periodontium Gum and bone tissues around the teeth.

Periodontitis Inflammation of the gum and bone tissues around the teeth that can progress and lead to the loss of teeth.

Periodontal pocket A space between a tooth and gum caused when periodontal disease detaches the gum from the root.

Plaque A mass of microorganisms and protein, food, and other matter that firmly adheres to all hard surfaces in the mouth; can only be removed from brushing and flossing.

Radiograph Sometimes called an "X ray," radiographs are images, usually recorded on film, that are produced by ionizing radiation.

Tartar Also called calculus, this is a hard, calcified collection of bacteria that adheres to solid surfaces in the mouth; can only be removed with a professional cleaning.

what does a periodontist do?

Periodontists treat diseases and conditions of the gum tissue, which is called periodontal tissue in dentistry. Without periodontal care, people with uncontrolled periodontal disease will have irreversible damage to their gums and supporting bone tissue. In advanced cases, teeth will become loose and may even begin to fall out. According to The American Academy of Periodontology, 75 percent of all Americans have some form of periodontal disease. Many don't know it.

People who have periodontal disease can be any age, from teenagers to older adults. The most common group of patients seen in the periodontal office are middle-aged. Smokers have periodontal problems more often than nonsmokers. And, those afflicted often have halitosis—bad breath from decaying gum tissue. The motivation for treating periodontal disease is usually cosmetic—to retain teeth. However, gum diseases can also result in crooked teeth and tooth loss, which can also create functional challenges for speaking and chewing. In addition, crooked teeth are harder to keep clean, and plaque and tartar build up are the biggest cause of periodontal disease.

Periodontal disease begins with gingivitis, a mild infection and inflammation of the gums from ineffective brushing and flossing, or from not visiting a dentist regularly for a dental prophylaxis (teeth cleaning). The toxins in plaque (bacteria) on teeth irritate gums. If they are allowed to remain irritated, the gums may separate from the teeth, which creates a pocket or space. Food debris and bacteria accumulate in the pockets between teeth and gums, accelerating the destruction to the gums and bone tissue beneath the gums. Simple gingivitis may or may not progress to periodontal disease. But because this disease is often painless, there are symptoms patients can look for: bleeding gums when brushing or flossing; halitosis (chronic bad breath); oozing, infected gums; receding, shrinking and loosening gums; and new space around or between teeth. Some patients notice these symptoms and get the name of a periodontist from a friend or the phone book. Most likely, however, patients are sent to a periodontist at the suggestion of their general dentist or other dental specialist who may have suspected a periodontal problem.When the patient comes to the office, periodontists take a complete medical and dental history to make sure they know what has affected or is influencing health in general and teeth in particular. Next, the mouth is carefully examined to look for oral evidence of disease. The health of teeth and gums are carefully evaluated.

During the examination, an periodontist judges whether the teeth fit together properly and if gums have receded. As part of the examination, periodontists place small measuring instruments in between patients' teeth and gums to determine depths of the periodontal pockets. By measuring periodontal pockets at each session, periodontists determine if gum health is stabilized, worsening or improving.

To further make a diagnosis, the periodontist needs to radiographically evaluate health of bone tissue (roots and surrounding jaw bone). X rays are one type of radiograph that reveal status of tissues that can't be seen by the eye, including not only problems with roots and supporting jaw bone, but problems inside the teeth and facial bones. To create a baseline of data on periodontal health, X rays are taken at the first appointment. By taking X rays at subsequent appointments, a periodontist can determine if the bone tissues have resorbed or deteriorated and receded. In some periodontal offices, computer programs are used to take detailed measurements of the changes in a series of X rays over time. Other techniques and strategies help periodontists diagnosis gum diseases, but periodontal probing and X rays are relied upon heavily.

Once a diagnosis is made, periodontists may give the patient an oral or written treatment plan. This plan includes the diagnosis, the recommended treatment specifics and cost estimate of treatment.

Early periodontal disease, where the beginnings of gum recession are seen, is treated by nonsurgical deep cleaning around the teeth below the gums. This procedure is called "scaling and root planing" and eliminates plaque and tartar buildup. After this procedure, the teeth above and below the gums are smoother, making it difficult for bacteria to latch onto them. The patients are carefully educated on how to keep their teeth clean and may be given a therapeutic mouthrinse. This may be all the periodontist needs to do to control or reverse the problem at this stage.

For moderate to advanced periodontal disease, periodontists need to perform other procedures such as open flap surgery or a gum tissue graft. Open flap surgery involves pulling back gum tissue and cleaning the infected side of the root and the bottom of the periodontal pocket. Then the flap is sutured back in place. Gum tissue grafts involve surgically removing a small piece of healthy gum tissue from the mouth, often the roof of the mouth, and placing it where gum tissue has receded.

Guided tissue regeneration is another exciting periodontal procedure. It is a technique for regenerating periodontal ligament and bone that involves placing a mesh-like barrier around a tooth root. The barrier keeps the gum tissue away while saving space for the ligament and bone to grow.

Additional periodontal procedures include doing osseous grafts. This is where the periodontist takes either the patient's bone tissue or that from a donor or synthetic source and surgically places it around the teeth where bone has been lost due to periodontal disease.

There are many other types of periodontal procedures, including surgical placement of dental implants. Implants function as anchors or tooth root replacements to which an artificial tooth or denture can be attached—an exciting development in modern dentistry for those who have lost teeth.

While private practitioners make up the majority of periodontists, other periodontists teach full- or part-time at universities, perform research at dental schools or for industry such as dental product manufacturers, work in the military as government employees, or for the U.S. Public Health Service.

what is it like to be a periodontist?

Sara Whitener has been a periodontist for four years. She is a partner in a group periodontal private practice in Belleville, IL. The group also has a satellite office in Mount Vernon, IL. The office is open five days a week. Office hours are 8 am to 5 pm and each of the three periodontists works four to five days a week. The senior partner started the practice twenty-one years ago and the other partner has been with the practice for twelve years. As the youngest periodontist to the practice, Whitener worked hard to prove herself. It paid off, and she was made a partner.

Whitener's schedule each week is structured. "I see patients Monday through Thursday, and I take Fridays off to teach periodontics at Southern Illinois University School of Dental Medicine. On the days I work in the office, one hour is devoted to paperwork. This involves writing diagnosis and treatment plan letters with copies of radiographs to send to patients' general dentists," Whitener said. Her husband understands that she needs to spend time on weekends to tackle other paperwork. She needs to communicate with general dentists regarding treatment plans or completed treatment for every patient.

To ensure the dental office is a safe place for employees and patients alike, Whitener shares the duties of regularly evaluating procedures and conditions in the office to be certain everything is in compliance with the federal Occupational Safety and Health Administration standards. This takes time, as well. And although staff members are in charge of taking inventory and ordering supplies, the periodontist oversees the process.

FYI

Widely considered to be the "Father of Periodontics," John Riggs was the first to have a paper published describing periodontal disease and the recommended therapy-treatment that is still valid now, more than a century later. "Suppurative Inflammation of the Gums and Absorption of the Gums and Alveolar Process" was published in the March 1876 issue of the *Pennsylvania Journal of Dental Science*.

Whitener must also meet with her partners on a regular basis to discuss patient treatment plans and consult on problems. These problems may involve bookkeeping and strategies for keeping track of the supplies, benefits, tax deductions, and setting salaries and raises. They must work together on the overall planning for the practice.

Remember Tom with braces and receding gums on his bottom teeth? He returned to the office for the gingival graft procedure. He was nervous about the shot he had to be given. Whitener, however, always places a gel anesthetic on gum tissue to numb it before patients receive anesthetic injections. So Tom didn't feel the pain many people associate with shots. The Novocaine so thoroughly numbed him, that Tom claims he never felt the surgery.

A week later when he returned, Tom was much more relaxed.

"Well, Dr. Whitener, it looks like you fixed me up. Its healing pretty well, you must know what your doing" Tom said with a grin.

Taking a look, Whitener said, "Why do you think we go to school for so long? It looks like its healing great. Now I'll show you how to brush properly so it continues to heal and so you'll have less chance of having more gum recession in the future," Whitener said.

Tom was visibly relaxed. "Thanks a lot, Doc. For awhile there, I thought I was going to be the only toothless twelve-year old!" Tom said, getting ready to get out of the dental chair.

"Not so fast, Tom. First let me show you how to floss under your braces," Whitener said.

Patients like Tom are the reason Whitener enjoys working as an periodontist. The former junior high school math and science teacher likes helping people understand concepts. "I enjoy teaching, not just dental students on Fridays, but patients in the practice. I get a great deal of satisfaction when I see them comprehend their situation and understand what they need to do to improve their oral health and fight their gum disease," Whitener said.

Another periodontist, Robert Pick, D.D.S., M.S., practices as a partner in a Naperville, IL, and in a Chicago university-based group practice. He, too, teaches one day a week. Pick also trains periodontal residents to be periodontists. In his spare time, he lectures to periodontists and dentists on practice management, periodontal surgical techniques, and how to best utilize high-tech innovations to improve the practice. For example, his practice files electronic claims using the Internet, has a Web site, an audio-visual room for patient education and consultations, intraoral cameras for taking photos inside the patient's mouth and projecting their teeth and gums on a TV screen.

"Once they see an 8 X 10 image of their puffy, receded and bleeding gums, they are motivated to receive treatment. We also use computer imaging to 'paint away' excess gum tissue or add additional tissue where the gums have receded. This gives the patient an idea of what they'll look like after the procedure," Pick said.

Pick, who has written a text book on lasers, uses them instead of scalpels where applicable. "With lasers there's no bleeding, swelling, scarring, suturing and pain is reduced," Pick said.

To be a successful periodontist, you should

- Have dexterity for detail work
- Be self-motivated
- Have excellent eye-hand coordination
- Communicate effectively with others-patients, colleagues and staff

have I got what it takes to be a periodontist?

Whitener was thoroughly trained in dental school and during her periodontal postgraduate program, and she obtained a master's degree in periodontics.

A periodontist must meet physical challenges. Manual dexterity and tactile sensitivity are necessary assets, along with good hand-eye coordination. Fingers, hands, wrists and arms are in controlled motion within small spaces throughout the day. There is little room for error in judgments when performing delicate gum surgery. This is also not a career for the squeamish as surgical procedures involving blood and bone are common.

Compassion and tolerance are good character traits in those who wish to be periodontists. People with gum disease often have bad breath and poor oral hygiene. It takes a great deal of patience to understand the complexities of human nature. As educators, Dr. Whitener and Dr. Pick are well-suited in this field because they can communicate complex ideas in simple terms that patients can understand.

To keep abreast of advancements in periodontics, periodontists must take continuing education courses every year. Some are required to maintain a dental license; other courses help the periodontist better manage the practice. Business skills help keep the practice running efficiently for maximized profitability while providing highest quality results.

Being a level-headed communicator while under time pressure is critical. Emergencies and other problems may arise early in the morning that need attention. In between seeing patients, phone calls must be taken and letters may need to be dictated quickly—it's all about being efficient and effective. If a periodontist gets behind schedule in the morning, all other patients are backed up for the rest of the day. Patients' time is valuable, too, and they can become angry if made to wait an unreasonable amount of time. Luckily, both Dr. Whitener and Dr. Pick are self-motivated and are good time managers—a highly advantageous skill.

Being able to hire and manage an excellent staff is another nonclinical skill that a successful periodontist needs. Each staff member represents the periodontal practice, so great pains should be taken to choose staff members who are knowledgeable and courteous. To make sure that procedures are done quickly and properly everyday, periodontists must delegate responsibilities to the staff and oversee their performance in completing them. If a problem or disagreement arises—a patient is angry at a staff member or staff members are in an argument, for example—the periodontist may need to draw upon diplomacy skills to arbitrate and smooth things out.

> "With lasers there's no bleeding and pain is reduced."

how do I become a periodontist?

education

High School

High school students interested in becoming periodontists should begin preparing for this career with a course load emphasizing, but not restricted to, math and science subjects. Courses such as algebra, calculus, chemistry, physics, trigonometry, biology and health are all solid baseline courses for college preparation.

Postsecondary Training

Getting admitted to dental school requires that students first complete three to four years of undergraduate college education. Maintaining a high grade point average is important while in college. Because gaining acceptance into a graduate program in periodontics is fiercely competitive, strong grade point averages are necessary. While a bachelor's degree is not strictly required, it is a standard that significantly heightens an applicant's chances of being admitted to a dental school.

Recommended college courses are similar to those suggested in high school. Often, students who are planning on becoming periodontists work toward obtaining a bachelor of science degree in biology. This may involve taking math courses such as algebra, calculus, trigonometry and geometry. Science courses may include biology, anatomy, physiology, anthropology, zoology, botany, and microbiology.

On the practical side, business classes such as marketing, economics, accounting, management and finance prepare periodontics students for owning and operating a business. Liberal arts courses such as psychology, sociology, English and drama may also help a future periodontist to become more comfortable in communicating with people. These types of classes prepare students to understand and relate to patients-a unique perspective.

A discussion with your college advisor, a university version of a secondary school guidance counselor, can help to identify required and suggested classes best suited for obtaining your degree and added skills for this career choice.

College students must score well on the Dental Admissions Test (DAT) before being admitted into a dental program. Doing well on the DAT helps dental schools determine whether or not students will succeed in dental school. Dental school courses are made up of advanced science, clinical and laboratory technique coursework. During the last two years of dental school, clinical treatment is emphasized and students begin supervised treatment of patients at university dental clinics. Graduates receive a Doctor of Dental Surgery (DDS) or Doctor of Dental Medicine (DMD) degree.

This would conclude the formal education if a student was planning on working as a general dentist. However, to be a dental specialist known as a periodontist, more schooling is needed. In fact, postgraduate programs, which are accredited by the American Dental Association Commission on Dental Accreditation, last three years.

certification or licensing

For new dentists to be allowed to practice, they must first pass a licensing examination in the state in which they are planning to practice. This test may include working on a patient. For those who wish to be periodontal specialists, a three-year postgraduate program that usually involves getting a master's degree is needed. In some states, they must also pass a specialty licensing examination. Board certification independent of, and above and beyond that which is required for licensing, is also available through the American Board of Periodontology (ABP). To achieve ABP diplomate status, periodontists must file an application with the ABP, be interviewed and approved as a candidate, pass written and oral examinations, and provide written periodontic case histories. ABP diplomate status is sought voluntarily by periodontists to show they've mastered excellence in their abilities.

Periodontists, as well as all dentists, also must plan on taking courses after they are practicing. These continuing education courses are taken to maintain a dental license. Other voluntary educational activities besides attending workshops and seminars include reading professional journals and participating in study clubs. This helps a practicing periodontist to acquire the most up-to-date skills and knowledge of the best materials on the market.

scholarships and grants

Scholarships and grants are often available from individual institutions, state agencies, and special-interest organizations. The book *Dollars for College: Medicine, Dentistry, and Related Fields* by Ferguson Publishing Company is an excellent source for this information. Many students finance their medical education through the Armed Forces Health Professions Scholarship Program. Each branch of the military participates in this program, paying students' tuitions in exchange for military service. Contact your local recruiting office for more information on this program. The National Health Service Corps Scholarship Program also provides money for students in return for service. Another source for financial aid, scholarship, and grant information is the Association of American Medical Colleges. Remember to request information early for eligibility, application requirements, and deadlines.

Association of American Medical Colleges
2450 N Street, NW
Washington, DC 20037
TEL: 202-828-0400
WEBSITE: http://www.aamc.org
Specific information on financial aid programs can be found at:
WEBSITE: http://www.aamc.org/stuapps/finaid

Ferguson Publishing Company
200 West Madison, Suite 300
Chicago, IL 60606
TEL: 312-580-5480

National Health Services Corps Scholarship Program
U.S. Public Health Service
1010 Wayne Avenue, Suite 240
Silver Spring, MD 20910
TEL: 800-638-0824

who will hire me?

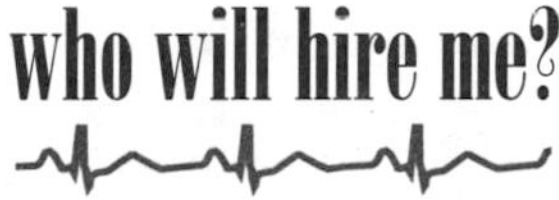

The American Academy of Periodontology (AAP) has 4,200 periodontist members in the United States; and more than 90 percent of them are in private practice. There are different types of private practices, such as solo or group. Periodontists may own their own practice or may work as an associate or a partner in another periodontist's practice. Information about private practice opportunities is available in the AAP News, the AAP membership newsletter. For those not joining an existing practice, the resources required to set up a private practice are considerable—typically a bank-financed endeavor.

Other opportunities for periodontists include teaching at universities, either full-time or part-time, while also practicing. Periodontists may volunteer to teach a class since university teaching is a respected endeavor in the field.

Some periodontists also work in a dental school environment, but choose to do research. Others perform research while testing new materials and procedures and writing about them for industry. Researchers may test new periodontal materials or techniques by working on anything from model mouths to animals.

Combining one or more aspects of clinical practice, teaching, and research, some periodontists are employed by the Federal Dental Health Services. These periodontists may be positioned all over the country via the Air Force, Navy, Army, the Veterans Affairs department, and Public Health Services. Those who work in the Pubic Health Service typically work with underserved populations, usually in low-income communities.

where can I go from here?

The primary career path for most periodontists in private practice is to build a reputation for the practice with the general dentists in the surrounding community who refer the majority of the periodontist's patients. Periodontists who can effectively communicate with a patient's general dentist and facilitate easy coordination of treatment are more likely to be trusted by the general dentist. These practitioners are more apt to build their practices.

Involvement in periodontal associations and study clubs may lead periodontists to active participation in organized dental events. Some periodontists even become officers and committee chairs of their professional associations. After many years of working, periodontists may slow down to part-time status or retire and teach at a university during their retirement years.

what are the salary ranges?

According to the American Dental Association Survey Center, the mean average net salary of periodontists who are under age forty is about $118,000. That's the lower end of the salary range.

The mid-range salary is the mean average income; and the average annual income from the primary private practice for all periodontists is approximately $138,000.

On the upper end of the range, periodontists who work more than thirty-two hours a week, work an average of 39.5 hours and make about $142,000. In addition, middle-aged periodontists earn more, on average, than younger periodontists. The average net income for periodontists over forty years old is $145,000.

The location of a periodontist's private practice may play a role in determining income, as well. Dentists in Pacific, Mountain, Northern and New England states typically have higher incomes than those in Southern states. Specialists' incomes are also affected by how many other specialists in their area of expertise are working in the community. In an area with few or no other periodontists, a periodontal practice may have "an edge" and find it easier to obtain referrals.

what is the job outlook?

The demand for periodontists should remain constant. The use of dental implants should remain steady, and even increase with the aging Baby Boomers who want to keep their teeth for as long as possible. And because periodontal services are needed to retain teeth and eliminate bad breath, and our society values physical attractiveness, desire for periodontal services is predicted to be strong. To make periodontal services as accessible as possible to patients, some offices accept charge cards or refer their patients to financing sources where instant, over-the-phone approval may be obtainable. Other offices work out long-range payment plans as long as a downpayment is made at the onset of treatment.

how do I learn more?

professional associations

Following are organizations that provide information on dental careers, accredited schools, and employees.

American Dental Association
211 E. Chicago Avenue
Chicago, IL 60611
TEL: 312-440-2500
WEBSITE: http://www.ada.org

The American Academy of Periodontology
737 N. Michigan Avenue
Suite 800
Chicago, IL 60611
TEL: 312-787-5518
WEBSITE: http://www.perio.org

bibliography

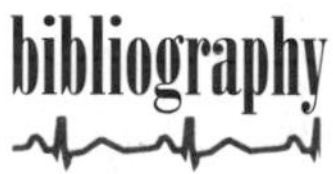

Following is a sampling of materials related to the professional concerns of periodontists.

Books

Burns, Joel M. *Understanding Periodontal Disease,* revised edition. Carol Stream, IL: Quintessence Publishing Co., 1993.

Manson, J. D., and B. M. Eley. *Outline of Periodontics,* 3rd edition. Newton, MA: Butterworth-Heinemann, 1995.

Seymour, Robin A., and Peter A. Heasman. *Drugs, Disease, and the Periodontium.* New York, NY: Oxford University Press, 1992.

Periodicals

International Journal of Periodontics and Restorative Dentistry. Bimonthly. Clinically oriented coverage of the relationship between a healthy periodontium and precise restorations. Quintessence Publishing Co., Inc., 441 Kimberly Drive, Carol Stream, IL 60188, 708-682-3223.

Journal of Periodontology. Monthly. American Academy of Periodontology, 737 N. Michigan Avenue, Suite 800, Chicago, IL 60611, 312-573-3220.

pharmacist

Definition

Pharmacists dispense drugs prescribed by physicians and other health practitioners. They also provide information to pharmacy customers about their medications.

Alternative job title

Druggist

Salary range

$29,000 to $53,500 to $76,000

Educational requirements

High school diploma; Bachelor of Science degree in pharmacy

Certification or licensing

Mandatory

Job outlook

Average

GOE
02.04.01

DOT
074

High School Subjects

Biology
Chemistry
Mathematics
Physics

Personal Interests

Health care
Helping people
Medicine

Calling from the front counter, the pharmacy technician asks, "Do you have a second, Mike?" Mike Schaeuble, pharmacist and manager of "The Medicine Shoppe," rises from his desk, where he was getting an order ready to phone in to the pharmaceutical wholesaler.

"What do you need, Deb?" he asks as he walks toward her.

"Linda Watson called in with a question on Paxil," Deb replies. "She's going in for elective surgery in a week, and her doctor wanted her to make sure she's been off the Paxil long enough. Apparently, it can cause complications with the anesthesia."

Mike pulls open a drawer and takes out a file. He flips through the contents slowly. "There's nothing in the literature on it," he says. "Get SmithKline Beecham, Paxil's manufacturer, on the phone for me so I can ask them about it. In the meantime, I've got to finish up my order and get it phoned in before 10:00."

what does a pharmacist do?

Pharmacists dispense drugs that have been prescribed by physicians, dentists, and other health care practitioners. They must have a thorough understanding of drug products and how they affect people, and they must counsel their customers about the proper uses of medications. This knowledge is very important because some drugs can be ineffective or even dangerous if they are taken with other drugs or with alcohol. Pharmacists must also warn their customers about such potential side effects as drowsiness, nausea, and increased sensitivity to sunlight.

lingo to learn

Compounding The mixing of ingredients to form powders, tablets, capsules, ointments, and solutions.

Contraindication Something, such as a patient's medical condition or a patient's use of another drug, that makes prescribing a particular drug inadvisable.

Pharmacokinetic Pertaining to the way a drug interacts with the human body, in terms of the drug's absorption, distribution, and excretion.

Pharmacology The study of the properties of drugs, including their therapeutic values.

Pharmacotherapy The treatment of disease, especially mental illness, with drugs.

Protocol A detailed plan for how a particular drug should be used for medical treatment.

Radiopharmacy The use of radioactive drugs for diagnostic or therapeutic purposes.

Suspension A type of medicine that consists of solid particles mixed with, but undissolved in, a fluid.

Pharmacists receive their customers' prescriptions in written form or over the telephone. They then fill the prescriptions with the proper drugs in the strengths indicated.

Pharmacists formerly had to mix many drugs together themselves. Today, most drugs are made and sold in ready-to-take forms by pharmaceutical companies. Because of this, compounding (mixing ingredients to form medications) is a very small part of a pharmacist's job.

Pharmacists keep records of prescriptions filled for each customer. Today, most pharmacies use computers to do this. Each customer has a file that contains pertinent data, such as his or her address, phone number, and insurance information. When filling each prescription, a pharmacist enters new information into the file, including the date, the prescribing doctor's name, and the type, strength, and dosage schedule of the medicine. By referring to customer records, a pharmacist can detect the possibility of negative reactions caused by taking one medicine in combination with others. Reference to customer records will also tell a pharmacist if a prescription is being refilled too soon or too often.

Most pharmacists work in community pharmacies, which may be either independent or affiliated with grocery or department stores. These pharmacists, in addition to selling prescription medicines, also sell such nonprescription items as vitamins, aspirin, cough syrup, and cold remedies.

Pharmacists who work in community settings often also function as pharmacy managers. They are responsible for purchasing and tracking inventory, keeping financial records, and billing insurance carriers. They also supervise other pharmacy workers. Among the workers that pharmacists supervise are *pharmacist assistants,* whose duties include compounding medications and submitting pharmacy reports, and *pharmacist technicians,* whose duties include filling bottles with tablets and typing labels.

Some pharmacists work in hospitals or other institutional settings. They fill prescriptions, stock pharmaceuticals, keep patient records, and prepare sterile solutions for IVs. In addition to these duties, hospital pharmacists often confer with doctors, nurses, and other staff members about patient treatments. In some cases, pharmacists work directly with physicians to help in drug therapy selection and monitoring.

A growing number of pharmacists today are choosing to work for pharmaceutical companies. Some of these pharmacists are involved in research and product development—conducting analyses and testing of products. Others work in production and quality assurance—evaluating procedures for manufacturing and packaging drugs. Still other pharmacists employed by pharmaceutical companies work in marketing or as sales representatives.

Finally, some pharmacists work for managed care organizations. In these settings, they work directly with physicians and other health care providers to ensure that pharmaceutical therapies are prescribed in the most appropriate and cost-effective way. This often involves reviewing medical literature to determine which medications are the safest and most effective. It can also involve gathering data from the organization's patient data base and analyzing it.

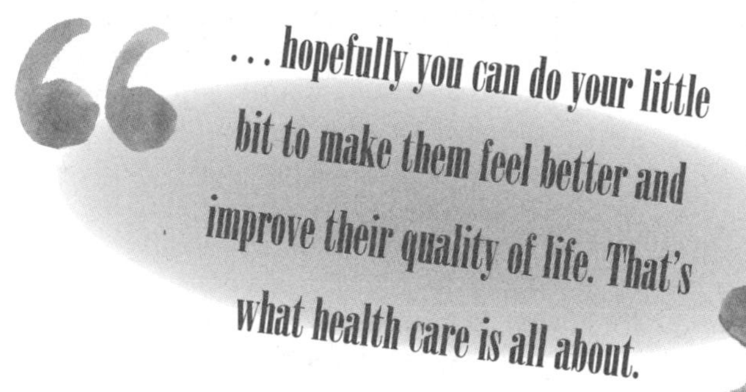

what is it like to be a pharmacist?

Mike Schaeuble is the owner and manager of a franchise pharmacy located a few blocks from a hospital in a mid-sized town. His pharmacy sells only health-related merchandise, instead of the lines of cosmetics and hygiene products often found in larger "drug stores."

His days start at 8:30 AM, Mondays through Fridays, with a quick check of phone calls that might have come in during the night. "A lot of times, we will have gotten calls in from doctors or patients needing prescriptions filled," Mike says. "That's the first thing we look at. Then we check our stock for anything we need, and we put together an order for delivery the next day."

Monitoring the pharmacy stock is an important part of Mike's job. Because pharmaceuticals are so expensive, he tries to keep excess product to a minimum. "That's well over $100,000 in inventory right there," he says, gesturing to the shelves behind his pharmacy counter. "Part of the business is trying to keep the stock as low as possible without running out." To do this, Mike doesn't "warehouse" product at all; he reorders only when he needs a particular medicine.

After the morning order has been placed and any other necessary paperwork done, he settles down to the main business of the day. "In this particular pharmacy, 99 percent of our business is filling prescriptions," he says.

Prescriptions are either brought in by patients or called in by the prescribing doctor or nurse. Before any prescription is filled, a certain amount of patient information must be gathered and put into a computerized file. "We need to have name, address, phone, and insurance information," Mike says. "And we try to have a history of the medications that each patient is on." When the new prescription information is keyed in, a computer software program scans the entire patient record for possible negative drug interactions. Mike also checks the patient record, using his own knowledge of pharmaceuticals to make sure that no harmful interactions will take place.

Once the necessary information has been entered, Mike fills the prescription. "We make sure that we are reading it accurately. If there's any question at all, we call the physician," he says. "Obviously, the doctors make the biggest part of the medication decisions. We don't have a lot of input into that, unless it's a product that has more than one manufacturer." If there is a generic version of a particular product, the pharmacist must get both the doctor's and the patient's permission before dispensing it.

Because virtually all medicines are now manufactured in ready-to-take form, the actual filling of the prescription is not difficult. It is, in almost every case, a matter of counting out tablets or capsules or measuring liquids. Occasionally, however, Mike must compound a medicine. "The dermatologists are the ones I most often compound a prescription for," he says. "And more frequently now, gynecologists order progesterone suppositories that have to be compounded."

At the same time Mike is filling a prescription, he is creating the label for the medicine bottle and sending the necessary information to the patient's insurance carrier for authorization. "We're online with most major carriers," he says. "When I fill a prescription, the information is automatically sent to the carrier, which either authorizes payment for the fill or tells us why they won't." On some occasions, the insurance carrier's records show that the patient is not due for a refill. In these cases, Mike may have to mediate between the carrier, the patient, and the prescribing doctor.

A large part of Mike's job consists of patient education. Many drugs have side-effects that can be serious if they are ignored. When a patient gets a prescription that he or she isn't familiar with, Mike explains to the patient the proper way to take the medication and the things to avoid while taking it. "The days of 'just take this' are in the past," he says. "We want to try to educate the patients so they know what they're taking, how they should be taking it, and why. A knowledgeable patient is a better patient."

have I got what it takes to be a pharmacist?

Pharmacists are an important link in the health care chain. They are responsible for making sure that the patient actually gets what the doctor ordered. There is no room for mistakes. The wrong drug or the wrong dosage could be dangerous or even fatal. For this reason, a high level of personal reliability is necessary for this job. "Basically, you have to be a perfectionist," says Mike. "What you do has to be done right every time. There's no real margin for error."

A pharmacist also needs to be ethical. Many of the drugs pharmacists deal with are addictive and must be closely regulated. The responsibility for dispensing drugs in strict accordance with doctors' orders is not to be taken lightly.

FYI

Pharmacy is an ancient science. It dates back almost 5,000 years to Egypt, where physician-priests were responsible for preparing remedies. One of the most famous Egyptian pharmaceutical records, the Ebers Papyrus, was compiled in about 1500 B.C. It contains descriptions of about 800 prescriptions.

A willingness to learn is vital to being a good pharmacist. New pharmaceutical products are constantly being created, and medical research continually suggests new approaches to drug therapy. A pharmacist must remain aware of new developments in the field. "You have to keep up," says Mike. "Our profession is in the knowledge of the medication. If you don't keep up, that's when mistakes are made."

Pharmacists who work with the public, as many do, need to have good people skills. "I think you have to like the interaction with the public," Mike says. "In fact, I consider many of my customers as friends." Even those pharmacists who do not work directly with the public need good communication skills for interacting with physicians, nurses, researchers, and colleagues.

Finally, a strong interest in health care is important for pharmacists. Mike especially likes the fact that he is helping others. "You see people come in and they're feeling poorly, and hopefully you can do your little bit to make them feel better and improve their quality of life," he says. "That's what health care is all about."

The down side of pharmacy, for Mike, lies in dealing with insurance companies. "The amount of time spent meddling with the carriers just seems to be increasing," he says. "That gets tedious."

Another problem with the career, he notes, can be irregular hours. "If you're in a department store setting, your hours may not be good. They can include evenings, weekends, and holidays," he says.

how do I become a pharmacist?

education

High School

Because so many college courses in the pharmacy curriculum are science-related, students should begin building their math and science skills while still in high school. A good background in chemistry is especially significant for prospective pharmacists. Other science courses, such as biology and physiology, are also good choices, as is mathematics.

Pharmacies, like most other businesses, are becoming increasingly dependent upon computers. Most pharmacists today use computers to maintain customer information, communicate with insurance carriers, and track inventory. Because they will need to use computers regularly, prospective pharmacists should be computer literate. Courses in keyboarding and other computer-related topics will increase familiarity and skill in this area.

Business, English, and communication classes, including speech, are important because they help develop skills that are useful throughout one's professional career. These skills are not only necessary for dealing with future customers, but they will also prove helpful during job interviews and college classes.

Postsecondary Training

A Bachelor of Science degree in pharmacy is the minimum education level acceptable for careers in drug stores and hospitals. To receive this degree, at least five years of college study are required. There are seventy-five accredited colleges and schools of pharmacy in the United States. Twenty-one of these are private schools, and the remaining fifty-four are in public universities.

In any of these schools, the course of study usually begins with one to two years of prepharmacy classes, including mathematics, chemistry, biology, physics, social sciences, and humanities. After taking the prepharmacy classes, the student must take the Pharmacy College Admissions Test (PCAT). Upon passing the PCAT, the student is admitted into an accredited pharmacy program. Classes in these programs are specific to the practice of pharmacy; they include organic and medicinal chemistry, biochemistry, pharmaceutics, physiology, pathophysiology, pharmacology, pharmacy law, and laboratory and clinical practice.

For pharmacists who plan to do research or administrative work, a master's degree is usually required. Course work for the master's degree builds and expands upon the information taught in undergraduate classes.

Today, many colleges of pharmacy are choosing to award a Doctor of Pharmacy (Pharm.D.) degree rather than a Bachelor of Science degree. For this degree, students first complete two years of prepharmacy study and then four years of professional study. A student who has a bachelor's degree in pharmacy can enter a Pharm.D. program, but this approach usually requires more than the normal six years of study.

An increasing number of pharmacy graduates are seeking residency training in pharmacy practice. There are over 400 of these pharmacy residencies offered across the country in hospitals, pharmacies, and other facilities.

To be a successful pharmacist, you should

- Have good communication skills
- Be accurate and detail-oriented
- Have a strong sense of responsibility
- Be flexible and willing to keep up on new developments in the field
- Have an interest in science and health care

New pharmacists may take residencies that focus on general pharmacy practice, clinical pharmacy, or other specialty areas. Some employers, particularly hospital pharmacies and pharmacy schools, require a pharmacist to have completed one of these residencies as a prerequisite for employment.

certification or licensing

All states and the District of Columbia require that pharmacists be licensed to practice. In order to become licensed, applicants must have either a B.S. in Pharmacy or a Pharm.D. degree. Most states also require a license applicant to have spent a specified amount of time in a supervised internship. Internships are usually incorporated into the college curriculum.

A pharmacy graduate must take a licensing examination to test his or her knowledge of the skills necessary to practice pharmacy. Licensing exams are administered on a state-by-state basis, by state boards of pharmacy. Although a pharmacy license is valid only in the state in which it is granted, most states grant licenses to pharmacists licensed in other states without extensive reexamination.

After being licensed to practice pharmacy, a pharmacist must continue his or her education. Most states require fifteen hours of additional education yearly in order to retain a license.

scholarships and grants

Financing the cost of a pharmacy education may be difficult. Tuition costs vary depending upon the size of the school, whether or not the school is in the state where the student resides, and whether the school is privately or publicly funded.

Perhaps the best place to start a search for scholarship information is with the Interorganizational Council on Student Affairs (ICSA), an organization that brings together representatives from various professional associations of pharmacists. ICSA compiles and maintains a current list of available scholarships, grants, loans, awards, and fellowships. These programs generally apply only to students who have completed at least one year of pharmacy school.

There are various loan programs available through the federal government; including Pell Grants, Stafford Student Loans, National Direct Student Loans, Health Education Assistance Loans, and Health Professions Student Loans. There are also grants, scholarships, and loans available through most pharmacy colleges.

The easiest way to explore the various financial aid possibilities is to write directly to the financial aid offices of pharmacy schools and request information and application forms.

who will hire me?

Mike was recruited for his first pharmacy position while he was still in college. "I went to South Dakota State," he says, "and in January of my senior year, the recruiters for the May graduates came on campus for interviews." He was offered a job with Osco, a chain of drug stores, as a staff pharmacist.

There are many employment possibilities for pharmacy graduates. Of the approximately 175,000 practicing pharmacists in the United States, more than half work in community or chain pharmacies. About one-quarter work in hospitals. The remainder work in pharmaceutical companies, wholesaling companies, health maintenance organizations (HMOs), and government and educational institutions.

Generally speaking, it is not difficult for new pharmacists to find jobs. Many, like Mike, will be recruited for entry positions while still in college. If a student does not secure a job with an on-campus recruiter, he or she may be able to find a job through the pharmacy school's placement office. In fact, this office is a good place to initiate a job search.

Another way of finding a pharmacist's position is to contact employers directly. The job seeker might send cover letters and resumes to pharmacies or pharmaceutical companies within the region where he or she wishes to work.

If the job seeker has access to a computer with an Internet service provider, performing a keyword search on "pharmacist" can lead to Web pages containing job listings. This approach, however, can be haphazard and time-consuming. The American College of Clinical Pharmacy has an online listing of job openings, which can be found at its website, http://www.pitt.edu/~gjb/accp.html.

where can I go from here?

Mike started his career as a staff pharmacist. He later moved into a position managing two pharmacies affiliated with a chain grocery store. After several years, he left the chain store and became the manager of an independent franchise pharmacy, where he now plans to remain.

"I like this," he says. "I like the steady hours and the fact that I only deal with health-related merchandise. It's nice not having to answer questions about where the paper towels or light bulbs are. I'm going to stay with it."

Advancement opportunities in pharmacy depend largely upon where the pharmacist is employed. In drug store chains, pharmacists may move into management positions. A common management position is district manager in charge of several pharmacies. With the necessary experience and capital, a pharmacist might open his or her own pharmacy.

In a hospital, the qualified pharmacist may advance to the position of chief pharmacist, or director of pharmacy services. In this position, he or she would be responsible for all the pharmaceutical needs of the hospital, including the supervision of the pharmacy staff.

Pharmacists who work for pharmaceutical manufacturers may be promoted to supervisory positions in sales, research, quality control, advertising, production, packaging, or general business management.

For the pharmacist who has a Pharm.D. or Ph.D. in Pharmacy, there is the option of teaching pharmacy or pharmacy-related classes at the college level. These pharmacists may also choose to go into pharmaceutical or pharmacological research.

what are the salary ranges?

The average salary for a pharmacist varies with the location and the size of the organization for which he or she works. Those working in chain drug stores generally earn the most, followed by those who work in hospitals and health maintenance organizations. With regard to location, pharmacists practicing in the western states tend to make the highest wages, while those in the southern and midwestern states generally make the lowest.

The average entry-level annual salary for pharmacists is $46,300. The overall median annual salary for pharmacists is $53,500, and it is reached relatively quickly. A pharmacist who has several years experience and who has a supervisory position might expect to earn around $60,000.

Pharmacists who teach at the college level earn anywhere from $50,000, for an assistant professorship, to $83,000, for a full professorship. Deans may make between $80,000 and $115,000 annually.

Pharmacists who work for the federal government generally make less than their private sector counterparts. Beginning salaries for government pharmacists start around $29,000. The overall average annual salary for pharmacists in the federal government is $37,250.

In addition to salary, most pharmacists are provided with a full benefits package, which includes paid vacation, medical and dental insurance, and extra pay for overtime. Some employers provide bonuses and profit-sharing plans.

Advancement Possibilities

Directors of pharmacy services supervise and coordinate the activities and functions of hospital pharmacies.

Pharmacy district managers manage several pharmacies in a certain geographic area, usually for a drug store chain, department store, or grocery store.

Pharmaceutical researchers develop and analyze new drugs.

Professors of pharmacy and **professors of pharmacology** teach classes to pharmacy students at the college and university level.

what is the job outlook?

Through 2005, employment opportunities for pharmacists should grow about as fast as the average for all occupations. A key reason for this expected increase is the growth in the nation's elderly population. The elderly are the main users of medical care, including prescription drugs. Therefore, as the number of elderly people increases, so does the need for pharmaceuticals and for pharmacists.

Another factor influencing the growth of employment is the rapid pace of medical research, which continually creates more drug products and new methods of administering them. As new methods of drug therapy become more widely-used, various pharmacy subfields are developing. For example, radiopharmacy involves the use of radioactive drugs, and pharmacotherapy involves the use of drugs to treat mental illness.

Yet another trend is the increasing involvement of pharmacists in drug therapy decision-making. Pharmacists are working more closely with physicians and health maintenance organizations to determine the most effective methods of treatment. The increasing involvement of pharmacists in this area should lead to more job openings in HMOs and in clinical settings.

There is, however, one factor that may negatively impact the growth of employment in pharmacy. A 1996 study by the Pew Health Professions Commission concluded that the United States is producing too many health care professionals. They recommended closing at least fifteen of the nation's seventy-five pharmacy schools by 2005 in order to help offset this trend. This study raised the possibility that pharmacists may face increasing competition for jobs.

how do I learn more?

professional organizations

Following are organizations that provide information on pharmacy careers, accredited schools, and employers.

American Association of Colleges of Pharmacy
1426 Prince Street
Alexandria, VA 22314
TEL: 703-739-2330
WEBSITE: http://www.aacp.org

American Pharmaceutical Association
2215 Constitution Avenue, NW
Washington, DC 20037
TEL: 202-429-7595
WEBSITE: http://www.aoa.dhhs.gov/aoa/dir/49.html

American Society of Consultant Pharmacists
1321 Duke Street
Alexandria, VA 22314
TEL: 703-739-1300
WEBSITE: http://www.ascp.com/

Academy of Managed Care Pharmacy
1650 King Street,
Suite 402
Alexandria, VA 22314
TEL: 703-683-8416

American Society of Health-System Pharmacists
7272 Wisconsin Avenue
Bethesda, MD 20814
TEL: 301-657-3000
WEBSITE: http://www.social.com/health/nhic/data/hr0100/hr0192.html

bibliography

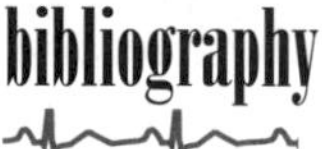

Following is a sampling of materials relating to the professional concerns and development of pharmacists.

Books

Frook, John, editor. *The Pfizer Guide: Pharmacy Career Opportunities,* 2nd edition. Old Saybrook, CT: Merritt Communications, 1994.

Gable, Fred B. *Opportunities in Pharmacy Careers,* revised edition. Lincolnwood, IL: VGM Career Horizons, 1997.

Stonier, P. D., editor. *Discovering New Medicines: Careers in Pharmaceutical Research and Development.* New York, NY: Wiley, 1995.

Periodicals

Drug Topics. Semimonthly. Publishes current trends and developments affecting the pharmacy field. Includes merchandising, government affairs, management, professional, and clinical news. Medical Economics Publishing Co., Inc., Five Paragon Drive, Montvale, NJ 07645, 201-358-7200.

Journal of Pharmaceutical Care in Infectious Disease Management. Quarterly. Provides information for pharmacists on the most recent advances in the management of infectious diseases. Haworth Press, Inc., 10 Alice Street, Binghamton, NY 13904, 800-342-9678.

Journal of Pharmacy Practice. Bimonthly. Devoted to exploring new practice areas and therapies, giving current information on new drugs, pharmacokinetics, drug administration, and adverse drug reactions. W.B. Saunders Co., The Curtis Center, 3rd Floor, Independence Square West, Philadelphia, PA 19106-3399, 215-238-7800.

Journal of Pharmacy Technology. Bimonthly. Aimed at pharmacists and technicians. Covers therapeutic trends, current research and organizational, legal, and educational activities. Includes information on new drugs and medical products and equipment. Harvey Whitney Books Company, Box 42696, Cincinnati, OH 45242, 513-793-3555.

Pharmacist's Letter. Monthly. Advises pharmacists on current drug therapy, including drug interactions, proper drug use, trends in therapy, new research findings, and new drugs. Therapeutic Research Center, 8834 Hildreth Lane, Box 8190, Stockton, CA 95208, 209-931-2923.

Pharmacy Cadence. Annual. Overview of pharmacy for students and others new to the profession in the U.S. and Canada. P A S Pharmacy Association Services, Box 6565, Athens, GA 30604, 706-613-0100.

Pharmacy Today. Monthly. Reports on current news and opinions, including pharmacotherapeutic, legislative, and socioeconomic news. American Pharmaceutical Association, 2215 Constitution Avenue, NW, Washington, DC 20037, 202-628-4410.

pharmacologist

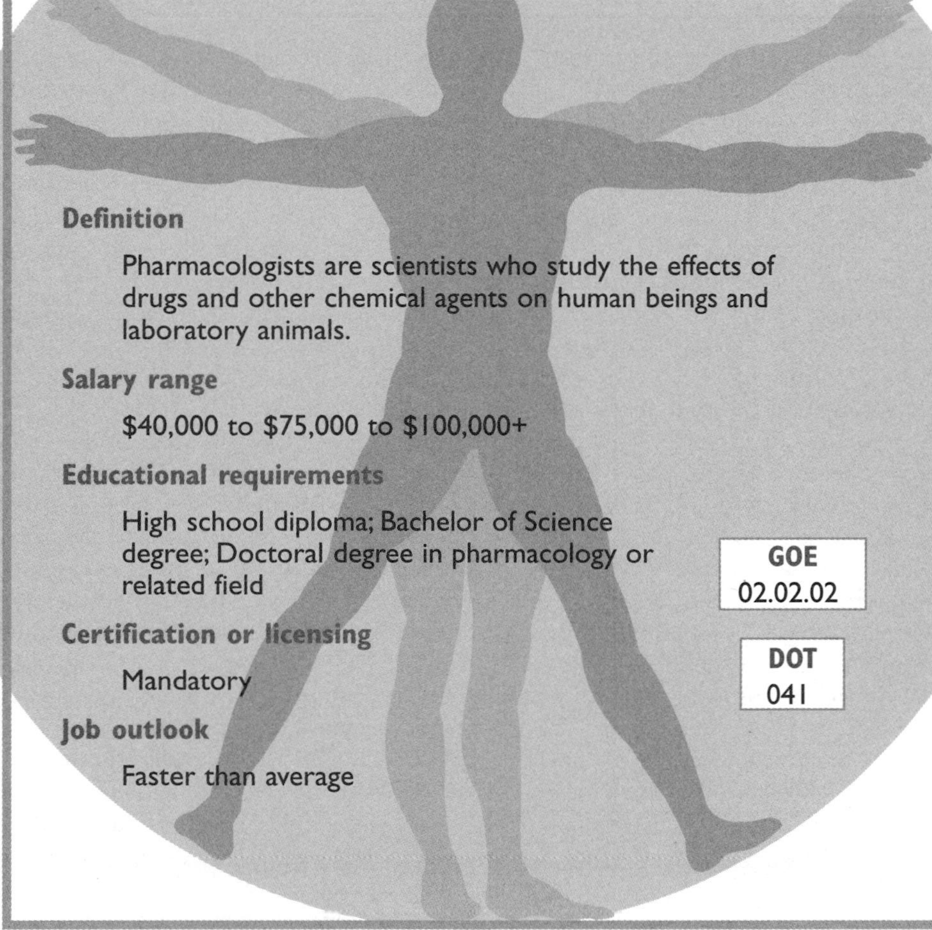

Definition

Pharmacologists are scientists who study the effects of drugs and other chemical agents on human beings and laboratory animals.

Salary range

$40,000 to $75,000 to $100,000+

Educational requirements

High school diploma; Bachelor of Science degree; Doctoral degree in pharmacology or related field

Certification or licensing

Mandatory

Job outlook

Faster than average

GOE
02.02.02

DOT
041

High School Subjects

Biology
Calculus
Chemistry
English
Physics

Personal Interests

Medicine
Science
Solving problems

The white rat is getting air blown into its face in Dr. Joe DiMicco's laboratory. The rat is in a device called a stress chamber, having its cardiovascular functions monitored with another device, called a telemetric receiver. Dr. DiMicco, clad in a white lab coat, is pointing to the rat while talking to a small group of pharmacology graduate students.

Referring to a three-dimensional model of the rat's brain, Dr. DiMicco points to the part of the brain that his research experiment is focusing on—the dorsomedial hypothalamus. "This is where we're going to be injecting the drug," he says. "We're going to be microinjecting bicuculline methiodide into this area to block the brain cells known as GABA receptors." He reaches for the syringe, and his students shift slightly to get a better view.

what does a pharmacologist do?

A *pharmacologist* is a scientist who studies the effects of drugs and other chemical agents on animals, including humans. One of a pharmacologist's main duties is to develop and test chemical agents that can cure, relieve, or prevent disease. A pharmacologist uses techniques from different sciences, including mathematics, chemistry, biology, physics, and physiology.

Pharmacologists usually conduct their research work in laboratories. The tools and materials they use vary, depending upon the experiment. They may use tissue samples, bodily secretions, body organs, or live animals as test subjects. They use computers and other electronic instruments, various chemical compounds, and radioactive and nonradioactive isotopes (types of atoms).

Different experiments call for different procedures. In some cases, for example, a pharmacologist might inject a chemical into a living tissue sample from a human donor. In other cases, the pharmacologist might inject a drug into a laboratory animal. During such experiments, the pharmacologist monitors the tissue sample or animal closely to see what results the drug has. Test animals are sometimes sacrificed so that necropsies, or autopsies, can be performed to determine the effects of particular drugs on various parts of the body.

Some pharmacologists work for pharmaceutical companies and are directly engaged in the development and testing of new drugs. Before any new drug is marketed to the public, it must be extensively tested and refined. Pharmacologists working on a new drug perform tests to determine what side effects it might have, what dosage is most effective, what is the best way to administer it, and how the body absorbs, distributes, and eliminates it.

Pharmacologists also work in academic settings. These scientists, in addition to conducting research projects, teach classes and seminars and direct graduate students in laboratory work.

Pharmacologists may specialize in how chemicals affect certain parts of the body. A *cardiovascular pharmacologist* works with chemicals that affect the cardiovascular and circulatory systems. An *endocrine pharmacologist* studies the effects of drugs on the hormonal balance of the body. A *neuropharmacologist* works with drugs that affect the brain, spinal cord, and nerves. A *psychopharmacologist,* or *behavioral pharmacologist,* works with drugs that affect behavior.

A *clinical pharmacologist* specializes in testing various drugs and other chemicals on humans. He or she studies how certain drugs work, how they interact with other drugs, how their effects can alter the patterns of disease, and how disease can alter the drugs' effects.

There are additional areas of specialization in pharmacology. A *molecular pharmacologist* specializes in studying the precise interactions between drug molecules and cells. A *biochemical pharmacologist* works to determine how drugs influence the chemical activities within organisms. A *veterinary pharmacologist* studies and develops drugs used to treat cats, dogs, and other animals.

A field that is closely associated with pharmacology is toxicology. Toxicology is the study of chemicals found in the environment and how they affect living organisms. A *toxicologist* uses many of the same research techniques and materials as a pharmacologist. Toxicologists study the effects of toxic substances in the workplace, analyze food preservatives and colorings, and test such common household substances as aerosol sprays and cleaning agents.

lingo to learn

Pharmacodynamics The study of the reactions between drugs and living systems.

Pharmacognosy The science concerned with the composition, production, use, and history of crude, or unrefined, drugs.

Pharmacokinetics The study of how drugs are absorbed, distributed, metabolized, and excreted.

Toxicology The study of the adverse effects of drugs and other chemical agents.

what is it like to be a pharmacologist?

Dr. Joe DiMicco works in the department of pharmacology of a large state university. His office, on the fourth floor of the Medical Sciences Building, adjoins a high-tech laboratory. Dr. DiMicco splits his time between the office, the lab, and the classroom.

"I co-direct a course for second-year med students in the fall," he says. "So, when that's in session, I tend to be heavily involved on a day-to-day basis with it." When teaching, Dr. DiMicco arrives at his office at 6:30 AM to check his E-mail and respond to questions from students. After that, he assembles the slides and reviews the notes for his lecture. At 8:00, his two-hour lecture begins.

He spends afternoons in the laboratory with his students, directing their research experiments. "That's the way my day goes when I'm heavily into teaching," he says.

Besides teaching, the other major part of Dr. DiMicco's work is research. His avenue of research is neuroscience. "I am looking at pathways in the brain that are responsible for generating the physiological changes engendered by stress," he says. "The focus is mostly on cardiovascular indicators, with some endocrine studies, some behavioral, and some gastrointestinal."

Dr. DiMicco has two graduate students in pharmacology working in his lab, and he directs them in the planning and conducting of research experiments. Earlier in his career, he did most of the experiments himself. "One of the ironic things about science is that the more successful you are, the less you get to do the actual science," he says. "You build a little empire of people and then you rarely get into the labs to do the research."

Dr. DiMicco's research work involves testing the stress response in rats. In order to prove his hypothesis that a certain area of the brain—the dorsomedial hypothalamus—is the source of physiological stress symptoms, Dr. DiMicco uses various chemicals to stimulate that part of the rat's brain. "We take a rat under anesthesia and, using a cannula (a tube through which fluids are introduced to or withdrawn from a small part of the body), microinject different drugs to see different results," he says.

After the rat has been injected with a drug, it is tested for stress response. "We've developed a model for stress that involves very minimal discomfort for the rat," says Dr. DiMicco. "What we've discovered is that we can take a rat and put him into a little tube and blow air into his face. They hate having air blown in their faces and they have the maximal stress response for that."

While the rat is in the stress chamber, Dr. DiMicco and his students monitor its physical functions. "We can monitor cardiovascular functions using telemetry," he says. "There are little transmitters we implant in the abdomen, with a sensor in the aorta. When we sit the rat on the telemetric receiver, we get a moment-by-moment reading of its cardiovascular functions."

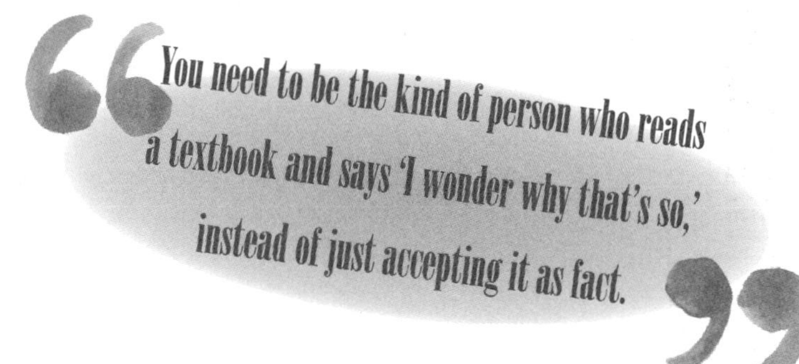

They also monitor the levels of stress hormones in the rat's blood by drawing blood samples. All the data collected for each experiment must be carefully documented and compiled. Dr. DiMicco takes the data from the experiments and enters it into a computer, where it can be analyzed and used to generate graphs and spreadsheets.

Another part of Dr. DiMicco's work involves reporting the results of his findings to the scientific community. He, like most academic scientists, publishes at least one research paper per year, explaining the nature and findings of his projects. Research papers are typically published in professional journals or as chapters for books.

In addition to his teaching and research activities, Dr. DiMicco has a number of administrative duties. Of these, the most significant and time-consuming is writing grant proposals. Securing grant money is the only way for him to insure that his research can continue. "It's a struggle to get funding these days because there's a lot of competition," Dr. DiMicco says. "I spend a lot of time writing grant proposals, which can be successful, but are more often not successful."

Other responsibilities include periodic trips to Washington, D.C., to work with the National Institutes of Health, the National Institute of Drug Abuse, and NASA. He also sits on a number of committees for his university, runs summer internship programs for local colleges, and occasionally does consulting work.

have I got what it takes to be a pharmacologist?

Curiosity and problem-solving skills are two vital qualities for pharmacologists, according to Dr. DiMicco. "It's important to question everything," he says. "You need to be the kind of person who reads a textbook and says 'I wonder why that's so,' instead of just accepting it as fact."

He also cites a keen eye for detail and excellent observational skills as important, saying that there is no substitute for being a good observer.

Because of the exacting nature of pharmacological experiments and the need for precision in performing them, it is important that pharmacologists be extremely thorough in their work habits. "If you get tired, you get frustrated, you leave out things, cut corners—those are the sorts of things that will do you in as a scientist," says Dr. DiMicco.

Good communications skills are also vital to success in this field. Although each scientist usually works alone on a specific project, he or she is nonetheless part of a team of researchers with whom it is necessary to communicate clearly. In addition, both oral and written communication skills are needed to present the results of research projects. "You've got to be able to communicate well," says Dr. DiMicco. "You could be doing the greatest science in the world, and if you can't communicate it, it's worthless."

Finally, pharmacologists need a great deal of patience and persistence in order to perform their work successfully. They spend months, and sometimes years, on experiments before they see the fruits of their labors. In some cases, the results of their research may never be used. This can be both frustrating and discouraging.

Dr. DiMicco says it is easy to get discouraged. "You may put together the most well-supported hypothesis, you can spend weeks in the library putting together all the information, you can feel sure that it's all going to work," he says, "then when you get in the lab, it may all fall flat."

Patience and persistence are especially helpful to pharmacologists (such as those working for universities or not-for-profit organizations) who rely on grant money to fund their projects. "There's so much competition for funding now," says Dr. DiMicco. "It's kind of ironic that as the breadth of our knowledge expands, and there's lots more science that should be done, the money gets tighter and tighter." It is necessary to keep looking for funding, even in the face of repeated turndowns.

Despite the sometimes discouraging and tedious nature of the work, most pharmacologists find their jobs to be very fulfilling. There is a sense of satisfaction in contributing to advances in medical science. There is also the thrill of proving one's hypotheses or discovering something new. "Most of us in this career find ourselves terribly spoiled, I think," says Dr. DiMicco. "To be able to do what fascinates you as your life's work is a tremendous privilege."

how do I become a pharmacologist?

When Dr. DiMicco was an undergraduate, he did not plan to become a pharmacologist. In fact, he wasn't even an enthusiastic science student at first. "I labored under the same misconception that most people have, which is that science is just a lot of facts," he says. It wasn't until he worked as a lab technician for a professor at MIT that he really grew to love science.

"Real science is going in the lab and asking 'What would happen if I did this?' It's getting a little glimpse into maybe something no one has ever seen or known about before," he says. "I realized that when I worked at MIT. And then the professor I worked for convinced me that I had a talent for doing science, that I could make a contribution."

education

High School

A high school diploma is the first essential step in becoming a pharmacologist. High school level science classes provide a foundation for future course work in college. Classes in biology, physics, and chemistry are especially helpful, as they provide information needed by the future pharmacologist and offer opportunities for laboratory research.

Mathematics courses, especially calculus, will help students develop the critical thinking skills needed in pharmacology. Math classes also help students by emphasizing the importance of precise measurements and calculations.

English and speech classes are also important to future pharmacologists, because jobs in this field are likely to include writing about and orally presenting research findings. Computer literacy is another valuable skill that should be acquired in high school. Computers are widely used in pharmacology to calculate and analyze research data.

Postsecondary Training

Because most colleges do not have pharmacology majors, a student who wants to become a pharmacologist usually earns a Bachelor of Science degree in chemistry or pharmacy. Recently, however, some colleges have added pharmacology programs for undergraduate students. Where these programs are available, they are certainly a wise choice.

Whichever undergraduate degree the student chooses, it will typically have a curriculum heavy in the natural sciences and mathematics. Students are required to take classes in organic and physical chemistry, biology, physics, molecular biology, mathematics, and statistics. Many of these classes include hands-on research experience.

In addition to science-related classes, students should take courses that help them communicate clearly. Classes in writing, literature, and humanities provide opportunities to develop communication skills.

After completing a bachelor's degree, a pharmacology student must complete four to five years of graduate study in pharmacology. Pharmacy schools, medical schools, schools of biomedical sciences, and schools of veterinary medicine usually have Ph.D. programs in pharmacology.

Pharmacology Ph.D. programs usually have curriculums that include cellular and molecular biology, biochemistry, physiology, neurology, statistics, and research design. Courses in the pharmacological sciences include basic pharmacology, molecular pharmacology, chemotherapy and toxicology. Students also take courses based on specific organ systems, such as cardiovascular pharmacology, renal pharmacology, and neuropharmacology.

The major component of graduate study in pharmacology is research. Graduate students conduct both supervised and independent research. The primary goal is to complete an original research study that yields new information.

Before taking a permanent position, a new Ph.D. graduate typically spends two to four years of further research training in a postdoctoral position. This provides the graduate with the opportunity to work on a second significant research project with an established scientist.

To be a successful pharmacologist, you should:

- Have excellent observational skills
- Be a critical thinker and good problem solver
- Be patient and willing to wait for results
- Have strong written and oral communication skills
- Have a strong sense of curiosity

scholarships and grants

Financing a Ph.D. in pharmacology can be very difficult. It can cost $12,000 a year to attend a public school, and private schools can cost up to $20,000 yearly.

Scholarships for graduate work are sometimes offered by individual universities to qualified candidates. These scholarships often cover all school-related expenses, including room and board. Many require that the recipient serve as an assistant to a professor in the classroom or laboratory. As an undergraduate student begins applying to graduate pharmacology programs, he or she should check with the universities for available scholarship or grants, application procedures, and deadlines.

The federal government offers several financial aid opportunities to college students. These programs include low-interest loans available to all students, and grants based on financial need and academic ability.

A good starting point for financial aid research is the National Association of Student Financial Aid Administrators (NASFAA). This organization maintains an extensive list of financial assistance opportunities.

NASFAA
1920 L Street NW
Suite 200
Washington, DC 20036
TEL: 202-785-0453
WEBSITE: http://www.finaid.org/nasfaa/

who will hire me?

Dr. DiMicco did two years of post-doctoral work at Georgetown University. While he was there, he was contacted for a job. He says it is not uncommon to find a job in this manner. "The vast majority of people with a new pharmacology degree do some kind of post-doctoral training," he says, "and networking is a very important feature of that whole process. A lot of people secure their initial positions through networking during their post-doc."

About 70 percent of the working pharmacologists in the United States are employed by medical, dental, or pharmacy schools, universities, the government, or non-profit organizations. The remainder work in pharmaceutical industries or related industries.

Most pharmacologists start looking for positions sometime before they complete their Ph.D.s. Pharmaceutical companies, universities, and governmental organizations frequently recruit pharmacologists who are earning their degrees. University placement offices may also help graduating pharmacologists find positions.

If the prospective graduate knows which subspecialty he or she is interested in, companies and universities concerned with that subspecialty should be contacted. Sending cover letters and resumes to the personnel directors of these companies and universities may bring results.

Pharmacologists interested in government work may look for employment in various agencies. They should contact the U.S. Department of Health and Human Services, the Nuclear Regulatory Commission, the Environmental Protection Agency, the U.S. Department of Agriculture, the U.S. Public Health Service, or the U.S. Department of the Interior for openings and application procedures.

where can I go from here?

New pharmacologists usually work with scientists experienced in research. They learn laboratory procedures, equipment operation and care, and how to perform tests on human and animal subjects for the specific projects they are assigned. They also learn how to comply with such governmental regulatory agencies as the Food and Drug Administration and the U.S. Department of Agriculture.

During their careers, pharmacologists gradually take on additional responsibilities. Eventually they get opportunities to work on their own projects. Advancement from this point usually involves coordinating major projects or supervising other scientists in laboratories. Supervisory positions and responsibilities are generally awarded to experienced pharmacologists who have proven themselves to be capable scientists.

Pharmacologists in academic settings can become tenured professors and department heads. Department heads supervise other professors and, in some cases, all the research projects being conducted within the department. Department heads are frequently asked to present papers and speak at conferences.

what are the salary ranges?

Pharmacologists' salaries are among the highest of all science occupations. A recent graduate can expect to earn about $40,000 per year by teaching or working in industry. As a pharmacologist's experience level and skill increases, so does his or her salary.

The average yearly salary of university professors of pharmacology is about $70,000. Pharmacologists who are senior faculty members in academic departments, or who supervise teams of people in large laboratories, earn the highest wages—sometimes substantially more than $100,000 per year. Pharmacologists who work for the government generally earn less than their private sector counterparts.

Benefit packages typically accompany salaried positions. Benefits may include paid vacations, sick days, and holidays, as well as health and dental insurance.

Before pharmacologists have completed their course work, paid opportunities may be available at colleges and universities. The stipend for these positions varies , but an average is $10,000 to $15,000 per year. Paid tuition is usually included as well.

what is the job outlook?

Employment of pharmacologists is expected to increase faster than the average for all occupations in the next several years. A significant factor in this is the continuing advancement of medical science and technology.

As medical scientists learn more about the human body and how it works, they uncover new possibilities for pharmaceutical treatments. Pharmacologists are needed to explore and experiment with these new treatment possibilities. Specifically, expanded research on such health issues as AIDS, cancer, organ transplants, and muscular dystrophy is likely to create jobs in pharmacology.

Another reason for the growth in jobs is the deepening concern about environmental toxins. Increasingly, pharmacologists are involved in researching the effects of atmospheric gases, household products, substances used in the workplace, and other environmental substances. This trend is expected to continue and to increase the demand for pharmacologists.

Other expanding pharmacological fields of research are drug abuse and gene therapy. Pharmacologists in the field of drug abuse are working to better understand the effects of abused substances on the fetus and on the body's organ systems. Research in gene therapy focuses on the development of gene products that alter the courses of disease. Both of these fields should provide good career prospects for pharmacologists.

Finally, the need for more pharmacologists involved in research will increase the need for teachers of pharmacology to train pharmacology students.

Despite the anticipated demand for pharmacologists, it is important to remember that much research and development is funded by the federal government. Therefore, budget cuts could lead to smaller increases in research and development expenditures, which would limit the dollar amount of each grant and slow the overall growth of research projects.

how do I learn more?

professional organizations

Following are organizations that provide information on pharmacologist careers, accredited schools, and employers.

American Society for Clinical Pharmacology and Therapeutics
1718 Gallagher Road
Norristown, PA 19401-2800
TEL: 610-825-3838
WEBSITE: http://oac1.oac.tju.edu/ASCPT/mainmenu.html

American Society for Pharmacology and Experimental Therapeutics
9600 Rockville Pike
Bethesda, MD 20814
TEL: 301-530-7060
WEBSITE: http://www.faseb.org/aspet

American Association of Pharmaceutical Scientists
1650 King Street
Alexandria, VA 22314
TEL: 703-548-3000
WEBSITE: http://www.aaps.org/

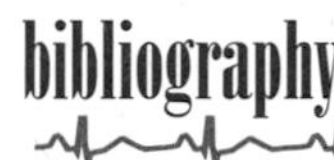

Following is a sampling of materials relating to the professional concerns and development of pharmacologists.

Books

Aspertheim, Mary K. *Pharmacology: an Introductory Text,* 8th edition. Philadelphia, PA: W.B. Saunders, 1996.

Eckler, Jody A., and Judy M. Fair. *Pharmacology Essentials*. Philadelphia, PA: W.B. Saunders, 1996.

Foster, R. W., editor. *Basic Pharmacology,* 4th edition. Newton, MA: Butterworth-Heinemann, 1996.

Hitner, Henry, and Barbara T. Nagle. *Basic Pharmacology for Health Occupations,* 3rd edition. Westerville, OH: Glencoe/McGraw-Hill, 1993.

Hollinger, Mannfred A. *Introduction to Pharmacology.* Bristol, PA: Taylor & Francis, 1997.

Levine, Ruth R., Carol T. Walsh, and Rochelle D. Schwartz. *Pharmacology: Drug Actions and Reactions,* 5th edition. Pearl River, NY: Parthenon Publishing Group, 1996.

Mutschler, Ernst, and Hartmut Derendorf. *Basic and Applied Principles of Drug Actions*. Boca Raton, FL: CRC Press, 1994.

Rice, Jane. *Principles of Pharmacology for Medical Assisting,* 2nd edition. Albany, NY: Delmar, 1994.

Stringer, Janet L. *Basic Concepts in Pharmacology: a Student's Survival Guide.* New York, NY: McGraw-Hill, 1995.

Theoharides, Theoharis. *Essentials of Pharmacology,* 2nd edition. Philadelphia, PA: Lippincott-Raven, 1996.

Woodrow, Ruth. *Essentials of Pharmacology in Health Occupations,* 2nd edition. Albany, NY: Delmar, 1996.

Periodicals

Clinical Pharmacology and Therapeutics. Monthly. Devoted to the study of the nature, action, disposition, efficacy, and total evaluation of drugs as they are used in man. American Society for Pharmacology and Experimental Therapeutics, Mosby, 11830 Westline Industrial Drive, St. Louis, MO 63146-3318, 314-872-8370, 800-325-4177.

Journal of Clinical Pharmacology. Monthly. Geared towards clinical pharmacologists and physicians concerned with and responsible for the appropriate selection, investigation, and prescribing of drugs. American College of Clinical Pharmacology, Lippincott-Raven Publishers, 227 E. Washington Square, Philadelphia, PA 19106, 215-238-4200.

Pharmacology and Therapeutics. Monthly. Presents authoritative review articles covering recent developments in pharmacology, including chemotherapy, toxicology, and clinical pharmacology. International Union of Pharmacology, Elsevier Science, 660 White Plains Road, Tarrytown, NY 10591, 914-524-9200.

pharmacy technician

Definition

Pharmacy technicians work with pharmacists in preparing medication and keeping patient records. This involves filling bottles with prescribed tablets and capsules, labeling the bottles, preparing IV packs, taking inventory, cleaning equipment, and entering patient data into a computer.

Alternative job titles

Pharmacy assistants
Pharmacy technologists
Pharmacy medication technicians

Salary range

$14,000 to $18,000 to $23,000

Educational requirements

High school diploma; six to twenty-four months of training

Certification or licensing

Recommended

Outlook

Faster than average

GOE
05.09.01

DOT
074

High School Subjects

Mathematics
Chemistry
Biology
English
Health

Personal Interests

Science
Computers
Health and fitness
Cooking

The Medical Center pharmacy is brightly lit. The fluorescent light bounces off the clean white shelves and counters, off the glass bottles and beakers. Like scientists in a laboratory, the pharmacy technicians in their white coats hover over vials and weights and measures. One tech prepares an IV, while another, wearing a special hood, carefully prepares an investigational drug.

A beeper pierces the quiet of the room, momentarily disturbing the order. A Code 5000, a call for the hospital emergency team, and Mike Holley moves into action. Emergency situations in the hospital occur every day, and Mike has become very familiar with emergency procedure. He takes the cart stocked with medications, equipment, and a monitor defibrillator and quickly makes his way through the hospital. At the end of the corridor, nurses, physicians, and an anesthesiologist stream into the patient's room. They all work hurriedly, yet smoothly and precisely. When Mike arrives with the cart, it becomes his responsibility to record all that happens, to maintain a legal record of the emergency scene. He listens and watches carefully, and also performs his other duties, preparing an IV or resuscitation equipment, as an important part of this emergency team.

what does a pharmacy technician do?

You've probably stood many times at a pharmacist's tall counter, waiting for a prescription to be filled. You've watched the pharmacist count out pills, or prepare capsules. You've been advised on how to use each medication safely and effectively. And you've probably noticed how much the pharmacist relies on his or her assistants. These assistants are known as *pharmacy technicians*, and they have become a recognized force in the health care industry.

Whether in a drug store, hospital, clinic, or nursing care facility, pharmacy technicians (usually referred to as pharmacy techs), perform a number of duties. As directed by a pharmacist, techs fill prescriptions and type and attach labels. They deliver medication to patients. A tech serves as record keeper, keeping patient files up-to-date by recording the prescribed drug and dosage in the pharmacy computer and on any necessary forms. So that the work area is kept orderly and organized, the tech stocks shelves and takes careful inventory. The pharmacy technician also cleans and sterilizes glassware and equipment.

In a hospital setting, these duties become particularly involved and complex. The tech prepares each patient's daily medications, individually labeling each tablet, capsule, suppository, and so on. Techs also take inventory on a daily basis, and daily restock the shelves in the pharmacy, in all the general nursing areas and in the operation theater. And a pharmacy tech sometimes acts as wholesaler, distributing medications to smaller, out-patient clinics.

Preparing medication for a hospital patient sometimes requires more than counting pills and filling bottles. Pharmacy techs work with a variety of substances and tools. A mortar and pestle, typically made of glass or porcelain, is used to grind crystalline or granular substances. Conical and cylindrical graduates are glasses used for measuring liquids. Techs use spatulas to prepare ointments, or to remove substances from the mortar and pestle. An experienced tech will work with investigational drugs—new drugs approved for human use, but with unknown side effects. Some patients agree to try these new drugs when all other prescribed drugs and treatments have failed. Preparing the investigational drugs sometimes requires special gloves and hoods. These experienced techs also work with chemotherapy agents and live bacteria, and prepare intravenous (IV) packs.

Pharmacy techs are responsible for the handling and safe delivery of controlled substances. In 1970, the Controlled Substances Act was passed by Congress. The purpose of the act is to improve the regulation of manufacturing, distributing, and dispensing of drugs necessary to control. Controlled substances are those drugs or substances with a high potential for abuse, which, when abused, may lead to severe dependence. Amphetamines, methamphetamines, codeine, and morphine are some of these substances.

Emergency situations are an everyday part of hospital work, and the pharmacy tech is an important part of the emergency team. Pharmacy techs prepare resuscitation equipment and keep a special cart stocked with medications and monitor defibrillator. In the case of an emergency in the hospital, the tech, along with

lingo to learn

Defibrillator A device for arresting chaotic contractions of the heart muscle.

Dosage The amount of medicine to be given.

Floor stock Medication kept in the drug cabinet or the nursing unit.

Intravenous An injection that involves inserting a needle or catheter into a vein to introduce a drug or solution.

Palliative A medicine that relieves without curing.

Parenteral Pertaining to drugs given by injection.

Pharmacopoeia A reference book of drug standards and dosages. Describes the drug's purity and the dosage forms in which it is available.

Therapeutic Pertaining to the treating or curing of disease or disorders.

available nurses, physicians, and anesthesiologists, is called to the site. The tech brings the cart and equipment and maintains a legal record of events.

what is it like to be a pharmacy technician?

In the Air Force, Mike Holley worked for eight years as a pharmacy technician. The extensive training he received in the military has helped him a great deal in his career. He currently works as a supervisor at the University Medical Center in Tucson, Arizona, where he coordinates the training for thirty-one techs. "I wish we had the funds for the kind of training I received," Mike says, adding that, in the military, he was required to put in three hundred hours of class time before he even picked up a medication.

To train pharmacy technicians, and to involve them with all aspects of the job, Mike devised a tech career ladder. This ladder is made up of the four main task areas of a hospital pharmacy. The technicians in the unit dose area prepare each patient's total medications for the day. These techs also handle incoming calls and prepare emergency equipment. In the controlled substances area, techs are responsible for the narcotics. They assure safe handling and delivery of the narcotics, and they correlate receipt slips. The techs who are responsible for floor stocking stock all shelves and take daily inventory.

The technicians-in-training are expected to be proficient in these three areas in six months. The more experienced techs are then assigned to the IV area, where they handle investigational drugs, chemotherapy agents, and live bacteria.

By rotating through these four task areas, a tech can take on the different responsibilities and become skilled at all aspects of the job. This variety of tasks is what keeps Mike interested in his career. "It's not repetitious," he says. "The chances of being bored are almost nil."

In the Medical Center pharmacy, a tech works one of three different shifts: 7:00 AM to 3:30 PM, 3:00 PM to 11:30 PM, or 11:00 PM to 7:30 AM. Mike generally works eight to ten hours a day, and sometimes works different hours to get a feel for all the shifts. Mike must also sometimes fill in for an absent tech. His other duties include addressing budget and disciplinary issues and attending committee meetings.

To be a successful pharmacy technician, you should

- Be able to work independently, and as part of a team
- Be responsible and reliable
- Be able to work in emergency situations
- Have good finger dexterity
- Have good hand-eye coordination

have I got what it takes to be a pharmacy technician?

Mike credits his management-mode of thinking to his success as a pharmacy tech supervisor. Training and supervising requires that he pay close attention to all the staff members and their work patterns. As a logically minded person, he is able to examine these work patterns and determine how to devise the most productive work place. These problem-solving skills are valuable to any pharmacy technician.

When hiring new technicians, Mike looks for people with a professional manner, people who exhibit a level of maturity. "I look for honesty and integrity," Mike says. Because pharmacy techs must work together in a variety of different ways, interpersonal skills are very important. A pharmacy should be a place of open communication, of careful watching and listening. Many people in a hospital—patients, nurses, physicians—rely on the pharmacy to run smoothly and efficiently. As a pharmacy technician, you work independently *and* as part of a team, and must be able to follow instructions, as well as give instructions clearly. These communication skills are important outside the pharmacy, also, as you are expected to advise patients in how to safely and effectively use the prescribed medication.

A hospital pharmacy technician must also act as part of the emergency team, which can mean performing duties in a stressful situation. Pharmacy techs are sometimes required to keep clear and precise legal record of the emergency situation, as well as offer necessary assistance.

Because pharmacy techs prepare drugs, and must handle needles and syringes, good hand-eye coordination and finger dexterity are necessary. Techs should also have good close-up vision, with or without glasses.

how do I become a pharmacy technician?

Mike Holley had not considered a career as a pharmacy tech before joining the Air Force, so his high school studies weren't directed toward pharmacy tech training. But his military training was extensive and helped him pass the pharmacy tech certification test with no problem. Mike believes a good community college program can also prepare you well for the test and a career as a pharmacy tech. Experience in a hospital setting is also valuable. Most pharmacy techs receive their training through community colleges, vocational/technical schools, and hospital community pharmacies throughout the United States. The length of the programs usually range from six months to two years, leading to a certificate or diploma, or an associate's degree in pharmacy technology.

education

High School

Most technical training programs require a high school diploma. To prepare for a training program, you should take high school courses that develop your basic skills in math, science (especially chemistry and biology), and language. Health courses can also help you. Involve yourself in extra-curricular activities, such as a business, drama, or journalism club, to develop communication and interpersonal skills.

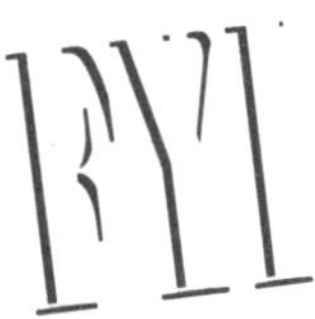

A little history

Rx, a symbol meaning *prescription*, was originally a symbol of the gods in early medical writings. The symbol was used as a prayer for healing.

A 5,000-year-old clay tablet, discovered in the Middle East, records drug remedies used by the Sumerians. Listed on the table are prescriptions for vegetable extracts, ointments, and solutions.

In ancient Mesopotamia, doctors tested drugs and poisons on slaves and prisoners.

Postsecondary Training

Many community college programs (usually called pharmacy technology programs) are designed to prepare you for the pharmacy technician certification exam, but can also prepare you for an associate of applied science program or a prepharmacy program. Some courses offered in these training programs include introduction to pharmacy and health care systems, pharmacy laws and ethics, medical terminology, anatomy, therapeutic agents, biology, and higher math. In addition, courses in microcomputers, writing, IV preparation, and interview and intercommunication skills are also part of some programs.

In addition to the class work, you may be required to perform an internship in a supervised clinical setting. The PTEC (Pharmacy Technology Educators Council) is working toward implementing a standardized curriculum across the United States. The Pharmacy Technology Educators Council publishes the *PTEC Directory,* a listing of pharmacy technician training programs throughout the United States and Canada.

certification or licensing

Though certification is not required of pharmacy technicians, it is highly recommended. To receive certification, you must pass a written exam—a standardized test recently adopted across the United States. "You won' t get the better jobs without certification," Mike says, pointing out that he prefers to hire certified techs. Certification shows employers you've received the training and gained the knowledge necessary for performing the duties of a technician. "A training program or hospital experience should prepare you adequately for the test."

scholarships and grants

Pharmaceutical companies offer scholarships to students pursuing pharmacy degrees, but these awards aren't generally offered to students in pharmacy technology programs.

who will hire me?

Upon leaving the Air Force and his first pharmacy tech job, Mike Holley looked to his county's Human Resources Department (sometimes referred to as Employment Services). Through this department, he learned of the job openings in local hospital pharmacies. A career as a pharmacy technician is best pursued on the local level. Check area newspaper ads for job listings, or use an employment agency. Some students of training programs may also move into tech positions with the hospital or clinics where they served as interns.

Pharmacy technicians can find work in hospitals (both in the in-patient and out-patient pharmacies), retail drugstores, nursing care facilities, and health care centers. A hospital provides the most varied experience and the opportunity for more specialized training. Because of these increased duties and responsibilities, a hospital pharmacy tech is generally paid more than a tech in a retail pharmacy.

More job opportunities are available in areas with an older population, because more medical services are generally required by the elderly. These areas typically include New York, Florida, California, Arizona, and New Mexico.

where can I go from here?

The career path for pharmacy technicians is not always clear cut. As supervisor, Mike has advanced as far as he can at the Medical Center. His position is actually rare—most pharmacies divide his supervisory duties between a lead technician and a pharmacist. Technicians may also move on to become data entry technicians, or technician managers.

Experienced pharmacy technicians may also choose to specialize in a particular area of pharmacy work, such as in narcotics control, or chemotherapy preparation. Others may choose to work primarily in the emergency room or operating room of a hospital or clinic. Some techs, having gained a few years' pharmacy experience, return to school to pursue a pharmacy degree.

what are the salary ranges?

Many retail pharmacies hire techs at minimum wage, with the possibility of future wage increases. But techs in hospital pharmacies can start at about $6.50 per hour, eventually working up to around $15.00 per hour. Sometimes a tech can make up to 50 percent of a pharmacist's salary. (The average pharmacist's salary is about $53,500 per year.)

what is the job outlook?

In efforts to reduce spending, many hospitals are developing managed care programs. Hospitals are also providing more treatment on an out-patient basis, to avoid the high costs of in-patient care. But employment in the health care field continues to grow, despite this cost cutting. As new technology and new medical treatments are developed, health care workers are needed to administer them. The U.S. government anticipates 4.2 million new jobs in health care by 2005.

Advancement Possibilities

Pharmacists compound and dispense prescribed medications, drugs, and other pharmaceuticals for patient care, according to professional standards and state and federal legal requirements.

Radiopharmacists prepare and dispense radioactive pharmaceuticals used for patient diagnosis and therapy, applying principles and practices of pharmacy and radiochemistry.

Directors of pharmacy services direct and coordinate, through subordinate supervisory personnel, activities and functions of hospital pharmacies.

Pharmacists are getting jobs with many different kinds of health care providers, which means more opportunities for pharmacy technicians as well. As techs continue to gain recognition for their skilled and specialized work, more career, training, and scholarship opportunities will arise. Those interested in pursing a career as a pharmacy tech should keep an eye on health care trends and government health care reform. Also watch for the changing role of hospitals, as hybrids between hospitals and nursing homes develop.

how do I learn more?

professional organizations

The following organization provides information on pharmacy technician careers.

American Association of Pharmacy Technicians
PO Box 1447
Greensboro, NC 27402
TEL: 910-275-1700

The following organization publishes *The Journal of Pharmacy Technology* and *The Pharmacy Technicians Education and Training Directory.*

Pharmacy Technology Educators Council
Harvey Whitney Book Publishing
PO Box 42696
Cincinnati, OH 45242
TEL: 513-793-3555

bibliography

Following is a sampling of materials relating to the professional concerns and development of pharmacy technicians.

Books

Durgin, Jane, and Zachary Hanan. *Pharmacy Practice for Technicians.* Albany, NY: Delmar, 1994.

Frook, John. *The Pfizer Guide: Pharmacy Career Opportunities,* 2nd edition. Old Saybrook, CT: Merritt Communications, 1994.

Gable, Fred B. *Opportunities in Pharmacy Careers.* Lincolnwood, IL: VGM Career Horizons, 1994.

Keresztes. *Manual for Pharmacy Technicians.* Philadelphia, PA: W.B. Saunders, 1997.

Moss, Susan K., and William A. Hopkins, Jr. *Pharmacy Technician Certification Quick-Study Guide.* Washington, DC: American Pharmaceutical Association, 1995.

Reilly, Robert, John Arross, and Kris Boyea-Sandberg. *The Pharmacy Tech: Basic Pharmacology and Calculations.* El Paso, TX: Skidmore-Roth, 1994.

Periodicals

ASHP Newsletter. Monthly. Covers society news and recent hospital pharmacy developments. American Society of Hospital Pharmacists, 7273 Wisconsin Avenue, Bethesda, MD 20814, 301-657-3000.

American Pharmacy. Monthly. Features coverage of drug research and pharmacy practice. American Pharmaceutical Association, 2215 Constitution Avenue, NW, Washington, DC 20037, 202-429-7557.

Hospital Pharmacy. Monthly. Devoted to technical and developmental aspects and the administrative procedures of hospital pharmacies. J.B. Lippincott Co., 227 East Washington Square, Philadelphia, PA 19106, 215-238-4200.

Inside Pharmacy. Monthly. Directed at pharmacy professionals who work in individual drugstores and drugstore and supermarket chains. Lebhar-Friedman Inc., 425 Park Avenue, New York, NY 10022, 212-371-9400.

Journal of Pharmacy Technology. Bimonthly. Aimed at pharmacists and technicians. Covers therapeutic trends, current research and organizational, legal and educational activities. Includes information on new drugs and medical products and equipment. Harvey Whitney Books Co., Box 42696, Cincinnati, OH 45242, 513-793-3555.

Pharmacy Times. Monthly. Covers research and developments in the pharmacy industry. Romaine Pierson Publishers, Inc., Box 911, 80 Shore Road, Port Washington, NY 11050, 516-883-6350.

Pharmacy Today. Biweekly. Provides association news and informational and legislative reports of interest to pharmacists. American Pharmaceutical Association, 2215 Constitution Avenue, NW, Washington, D.C. 20037, 202-628-4410.

phlebotomy technician

Definition

Phlebotomy technicians draw blood from patients or donors in hospitals, blood banks, clinics, physicians' offices, or other facilities. They assemble equipment; verify patient identification numbers; and withdraw blood either through a finger puncture or with a needle syringe. They label, transport, and store blood for analysis or for other medical purposes.

Alternative job titles

Blood technicians
Phlebotomists

Salary range

$15,344 to $17,166 to $22,339

Educational requirements

High school diploma; ten weeks to twelve months technical training through an accredited program, or on-the-job training.

Certification or licensing

Certification recommended. Licensing required in some states.

Outlook

Average

GOE
02.04.02

DOT
079

High School Subjects

Biology
Health
Physics
Computer science
English
Speech

Personal Interests

Socializing
Health, fitness, and exercise
Caring for people

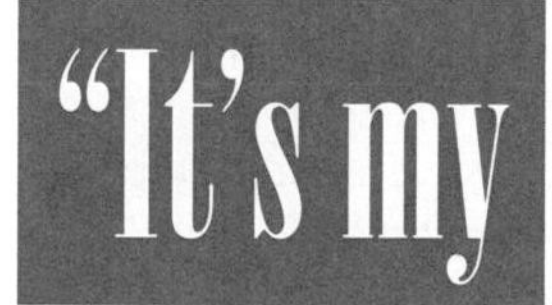

job to draw blood from donors," says Sherry Southerland. She works as a phlebotomy technician at a branch office of the Bonfils Blood Center, a blood bank that supplies most of the hospitals in Colorado. "I go over the donors' medical histories, ask them additional questions, scrub the skin, find the vein, collect, and label the blood. Like any job, after a while, things can get pretty routine." She sighs and adds, "But when my dad got sick and I saw him being transfused, I realized that phlebotomy technicians are not just some cog in a machine. I could see the other end of the process and it made a real difference."

Sherry stresses the vital role phlebotomy technicians serve in the collection of the nation's blood supply. "We've got to have this resource," she says, "and it must be screened well. When my dad was sick, I hoped that the phlebotomy technicians who had drawn the blood that he was receiving had done a good job screening donors. Did they ask enough questions, I wondered. Did they take time to explain why those questions were necessary? The importance of what I was doing as a phlebotomy technician suddenly came through."

what does a phlebotomy technician do?

Ancient people did not understand the role of blood, but they knew it was vital. Some believed that it might even be the home of the soul. Early Egyptians bathed in blood, hoping this act would cure illness or reverse the aging process. Some Romans drank the blood of dying gladiators in order to acquire the athletes' strength and bravery.

lingo to learn

Autologous donation A blood donation that is stored and reserved for return to the original donor during surgery.

Blood bank A facility responsible for collecting blood from donors, separating blood into its components, typing, and matching blood in order to ensure safe transfusions.

Blood components The red cells, white cells, platelets, and plasma that constitute blood.

Hematology The science of blood and blood diseases.

Plasma The liquid portion of blood, including protein, but excluding cellular components.

Platelets The cells in blood that are involved with clotting.

Transfusion A medical procedure to transfer blood from one body into another.

Typing A procedure to determine the blood group (A, B, AB, or O) within a particular sample.

Venipuncture The puncture of a vein with a hypodermic needle, commonly known as a needle stick.

Over time, scientists began to understand how blood functioned and they searched for ways to collect it or transfer it from one person to another. Quills or silver needles were attached to silver tubing and the tubings were attached to animal bladders in order to construct blood collection devices. Arteries were punctured and blood gushed out. Sometimes the donor died, as well as the patient. Little care was taken with the cleanliness of instruments. No one understood why blood sometimes failed to coagulate or coagulated too quickly. No one could explain why blood could not always be transferred successfully from one person to another.

Modern techniques of blood collection, typing, and transfusion developed only within this century. Today blood is drawn by professionals called *phlebotomy technicians* or *phlebotomists.* They work in clean, well-lighted laboratories, hospitals, and clinics.

Blood is used for a variety of medical tests, or is stored in blood banks for future use. There are three main methods by which blood can be drawn: venipuncture, arterial puncture, and capillary collection. Collecting through veins is the most common method, followed by artery collection, and capillary collection which involves punctures of the fingers or heels.

The first steps in drawing blood are to take the patient's medical history and match the physician's testing order with the amount of blood to be drawn. Then the patient's temperature and pulse are taken. Next, the site of the withdrawal is located. Typically, the large vein that is visible on the underside of the arm near the elbow is used.

Finding a suitable vein, however, is not always easy because there is a great deal of anatomical difference among people. Once a suitable site is located, a tourniquet is wrapped high on the patient's upper arm, as far from the elbow as is convenient. The phlebotomy technician checks the site for lesions, other needle marks, and any skin disorders that might interfere with the collection process. Then the site is cleansed by swabbing with a sterile solution. The phlebotomy technician grasps the patient's forearm and retracts the arm downward in order to immobilize the soft tissue and steady the vein. Sometimes the patient is asked to open and close his or her hand a few times to make the vein more prominent. Making a proper puncture takes practice. After the sterile needle is uncovered, it must be grasped tightly, but passed through the skin gently. The needle is inserted almost horizontal with the vein and as parallel to the skin as possible. Then the hub of the needle is raised and the angle toward the skin increased so that the needle can pierce the wall of the vein. After the needle is advanced slightly into the vein itself, blood may be withdrawn. Generally this is done by releasing a clamp attached to the blood collection device or to the tubing. When the required amount of blood is collected, the needle is removed and sealed, the site covered, and the tourniquet removed.

After collection, the phlebotomy technician labels the blood, coordinates its number with the worksheet order, and transports the blood to a storage facility or to another laboratory worker. The phlebotomy technician also checks to make sure that the patient is all right, notes any adverse reactions, and administers first aid or other medical assistance when necessary.

Specialists in blood bank technology are professionals who perform a variety of tasks associated with blood banking. They test blood for compatibility, type and match it, and store it until needed. Phlebotomy technicians who are employed by blood banks may be supervised by specialists in blood bank technology. Phlebotomy technicians who work in hospitals or clinics are supervised by other laboratory personnel.

what is it like to be a phlebotomy technician?

"When I come to work," says Sherry, "I never know whether the lobby of the blood bank will be full or whether no one will show up for an hour or two. The day after a disaster occurs anywhere in the U.S., however, we're always mobbed by donors. Regardless, eighty percent of the people we see are repeats, folks who come here every fifty-six days because they know how great the need is for blood. They know that blood banks like ours are on the front lines and that together, we're the ones fighting this war to keep people healthy."

Sherry's job as a phlebotomy technician begins by greeting donors when they arrive at the Bonfils Blood Center branch office in Lakewood, Colorado. If they are first time donors, she enters their names and medical information into the computer and if they are repeats, she pulls up their medical history cards. To give blood, donors must weigh over 110 pounds, not have infections such as colds or

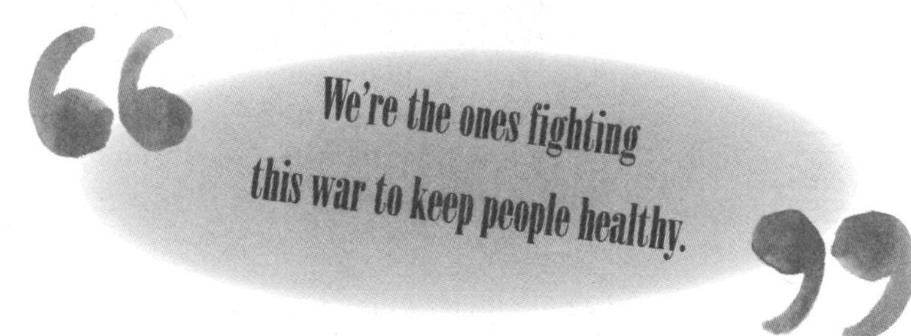

the flu, not be taking certain medications, and not be engaging in a variety of at-risk behaviors. At-risk behaviors include illegal, intravenous drug use and unprotected sex.

Sherry asks each donor several questions, some of which are repeats of medical history information. "People skills are very important in this job," she says. "I'm not trying to be nosy when I ask these questions. We're trying to retain donors and yet we need to weed out the high-risk volunteers too. You have to be dedicated to the donors and to putting out a safe product."

Updating medical histories and asking questions helps screen out people with illnesses or behaviors that might jeopardize the safety of the blood supply. In particular, phlebotomy technicians try to screen donors who might have active cases of, or have been exposed to, tuberculosis, malaria, hepatitis, syphilis, and HIV virus.

If the donors' medical histories are satisfactory, Sherry checks their temperatures and then, using a small centrifuge, does a quick blood test to verify iron levels. A low iron level indicates that the donor's body is in a weakened condition and there isn't enough hemoglobin present—the iron-containing proteins within red blood cells that carry oxygen. If a patient should receive such hemoglobin-poor blood, there wouldn't be enough red blood cells to perform vital functions within the body. If, however, iron levels are sufficient, Sherry directs the donors to a reclining bed where she takes their pulse and blood pressure, and swabs the skin with antiseptic.

Next comes the needle stick. "I can't look when it's my turn to give blood," she says. "And the first time I had to make a needle stick on someone else, I was so nervous. It's still a bit scary. You don't want to hurt people. Practice—that's the only way to learn." It takes about five minutes to collect a pint of blood. When the required amount is collected, Sherry uses a hematron, a device that heat-seals the tubing that extends from the needle in the donor's arm to the collection bag. Then the needle is removed and disposed of, and the blood is transported to the laboratory where it is typed by other workers. Next, she makes sure that the donor drinks some juice, eats cookies or crackers, and rests for ten to fifteen minutes before leaving the blood center. "Everybody reacts a bit differently to giving blood," she says. "Here, it's not like in a doctor's office where phlebotomy technicians draw only a small vial of blood. Taking a pint of blood makes some people turn white, others break out in cold sweats, and some people pass out completely. Still, only one percent of donors have any adverse reactions, at all.

Phlebotomy technicians are trained to watch for a range of responses from mild lightheadedness to loss of consciousness. Each year Sherry renews her First Aid and CPR training. She also has emergency medical training and a certificate that enables her to set up IVs, intravenous drips used to replace body fluids. Other portions of her day are spent performing quality checks on equipment, inventorying supplies, and attending meetings.

Specialists in blood bank technology (persons who have advanced degrees) process the blood collected, type it, make cross matches with patients, check the blood for communicable diseases and infections, and store it for future use.

have I got what it takes to be a phlebotomy technician?

"Being a phlebotomy technician is challenging work," says Sherry. "You're constantly working with people. Good communication skills are essential because you have to stick the patient or donor with a needle in order to draw blood. Yes, you're following orders and doing routine work, but a sense of humor helps too."

Mary Anderson, program director at the Wichita Area Vocational Technical School in Wichita, Kansas adds, "The patients have to feel like they are the most important thing in your world at that moment. Even when you have to work at a quick pace, you should not make the patients feel like they're on an assembly line. That's not always easy," she says, "particularly for phlebotomy technicians who work in hospitals. They have to deal with a variety of people under difficult circumstances. Often you're called to the bedside of a patient to draw blood and, not only are you dealing with a sick person who doesn't want to have another needle stuck in them, the doctors, the nurses, and sometimes the families, are after you to hurry up and finish your work."

According to the American Society of Phlebotomy Technicians, phlebotomy technicians are "often the only part of the lab staff that a patient sees. . . . Yet, phlebotomists work difficult hours, the pay is low, the turnover rate high, and they often find themselves faced with cantankerous patients. . . . Although phlebotomists serve as valuable liaisons between the patient and the clinical laboratory, many times they suffer low professional esteem."

"No matter what the working situation," says Mary, "phlebotomy technicians have to be patient and not get upset. This is essential because the blood test won't be any better than the samples they collect."

Phlebotomy technicians need to have excellent interpersonal communication skills. They should be good listeners and able to speak precisely and clearly. They should be able to reassure patients as well as be able to explain medical procedures. Some shift work may be required. Those working in hospitals, in particular, can expect to work some weekends and holidays as well. People in this profession work with precise, often small, medical supplies. Good manual dexterity is essential.

Persons who are squeamish at the sight of blood or have difficulty working with needles would find it hard to succeed as a phlebotomy technician. There is a small risk of exposure to contaminated blood and other illness in this profession, but phlebotomy technicians always wear gloves and, when necessary, additional protective clothing. This, along with common sense and attention to procedure, minimizes risk.

To be a successful phlebotomy technician, you should

- Enjoy working with people
- Be patient
- Be able to work under pressure
- Be attentive to detail
- Be an effective communicator and a good listener
- Have good manual dexterity

Advancement Possibilities

Phlebotomy supervisors oversee the work of other phlebotomy technicians, coordinating schedules and making certain the strict safety guidelines of the field are followed.

Training instructors work in technical school, community colleges, and hospital educational programs to train phlebotomists in their duties. They might also supervise the clinical practice portion of the training in a hospital.

Blood bank technologists are responsible for all the activities within blood banks, including the collection, testing, storage, and transportation of blood.

how do I become a phlebotomy technician?

Sherry had been a home health care aide and a hospice volunteer before she started working for Bonfils Blood Center. "I was trained on the job. That was a common practice then," she says. Now, in order to achieve certification and to move ahead professionally, formal training programs are highly recommended.

education

High School

Biology, health, and other science courses are helpful for students wishing to become phlebotomy technicians after graduation. Computer science, English, and speech classes are also important. In addition, students planning on entering formal phlebotomy training programs should be sure to fulfill the entrance requirements for thc program they plan to attend.

Postsecondary Training

Until recently, on-the-job training was the norm for phlebotomy technicians. Now formal programs are offered through independent training schools, community colleges, or hospitals. Most programs last from ten weeks to one year. They include both in-class study and supervised, clinical practice. Coursework includes anatomy, physiology, introduction to laboratory practices, communication, medical terminology, phlebotomy techniques, emergency situations, and CPR training.

certification or licensing

Certification and licensing for phlebotomy technicians varies according to state and employer. Several agencies grant certification. To be eligible to take the qualifying examination from the Amcrican Society of Phlebotomy Technicians, or from the Board of Registry of the American Society of Clinical Pathologists, applicants must have worked as a full-time phlebotomist for six months or as a part-time phlebotomist for one year, or have completed an accredited phlebotomy training program.

scholarships and grants

Many community colleges offer general scholarships and financial aid as do some hospitals and training programs. In addition, institutions with specific phlebotomy programs are sources of information on work-study and student internships.

Related Jobs

The U.S. Department of Labor classifies phlebotomy technicians under the headings Occupations in Medicine and Health, Not Elsewhere Classified (DOT) and Laboratory Technology: Life Sciences (GOE). Also under these headings are physician assistants, who work under the direction of doctors to provide health care services such as administering diagnostic tests, performing injections, suturing wounds, and providing family planning counseling; medical record technicians who compile, maintain, and retrieve medical records; and dental assistants who sterilize instruments, prepare patients, and assist dentists during examination and treatment

American Medical Technologists
710 Higgins Road
Park Ridge, IL 60068-5765
TEL: 847-823-5169

American Society of Clinical Pathologists
2100 West Harrison
Chicago, IL 60612
TEL: 312-738-1336
WEBSITE: http://www.ascp.org

American Society of Phlebotomy Technicians, Inc.
PO Box 1831
Hickory, NC 28603
TEL: 704-322-1334

National Accrediting Agency for Clinical Laboratory Sciences
8410 West Bryn Mawr
Suite 670
Chicago, IL 60631
TEL: 773-714-8880

bibliography

Following is a sampling of materials relating to the professional concerns and development of phlebotomy technicians.

Books

Davis, Bonnie K. *Phlebotomy: a Client-Based Approach.* Albany, NY: Delmar, 1996.

Garza, Diana, and Kathleen Becan-McBride. *Phlebotomy Handbook,* 4th edition. New York, NY: Appleton & Lange, 1996.

Periodicals

American Journal of Hematology. 8 per year. Provides investigative reports concerning various aspects of hematology, including the area of blood banking. Wiley, 605 Third Avenue, New York, NY 10158, 212-850-6000.

Blood Bank Week. Weekly. Newsletter focusing on issues of blood banking, transfusion medicine, and related health topics. American Association of Blood Banks, 8101 Glenbrook Road, Bethesda, MD 20814, 703-528-8200.

CCBC Newsletter. Weekly. Newsletter reporting on recent developments in the medical, regulatory, and management areas of the blood bank community. Council of Community Blood Centers, 725 15th Street, NW, Suite 700, Washington, DC 20005, 202-393-5725.

News Briefs. Monthly. Newsletter featuring issues related to blood banking transfusion medicine. American Association of Blood Banks, 8101 Glenbrook Road, Bethesda, MD 20814, 301-907-6977.

The Tourniquet. Annual. Newsletter providing reports on research and listings of employment opportunities. National Phlebotomy Association, 2623 Blakesberry Road, NE, Washington, DC 20018, 202-636-4515.

physical therapist

Definition

Physical therapists help alleviate pain, prevent disability, and restore mobility and function in patients with injuries, diseases, or birth defects. They also help improve the physical conditions of healthy people.

Alternative job title

Physiotherapist

Salary range

$20,000 to $42,000 to $62,000+

Educational requirements

Bachelor's degree in an accredited four-year physical therapy program; or bachelor's degree in a related four-year college degree program plus a master's degree in an accredited physical therapy program

Certification or licensing

Mandatory

Job outlook

Much faster than average

GOE
10.02.02

DOT
076

High School Subjects

Biology
Business and accounting
English
Physical education
Physiology
Speech

Personal Interests

Health care
Helping people
Sports

"There's no hope," the patient said in despair. For two weeks, his leg had been in constant pain, the result of a displaced disc in his spine. "I've taken painkillers, but they haven't helped. My doctor says I'll have to be operated on next. But I'm a waiter. How can I do my job if I can't walk?"

Gabor Sagi, the physical therapist assigned to the young man's case, helped him onto a mat on the floor. "Don't give up just yet. I'm going to lead you through a series of positions. I want you to tell me how each one feels."

Gabor pushed on the patient's shoulders and shifted the patient's pelvis forward. The young man cried out, "Wait!"

Then he started to laugh. "Gabor, this is incredible! What did you do? It's gone! The pain, I mean. Like you just shut it off. "

Gabor smiled. "So there's hope for you after all? Okay, now I'm going to show you some exercises to do at home. I'll bet you'll be back at the restaurant in a week."

"You'll come in then," the young waiter said, "and I'll serve you the biggest meal you've ever had!"

what does a physical therapist do?

Many illnesses, injuries, birth defects, and other health conditions can have a drastic effect on a person's mobility and overall quality of life. *Physical therapists* work with patients to help to relieve their pain and restore them to full function, if possible; or to help them adjust to life after disabling illnesses or injuries so that they can live independent lives. Physical therapists work as part of a team of health care professionals, which may include general practitioners, specialists, radiologists, occupational therapists, and social workers.

A physical therapist first consults a patient's medical history. The physical therapist may then speak with the patient's physician to discuss the patient's health and treatment options. The physical therapist also speaks to the patient to learn about the kind and amount of pain the patient feels. The therapist seeks to identify aspects of the patient's behavior, activity, and lifestyle that cause an onset of pain.

The next step is to conduct clinical tests to measure the patient's strength, range of motion, and ability to function. The physical therapist may observe the patient as he or she performs certain tasks, such as walking up and down stairs, walking on a treadmill, bending and stretching, and lifting objects. Once the patient's problems have been identified, the physical therapist will discuss them with the patient and with a team of health care professionals in order to set treatment goals and design a plan that will help the patient accomplish these goals.

Treatment is specifically designed according to the patient's needs and abilities. A physical therapist treating a patient who is paralyzed or otherwise immobilized may begin with passive exercises, such as stretching and manipulating joints and muscles. The therapist may use electrical stimulation, hot or cold compresses, or ultrasound in order to stimulate muscles and relieve pain. Traction and deep-tissue massages can also help relieve a patient's pain and restore function. As treatment progresses, the therapist may design a program of movements and exercises that help the patient regain strength and mobility.

For certain patients, such as a person who has suffered a stroke or lost a limb, a return to full function is not possible. Physical therapists work with such patients to help them adjust to their new conditions. They may help a patient adapt to wearing a prosthetic device such as an artificial limb, or to using crutches or a wheelchair. Other patients must relearn certain activities, such as walking, dressing, and climbing in and out of bathtubs, in order to return to independent lives. Physical therapists work with cardiac patients to increase their endurance and minimize the risk of further heart problems. Burn patients require treatment that will reduce scarring and maintain flexibility.

Physical therapists also work with athletes and other people who seek to improve their physical conditions. A physical therapist may devise an exercise program designed to enhance a person's athletic performance. The therapist will observe the person's movements and suggest ways of improving posture and technique to achieve the person's goals. Other professionals besides physical therapists do

Modalities are the various technical procedures used in physical therapy during treatment. They include the following:

Cryotherapy The therapeutic use of cold.

Diathermy The production of heat in parts of the body, using electric currents, microwaves, or ultrasound.

Hydrotherapy The therapeutic use of water on the outside of the body, including the use of exercise pools, whirlpools, and showers.

Laser therapy The use of lasers to reduce pain, inflammation, and swelling.

Traction A therapeutic procedure in which part of the body is placed under tension, as by the attachment of a weight.

Ultrasound The use of sound waves to treat soft tissues.

this type of work; these professionals include *athletic trainers, personal trainers,* and *physical instructors.*

The American Physical Therapy Association recognizes seven specialty areas within physical therapy: cardiopulmonary, clinical electrophysiology, geriatrics, neurology, orthopedics, pediatrics, and sports physical therapy.

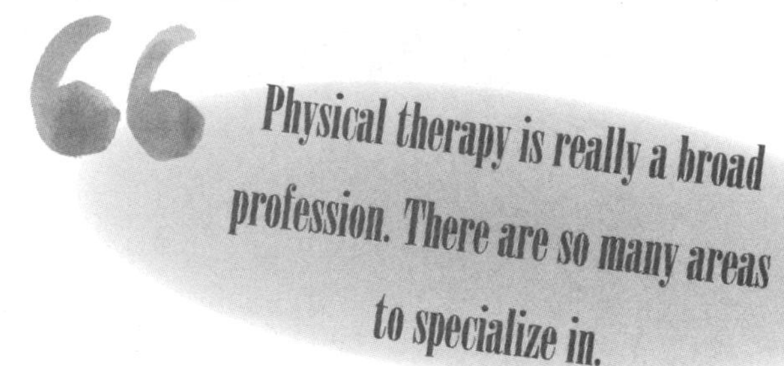

what is it like to be a physical therapist?

Gabor Sagi has been a physical therapist for ten years. He works as a full-time therapist at Mercy Hospital and Medical Center in Chicago, Illinois. "I was attracted to physical therapy as a career because of my interest in sports. In high school, I started lifting weights, and that made me more aware of my muscles and how the body works," Gabor says. "I became interested in the mechanics of the body and how it works." An injury to his back increased his interest. "I had to undergo therapy myself. What I liked was that physical therapy would give me a chance to work with both my mind and my hands."

Gabor generally works four full days (nine hours each) and one half day each week. "I set my appointments with my patients, so that gives me a lot of flexibility for setting my own schedule," he says. "But I usually put in at least a forty-hour week."

A typical day for Gabor begins at 8:30 AM. "I spend the first half-hour or so sending reports on my patients to their physicians and updating and reviewing notes on my patients. Then I'm ready to receive my first patient of the day," Gabor says. During the day, Gabor may see as many as twenty different patients. "I'll see a patient two or three times a week, for about thirty minutes each session. A patient's therapy program may last anywhere from two weeks to three months or more."

When Gabor receives a new patient, he performs an initial assessment of the patient's condition and what the patient expects to achieve from physical therapy. The initial assessment generally lasts from forty-five minutes to an hour. "The first thing I explore is the history of the patient's complaint. I want to know what his or her life is like. Usually, patients come to me because they're having trouble functioning. So I want to see what their functions are—their jobs or hobbies—and I set goals with them to return them to full function." Gabor speaks with patients at length about their conditions. "I learn the details of how their conditions affect them. I want to know what makes them feel better and what makes them feel worse. I try to find the pattern in a patient's behavior."

After this assessment, Gabor performs a physical examination of the patient. "I need to make sure that whatever treatment I use won't be dangerous or detrimental to a patient. The first thing I do is observe the patient's condition. I look for any deformities, swelling, muscle wasting, or scars. I'll palpate the patient, which means I'm touching the patient to look for tender areas and checking the quality of tissue texture.

Then I'll examine the patient's movement. I look at the range of movement the patient is able to achieve and the quality of the movement. I'll test muscles, overall strength, and speed and endurance. I'll also do a neurological exam to look for any motor or sensory deficits."

Once this examination is completed, Gabor and his new patient move on to more specific physical tests to better evaluate the patient's particular condition. Gabor says, "I also observe the patient performing certain tasks, like dressing and undressing, climbing stairs, using the treadmill, or reaching up or down and picking up objects."

After Gabor has completed examining his patient, he devises a treatment program. "It's important to set goals with a patient to bring back full physical function, if that's possible. I try to make each patient responsible for his or her own progress." Gabor prescribes an exercise or movement program, and other treatments the patient may need. He also schedules follow-up appointments with the patient. "I'm constantly assessing the patient. If something's not working, I need to know that so I can adjust the treatment plan."

have I got what it takes to be a physical therapist?

Physical therapists have become respected members of the team of health care professionals involved in a patient's treatment and rehabilitation. "When I first started working as a PT," Gabor says, "a lot of physicians still took the old approach to physical therapy. That is, the physician would prescribe the treatment and the physical therapist would be expected to carry it out. They'd tell you what to do even if they didn't really know anything about physical therapy! But nowadays the relationship has changed a lot. It's become much more of a two-way communication." Because physical therapists work not only with patients but also with other health care professionals, good communication skills are essential to this career. "I have to be able to explain things to my patients in ways they can understand," Gabor says. "It's important to be clear about what I expect of them and what they must expect of themselves."

For Gabor, his relationship with his patients is very rewarding. "You really get to work one on one with people. You get pretty involved in their lives and you become close to them on a pretty intimate level. But there's always a limit to that closeness. It's pretty much confined to the therapy center. And I like that, too." Physical therapists usually work with people who are in pain or who are undergoing a particularly stressful period in their lives. "There's a nice sense of responsibility, of taking charge, and of taking care of people and having them trust you," Gabor says. "But there's a downside to that, too. It can be quite overwhelming. A lot of the patients I see have pretty much given up. They'll be dependent on me. But it's important to help them take responsibility for themselves. I have to give the responsibility for their treatment back to them. And that can be difficult."

Physical therapy requires a great deal of creativity on the part of the therapist. No two patients are alike, and no two will respond the same way to the same treatment. The physical therapist must be aware of a patient's needs and condition, and be flexible enough to adapt therapy specifically to the patient. "But that's the part of physical therapy I like the most. Not only do I get to work with my hands, but I'm constantly working with my mind," Gabor says. "In a way, examining a new patient, especially someone with spinal problems, is like detective work. Often, a patient will be referred to me with a general diagnosis, like 'sciatica,' which just means the patient has pain in his or her leg. So it's up to me to know what kinds of questions to ask, like questions about the patient's symptoms and behavior, to track down the source of the pain and map out a treatment plan."

Gabor enjoys coming into contact with people. "I meet lots of different people in my job. I've treated chairmen of companies, politicians, police officers, people who haul garbage, you name it. Each patient is entirely new." Being a physical therapist has also given Gabor a chance to travel. "I've worked in maybe twenty different settings in the last ten years. I trained as a physical therapist in France, where I was born. But I worked for years in London, England before coming to work here. Everywhere that there are people, there's a need for physical therapists."

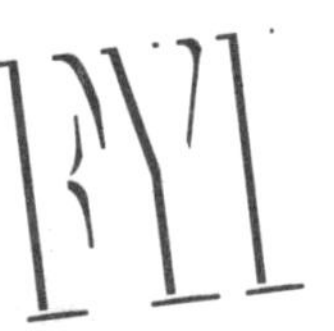

Physical therapist assistants assist physical therapists in the implementation of treatment programs. Under the supervision of physical therapists, they conduct treatments and train patients in exercises and other activities.

Physical therapist assistants have two-year associate's degrees. Some states require licensing; others don't.

how do I become a physical therapist?

Physical therapists undergo rigorous educational and clinical training to prepare for their careers. There are two primary paths for becoming a physical therapist. The first is to enroll in a four-year bachelor's degree program in physical therapy. The second path is to enroll in a two-year master's degree program. In 1995, there were more than 145 accredited physical therapist programs in the United States.

Pam Johnson, who works as a physical therapist at Swedish Covenant Hospital in Chicago, completed her master's degree in June, 1996. "I have a bachelor's degree in biology. After college, I volunteered in the physical therapy department of a hospital. That led to my being trained as a physical therapy aide," Pam says. "I think that experience helped me get into the master's degree program. It definitely gave me a good picture of what physical therapy is all about."

To be a successful physical therapist, you should

- Like working with people
- Have strong communication skills
- Be able to work independently and as part of a team
- Be creative
- Be in good physical condition

education

High School

Competition for entering both master's degree and bachelor's degree physical therapy programs is intense, so students should begin planning their careers while still in high school. Courses in mathematics, biology, chemistry, and other sciences should be part of a student's curriculum. "Taking physics is really important," Gabor Sagi says, "because physical therapy is really all about mechanics, the way things move." Students should also work on developing strong communication skills. "You have to be able to write reports and speak to other members of the medical and health care staff," Gabor says. "And you also need to be able to communicate with your patients."

An interest in sports and physical education will give a student more insight into the function of the body. Social sciences and psychology courses will also bring the student more understanding of people. A physical therapist works with many different people from a variety of cultures, and therapists should be sensitive to each individual's concerns. Volunteer work at local hospitals, health clinics, retirement homes, and other places that involve contact with both health care professionals and their patients will also help prepare students for this career. "It isn't like you see on television at all," Pam says. "Patients aren't always easy to work with. Sometimes they're not cognitively aware. And in real life you're dealing with people on respirators, catheter bags, IV lines, and other equipment. I admit I was uncomfortable with that as a student. But volunteering and working as an aide meant that I knew what I was getting myself into."

Postsecondary Training

A bachelor's degree program in physical therapy generally begins with courses in biology, chemistry, and physics. Students will follow specialized courses in biomechanics, neuroanatomy, manifestations of disease and trauma, human growth and development, evaluation and assessment techniques, and therapeutic treatment techniques. Students also receive laboratory and clinical experience. They visit hospitals to observe physical therapy treatments, and they begin supervised treatment of patients. While in college, students can volunteer in physical therapy departments of hospitals or clinics. They can also participate in meetings and lectures organized by the American Physical Therapy Association.

Students interested in supervisory, administrative, research, or teaching positions, should continue their education in master's degree programs in physical therapy. Physical therapist master's degree programs are also open to people who hold bachelor's degrees in related fields.

A master's degree program provides intensive education in physical therapy. "I'd say one of the hardest parts was being in class or in the lab all day, from eight in the morning to five in the evening," Pam says. "I think the bachelor's degree program is less intense that way. But the toughest of all was what are called 'practicals.' That's when you are given a case from an actual patient history. The professor plays the patient, and you have to go through an evaluation and assessment, give your diagnosis, develop goals for treatment, and suggest a treatment plan. The professor will then tell you how you did. It really forces you to think on your feet and confront things that aren't clear-cut. Practicals were a great learning experience."

certification or licensing

After graduation, a physical therapist is required to pass a licensing exam. Gabor says, "Because I was trained overseas, I had to first take an exam to have my training recognized, even though I'd already worked as a professional physical therapist for many years. I was given a provisional license to practice while I prepared to take the actual licensing exam." Licensed physical therapists should also expect to continue their education. "I've taken a lot of practical courses to learn specific techniques," Gabor says. "These are usually short courses lasting a few days."

A physical therapist is encouraged to become certified as a clinical specialist in one of the seven specialty areas recognized by the American Board of Physical Therapy Specialists. Certification is available to any physical therapist with several years of clinical experience and postgraduate education in a specialty area.

who will hire me?

Physical therapy offers a broad range of employment opportunities. About 30 percent of physical therapists work in hospitals. Others work in rehabilitation centers, health care clinics, physical therapy centers, community health centers, nursing homes, schools, pediatric centers, sports facilities, and research institutions. Many companies in manufacturing and other areas employ physical therapists in corporate and industrial physical therapy departments.

Pam Johnson performed her internship at the Rehabilitation Institute of Chicago. "That was a pretty intense place to work," Pam says. "I was offered a permanent job there, but I didn't want to specialize yet. So I went to a physical therapy job fair, and that's where I found out about Swedish Covenant. I also spoke to the people I was working with at RIC, and they recommended Swedish Covenant, too. So I applied for a position and was given an interview. They also let me come in and observe the physical therapy department, which was very helpful. I got to see what kind of atmosphere they had." Pam was lucky enough to have several job offers within a couple of weeks. "There still are jobs out there, but it's not as easy as it was, say, ten years ago. A friend of mine in San Francisco, for example, has had a horrible time of finding work."

Pam's choice of Swedish Covenant came because of the flexibility the hospital environment offered. "They have us on a rotating schedule. Every three months we're assigned to a different area of the hospital. Right now, for example, I'm assigned to the acute care unit, treating patients who are just out of surgery. It gives me exposure to the whole range of physical therapy, so I'll be able to choose a specialty later on. Working in a hospital also gives you a chance to move up to senior positions, something that isn't always available in other places. And here at Swedish Covenant, we have a very international staff. This gives me exposure to physical therapy techniques all over the world."

Gabor Sagi's career path has been different from Pam's. "My first jobs were as a contract PT in France. I'd fill in full-time for vacationing physical therapists who had their own private practices. After a year of that, I moved to Eng-

The Seven Specialties of Physical Therapy

Cardiopulmonary physical therapy is concerned with the heart and lungs.

Clinical electrophysiology physical therapy is concerned with the effects of electrical stimulation on the body.

Geriatrics physical therapy is concerned with elderly people.

Neurology physical therapy is concerned with the nervous system.

Orthopedics physical therapy is concerned with the skeleton.

Pediatrics physical therapy is concerned with children.

Sports physical therapy is concerned with athletics and exercising.

land, where I was self-employed. I worked on a part-time contract with a medical center, and another part-time contract with a hospital in the National Health System there." Gabor came to the United States after being offered his current position. "For a long time, there was a shortage of physical therapists in the States," Gabor says, "but that's changing."

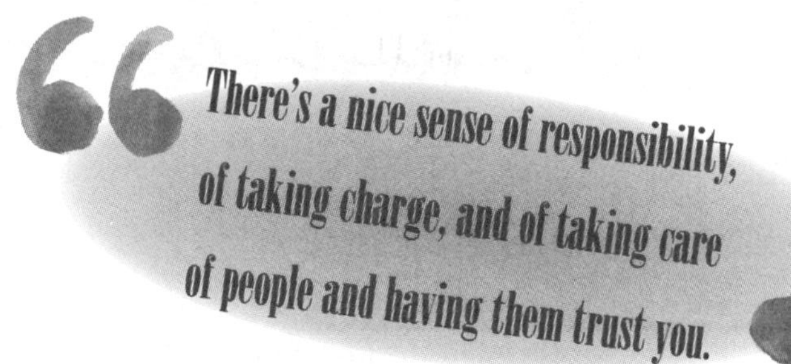

where can I go from here?

"Physical therapy is really a broad profession," Gabor says. "There are so many areas to specialize in. Right now, I tend to specialize in backs. But one day I could decide to move into a different area."

Gabor's interests include several areas. "I plan to go back to France eventually and start up my own private practice or a group practice with a couple of others. I also want to continue my interest in the spine and become more expert in that field. Then I'd like to teach others interested in that specialty." Gabor also plans to conduct clinical research; he is actively involved in studying a physical therapy technique called the McKenzie Approach. "I'm training to be an instructor now. Then I'll be bringing McKenzie to France," Gabor says.

For Pam Johnson, the future is still wide open. "I'm just starting out, so it's great that I get exposed to so many different areas of physical therapy," she says. "In the future, I might decide to get into aquatic therapy. Another area I'm interested in is working with spinal cord injuries. These patients tend to be pretty young. So the work I'd do would really have an impact on the rest of their lives."

Physical therapists with bachelor's degrees may consider earning master's degrees in order to achieve senior positions or become teachers. Some physical therapists go on to earn doctorate degrees in physical therapy and conduct research.

what are the salary ranges?

The average starting salaries for physical therapists range from $33,000 to $35,000 per year, although starting salaries for physical therapists working for the federal government are around $20,000. Average salaries for experienced physical therapists are around $42,000. Salaries vary according to location, setting, and position. Supervisory and administrative personnel earn more than the average, as do many physical therapists who operate their own private practices. The top 10 percent of physical therapists earned more than $62,000 per year.

what is the job outlook?

In the mid-1990s, there were an estimated 83,000 active physical therapists. Physical therapy has been one of the fastest growing health care professions. It is expected to grow by as much as 75 percent by 2005, though the number of persons entering the profession has also been increasing. Advances in surgical, medical, and therapeutic techniques have spurred the profession's growth. These techniques have enabled many people to overcome their disabilities, injuries, and illnesses. For example, babies born prematurely or with birth defects have a better chance of survival today than in previous times. These children often need physical therapy as they grow.

The aging of the population has also affected the growth of this career. More physical therapists are required to address the needs of the increasing number of elderly people. "Baby boomers," now in middle-age, will require more physical therapy as they develop the problems and injuries associated with getting older. The fitness boom has led more people into sports and other recreational activities, which have, in turn, led to an increase in sport-related injuries requiring physical therapy. The science of sports has increased rapidly, and more physical therapists specializing in advanced sport training techniques will be needed.

how do I learn more?

professional organizations

The following organization provides information on physical therapy careers, accredited schools, and employers.

American Physical Therapy Association
1111 North Fairfax Street
Alexandria, VA 22314
TEL: 800-999-2782
WEBSITE: http://www.apta.org

bibliography

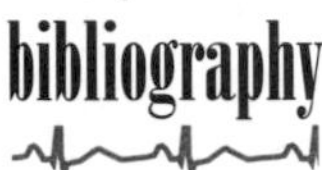

Following is a sampling of materials related to the professional concerns and development of physical therapists.

Books

Csengody, Patricia. *Essentials for Physical Therapists*. Thorofare, NJ: Slack, 1997.

Downer, Ann H. *Physical Therapy Procedures: Selected Techniques,* 5th edition. Springfield, IL: C.C. Thomas, 1996.

Hunter, Skip, and Lori Whitlow. *How to Become a Physical Therapist.* Alameda, CA: Hunter House, 1996.

Krumhansl, Bernice. *Opportunities in Physical Therapy Careers*. Lincolnwood, IL: VGM Career Horizons, 1994.

Miller, Mary, Lewis Baratz, and Jean Rosenbaum. *Opportunities in Fitness Careers,* 2nd edition. Lincolnwood, IL: VGM Career Horizons, 1997.

Perinigian, Lynda. *Physical and Occupational Therapists' Job Search Handbook: Your Complete Job Search Strategy: How to Hire; How to Be Hired.* Southfield, MI: Therapy Careers Press, 1989.

Shepard, Katherine F., and Gail M. Jensen. *Handbook of Teaching for Physical Therapists*. Newton, MA: Butterworth-Heinemann, 1997.

Sherman, Margie. *Your Opportunities as a Physical Therapist.* Salem, OR: Energeia, 1997.

Periodicals

NAPT Journal. Bimonthly. Provides reports on association news, legislation, courses, and articles of interest to members. National Association of Physical Therapists, Inc., 12602 Strathmore, Garden Grove, CA 92640, 818-332-7755.

Physical Therapy. Monthly. Features reports on clinical and testing procedures, research, educational programs, and professional philosophy. American Physical Therapy Association, 1111 North Fairfax Street, Alexandria, VA 22314, 703-684-2782.

Physical Therapy Forum. Weekly. Covers current research and development as well as reports on philosophical and ethical questions confronting those working in the field of physical therapy. Forum Publishing, Inc., 251 West Dekalb Pike, Suite A-115, King of Prussia, PA 19406, 215-337-0802.

Physical Therapy Progress Report. Monthly. Newsletter for association members containing general industry news and government reports. American Physical Therapy Association, 1111 North Fairfax Street, Alexandria, VA 22314, 703-684-2782.

Physical Therapy Today. Quarterly. Addresses business and clinical concerns of physical therapists in private practice. American Physical Therapy Association, Private Practice Section, 1111 N. Fairfax Street, Alexandria, VA 22314-1408, 703-684-2782.

PT Job News. Monthly. Newspaper providing job-related information for physical therapists. Prime National Publishing Corp., 470 Boston Post Road, Weston, MA 02193, 617-899-2702.

PT Magazine of Physical Therapy. Monthly. Addresses all areas of the physical therapy industry. American Physical Therapy Association, 1111 North Fairfax Street, Alexandria, VA 22314, 703-684-2782.

physical therapist assistant

Definition

Physical therapist assistants work under the supervision of physical therapists to improve the mobility and functionality of patients with injuries, illnesses, and other disabling conditions to restore them to an independent lifestyle and to improve their quality of life.

Alternative job titles

Physical therapy assistants
Physical therapy technicians

Salary range

$20,000 to $28,000

Educational requirements

High school diploma; associate's degree from an accredited two-year physical therapist assistant program

Certification or licensing

Required in most states

Outlook

Much faster than average

GOE
10.02.02

DOT
076

High School Subjects

English
Physical education
Biology
Physics

Personal Interests

Working with people
Dance or sports
Yoga
Relaxation techniques

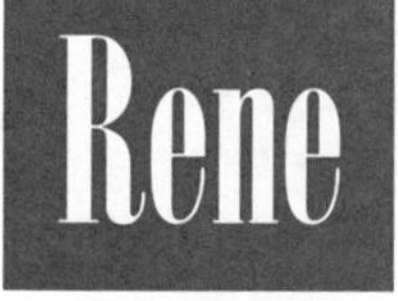

Freiwald waited in the hospital gymnasium for "Jim," her most difficult patient since she became a physical therapist assistant.

A month earlier, "Jim's" body had been so rigid he could barely move. Years of alcohol abuse had given him a condition more usually seen in elderly Parkinson's disease patients.

But "Jim" was only fifty years old.

"It's no use." Tears of frustration rimmed "Jim's" eyes. His jaw was so stiff he could hardly speak. "I won't get better. I'll never walk. The rest of my life I'll eat through a tube."

"Jim's" therapy called for stretching exercises to disassociate his joints and slowly counteract their stiffness. Briefed by his physicians, Rene knew that "Jim" was receiving medication to alleviate his rigidity.

But his depression remained an obstacle. He needed to believe in himself. That first day when "Jim" was wheeled into the gymnasium, Rene saw his pain, his hopelessness.

She had placed her hand in his. "We'll work together. We'll make you better. You'll see."

That was a month ago.

The door opens. Hallway light joins the sunlight from the gymnasium windows. Slowly, "Jim" walks unassisted into the room. He greets Rene with a smile.

what does a physical therapist assistant do?

Many diseases, injuries, and other medical conditions have a profound impact on the performance and mobility of the human body. For centuries, even in ancient times, forms of exercise, massage, and the use of heat and other techniques have been used to treat these conditions. Modern physical therapy has evolved to include not only the restoration of mobility and alleviation of pain and suffering as its goal, but also the prevention of permanent disability. Under the supervision and direction of a physical therapist, the *physical therapist assistant* works with patients to instruct and assist them in achieving the maximum functional performance of their bodies.

Injuries to the back, a common source of pain and immobility, often respond well to physical therapy. For some conditions, such as stroke, therapy may involve relearning such basic tasks as standing, eating, bathing, and walking. Other patients may be required to adapt to the permanent use of a wheelchair or an artificial limb. Patients with such severe impairments are often emotionally overwhelmed by these limitations of their bodies. A physical therapist assistant must also work with them to improve their state of mind. Ultimately, the goal of a physical therapist assistant is to help patients regain a maximum degree of independence.

As part of a team including the patient's physician, nurses, physical therapist, and, often, a psychologist and social worker, the physical therapist assistant participates in the evaluation of a patient's condition. An evaluation can include measuring the patient's strength, range of motion, and functional ability—that is, how well the patient performs certain physical tasks. If the patient is receiving medication, the physical therapist assistant considers such factors as the medication's side effects, its effect on the patient's condition, and the most appropriate times for therapy. Once the physical therapist has developed a treatment plan, it is the responsibility of the physical therapist assistant to carry out the therapy, to take notes on the patient's progress, and to report observations, particularly if he or she perceives that a patient is having severe difficulties or experiencing problems with his prescribed therapy. During complicated therapeutic procedures, the physical therapist assistant works along with the physical therapist; more routine procedures are usually carried out by the physical therapist assistant alone.

An important role of the physical therapist assistant is teaching patients the use of canes, walkers, crutches, or wheelchairs, and how to apply, remove, care for, and live with devices such as braces, or artificial limbs and joints. Many patients, especially geriatric (elderly)

lingo to learn

Disassociation Passive exercises, performed on the patient by the physical therapist or PTA, involving stretching parts of the body so as to loosen rigid or locked joints.

Quality of life In medicine, quality of life refers to the overall nature of a patient's physical and psychological well-being.

Traction A therapy involving specialized mechanical equipment. It is used to stretch, pull, or hold into position patients with fractures, other injuries, or muscle spasms, as a means to provide proper healing and relief of pain caused by physical pressure.

Ultrasound Refers to sound having a frequency greater than 30,000 Hz., which is beyond the range of human hearing. Ultrasound is commonly used in physical therapy as a means of relieving pain and swelling of joints and improving muscle condition.

Vestibular stimulation The vestibular nerve in the ear is related to the human sense of balance; some patients require therapy to stimulate and/or restore their sense of balance.

patients, need to learn how to climb stairs, or to transport themselves from bed or from a wheelchair to the shower or toilet. "Since the elderly are prone to falling," Rene says, "they need to learn how to get up again on their own. Many elderly don't know how to do that, and they end up lying where they fall until someone finds them. Part of my job is to teach them how to help themselves in these situations."

Improving the emotional and psychological condition of a patient is often a key element of their response to therapy. A physical therapist assistant plays a part in helping their patients overcome the feelings of hopelessness, loss, and fear that often accompany illness and disability.

In addition to these functions, a physical therapist assistant may also perform clerical duties, such as filling out reports, devising schedules, maintaining patient records, and coordinating inventory and supplies. A physical therapist assistant may also be responsible for coordinating the patient's treatment with the patient's insurance plans. "I have to know what will be covered and what won't," Rene says, "and I have to be able to justify the patient's progress. Insurance companies are not always as interested in whether, say, a patient can move his arm fifteen degrees. They want to know if they'll be able to move enough to reach a cupboard or climb the stairs to their home." Working with physicians and physical therapists, Rene helps to develop the best possible care within the patient's means.

what is it like to be a physical therapist assistant?

Rene has been a physical therapist assistant for three years. She works at Grant Hospital in Chicago, Illinois, where she is assigned to the skilled nursing facility. Rene, who is twenty-nine years old, came into this field after a career as a child care worker. "I like working with people," she says. "I like helping them. There's a lot of satisfaction at the end of a day."

The day begins for Rene at 8:00 AM. "But I prepare my schedule the night before. I know who I'll be seeing, what types of therapy I'll have to do." In the morning, Rene also consults with the physical therapists on evaluations of new patients, helping to develop the appropriate therapy. She then visits her patients, bringing them to the occupational therapy center of

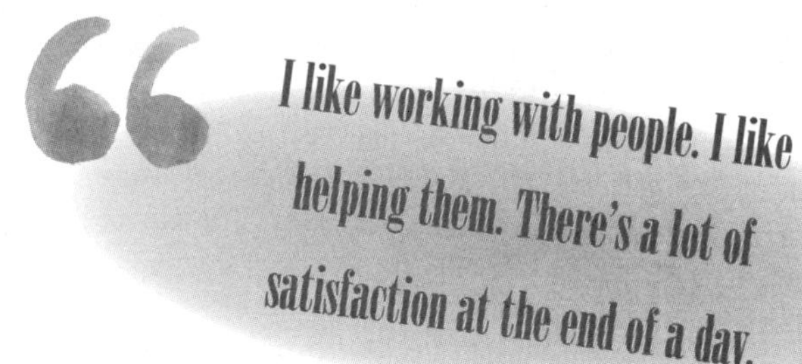

the hospital. "Some hospitals have transporters: people whose job it is to bring the patients to their therapy. But here that's part of my job too."

Patients are generally treated in half-hour sessions, although these may be flexible according to the patient's needs and abilities, and the fullness of the day's schedule. "Some days, I'll have a lot of patients to see. Other days are lighter, and I'll have more time for working with my patients, writing my notes, and reporting to the physical therapist and the patient's physician." This too is an important part of Rene's day. It is her responsibility to keep detailed records on each patient's progress and response to treatment.

Physical therapist assistants are trained in a variety of techniques and therapies. These may include the use of heat, cold, ultrasound, electricity, and water exercises to stimulate the patient's muscles, or to improve the mobility of their joints. Massage therapies, stretching and weight exercises, and traction may also be called for in a patient's treatment. Each patient's therapy is individually designed for that patient's particular needs. Combinations of therapies are usual, often including both active exercises, in which the patient performs various training and strength movements, and passive exercises, such as stretching, in which the physical therapist assistant moves the various parts of the patient's body to increase mobility and functionality.

Because Rene is assigned to the skilled nursing facility, she sees many geriatric patients. Elderly patients require special care, as many need help in adjusting to the limitations of age. Rene works with these patients to help them learn the proper use of walkers or canes, or to teach them techniques for activities that younger people take for granted, such as rising from a chair. Many elderly stroke victims, for example, will need to relearn how to walk, speak, and eat, and other routine daily activities. Other conditions, such as Parkinson's disease, heart disease, amputations, or injuries such as fractures, may require the patient to learn ways of accommodating new physical limitations. Part of Rene's work is to help her older patients to continue to lead active, independent lives. "I've learned a great respect for age," Rene says, "especially because I'll be old one day too. Respecting my patients is very important to me, and for them too."

During the day, Rene also prepares reports based on her observations of her patients. These reports are an important tool for the patients' physicians and physical therapists, allowing them to modify treatment to respond to each patient's immediate needs. Rene also meets with the hospital's psychiatric staff and social workers, giving them insight into each patients' emotional status, and alerting them to any special requirements patients may have upon returning to their homes. In some cases, Rene will also meet with the patients' families, in order to discuss with them any special needs the patient will have. Finally, Rene works with physicians and physical therapists to keep them aware of their patients' insurance requirements and limitations. She also participates in deciding when a patient is ready to be discharged from the hospital and allowed to go home.

have I got what it takes to be a physical therapist assistant?

A physical therapist assistant works with people who, whether because of injury, disease, or advancing age, are undergoing an extremely stressful time in their life. When a condition will not permit patients to regain full use of their bodies, the physical therapist assistant helps them to adjust to this, and to discover ways to become as self-sufficient as possible. "I never lie to my patients," Rene says. "I'm straightforward with them about what they can expect from therapy, and what they can't."

A physical therapist assistant is often responsible for many patients in a day. This requires him or her to be organized, efficient, and realistic about what can be accomplished. "Rene is very organized and self-motivated, and she's an excellent decision-maker," says Joseph Vibert, manager of physical therapy at Grant Hospital, and Rene's supervisor. "She knows the system very well, too. It's important that we have confidence in our assistants, since they often work the closest to our physical therapy patients."

A strong knowledge of all of the many therapy techniques is essential. And a physical therapist assistant must also have good observational skills in order to recognize what is and is not working for a patient. These observations must be communicated properly to the patient's physical therapist and physician. "I like it that Rene is not at all afraid to talk to the doctors," Joseph Vibert continues. "That's important, because she'll often be aware of things that they're not."

A physical therapist assistant is constantly challenged in his or her work. Not only does this career require a great deal of stamina and physical strength, but, because of the often slow healing process and the repetitive nature of many therapy techniques, the therapist assistant must have patience as well. The ability to communicate enthusiasm and encouragement is a great asset to the physical therapist assistant. "Often, patients are very depressed. And the hospital can be such a cold setting. That can be very difficult, for me too," Rene admits, "but I bring a lot of compassion to the people I work with. I try to put them at ease so that they can achieve the most possible benefit from their therapy. It's part of my job to help them gain a positive attitude. Because that way, they'll heal quicker too."

To be successful physical therapist assistant, you should

- Like to work with people and have an outgoing personality and strong communication skills
- Be patient, encouraging, and creative
- Have stamina, good physical dexterity and coordination, and enjoy physical activity
- Have good decision-making abilities, and be able to follow directions
- Be organized and self-motivated

how do I become a physical therapist assistant?

Physical therapist assistants must receive a degree from an accredited PTA program, available at many community and junior colleges, vocational schools, and universities. These programs usually last two years and combine academic instruction with a period of clinical practice, or "rotations," in which time the student may be exposed to a variety of physical therapy environments. During her clinical rotations, for example, Rene was assigned to the clinical nursing facility at Grant Hospital, and, after three months there, was offered a permanent position. "It was the right environment for me," Rene says.

education

High School

High school students interested in becoming a physical therapist assistant should take courses in biology, health, math, psychology and social science, and courses that will help them develop strong communication skills, such as English. Ability in using computers, writing, and having both physical dexterity and fitness will also be helpful. Some high schools offer class programs in health, which may combine preparation for specific job skills in the health and medical areas with practical work experience.

Volunteering at a local hospital is an excellent way to explore the hospital environment and to become familiar with aspects of this career. Working with children, the physically disabled, or the elderly is another way to prepare for a career as a physical therapist assistant. "I worked at a summer camp for disabled kids," Rene says, "so I already had an introduction to what I'm doing now."

Postsecondary Training

Students must attend an accredited physical therapist assistant program. The American Physical Therapy Association (APTA) sets the standards for accreditation and educational requirements for these programs.

Physical therapist assistant programs include courses in general education, anatomy, physiology, biology, the history and philosophy of rehabilitation, human growth and development, and psychology, as well as courses in mathematics and applied physical sciences, which will help give the student an understanding of the apparatus and the principals behind the therapeutic procedures they will use. Students will also receive training in the variety of physical therapy techniques, including massage, therapeutic exercise, and heat and cold therapy. During their clinical rotation period, students will apply the education, techniques, and skills they have learned in various hospital facility settings, under the supervision of senior physical therapist assistants and physical therapists.

certification or licensing

Upon graduation, most states require that a candidate pass a written examination administered by the state in order to become a licensed physical therapist assistant. The process for renewing the physical therapist assistant license also varies by state.

scholarships and grants

There are a variety of awards available to physical therapists and physical therapist assistants, offered through the APTA and other professional physical therapy organizations. Many of these awards are given in recognition of superior performance, or in order to support investigative and research efforts in the field of physical therapy. The APTA also offers the Mary McMillan Scholarship to students enrolled in physical therapist assistant programs accredited by the APTA. This award is for $1,000, and is given to outstanding students on a competitive basis.

internships and volunteerships

Students interested in becoming a physical therapist assistant can find summer and part-time jobs, or positions as volunteers in the physical therapy department of a hospital or clinic. This is particularly important because some schools require prospective students to have completed up to 150 hours of volunteer work in a hospital physical therapy clinic in order to be eligible for admission into a physical therapy assistant program. Many public and private schools may also accept volunteers to assist with their disabled student population. As Rene discussed, jobs at summer camps for disabled children are also an excellent experience for the prospective physical therapist assistant. Nursing home and other elderly facilities are another source for work experience and volunteerships. Such hands-on activities are helpful in exploring your abilities, and in determining whether you have the personal qualities needed for this career. As another way to gain more knowledge about this field, you can arrange to speak with physical therapists and physical therapist assistants at your high school's Career Day, or by contacting the physical therapy department at your local hospital or clinic.

Armed forces training programs, which generally do not offer degrees or meet state requirements for physical therapist assistant programs, nonetheless provide a good introduction to the field.

Speak to your high school guidance counselor for help in locating these and other opportunities for experience in and knowledge about this career.

who will hire me?

Physical therapist assistants are employed in a variety of settings. The school placement office is the best place for a graduating physical therapist assistant to find employment. Part of a school's reputation rests on how many of its graduates find work in their field. The placement office will be able to offer listings of available positions in the area and advice on the particular physical therapy environment. As with Rene, the clinical rotation segment of the PTA program is also a good path to a permanent job and allows prospective PTAs insight into the various settings for physical therapy. This is helpful in choosing the area of physical therapy that feels most right to them. PTAs can also apply for positions at local hospitals, rehabilitation centers, extended-care facilities, schools for physically and emotionally disabled children, nursing homes, and private physician and physical therapy offices. The classified ad section of newspapers and professional journals will also have announcements for jobs, as will public and private employment agencies.

PTAs work with a variety of patients. In an acute care hospital, the PTA may see patients with back problems, severe burns, forms of cancer and other debilitating diseases, and people involved in motorcycle and car accidents. In a rehabilitation facility, the PTA works even more closely with patients to restore them as fully as possible to an independent lifestyle. Rehabilitation therapy can be more intensive, focusing on adjusting the patient to a new disability, often helping the patient relearn the basic tasks of life. Therapy sessions in such a setting can last three hours or more, including occupational and speech therapy, as well as physical therapy techniques and exercises.

Home health therapy allows still more individual contact with the patient. The PTA visits the patient in his or her home, developing a personal relationship in a nonclinical setting; this also allows the PTA to assess the patient's abilities for performing real-life tasks, even simple chores like sweeping, doing the dishes, cleaning, or making the bed. The PTA will work with the patient to teach him or her different techniques for accomplishing these tasks safely. Many home health patients are elderly and often confined to their homes. The PTA forms an important link for these patients to the outside world.

Advancement Possibilities

Physical therapists plan and administer medically prescribed physical therapy treatment for patients suffering from injuries, or muscle, nerve, joint, and bone diseases, to restore function, relieve pain, and prevent disability.

Physiatrists are medical doctors who specialize in clinical and diagnostic use of physical agents and exercises to provide physiotherapy for physical, mental, and occupational rehabilitation of patients.

PTAs are also employed by many school districts to work with developmentally disabled children. For many of these children, therapy begins as early as the age of three and can continue until they are twenty-one years old. The PTA works with these children through play, concentrating on motor planning, vestibular stimulation, balance and coordination. The PTA will help children learn to walk, crawl, sit, or stand, and, through the years, help them achieve the most possible independence.

where can I go from here?

A physical therapist assistant's responsibilities may increase as his or her level of experience increases. Depending on the size of the facility at which one works, a physical therapist assistant may, at a larger facility, receive promotions to a supervisory position, or, in a smaller facility, gradually receive more and more responsibility for the coordination of the physical therapy office. As a physical therapist assistant develops greater experience and responsibilities, he or she may expect to receive corresponding raises in pay.

PTAs may also choose to advance by changing facilities, moving from a hospital setting to a home health setting, for example, or from the acute care facility to the outpatient unit of a physical therapy department. Each area of physical therapy brings its own challenges, and rewards.

Many PTAs return to school in order to become fully qualified physical therapists. Many universities and colleges offer bachelor's and master's level programs in physical therapy. Competition for placement in a physical therapy program is expected to remain keen; a physical therapist assistant with a degree from an accredited program, good grades, and strong work experience may find acceptance into a physical therapy program easier than those with no prior experience in this field. Some physical therapists and physical therapist assistants may find opportunities for conducting research into the effectiveness of physical therapy techniques, or participating in the development of new therapies. Still others may develop a desire to continue on into other health and medical careers.

Related jobs

A variety of professions work with the physically or mentally disabled to help them improve their quality of life. The U.S. Department of Labor classifies physical therapist assistants under the headings Therapists (DOT) and Nursing, Therapy, and Specialized Teaching Services: Therapy and Rehabilitation (GOE). Also listed under these headings are people who work as occupational therapists and occupational therapist assistants, orientation therapists for the blind, art therapists, corrective therapists, music therapists, dialysis technicians, recreational therapists, athletic trainers and physical education instructors, manual arts therapists, and radiology technologists.

what are the salary ranges?

Physical therapist assistant salaries vary according to type of facility, geographical location, the employer, and the PTA's level of experience. Recently graduated PTAs will typically receive salaries ranging from $20,000 to $23,000 per year. Experienced PTAs can earn between $21,000 and $28,000 per year. Benefits will also vary, but usually include paid holidays and vacations, health insurance, and pension plans.

what is the job outlook?

The outlook for job growth in physical therapy is expected to be very good into the next century. Demand for physical therapist assistants will likely outpace the average growth for all occupations, and the high turnover rate within the profession will mean a continual need for new physical therapist assistants.

The high growth of jobs in this field is attributable to a variety of factors. As medical technology advances, more patients will be saved and will be in need of physical therapy. New abilities to treat disabling conditions will also provoke more demand for PTAs to work with these patients. Also, as the population continues to age, and as more and more people survive into advanced age, the numbers of elderly with chronic and debilitating conditions will also increase and will require physical therapy. The large baby boomer generation is also aging; as more and more fall victim to heart attacks and strokes and other conditions of age, they too will increase the demand for physical therapists and physical therapist assistants. The technologies that also permit more infants and young children to survive severe birth defects are also a factor in the forecast for strong growth in jobs in the field.

An additional factor in the growth of the number of jobs for physical therapist assistants is the need for containing the rise of medical costs: many hospitals will look for physical therapist assistants to fill out their physical therapy staff, rather than increasing the number of higher-paid physical therapists.

how do I learn more?

professional organizations

Following are organizations that provide information on physical therapist assistant careers, accredited schools, and employers.

American Physical Therapy Association
1111 North Fairfax Street
Alexandria, VA 22314
TEL: 800-999-2782
WEBSITE: http://www.apta.org

Orthopaedic Section, American Physical Therapy Association
505 King Street, Suite 103
La Crosse, WI 54601
TEL: 608-784-0910

bibliography

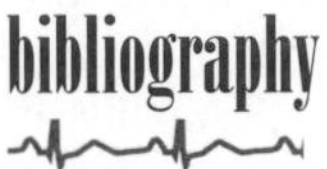

Following is a sampling of materials relating to the professional concerns and development of physical therapist assistants.

Books

Brister, Shirley J. *Mosby's Comprehensive Physical Therapist Assistant Board Review.* St. Louis, MO: Mosby, 1995.

Krumhansl, Bernice. *Opportunities in Physical Therapy Careers.* Lincolnwood, IL: VGM Career Horizons, 1994.

Luken, Marianne. *Documentation for Physical Therapist Assistants.* Philadelphia, PA: F.A. Davis, 1996.

Minor, Mary A., Lynn Lippert, and Scott D. Minor. *Kinesiology Laboratory Manual for Physical Therapist Assistants.* Philadelphia, PA: F.A. Davis, 1997.

Ratliffe, Thomas. *Pediatric Physical Therapy for the Physical Therapist Assistant.* St. Louis, MO: Mosby, 1997.

Shankman, Gary. *Fundamental Orthopaedic Management for the Physical Therapist Assistant.* St. Louis, MO: Mosby, 1996.

Weiss, Roberts C. *The Physical Therapy Aide: a Worktext.* Albany, NY: Delmar Publishers, 1993.

Weiss, Roberta C. *Your Career as a Physical Therapy Aide.* Albany, NY: Delmar Publishers, 1993.

Periodicals

PT Magazine of Physical Therapy. Monthly. Addresses all areas of the physical therapy industry. American Physical Therapy Association, 1111 North Fairfax Street Alexandria, VA 22314, 703-684-2782.

physician assistant

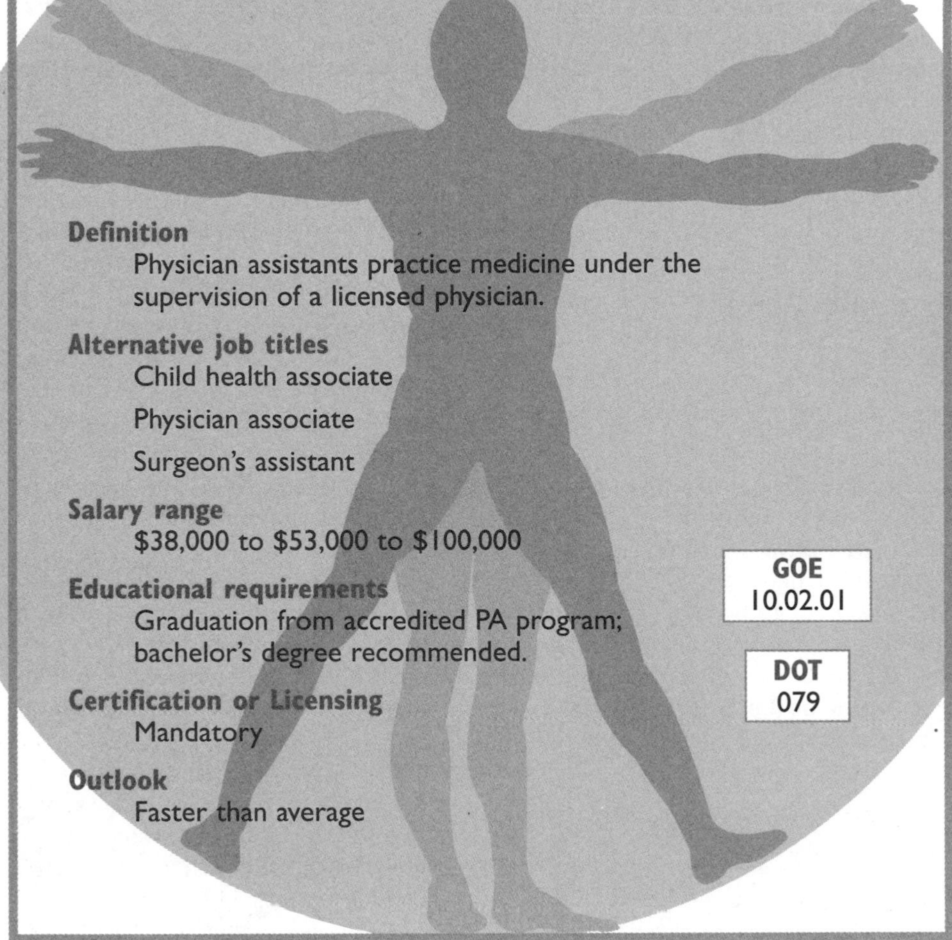

Definition
Physician assistants practice medicine under the supervision of a licensed physician.

Alternative job titles
Child health associate
Physician associate
Surgeon's assistant

Salary range
$38,000 to $53,000 to $100,000

Educational requirements
Graduation from accredited PA program; bachelor's degree recommended.

Certification or Licensing
Mandatory

Outlook
Faster than average

GOE
10.02.01

DOT
079

High School Subjects

Biology
English
Chemistry
Math

Personal Interests

Health care
Working with people
Hospital volunteer work

As soon as she arrives at the hospital, Mary Murray checks the list of patients she will see that day. As a physician assistant, she will spend time with each one, taking the patient's medical history, doing a physical exam, listening to each patient's medical problem. Then, she will order any necessary tests, make a diagnosis, and prepare a treatment plan.

If she has any questions about a patient's medical problem, she will discuss them with her supervising physician. "Physician assistants see patients on their own, but the supervising physician is available in case there is any question about a diagnosis," Mary said. If the supervising physician is not on the premises, questions may be resolved by phone. For instance, a patient with a questionable rash may show up. If Mary is not sure how to treat it, a quick phone call will resolve her questions.

Mary likes working with people. She enjoys the challenge each day brings with new patients to diagnose and help to feel better. She sees patients with any number of medical problems, from lacerations to abrasions to burns to high blood pressure. She says she does not treat as many patients as a physician does, and she cannot work completely independent of a physician. Mary spends some of her time counseling patients and discussing preventive health care with them. When she was in the physician assistant program, her goal was to work in a family practice clinic. She has achieved her goal by working in a hospital family practice/urgent care setting.

what does a physician assistant do?

Physician assistants, or PAs, are licensed health professionals who practice medicine under the supervision of a physician. They provide some of the skilled patient care usually done by physicians, allowing the physicians to spend their time on more serious medical care. Much of the patient care physician assistants provide used to be limited to physicians. The profession was started in the 1960s to relieve a physician shortage in some areas of the country and to improve access to high-quality care. The first physician assistant program began at Duke University in North Carolina with a class of four military corpsmen.

Physician assistants practice as part of a team, always under the supervision of a licensed doctor of medicine or osteopathy. Physician assistants perform many essential but time-consuming tasks. They are educated to recognize when patients need the attention of a supervising physician or another specialist. They provide a wide variety of routine diagnostic, therapeutic, and preventive health care services. They take medical histories, examine patients, order and interpret laboratory diagnostic tests and X rays, diagnose common illnesses and disorders, develop treatment plans, provide counseling, manage infections, and treat minor problems, such as burns and abrasions. They suture wounds and set simple fractures. They prescribe medications in most states. Some physician assistants perform surgical procedures. They may also perform managerial duties, and some supervise technicians and assistants.

Physician assistants are also trained to provide medical emergency care. They deal with such emergencies as severe drug reactions, heart attacks, psychiatric crises, or uncomplicated deliveries until a physician becomes available.

The type of tasks they handle depend on their education, experience, state laws, and the type of practice they are in. In some states, the state regulatory agency determines what duties they may perform; in others, the supervising physician does. Physician assistants have to know the laws and regulations in the state in which they practice. Not being independent practitioners, physician assistants do not work in solo practice, though they do many of the same things that physicians do. They are like physicians in many ways, but they are not physicians.

"The practice lends itself to what the physician feels comfortable letting the physician assistant do," explained Mary. "For example, I haven't had much experience in splinting and casting, so a supervising physician is not likely to give me this type of work. Instead, the physician will give this duty to a physician assistant who has this type of experience, perhaps someone who has worked in orthopedics."

In supporting physicians, physician assistants help cut waiting time for patients and spend more time examining patients and

lingo to learn

Ambulatory care centers Doctor's offices, clinics, hospitals, or other "walk-in" health care facilities that provide medical care.

Chart A collection of written materials relating to the health care of a patient.

Clinical rotation Supervised clinical training in family medicine, emergency medicine, pediatrics, surgery, and other areas.

Family practice An area of medicine that provides general health care to patients of all ages.

Primary care A specialty that includes family practice, internal medicine, pediatric care, and ob/gyn.

answering their questions than physicians usually do. They also help relieve the physician shortage in rural areas where access to health care is a problem. Physician assistants working in rural or inner-city clinics may provide most of the patient care there and consult with the supervising physician by telephone, as needed and as required by law. A physician may be available in a clinic only one or two days a week. Or physician assistants may work in a satellite clinic that has no physician on site. In that case, they use telecommunications to maintain contact with the supervising physician. Physician assistants may also visit patients in their home or in hospitals and nursing homes, again consulting with the supervising physician.

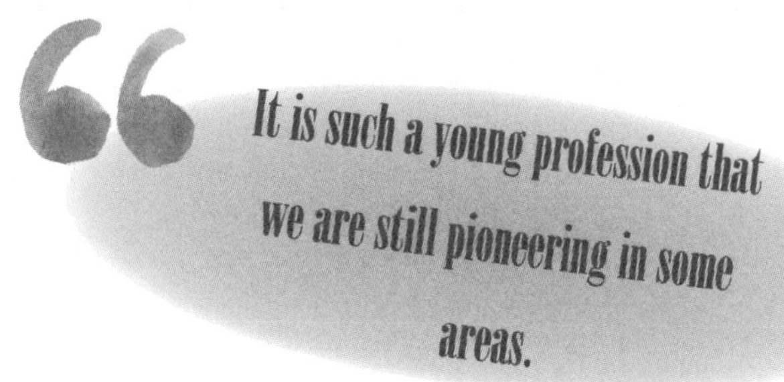

In hospitals, physician assistants' duties include making patient rounds, recording patient data in charts, counseling patients, interpreting test results, and offering treatment.

Most physician assistants work in primary care areas such as internal medicine, family medicine, and pediatrics. Increasing numbers work in surgery. They also work in specialized areas such as obstetrics/gynecology, emergency medicine, occupational medicine, psychiatry, orthopedics, and geriatrics.

what is it like to be a physician assistant?

Mary Murray has been a physician assistant for ten years, working mainly in a family practice clinic and in family practice/urgent care in hospitals. After she graduated from high school, she went to college and received a bachelor's degree in nursing. After working as a nurse, she decided she wanted to do more in patient care, but she did not want to make the time commitment required to attend medical school and practice as a physician.

"Becoming a physician assistant seemed to be the answer," Mary said. "It allowed me to learn more and become more involved with patient care. I'm happy with it."

Physician assistants work in a wide variety of health care settings. They may work in physicians' offices or medical group practices, hospitals, clinics, nursing homes, long-term care facilities, prisons, and rehabilitation facilities. Often, physician assistants have to stand for long periods, especially those who work in surgery, and they may do a lot of walking. They usually work in comfortable, well-lighted environments and deal directly with patients. On the downside, they may be exposed to infectious diseases. Their hours vary, depending on the setting, duties, and medical practice. Physician assistants who work in hospital emergency departments may work long shifts, such as twenty-four-hour shifts twice a week or twelve-hour shifts three times a week. Those who work in physicians' offices, group practices, or hospitals may have to work weekends, nights, and holidays. They may be on-call. Physician assistants employed in clinics generally work forty-hour, five-day weeks. They may wear lab jackets or operating room scrubs.

"You can choose the type of setting you want to work in," Mary said. "The type of setting you're in, determines the hours you work. You will work longer hours in a hospital or in obstetrics/gynecology."

A few years ago, Mary added teaching to her professional duties. She now teaches in the physician assistant program at Midwestern University in Downers Grove, Illinois. Initially, Mary was an adjunct instructor for a couple of years, teaching part-time. She has been a full-time clinical instructor there for a year and a half. She teaches medical Spanish to those who plan to practice with a Spanish-speaking population. In addition, she still works part-time as a physician assistant in family practice/urgent care at MacNeal Hospital in Berwyn, Illinois, and in urgent care one day a week in the emergency depart of another hospital. The patients she treats are not as seriously ill as those seen by physicians.

"As faculty, we are trying to keep our clinical skills as up to date as possible, so we can keep abreast of medical advances in order to teach them," Mary said of her dual roles as both teacher and practitioner. "It adds credibility when you are practicing and keeping up on changes in the medical field so you can keep teaching students about current topics, such as AIDS."

The amount of supervision that physician assistants have is up to the supervising physician. Some physician assistants work in clinics where a physician is not present, so supervision has to be via telecommunications. Supervision is greatest for practitioners who are recent graduates, Mary explained. "As soon as you graduate and are certified, you can practice," she said. "The supervising physician is available to answer questions or deal with issues that you do not feel prepared for."

With experience, the physician assistants practice more independently, but we are not independent practitioners. We could never hang up our shingle and practice by ourselves. Supervising physicians are there to lend us assistance and share the experience and knowledge they get through medical school and residency."

have I got what it takes to be a physician assistant?

Because they deal directly with patients, physician assistants must enjoy working with people and must be able to relate to people effectively. They need good communication skills, so they can inform and motivate patients at a level that the patients will understand. They have to demonstrate self-confidence and good judgment. They also need to be conscientious and patient, always treating people tactfully and respecting their confidentiality. They have to be able to respond to emergencies calmly and be able to make decisions quickly. Of course, they must also be interested in health care and science.

"People skills, interpersonal skills are necessary. Communication skills are vital. You also have to like working with people," Mary said. She added that "shadowing" is encouraged for those interested in a physician assistant career. That is, people who think they would like to work as a physician assistant are often advised to spend some time with one so they will see what the job involves and find out if they would really like doing that, she explained. In this way, they can determine whether they have an interest in this type of work.

Mary enjoys the challenge and satisfaction in helping others that being a physician assistant brings her. "When you see a patient and take the history, and do the physical exam, you have to come up with a diagnosis and make them feel better," she said. "I think the appeal I find in the profession is in the education of patients, in helping them understand why you are doing what you are doing."

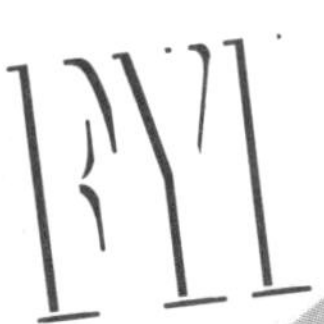

There were 78 programs accredited to train physician assistants in 1997. The average program lasts 108 weeks.

how do I become a physician assistant?

Most states require physician assistants to complete course work in an accredited educational program. In 1996, there were more than seventy accredited programs throughout the United States. When they finish the program, physician assistants receive a certificate of completion or an associate's, bachelor's, or master's degree, depending on which type of school they attended. Most of the programs offer a bachelor's degree. All states require physician assistants to be certified by the National Commission on Certification of Physician Assistants. Only physician assistants with current certification may use the designation Physician Assistant-Certified (PA-C). Most states also require physician assistants to register with the state medical board.

education

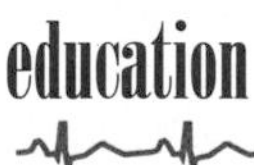

Physician assistants perform many types of patient care:

- Examine patients
- Take medical histories
- Order and interpret laboratory tests
- Order X rays
- Diagnose common illnesses
- Treat minor injuries
- Promote disease prevention

High School

While in high school students should take college prep courses. Biology, chemistry, and physics are important science classes. English and speech classes can help develop communication skills. If possible, students should find part-time or volunteer work in a hospital, nursing home, or clinic.

Postsecondary Training

Most physician assistants educational programs are affiliated with two- and four-year college and university schools of medicine and allied health. Some are offered in hospitals; others in the armed forces. Most of the programs require two years of college and some work experience in the health care field for admission. More than half of the applicants already hold a bachelor's or master's degree. Prerequisite courses for admission usually are English, biology, chemistry, math, psychology, and social sciences. Most of the physician assistant programs last two years. Many applicants have studied and worked in the health care field, usually as registered nurses, medical technologists, or other allied health professionals. Competition for admission to physician assistant programs is intense. "At Midwestern University, we have 1,300 applicants for ninety positions," Mary said.

Midwestern University, where Mary teaches, offers a two-year physician assistant program. "Most of the PA programs are eighteen to twenty-four months in length," she said. "It is a rigorous, very intense twenty-four months. The programs are scheduled twenty-four months straight. Students do not get a summer break. Working full-time while going to school is out of the question. Working part-time is difficult." Those planning to enter the program should make any financial arrangements in advance, such as applying for grants, scholarships, or loans.

The educational program includes classroom instruction and clinical training. The classroom instruction, which usually lasts from six to twenty-four months, includes biochemistry, human anatomy, physiology, pharmacology, microbiology, physiology, medical ethics, pathology, clinical laboratory, and health promotion. Mary likened the program to a "mini medical school." "It is almost like taking medical school in one year. Students take sixty some credit hours the first year," she said. "There are courses in neuroscience, introduction to clinical medicine, agricultural medicine, and corrective medicine."

The supervised clinical work, which lasts nine to fifteen months, includes training (called clinical rotations) in areas such as family medicine, internal medicine, emergency medicine, pediatrics, geriatric medicine, obstetrics/gynecology, surgery, orthopedics, psychiatry, radiology, and general surgery. Students take these clinical rotations in private medical practices or hospitals, and many students receive a job offer from the supervising physician they worked under during a rotation.

Four-year programs generally include liberal arts courses with the biological and behavioral sciences.

Postgraduate residency training programs, which are not accredited, are available in gynecology, geriatrics, surgery, pediatrics, neonatology, and occupational medicine. Candidates must have graduated from an accredited program and be certified by the National Commission on Certification of Physician Assistants.

"The field has become so competitive that having a background and experience in health care will help those applying to physician assistant programs," Mary said. "Science-oriented classes will help as will anything they can do to expose themselves to health care careers, such as volunteering at a hospital."

certification or licensing

State laws and regulations control the scope of the physician assistant's duties. Before they can practice, physician assistants must complete an accredited training program and take a national certifying examination developed by the National Board of Medical Examiners and administered by the National Commission on Certification of Physician Assistants. "After I graduated, I had to wait a month and a half to sit for the boards," Mary said.

Certification is required for licensing, and all states require PAs to be licensed. They can then start working under the supervision of a licensed physician. They do not have to serve a residency, as physicians do. Physician assistants are required to complete one hundred hours of continuing medical education every two years and pass a recertifying examination every six years. Recertification ensures that physician assistants keep up with medical advances.

Mary said the continuing education requirement can be met by attending conferences and seminars and reading professional journals. She belongs to the American Academy of Physician Assistants and the Illinois chapter of the AAPA. Through these organizations, she receives professional journals to help her meet the continuing education requirement. These organizations also sponsor continuing education seminars.

scholarships and grants

Scholarships and grants are often available from individual institutions, state agencies, and special-interest organizations. The book *Dollars for College: Nursing and Other Health Fields* by Ferguson Publishing Company is an excellent source for this information. Many students finance their medical education through the Armed Forces Health Professions Scholarship Program. Each branch of the military participates in this program, paying students' tuitions in exchange for military service. Contact your local recruiting office for more information on this program. Another source for financial aid, scholarship, and grant information is the Association of American Medical Colleges. Remember to request information early for eligibility, application requirements, and deadlines.

Employment of Physician Assistants by Speciality

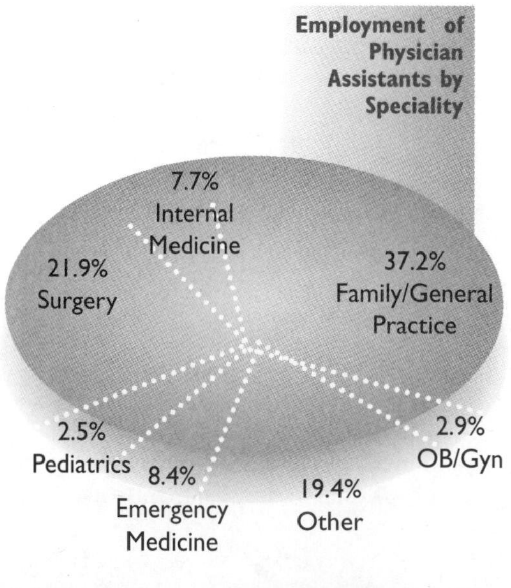

7.7% Internal Medicine
21.9% Surgery
37.2% Family/General Practice
2.5% Pediatrics
8.4% Emergency Medicine
19.4% Other
2.9% OB/Gyn

Association of American Medical Colleges
2450 N Street, NW
Washington, DC 20037
TEL: 202-828-0400
WEBSITE: http://www.aamc.org
Specific information on financial aid programs can be found at:
WEBSITE: http://www.aamc.org/stuapps/finaid

Ferguson Publishing Company
200 West Madison, Suite 300
Chicago, IL 60606
TEL: 312-580-5480

National Health Services Corps Scholarship Program
U.S. Public Health Service
1010 Wayne Avenue, Suite 240
Silver Spring, MD 20910
TEL: 800-638-0824

who will hire me?

Working in a family practice clinic was Mary Murray 's goal when she was in school. The first job she landed right out of school, however, was working in open-heart surgery in a hospital. That setting was more technical than most. It was focused on spending time in the operating room, she said, rather than on preoperative and post-operative care. After nine months, she moved into an internal medicine practice at a health maintenance organization for a couple years. She also worked in a family practice clinic full time. Currently, she teaches in a physician assistant program and practices in hospital settings.

Many students get job offers as a result of their clinical rotations, but additional job placement resources are available. Most schools have placement offices that offer their students information about job openings.

Because they were required to have work experience in the health care field when they applied to the training program, physician assistants can contact their former employers for information about job availability. In addition, many schools sponsor job fairs for physician assistants.

"Recruitment is phenomenal as the profession grows," Mary commented.

Physician assistants work in a variety of settings. Historically, they have worked in areas where there is a shortage of physicians and residents lacked access to high-quality health care. They work in major cities as well as rural areas in most health care settings. More than half work in medical offices, but many others work in hospitals, academic medical centers, public clinics, nursing homes, and health maintenance organizations. Nationally, women comprise about 40 percent of physician assistant positions.

The federal government employs physician assistants in the military, Veterans hospitals, prisons, the Public Health Service, and other agencies.

One value in belonging to professional organizations, Mary pointed out, is that in addition to the continuing education that is available through them, members also network with colleagues in the field. "Networking is very important in such a fast-growing profession," she said. Professional organizations enable members to learn what their colleagues are doing, what advances are occurring in various types of work settings, and where jobs are available. Some trade publications contain job listings.

where can I go from here?

"I'm very clinically minded, so I do not plan to move into management," Mary said. "I enjoy providing patient care. However, opportunities exist for physician assistants who are interested in moving into management positions. Their health care skills are an asset. Clinical areas need managers with a health care background to perform managerial duties. Also, employers who are increasing their physician assistant staffs will need coordinators and supervisors for those staffs. Physician assistants can move into these positions."

The physician assistant profession is still relatively young, and there are no formal lines of advancement yet. Physician assistants can find some career advancement by taking on greater responsibility with higher salary, completing graduate study and practicing in a specialty, or moving to a larger hospital or clinic. Some physician assistants join a private partnership practice. Others teach in a program for physician assistants or administrators in hospitals or clinics.

what are the salary ranges?

Salaries vary by employer, amount and type of training, experience, geographical location, and specialty. A University of Texas Medical Branch survey of hospitals and medical centers showed a median annual salary of $48,264 in 1994 for physician assistants working a forty-hour week. The average minimum salary was $37,639, while the average maximum salary was $57,005.

Physician assistants working in hospitals and medical offices earn more than those in clinics. According to the American Academy of Physician Assistants, the median annual income for all physician assistants in 1994 was $53,284. Median income for first-year graduates was $44,176 a year. Physician assistants working for the federal government are paid slightly less. Some physician assistants report earning $100,000 or more.

what is the job outlook?

Employment of physician assistants is expected to grow faster than the average for all occupations through the year 2005. Demand far outpaces supply. Employment opportunities are expected to be excellent, especially in locations where physician shortages exist. As physician assistants take on greater responsibilities and move into diverse work settings, they are being increasingly recognized as providers of high-quality patient care. Health care organizations are being restructured for cost economies, and the restructuring of health services is expected to bring standardized regulations for physician assistants. The continued growth of the profession depends on their acceptance by physicians.

"The profession is growing by leaps and bounds," Mary said. "Nationally, there are six jobs for every physician assistant. The field is very competitive."Anticipated job growth is based on expected expansion of the health services field and an emphasis on controlling costs. As managed care grows, employers, physicians, and health care institutions continue to look for ways to keep health care costs down. Employing physician assistants helps because they perform essential but time-consuming patient care services, freeing physicians to perform more complicated, revenue-generating activities. physician assistants meet the needs of patients in a variety of medical settings and are cost-effective.

"Everyone has to go to the doctor sometime. Seeing patients gives physician assistants an opportunity to let people know what they do and helps increase the visibility and acceptance of the profession. Physician assistants can get the message out that way," Mary said. "The more educating we do, the more aware people will be of what we can do. We should try to get as much correct information out there as we can. It is such a young profession that we are still pioneering in some areas."

Insurance companies are increasingly paying for the use of physician assistants, and the public's acceptance of them is growing. Medicare now lets physicians bill the government for services provided by physician assistants in hospitals and nursing homes. The best job opportunities for physician assistants will be in states where they have a wider scope of practice, such as prescribing medications.

how do I learn more?

professional organizations

Following are organizations that provide information on physician assistant careers and accredited schools.

American Academy of Physician Assistants
950 North Washington Street
Alexandria, VA 22314
TEL: 703-836-2272
WEBSITE: http://www.aapa.org/gandp

Association of Physician Assistant Programs
950 North Washington Street
Alexandria, VA 22314
TEL: 703-548-5538
WEBSITE: http://www.apap.org

National Commission on Certification of Physician Assistants, Inc.
6849-B2 Peachtree Dunwoody Road
Atlanta, GA 30328
TEL: 770-399-9971

bibliography

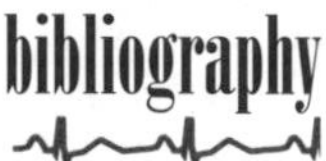

Following is a sampling of materials relating to the professional concerns and development of physician assistants.

Books

Labus, James. B. *The Physician Assistant Surgical Handbook.* Philadelphia, PA: W.B. Saunders Co., 1997.

Sacks, Terence J. *Opportunities in Physician Assistant Careers.* Lincolnwood, IL: VGM Career Horizons, 1995.

Periodicals

A A P A News. Biweekly. Newsletter. News on physician assistant programs, AAPA's activities, and employment information and opportunities. American Association of Physician Assistants, 950 W. Washington Street, Alexandria, VA 22314, 703-836-2272.

American Academy of Physician Assistants Journal. 10 per year. Focuses on the clinical conditions seen in the primary care and specialty settings where physician assistants practice. Medical Economics Publishing Co., Inc., Five Paragon Drive, Montvale, NJ 07645, 201-358-7200.

physiologist

Definition

Scientists who conduct research on living organisms to understand their systems and determine the effects that stress and environmental changes can have on the organisms.

Salary range

$16,300 to $37,900 to $67,000

Educational requirements

Doctorate for medical physiologists; Master's recommended for exercise physiologists

Certification or Licensing

Recommended for exercise physiologist

Outlook

Faster than average

GOE
02.02.03*

DOT
041*

*Shown are the U.S. Department of Labor classifications for medical physiologists. The classifications for exercise physiologists are: GOE: 10.02.02; DOT: 076

High School Subjects

Biology
Chemistry
Health/Nutrition
Physical Education
Physics

Personal Interests

Athletics
Helping others
Laboratory work
Physical fitness
Research
Teaching

His doctors told him to use a cane but he refused. John was a proud man, and he wanted to remain independent, but he had become frail and was having trouble keeping his balance when he walked.

"I'm going to get stronger," said John determinably to his exercise physiologist, Fred Kronk. So, Fred began working with him two to three times a week, designing and monitoring his exercise regimen. After several months he saw John progress from not being able to walk more than a tenth of a mile to walking a full mile. Regaining his independence made John proud, "I can make it around myself. I can make it to the bus. I can make it to work." Watching John recover also made Fred proud. "When I see something like that, I think I was a tool that came into play to help him do that. And when I see something like that happen, I know that everything is going right in my life."

what does a physiologist do?

Physiologists study the bodily systems of living organisms, especially how stress and environmental changes affect them. They try to understand how these systems work, how they might work better, and how they are related to things around them.

lingo to learn

Aerobic exercise A form of exercise that promotes cardiovascular fitness. An aerobic exercise sustains activity long enough to require the cardiovascular system to fuel muscles with oxygen. Aerobic exercises including running, bicycling, and cross-country skiing.

Anaerobic exercise A form of exercise in which the muscles are able to provide energy through a chemical process that does not involve oxygen. These exercises are usually used to build strength. Weightlifting is a form of anaerobic exercise.

Electron microscope A microscope that uses beams of electrons to scan cell surfaces. The final image is viewed on a monitor or photographic plate.

Magnetic resonance imaging (MRI) A medical imaging device that uses magnetic fields to produce images of internal organs.

Oscilloscope An electronic instrument that graphically displays an electrical signal as a glowing line on a fluorescent screen. The pattern on the screen is actually a rapidly moving point of light.

Target heart rate (THR) The ideal pulse rate to strive for during aerobic exercise. The rate varies according to age and is generally between 70 and 85 percent of your maximum heart rate. One method of calculating your maximum heart rate is by subtracting your age from 220.

There are two general types of physiologists that are closely associated with health care: medical physiologists and exercise physiologists. This chapter discusses both.

Medical physiologists conduct research with the aim of increasing scientific knowledge about the functions of the human body. A medical physiologist may often study the systems of other animals and plants with the ultimate aim of applying this knowledge to humans. For instance, a medical physiologist may study the cardiovascular system of a baboon to answer questions pertaining to heart disease in humans. Medical physiologists are subdivided into many specialties, most of which deal with a specific bodily system (e.g. respiratory, endocrine, neurological, and circulatory) or a specific anatomic level (cellular or molecular).

In an experiment at Northwestern University's Medical School, in Chicago, Professor Don McCrimmon is trying to determine how the brain controls an animal's breathing. "I work on neuro-control breathing. So we look at mechanisms for generating basic respiratory movement, the way the brain does that. We look at mechanisms that the body has for controlling breathing so we have to adjust breathing as we change our level of activity. . . . How does all of that happen? It turns out it looks like some of the interesting aspects of the control in much of the way we breath during exercise appears to be actually a learned response."

Research consumes a large portion of the careers of medical physiologists. It is difficult to determine the expected length of an experiment because the findings of one experiment may lead to many subprojects. In fact, an experiment may last from a few months to several years before it is completed. The number of projects being conducted in a particular laboratory can vary greatly as well.

Currently, Dr. McCrimmon has a staff of four assisting him with his experiments. In addition to his research, Dr. McCrimmon also teaches physiology to students from the medical school, dental school, and students studying physical therapy.

The responsibilities of *exercise physiologists* vary greatly depending on their place of employment. When working in a clinical setting, exercise physiologists will conduct research on both human and animal subjects to measure their physical responses before, during, and after exercise. When working in a non-clinical setting, such as a health club or a Y, exercise physiologists will work with their clients to develop exercise programs that help their clients stay physically fit.

During his initial interview with new members, Fred Kronk, an exercise physiologist at Gold Coast Multiplex, in Chicago, will try to develop a clear understanding of their fitness goals, as well as learn their medical history and vital statistics. "If somebody comes in and says, 'Oh, I just want to tone up' well . . . that means a lot of different things to a lot of different people. So I need to really dive down and find out. What's your background like, outside your medical history? Do you like exercise? Do you like fitness? Does it work for you?"

If necessary, exercise physiologists will work with their client's physicians to devise a program that is best for each client. For example, when people join Fred's club they are required to complete a physical activity readiness questionnaire. With the answers from the questionnaire, exercise physiologists will learn if members have any health problems that may pose a potential risk when they exercise. In some cases, Fred will ask members to get permission from their doctors before they can begin their programs. Fred will also contact the physician's office notifying the doctor that their patient has joined the club and inquire if there are any restrictions that the physician would advise.

In addition, as Director of Health and Fitness, Fred is responsible for ensuring that all the equipment on the floor is well maintained and that members are receiving adequate instructions on use of the equipment. His responsibilities also include: supervising any athletic leagues, such as volleyball or softball, that may be organized by the club; managing group exercise classes; and acting as a personal trainer for clients requesting one-on-one biomechanical analysis of their exercise routines.

The responsibilities for exercise physiologists working in a clinical setting are somewhat different. They generally work under a physician's supervision. They may be required to do a great deal of stress testing—a test that measures a patient's heart activity while running on a treadmill. They study the amount of fat in the body, analyze the patient's blood for cholesterol, and update the patient's charts.

Because the health club is a non-clinical setting, fitness testing is not as extensive. "We do things like measure their resting heart rate and blood pressure. We look at their upper body strength, their endurance levels. How many sit-ups can they do? We estimate their oxygen consumption. . . . It's a good indicator of general health and that we can do without a physician present."

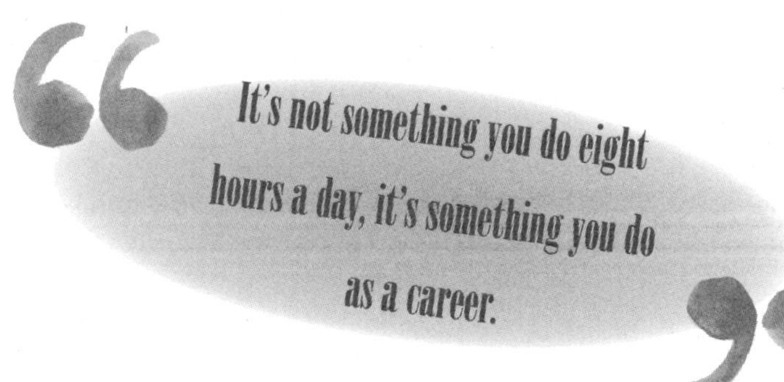

what is it like to be a physiologist?

Medical physiology generally involves work in a laboratory, including those in hospitals, universities, government agencies, and private industry. Some medical physiologists may venture outside the confines of the laboratory to pursue their research "in the field." In other words, they will work in the natural habitat of the subjects they are studying.

For a medical physiologist working at a university, there are rarely two days in a row that are the same. Professor McCrimmon's typical day includes a fair bit of juggling of responsibilities. In the morning he may begin an experiment that will run from eight to ten hours. However, with the assistance of his research associate, who will perform a great deal of the basic preparations, Dr. McCrimmon will be able to focus on his teaching responsibilities, as well as any administrative work that he may need to complete.

Dr. McCrimmon finds the research and teaching very rewarding. The research is rewarding because it gives him an opportunity to satisfy his natural curiosity and advance scientific understanding. He sees teaching as an added benefit, ". . . students with a scientific curiosity in particular are fun to work with, and it's particularly rewarding when you can help them understand some concepts and can actually work through problems that aren't already solved."

However, while working in an academic environment offers medical physiologists the opportunity to conduct research and help their students, they must also set aside time in their schedules to attend to any administrative duties they may have. This may also include spending time in organizational and departmental meetings.

Fred Kronk believes a career as an exercise physiologist offers many different challenges everyday and that it is always interesting and new. As he explains, "it can be really varied, and that's why I like the job, because you can do so many things."

Throughout the day, exercise physiologists will work with many different people on both an individual or group basis. During a typical day Fred will meet with clients to discuss their exercise goals and schedules and then create specific exercise programs that meet the needs of his client. Fred believes that to achieve their goals, clients must concentrate on the process rather than the end results. As he explains, ". . . if your mind is on a goal, I don't believe you're going to get there. I believe you're going to get there sooner if you focus on the process and that you're going to find things about yourself that you don't even know."

Exercise physiologists are limited in the types of fitness testing they can conduct at health clubs without a doctor being present. However, they can test for the client's resting heart rate, blood pressure, upper body strength, and endurance level. They can also analyze the client's oxygen consumption to determine how efficiently the client's heart muscles and lungs are using oxygen.

A good exercise physiologist has to be a good teacher. Clients come into health clubs with questions regarding the latest trends in diet and exercise they have read about in a magazine or seen on television. Exercise physiologists need to be able to separate fact from fiction for their clients and explain the correct ways to achieve fitness goals. In addition, they need to ensure a safe workout environment.

have I got what it takes to be a physiologist?

Medical physiologists are born with a great deal of curiosity. They are the detectives of the natural world. They want to know how organisms work. How different organisms are related. Their research, though dealing with different plants and animals, is ultimately pursued to benefit humans.

There is a certain level of interaction between medical physiologists and their experiments. Professor McCrimmon explains the relationship between physiologists and their research this way: "[medical physiologists] have to treat the science and the experiments the same way a musician treats the instrument he works with. . . ." Their work becomes more of a vocation rather than just a career. It is a way of life, a way of thinking. "It's not something you do eight hours a day, it's something you do as a career. You think about it on weekends, and evening, pretty much on and off all the time," states Dr. McCrimmon.

Like medical physiologists, exercise physiologists must be dedicated to their career to succeed. When Fred Kronk is working with a client he directs all of his attention to the client. For example, after the fourth or fifth session he will be able to tell if clients have progressed at all just by their posture or the way they walk.

However, beyond dedication and an attention to detail, one of the most important characteristics of competent exercise physiologists is their ability to be a caregiver. Exercise physiologists must have the nurturing instinct that immediately tells the client that they are there to help the clients feel better. Exercise physiologists who can not become caregivers usually end up changing careers. As Fred states, "people who aren't comfortable with that don't last in the field."

Being a good communicator is a necessity for exercise physiologists because they spend a great deal of time teaching their clients. They must explain and provide the correct instructions to use the exercise machines effectively. Furthermore, exercise physiologists must weed through the latest exercise trends and diet fads to teach their clients the safest ways to become fit.

Also, while speaking with their clients they must be completely honest. If Fred believes that a client is not progressing as he would like he will ask the client to sit down and speak with him about it. Fred sees this dialogue as an opportunity for the client to express any thoughts they may have regarding their exercise programs.

how do I become a physiologist?

Professor McCrimmon was introduced to the subjects of physics and chemistry in high school. He was immediate intrigued by physics. He received his undergraduate degree in Canada. He earned a Ph.D. at the University of Wisconsin at Madison. It was while he was at graduate school that he attended a physiology class taught by two professors who made the subject so interesting that he continued to study physiology. He completed his postdoctoral work at Northwestern University's Medical School in Chicago where he now teaches and conducts research.

Fred Kronk received an undergraduate degree in the fine arts. However, to earn money while he was working toward his degree, he worked at health clubs in his area. He found he liked working at clubs and that the members seemed to like him. He decided to attend Northeastern Illinois University's graduate program in physiology where he earned a master's degree in physiology.

To be a successful medical physiologist you should

- Have a great deal of curiosity
- Be a meticulous researcher
- Enjoy laboratory work
- Have very good observation skills
- Be a good teacher
- Be adept at using scientific instruments

education

High school

High school students interested in careers in physiology should take as many science classes as possible. These should include biology, chemistry, and physics. In addition, if students believe that they will want to work in the area of exercise physiology, they should also take classes in physical education and health.

While attending high school, students interested in careers in physiology should seriously consider what subfield they ultimately will pursue. Most colleges that offer undergraduate degrees with majors in physiology also have different special areas of study within the subject. In addition to exercise, these may include cellular, environmental, or nutritional physiology. Once students figure out what subfield they are most interested in, they should enroll in the college that offers a degree in that subfield. Students should contact the American Physiological Society. The society offers a booklet that lists the various institutions across the country that award academic degrees with a major in physiology and the special areas of study they have.

Postsecondary Training

To be competitive in the job market, students interested in working in exercise physiology need to earn a master's degree. Even though some health clubs employ people with bachelor's degrees, exercise physiologists must have an advanced degree to have the potential to move into any independent or administrative position.

There are few fields that require a doctorate for entry-level positions, but medical physiology is one of them. Students interested in teaching in any area of medical physiology programs at the college level or in pursuing independent research must earn a Ph.D. Researchers with only bachelor's or master's degrees in physiology generally work under the supervision of a physiologist with a doctorate. Most medical physiologists with bachelor degrees work as technicians or assistants.

The course work will differ depending on the prospective employment field. All physiologists must take a concentration of science courses, including biology, anatomy, chemistry, and physics. Also important are classes in composition, statistics, and mathematics. Those wishing to be exercise physiologists should take courses in physical education, nutrition, kinesiology, and physical therapy.

Physiologists begin to focus more closely on their chosen area at the masters and doctoral levels. The course work and research will reflect the individual's focus. Because acquisition of an advanced degree requires several more years of study, you must have a strong commitment to your area of study.

certification and licensing

There is no certification or licensing for medical physiologists. For exercise physiologists, however, the American College of Sports Medicine offers two certification programs. The first program is called the Health and Fitness Track Certification program and includes certifications for ACSM Health Fitness Director,

To be a successful exercise physiologist you should

- Have an intense interest in fitness
- Be a good teacher
- Have excellent people skills
- Be a committed caregiver
- Be a team player
- Be a good motivator
- Have the ability to understand and use a wide variety of exercise equipment

Health Fitness Instructor, and Exercise Leader. The second program is called the Clinical Track Certification and includes certifications as Program Director, Exercise Specialist, and Test Technician.

Fred Kronk has received certification as a test technician and health fitness instructor. A certified test technician can analyze the gasses a person exhales while exercising on a treadmill. Certification as a Fitness Instructor is evidence that Fred knows how to work well with people when they are working out on the club floor. To be certified by the American College of Sports Medicine is considered a hallmark within the exercise physiology industry. As Fred states, "ACSM tends to be considered by some as the gold standard. . . ."

It is a requirement of ACSM that members accumulate a certain number of hours of continuing education to retain their certification. This is done to help ensure that exercise physiologists are up to date with the latest research on exercise physiology.

internship and volunteerships

In the fields of medical and exercise physiology there are several opportunities to gain practical experience as either an intern or as a volunteer. An internship or volunteership provides a great chance for you to learn about the many different types of employment opportunities available and to help you decide which area will be your specialty. Furthermore, through internships and volunteer work, you can speak with professionals within the field and gain by their experience. It is an opportunity to find out what the people who are working in physiology like and dislike about their careers.

Many teaching hospitals across the country have excellent volunteer programs. Those interested in physiology should contact the hospital in their area and inquire about volunteer opportunities. There is an excellent volunteer program at Northwestern Memorial Hospital. In some instances, it may even be possible for volunteers to work in the laboratories as a technician for a term. This opportunity gives students the chance to learn from basic researchers. Students should also contact the American Physiological Society, which has outreach programs to help students interested in physiology.

Students interested in exercise physiology should contact the health club in their area and ask to speak to the exercise physiologist on staff. If they do not have a physiologist on staff try a different club. The internship process should be formalized and managed through the student's college. Some health clubs, like Fred Kronk's, have internship programs with the colleges in their area. These are formal internships set up with the student's internship department. When working with an intern, Fred receives a syllabus from the college and there is a formal review at the end of the internship. An internship can last a few days or a few weeks but it offers valuable information because as Fred states, ". . . the most valuable experience is to see what actually goes on at a club."

who will hire me?

Exercise physiologists can find work in a variety of places, including health clubs, hospitals, universities, athletic organizations, and large corporations that have exercise programs available for employees. They may also be employed as research scientists at private laboratories. Self employment, as a personal trainer, is also a possibility for an ambitious exercise physiologist. Because of their advanced training and clinical understanding of the human body, exercise physiologists have an advantage over many other fitness experts when it comes to becoming a personal trainer.

The majority of medical physiologists today work for colleges and universities or for the federal government. There are hundreds of educational institutions across the country offering degrees in physiology. Furthermore, within each department there may be over twenty different special areas of study that need qualified physiology professors. Half of the 62,000 biological scientists working in 1990 held teaching positions. At most of these colleges they are responsible for both teaching and research. They may also be responsible for acting as advisors to students who are trying to earn their doctorate.

Medical physiologists may also find employment opportunities with pharmaceutical companies in research and testing labs. They may also be employed at hospitals and doctor's offices.

Future, job growth will come primarily from the private sector for both medical and exercise physiologists.

where can I go from here?

Because of academic demands, an entry-level position as a medical physiologist at a university requires a doctorate in physiology. After earning their doctorate, medical physiologists will then complete a post doctoral fellowship at a different institution. By changing lab settings, beginning physiologists can increase their basic skills as well as increase their knowledge of techniques and gain more insight into different scientific problems and issues. After their fellowships are complete, physiologists will move into careers either in the commercial area or at academic institutions.

Entry-level positions for exercise physiologists can be called different things at different clubs. At Fred Kronk's health club the entry-level position is referred to as a fitness specialist. When Fred began working he was required to attend an orientation session where he received instructions regarding the club's equipment and testing procedures. As fitness specialists, physiologists not only work with members in the health club and conduct programming, but they also gain the practical experience in the business of exercise. Fitness specialists are supervised and are reviewed first after ninety days and then after a year. They also receive feedback constantly from their departmental managers.

To move into management positions, exercise physiologists must have proven technical skills, must exhibit a firm commitment to customer service, and must work well as a team player. Furthermore, health and fitness directors want creative people on their staff who will approach problems from a new perspective to help work with their members.

Exercise physiologists who establish an excellent reputation and become well-known may decide to open a business as a personal trainer or may be hired by a professional sports organization.

what are the salary ranges?

Medical physiologists breaking into the field with a bachelor's degree, in private industry, can expect to earn approximately $23,000. Physiologists who hold master's degrees may earn as much as $30,000 and physiologists who have earned a doctorate may have a salary of $48,000 a year. The median income was approximately $38,000 in 1994. At the lowest level, physiologists earned a little more than $16,000 a year, while some highly skilled physiologists with many years of experience earned $67,000.

Physiologists working for the Federal Government in the early nineties earned almost $62,000.

The annual salary of exercise physiologists depends on many things, including the area of the country they work in, their years of experience, and the degree they hold. In some cases, if they work in administrative or managerial positions, their annual salary will be higher.

what is the job outlook?

There has been an explosion in the knowledge of genetics and molecular biology recently, largely due to the research that is presently being conducted in those subjects. These changes may have a great effect on the overall field of medical physiology. Being able to manipulate and analyze an organism at a genetic level helps with the ability to understand what is going on with the organism systematically. As Dr. McCrimmon explains "We can manipulate DNA and alter an animal and find out how their alterations affect the ability of that animal to adapt to various situations. . . ." These new discoveries will lead to the future demand for medical physiologists.

The future for exercise physiologists is quite healthy. As the baby boom generation ages, by the year 2000, 74 percent of the population is expected to be over forty years old, the demand for qualified experts in the fitness business will be quite high. Research is presently being conducted aimed at investigating different ways the aging process can be slowed down with a good exercise program. Another positive effect on exercise physiology has been the development of wireless computers that allow people to monitor their activity while they exercise. Additionally, more insurance companies are considering a good fitness program to be a form of preventative care and are considering reimbursing their members for their health club costs. All of these reasons combined point to a healthy future in the field of exercise physiology.

how do I learn more?

professional organizations

Following are organizations that provide information on medical and exercise physiologist careers, accredited schools, and possible employers.

American College of Sports Medicine
P.O. Box 1440
Indianapolis, IN 46202-1440
TEL: 317 637-9200
WEBSITE: http://www.acsm.org/sportsmed

American Physiological Society
9650 Rockville Pike
Bethesda, MD 20814-3991
TEL: (301) 530-7164
WEBSITE: http://www.faseb.org/aps/

bibliography

Following is a sampling of materials relating to the professional concerns and development of physiologists.

Books

Heron, Jackie. *Careers in Health and Fitness,* revised edition. New York, NY: Rosen Group, 1989.

Johnson, Leonard R., editor. *Essential Medical Physiology.* Philadelphia, PA: Lippincott-Raven, 1991.

MacKenna, B. R., and R. R.Callander. *Illustrated Physiology,* 5th edition. New York, NY: Churchill Livingstone, 1991.

Poder, Thomas C. *Basic Concepts in Physiology: a Student's Survival Guide.* New York, NY: McGraw-Hill, 1997.

Sugar-Webb, Jan. *Opportunities in Physician Careers.* Lincolnwood, IL: VGM Career Horizons, 1994.

Tortora, Gerard J., and Sandra R. Grabowski. *Principles of Anatomy and Physiology.* Reading, MA: Addison-Wesley, 1993.

Periodicals

American Journal of Physiology. Monthly. Consolidates papers published in eight subject-specific journals making up the *American Journal of Physiology* series. American Physiological Society, 9650 Rockville Pike, Bethesda, MD 20814-3991, 301-530-7164.

The Physiologist. Bimonthly. Newsletter. Contains book reviews, employment opportunities, statistics, and abstracts of annual meetings. American Physiological Society, 9650 Rockville Pike, Bethesda, MD 20814-3991, 301-530-7164.

plastic and reconstructive surgeon

Definition

This surgeon deals with the repair, replacement, and reconstruction of defects of the form and function of the skin and its underlying musculoskeletal system.

Alternative job title

Plastic surgeon

Salary range

$31,000 to $150,000 to $250,000+

Educational requirements

Bachelor's degree, M.D., three-year residency in general surgery, two-year residency in plastic and reconstructive surgery, optional fellowships

Certification or licensing

Certification is highly recommended; licensing is mandatory.

Outlook

Much faster than average

GOE
02.03.01

DOT
070

High School Subjects

Biology
Chemistry
Computer science
English
Mathematics
Physics

Personal Interests

Creative problem solving
Design and appearances
Helping people
Working with your hands

The team of plastic surgeons, anesthesiologists, and nurses arrived in Guatemala City, Guatemala, to find that three boxes of their surgical equipment had been lost by the airline. Working with the nonprofit group Casa de Guatemala, the team had come to perform surgery on underprivileged children. Now one of their precious operating days was lost in the effort to replace the missing equipment. The medical team was donating their time and talent. They realized that the experience would not be like doing surgery at a hospital back home. The loss of one operating day, however, was a disappointment. Dr. Mimis Cohen of Chicago, Illinois, has taken these trips for years. "With work like this," he says, "you have to be prepared for the worst. If you go with the attitude that it's going to be like operating in Chicago—it won't succeed."

Dr. Cohen explains the set up, "On the first day, we have a clinic and we sort the kids out. We treat primarily birth defects. Often the parents will travel for twenty-four hours from remote villages, and it's heartbreaking when you have to turn kids down." Parents and children filled the clinic, waiting to be helped. Dr. Cohen began his day by operating on a small boy with a cleft lip and palate. "We each operate on between fifteen and sixteen children a day," he says. "Many with double- and triple-procedure surgeries." Despite the long hours and limited resources, these professionals believe their work is well worth the effort. They know that the corrective surgeries they preform have the potential to greatly improve the quality of the children's lives.

lingo to learn

Alloplasty In plastic surgery, implanting synthetic materials to replace or build up a tissue or organ.

Blepharoplasty Surgery of the eyelid.

Excisional surgery Surgery that "cuts out" something, such as a tumor.

Flap A section of living tissue that carries its own blood supply and is moved from one area of the body to another.

Maxillofacial Having to do with the jaw and face.

Skin graft A patch of healthy skin that is taken from one area of the body, called the "donor site," and used to cover another area where skin is missing or damaged. The three basic types of skin grafts are the split-thickness graft, the full-thickness graft, and the composite graft.

Tissue expansion A procedure that enables the body to "grow" extra skin by stretching adjacent tissue. A balloon-like device called an expander is inserted under the skin near the area to be repaired and then gradually filled with saltwater over time, causing the skin to stretch and grow.

what does a plastic and reconstructive surgeon do?

A *plastic and reconstructive surgeon* deals with the repair, replacement, and reconstruction of defects in the form and function of the skin and its underlying musculoskeletal system. The plastic and reconstructive surgeon is especially skilled in working on such areas of the body as the head, neck, and face; upper and lower limbs; breasts; and external genitalia. Besides performing surgery to correct medical problems, the plastic and reconstructive surgeon also can preform surgery for purely cosmetic results.

Special knowledge and skill in the design and transfer of skin flaps, in the transplantation of tissues, and in the replantation of structures are vital to the performance of plastic surgery. The plastic surgeon must also possess excellent skills in the performance of excisional surgery, in the management of large wounds, and in the use of synthetic materials. In addition, a vast knowledge of surgical instruments and how to use them is necessary for this specialty.

Some the most commonly performed procedures include surgery to correct cleft lip and cleft palate; surgery to the outer ear (otoplasty); scar revision; dermabrasion; breast reconstruction; hand surgery; abdominoplasty ("tummy tuck"); rhinoplasty ("nose job"); liposuction; chemical peel; and hair replacement surgery. Surgeons working on trauma victims may perform several of these surgeries at once, or in stages to allow for proper healing.

The profession breaks down into two areas of expertise—plastic (also called cosmetic) surgery and reconstructive surgery. Physicians complete training in both disciplines, although some surgeons may specialize in one area by taking additional years of fellowships in one or more areas.

The main goal of reconstructive surgery is to restore, or allow for, normal function of an abnormal body structure. Abnormalities are caused by such things as birth defects, injuries, infections, tumors, or diseases. A secondary result of reconstructive surgery may be an approximation of normal appearance. The goal of cosmetic surgery, on the other hand, is to reshape normal structures of the body to improve the patient's appearance and self-esteem.

Plastic and reconstructive surgeons must have extensive knowledge of wound treatment and closure. A wound may be the reason for a procedure or the byproduct of the procedure. In either case, treatment is necessary and can be accomplished in several ways, depending on such factors as amount of skin missing and extent of nerve damage. Skin grafts, tissue expansion, and skin flaps are among the commonly used methods of closing, "growing," and transplanting skin. Plastic surgeons take great pains to render the surgical areas as scar-free and aesthetically pleasing as possible, although scarring is sometimes unavoidable. Many patients having reconstructive surgery often return to have scarring reduced or to have cosmetic surgery performed to improve their post-reconstruction appearance.

Plastic and reconstructive surgeons routinely use a variety of lasers to preform reconstructive surgery. The carbon dioxide laser is used to cut tissue and seal blood vessels simultaneously. The YAG laser is effective in treating skin growths with heavy concentrations of blood vessels. The YAG delivers its highly-focused beam right to the skin's surface, allowing the surgeon to use it like a scalpel. Argon and copper vapor lasers are used, respectively, to treat abnormalities with a proliferation of blood vessels, such as bulky vascular tumors, and brown or red pigmented areas.

Cosmetic surgery is usually done to correct minor defects and should not leave large, visible scars. Surgeons frequently perform endoscopic surgery for cosmetic procedures. In a typical endoscopic surgery, only a few small incisions, each less than one inch long, are needed to insert the endoscope and other instruments. The endoscope is a flexible, fiber-optic instrument that allows the surgeon to see the interior of a hollow organ. Because incisions for endoscopic surgery are small, bleeding, bruising, and swelling may be reduced, as is the patient's recovery time. Endoscopic surgery is commonly used in abdominoplasties, breast augmentations, facelifts, and forehead lifts.

The future of plastic surgery may also include the use of lasers to resurface the skin. Lasers remove old layers of skin in a manner that is less harsh and aggressive than deep chemical peels or abrasions. This is a new technique and long-term data on results are not yet available.

To be a successful plastic and reconstructive surgeon, you should

- Be both a good listener and a good communicator
- Pay close attention to detail
- Have a compassionate nature and enjoy helping people with aspects of their bodies about which they may feel sensitive and/or self-conscious
- Have good hand-eye coordination and manual dexterity

what is it like to be a plastic and reconstructive surgeon?

For the last six years, Dr. Mimis Cohen, the Chief of Plastic Surgery at Cook County Hospital and the University of Illinois, both in Chicago, and Professor of Surgery at the University of Illinois, has taken a team of surgeons, anesthesiologists, and nurses with him to Guatemala to perform reconstructive plastic surgery on disadvantaged children. "There are such a huge number of problems, I could have a full-time job down there," he says.

Months and months of planning go into one of Dr. Cohen's trips. He arranges for a hospital in Guatemala City to screen surgery candidates. "They have scattered clinics, so if a candidate for surgery comes along, they make sure he or she gets to us," he explains. "Then we fly down with our equipment: computers, lasers, syringes, gowns, IVs." Dr. Cohen takes two to three other surgeons, three pediatric anesthesiologists, and six to seven operating room and recovery nurses. All of the surgeons are highly experienced. Dr. Cohen says, "I don't use the trip as a training ground. These kids only have one shot." The doctors donate their time and expertise, and pay for the hotel, food, and transportation of the nurses.

The first day the children are sorted into three groups headed by one of the three surgeons. Each surgeon will operate on thirty to forty patients. They only have one week to get there, set up, screen the children, and then perform the surgeries and provide as much postoperative care as they can before leaving for the United States. "The surgeon examines the child with the parents, and then the anesthesiologist examines the child to make certain there aren't any complications, like a heart condition," Dr. Cohen explains. "If the child is okay, we accept him or her for surgery. After we've finished screening all the kids, we have a priority conference to determine the order of the surgeries." Generally, those who need to stay under the longest postoperative care will go first. "So, newborn babies go first, complex patients go next. We don't want to have some complication develop after I've left," says Dr. Cohen. "The local doctors are involved in the postoperative and follow-up care, but we want to make certain we leave them in the best shape."

When Dr. Cohen is not planning one of these trips to Guatemala—or on one—his time is taken up with his responsibilities as Chief of Plastic Surgery at Cook County Hospital and the University of Illinois. "At the university, I do a fair amount of reconstruction on children with deformities. Mainly facial, but also hands and birthmarks. I do a fair amount of cancer reconstruction on the breast and face," he says. "At [Cook] County [Hospital] I do a lot of trauma, maxillofacial work," he says. "And I also do a fair amount of cosmetic surgery." Teaching responsibilities, conferences, and presentations also take up a great deal of Dr. Cohen's time and attention. "Some people have the notion that you just teach in classrooms, but that's not true. You teach surgery in surgery," he says. "You teach through patient care."

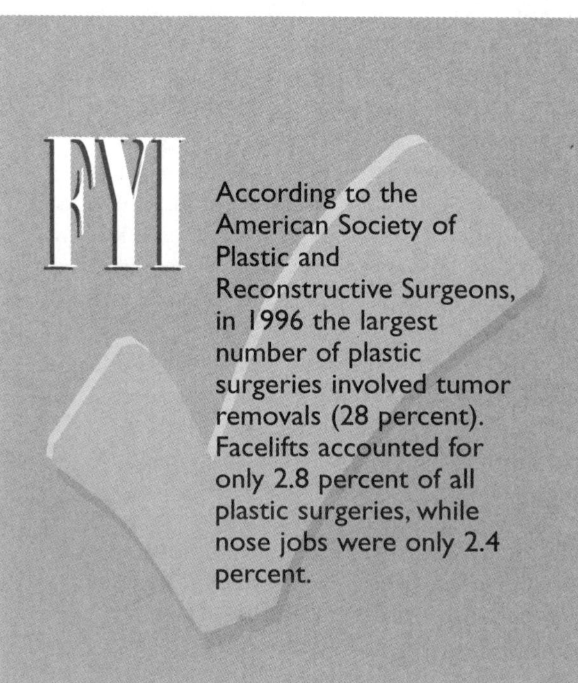

According to the American Society of Plastic and Reconstructive Surgeons, in 1996 the largest number of plastic surgeries involved tumor removals (28 percent). Facelifts accounted for only 2.8 percent of all plastic surgeries, while nose jobs were only 2.4 percent.

Dr. Roxanne Guy, a plastic and reconstructive surgeon who practices in Melbourne, Florida, estimates that half of her practice is reconstructive and the other half is cosmetic. "Breast reconstruction after mastectomy, breast reductions, skin cancer resections, and trauma cases, facial fractures and burns," she lists the reconstructive surgeries she frequently performs. "Accidents where the patient has lost part of an ear, or a cancer that takes part of the patient's face—no surgery is ever the same. The defects are all different and individual. It's sort of like a puzzle, somewhat exciting and different. As a surgeon, you have to use imagination and skills and the principles of wound healing and grafting to fill in the puzzle."

For new patients, Dr. Guy says, "We send information, a brochure on the problem, to the prospective patient to help educate him." On the day of the appointment, the patient fills out a brief questionnaire about his or her medial history, which Dr. Guy will add to when she meets with the patient. "A nurse would take the patient's history—allergies, et cetera—and show the person an informational video on the problem and the various options for treatment, including the surgical procedure. Then, I meet with the patient and review the patient's history, as well as the procedure, including any complications, risks, and the prescribed postoperative care. Afterwards, I would examine the patient and decide what would be the best solution for that patient."

Dr. Guy then provides the patient who wants cosmetic surgery with a cost-sheet outlining the costs of the various procedures. For patients who are seeking reconstructive surgery, insurance pre-approval forms are provided to be completed and sent to their health insurance company. If the patient decides to go ahead with the surgery, he or she comes back for a detailed health history and physical. Dr. Guy sends the patient's blood work to the lab to rule out any further complications, schedules the surgery, and explains any preoperative care instructions to the patient. A procedure may be performed in her office, in an ambulatory surgery center, or in a hospital; it all depends on the complexity of the surgery and whether or not a one- to two-night stay in the facility is necessary. "Microsurgery cases I do at the hospital, for example," she says. The day of the surgery, Dr. Guy sees the patient in pre-op and then performs the surgery.

have I got what it takes to be a plastic and reconstructive surgeon?

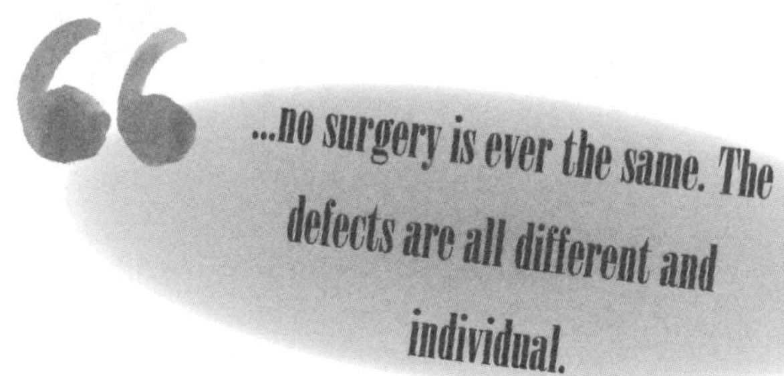

> ...no surgery is ever the same. The defects are all different and individual.

"It's drama, it's theatre, it's fun, it's positive," Dr. Guy says of her work. "And I like providing something that is a happy experience. If it's a reconstructive case, I'm fixing something damaged, and if it's an aesthetic case, I'm helping to create or fix something." Dr. Guy explains, "Plasticos is Greek for 'to shape or remold.' People who have cosmetic surgery experience a positive rise in self-esteem following the procedure."

Plastic surgeons must possess excellent manual dexterity skills and the ability to make and execute decisions promptly. Any operation involves risks, and during surgery a plastic surgeon may have to deal with the unexpected, such as a patient's sudden drop in blood pressure or a bad reaction to the anesthesia. The surgeon must be able to cope with such situations, while maintaining his or her composure.

Another essential quality in surgeons is a genuine concern for people. Those who aspire to be plastic surgeons must be able to deal compassionately with patients and their families. Surgeons should be effective communicators, able to address any fears, questions, and needs their patients have. Plastic surgeons must also have good judgment and know when to refuse to perform a surgery that would not benefit the patient.

how do I become a plastic and reconstructive surgeon?

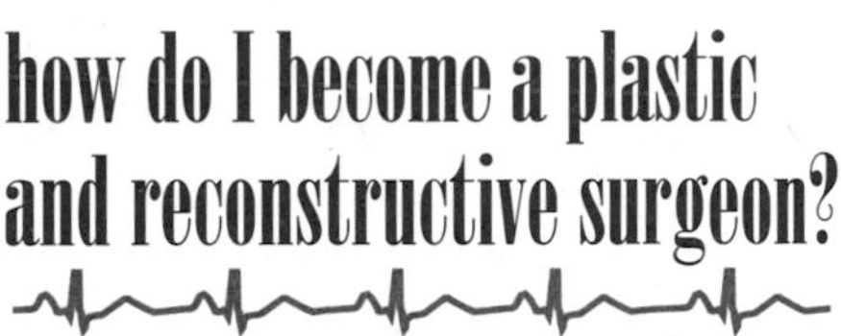

education

High School

If you are interested in pursuing a medical degree, a high school education emphasizing college preparatory classes is a must. Science courses, such as biology, chemistry, and physics, are necessary to take, as are math courses. These classes will not only provide you with an introduction to basic science and math concepts, but also allow you to determine your own aptitude in these areas. Since college will be your next educational step, it is also important to take English courses to develop your research and writing skills. Foreign language, social science, and computer classes will also help make you an appealing candidate for college admission as well as prepare you for your future undergraduate and graduate education. High school juniors or seniors should also be aware that some colleges or universities are associated with a medical school and can offer a medical degree through an accelerated program. You may want to consider applying to one of these schools. High school guidance counselors should be able to provide you with information about such schools.

Postsecondary Training

Following high school, your next step to becoming a plastic surgeon is to receive your bachelor's degree from an accredited four-year college or university. Often those planning to attend medical school major in a science. No matter what your major, however, the typical college courses that may help you prepare for medical school include biology, chemistry, anatomy, psychology, and physics. English courses will help you to hone research and communication skills. Social sciences and ethics courses will help prepare you for a people-oriented career.

If you choose to attend a college or university associated with a medical school that offers the accelerated medical program, your undergraduate education will be slightly different from that of other undergraduates. An accelerated program typically reduces or consolidates the number of years you spend as an undergraduate, thereby speeding up the your entrance into medical school. A six- or seven-year medical student is actually enrolled for two or three years, respectively, of undergraduate school, plus the requisite four years of medical school.

After receiving an undergraduate degree, you must then apply to and be accepted by a medical school. Most students apply to several schools early in their senior year of college. Admission is competitive; only about one-third of the applicants are accepted. The admissions process takes into consideration grade point averages, scores on the Medical College Admission Test (MCAT), recommendations from professors, and extracurricular activities, such as volunteering at hospitals. Often schools also conduct interviews with prospective students.

In order to earn the degree doctor of medicine (M.D.), a student must complete four years of medical school study and training. For the first two years of medical school, students attend lectures and classes and spend time in laboratories. Courses include anatomy, biochemistry, physiology, pharmacology, psychology, medical ethics, and laws governing medicine. They learn to take patient histories, perform routine physical examinations, and recognize symptoms of diseases.

In their third and fourth years, students are involved in more practical studies. They work in clinics and hospitals supervised by residents and physicians and they learn acute, chronic, preventive, and rehabilitative care. They go through rotations (brief periods of study) in such areas as internal medicine, obstetrics and gynecology, pediatrics, psychiatry, and surgery. Rotations allow students to gain exposure to the many different fields within medicine and to learn firsthand the skills of diagnosing and treating patients.

After graduating from an accredited medical school, physicians must pass a standard examination given by the National Board of Medical Examiners. Most physicians complete an internship, also referred to as a transition year. The internship is usually one year in length, and helps graduates to decide what will be their area of specialization.

Following the internship, the physicians begin what is known as a residency. Physicians wishing to pursue the surgical specialty of plastic and reconstructive surgery, must first complete a minimum of three years in a general surgery residency. This general surgery training is followed by two years of training in plastic surgery. Most physicians add another six to twelve months of training to focus on a particular field of interest. At this point, for example, a surgeon may choose to focus on one of the subspecialties of plastic surgery, such as hand surgery.

certification or licensing

In order to receive certification from the American Board of Plastic Surgery, a candidate must have successfully completed the approved residency program in plastic surgery. The plastic surgeon then applies to the ABPS and, once the application is approved, take the qualifying written examination. After passing the written examination, the applicant must then pass the oral examination.

In order to become certified, the plastic surgeon must also practice the specialty of plastic surgery for two years. The candidate can take the written examination any time during the two year's of practice, but the oral examination cannot be taken before the candidate has finished the two-year practice requirement.

Licensing is a mandatory procedure in the United States. It is required in all states before any doctor can practice medicine. In order to be licensed, doctors must have graduated from medical school, passed the licensing test of the state in which they will practice, and completed their residency.

scholarships and grants

Scholarships and grants are often available from individual institutions, state agencies, and special-interest organizations. The book *Dollars for College: Medicine, Dentistry, and Related Fields* by Ferguson Publishing Company is an excellent source for this information. Many students finance their medical education through the Armed Forces Health Professions Scholarship Program. Each branch of the military participates in this program, paying students' tuitions in exchange for military service. Contact your local recruiting office for more information. The National Health Service Corps Scholarship Program also provides money for students in return for service. Another source for financial aid, scholarship, and grant information is the Association of American Medical Colleges. Remember to request information early for eligibility, application requirements, and deadlines.

Association of American Medical Colleges
2450 N Street, NW
Washington, DC 20037
TEL: 202-828-0400
WEBSITE: http://www.aamc.org
Specific information on financial aid programs can be found at:
WEBSITE: http://www.aamc.org/stuapps/finaid

Ferguson Publishing Company
200 West Madison, Suite 300
Chicago, IL 60606
TEL: 312-580-5480

National Health Services Corps Scholarship Program
U.S. Public Health Service
1010 Wayne Avenue, Suite 240
Silver Spring, MD 20910
TEL: 800-638-0824

who will hire me?

Many plastic surgeons go into private practice. Others work full-time in academic and research institutions. Still others combine a private practice with academic and research work.

A private practice in plastic surgery can be devoted to one area of expertise—such as hand surgery—or the practice can be considered general. In a general practice, the plastic surgeon performs a wide range of cosmetic and reconstructive procedures. Most plastic surgeons in private practice divide their time between cosmetic and reconstructive work, simply because their work is more interesting if it is varied. It is possible, however, to have a private practice devoted entirely to cosmetic surgery, since these procedures can easily support an entire practice.

where can I go from here?

Plastic surgeons can advance by attending conferences featuring discussions of new procedures or by reading about and learning new techniques. Surgeons must also continue to master new technologies that will improve the operations they perform. They may also advance their careers by conducting research, teaching, and developing a larger client base.

Plastic surgeons may go back to school to train in a subspecialty through a fellowship. Many plastic surgeons, however, achieve a level of expertise simply by doing something better than anyone else. This, of course, is accomplished through practice and much refinement of technique. Publishing articles in respected medical journals, such as *JAMA*, is another way to increase one's professional stature.

what are the salary ranges?

The national average salary for first-year residents in the mid-1990's was approximately $31,000. That average increased to $41,800 by the final residency year. Salaries will vary depending on the kind of residency, the hospital, and the geographic area.

Once a plastic surgeon is out of residency and in private or academic practice, his or her salary rises considerably. A plastic surgeon in the first five years of private practice can earn between $75,000 and $150,000. Someone who has been practicing five to ten years can earn between $150,000 and $250,000. A few plastic surgeons with much specialty experience can earn between $250,000 and $300,000. Some surgeons earn $400,000 or more. Incomes will vary, depending on such factors as a surgeon's reputation, the geographic location, and the types of procedures the surgeon preforms. Currently, plastic surgeons in private practice tend to earn more than those in academic and managed care settings.

what is the job outlook?

The job growth for plastic surgeons is expected to increase at a much faster than average rate into the twenty-first century. Both men and women will continue to want cosmetic surgery. Reconstructive surgery will continue to be performed on anyone—young or old, male or female—who needs it. If health insurers do not pay for certain procedures, individuals will cover the cost themselves. In addition, as technology advances, plastic surgeons develop new increasingly safe and easy ways to eradicate deformities and improve appearances. With such advances, many people will seek out the plastic surgeon's services.

how do I learn more?

professional organizations

Following are organizations that provide information on the profession of plastic and reconstructive surgery.

American Board of Plastic Surgery
Seven Penn Center, Suite 400
1635 Market Street
Philadelphia, PA 19103
TEL: 215-587-9322

American Society for Aesthetic Plastic Surgery
444 East Algonquin Road, Suite 110
Arlington Heights, IL 60005
TEL: 847-228-9905

American Society of Plastic and Reconstructive Surgeons
444 East Algonquin Road
Arlington Heights, IL 60005
TEL: 847-228-9900
WEBSITE: http://www.plasticsurgery.org

bibliography

Following is a sampling of books and periodicals relating to the professional concerns and development of plastic and reconstructive surgeons.

Books

Finley, John M. *Considering Plastic Surgery?* Gretna, LA: Pelican Publishing Co., 1991.

Marks, Malcolm W., and Charles Marks. *Fundamentals of Plastic Surgery*. Philadelphia, PA: W.B. Saunders Co., 1997.

Michaels, Katherine. *Crashing into the Wall of Vanity: Cosmetic Surgery: Is It for You?* New York, NY: Avon Books, 1992.

Spira, Melvin. *Essentials of Plastic Surgery*. St. Louis, MO: Quality Medical Publishing, 1996.

Periodicals

American Journal of Cosmetic Surgery. Quarterly. Covers thought, experience, opinion, technique, research, legal aspects, patient relations, office protocol, and any other subject relating to cosmetic surgery. American Academy of Cosmetic Surgery, Inc., 401 N. Michigan Avenue, Chicago, IL 60611, 312-527-6713.

Annals of Plastic Surgery. Monthly. Forum for the latest in surgical techniques, interesting cases, and practical briefs on surgical devices. Little, Brown, Medical Journals, 34 Beacon Street, Boston, MA 02108, 617-859-5500.

Operative Techniques in Plastic and Reconstructive Surgery. Quarterly. Each issue focuses on a particular restorative surgical procedure or clinical condition. W.B. Saunders Co., Curtis Center, 3rd Floor, Independence Square West, Philadelphia, PA 19106, 215-238-7800.

Plastic and Reconstructive Surgery. 14 per year. Examines plastic and reconstructive surgery techniques. American Society of Plastic and Reconstructive Surgeons, Williams & Wilkins, 428 E. Preston Street, Baltimore, MD 21202, 410-528-4000, 800-638-6423.

podiatrist

Definition

Podiatrists diagnose, prevent, and treat foot disorders by prescribing medication, performing surgery, and fitting corrective orthotic devices.

Alternative job titles

Doctor of podiatric medicine

Foot doctor

Salary range

$30,000 to $53,000 to $120,000

Educational requirements

High school diploma; bachelor's degree from an accredited college or university; four-year degree from an accredited college of podiatric medicine; one-year residency

Certification or licensing

Mandatory

Job outlook

Average

GOE
02.03.01

DOT
079

High School Subjects

Biology
Chemistry
Physics
Physiology

Personal Interests

Health care
Helping people
Medicine

The bright lights of the operating room shine on Gerry Hash as he pulls latex gloves over his hands, preparing for the morning's first surgical procedure. "Is she ready to go?" he asks the anesthesiologist as he nears the operating table. The patient on the table, who has received general anesthetic, is a sixty-year-old woman and a longtime patient of Gerry's.

The anesthesiologist looks up from the monitor on which he is closely observing the patient's vital signs. "She's stable," he says. "You're ready to go."

Gerry assesses different sites on the patient's left foot to determine the best place to make the incision. "Scalpel," he says to the scrub nurse standing beside him.

Taking the scalpel from the nurse, Gerry leans forward slightly and makes a small incision on the inside of the patient's foot. As the scrub nurse blots the incision site with a sterile sponge, Gerry hands the scalpel back to her.

The surgical procedure is a relatively uncomplicated one that Gerry has performed many times before. He proceeds in a relaxed and confident manner, and he chats with the nurse as he operates. "So what happened on 'ER' last night?" he asks her.

what does a podiatrist do?

Podiatrists, or *doctors of podiatric medicine,* are to feet what dentists are to teeth and ophthalmologists are to eyes. They are specialists dedicated to treating disorders of the foot and ankle.

lingo to learn

Achilles tendon The tendon connecting the heel bone to the calf of the leg; the strongest tendon in the body.

Athlete's foot A skin disease, usually occurring between the toes, caused by ringworm fungi.

Bunion An inflamed swelling of the joint at the base of the big toe. A bunion often results from wearing narrow, high-heeled shoes.

Closed reduction Realignment of a fractured bone by manipulation (without incision).

Corn A cone-shaped mass of thickened skin on a toe; it is caused by long-term friction and pressure.

Flatfoot Lack of an arch in the foot. Though almost everyone is born with flat feet, arches usually develop by age six.

Metatarsals The bones between the toes and the ankle.

Open reduction Realignment of a fractured bone after incision into the fractured site.

Phalanges The bones that make up the toes and the fingers.

Plantigrade Walking with the heel touching the ground—as humans, bears, and raccoons do.

Tarsals The bones that make up the ankle.

Podiatrists see patients who are having problems with their feet. To determine the nature of foot problems, podiatrists talk with patients and visually examine their feet. Sometimes, in order to make diagnoses, podiatrists take X rays, perform blood tests, or prescribe other diagnostic tests.

Podiatrists treat many common disorders, including corns, calluses, warts, ingrown toenails, and athlete's foot. Bunions, deformed toes, arch problems, and cysts are other examples of common foot disorders treated by podiatrists. Among the relatively uncommon foot disorders treated by podiatrists are infections and ulcers related to diabetes. Podiatrists also treat injuries to the foot and ankle, such as breaks and sprains.

The method of treatment varies considerably depending on the patient's problem. For some patients, podiatrists prescribe physical therapy sessions or give instructions on how to perform certain exercises. For other patients, podiatrists prescribe medications, either to be injected, taken orally, or applied in ointment form.

Some foot disorders, such as ingrown toenails or warts, may require minor surgical procedures. Podiatrists typically perform these kinds of procedures in their offices. Other disorders require more extensive surgery, for which patients may be anesthetized. For this kind of surgery, a podiatrist must use a sterile operating room, usually either in a hospital or an outpatient surgery center.

Another responsibility of podiatrists is to fit patients with corrective *orthotic devices,* or *orthoses,* such as braces, custom-made shoes, lifts, or splints. For a patient who needs an orthotic device, a podiatrist makes a plaster cast of the patient's foot, determines the measurements and other characteristics needed to make the device, and sends the information to a manufacturing plant called a "brace shop." When the device is complete, the podiatrist fits it to the patient and makes follow-up evaluations to ensure that it fits and functions properly. The podiatrist may also make any modifications or repairs that are needed.

Podiatrists frequently treat patients who have injured their feet or ankles. A podiatrist may wrap, splint, or cast a foot to keep it immobile and allow it to heal. In more complicated cases, podiatrists may perform corrective surgery.

A key responsibility of podiatrists is recognizing serious health disorders that sometimes show up first in the feet. For example, diabetics are prone to foot ulcers and infections because of their poor blood circulation. Symptoms of kidney disease, heart disease, and arthritis also frequently appear first in the feet. A podiatrist must be alert to symptoms of these diseases in his or her patients, and refer them to the appropriate doctors and specialists.

There are three subspecialties of podiatric medicine recognized by the American Association of Colleges of Podiatric Medicine—orthopedics, surgery, and primary medicine. Although any licensed podiatrist is considered qualified to address all areas of podiatric medicine, certification as a specialist in one of these three areas requires completion of specialized training.

Podiatrists who specialize in *orthopedics* use mechanical devices, physical treatments, medications, and exercises to treat structural disorders of the foot. Podiatrists who specialize in *podiatric surgery* are trained in the use of prosthetic joint implants, plastic surgery, and other surgical techniques to correct foot deformities. Podiatrists with a specialization in *primary podiatric medicine,* or *general podiatric medicine,* focus on prevention, diagnosis, and general care of the foot and ankle.

The average workweek for a podiatrist is thirty-five to forty hours long. Most podiatrists work in private offices, and see their patients in examining rooms. Some podiatrists work in outpatient clinics, nursing homes, or hospitals.

Some podiatrists are helped by *podiatric assistants.* A podiatric assistant prepares patients for treatment and assists the podiatrist in administering treatments. A podiatric assistant also develops X rays, sterilizes instruments, and performs general office duties.

what is it like to be a podiatrist?

"My day starts like almost anyone else's workday," says Gerry Hash, a podiatrist in a midsized midwestern city. "I come in and look at my schedule, return phone calls, and catch up on paperwork." Gerry works as a private practitioner. As such, he is basically the owner and manager of his own business, in addition to being a doctor.

"I don't have a business manager, so I do all the business stuff," he says. "I pay the phone

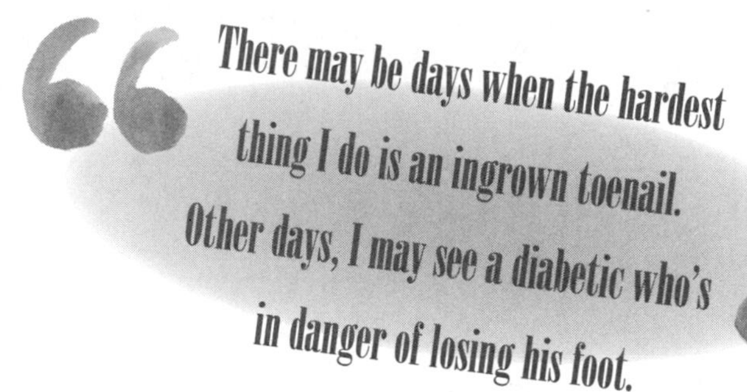

bills, the nursing staff, the lease on the office, the yellow page ads." The only part of the business that he does not deal with directly is billing. For that, he has a contract with a company that bills both patients and insurance carriers.

After the phone calls and paperwork have been taken care of, Gerry begins seeing his patients. On Mondays, Tuesdays, and Wednesdays, he sees patients in the office, with appointments scheduled fifteen minutes to a half-hour apart. Thursdays are set aside for surgeries. On Fridays, he visits local nursing and retirement homes to see patients who can't come into the office.

Gerry's days are extremely varied. "The thing about podiatry is that even though it is a limited area, there is such a wide variety of things you see and do on a daily basis," he says. "There may be days when the hardest thing I do is an ingrown toenail. Other days, I may see a diabetic who's in danger of losing his foot."

"There are so many different things and so many different methods of treatment," he says. "I write prescriptions, drain abscesses, remove nails, prescribe home exercises, give injections, order X rays or bone scans...on and on." The only surgeries that Gerry performs in his office are wart removals and procedures involving toenails. All other surgical procedures require sterile operating rooms, and are done in either hospitals or outpatient surgery centers.

Surgeries that must be done in operating rooms are scheduled for Thursdays. Surgery may last anywhere from thirty minutes for minor procedures to four hours for more complicated cases. Injuries and problems with the back part of the foot typically require the most time to correct.

"Today, for example, was my surgery day," Gerry says. "I reduced a dislocated toe. That means that I made an incision, put the toe back in place, and fixed it in place with a pin.

Then, I did an bunionectomy, in which I reduced the bone on the inside of the foot. After that, I corrected a hammertoe, a toe that curls under." While the surgical lineup varies from week to week, the procedures he describes are fairly common ones.

Gerry prescribes orthotic devices for some of his cases. "Orthoses don't necessarily correct the problem, but they accommodate for it by increasing the efficiency and mechanics of your foot." When a patient needs an orthotic device, Gerry measures the joint motion in the foot and ankle, as well as the leg length. He also analyzes the patient's gait, or manner of walking. Finally, he makes a plaster cast of the foot. Using the cast, measurements, and results of the gait analysis, he fills out a prescription form that tells the brace shop how to make the device. After the device is made, Gerry fits it to the patient and makes periodic adjustments and evaluations of its effectiveness.

Gerry's job frequently requires him to work closely with other medical specialists. "Diabetes and vascular or neurological problems often manifest themselves first in the feet, so I may be the first doctor that patient comes to," he says. "For example, a patient might come in with her feet getting numb. This could mean she's got compression of some nerve group. It could mean she's got diabetes. I've got to recognize the problem and know who to send her to."

FYI

The legend of Achilles

Achilles is a legendary character of ancient times who was the greatest Greek hero in the Trojan War. When he was a baby, his mother dipped him in the River Styx to make his body safe from all wounds. Unfortunately, because the water did not touch the heel by which his mother held him, he was vulnerable in that one spot. And in this spot, a poisoned arrow ultimately hit him and killed him. "Achilles' heel" is the term used today to identify a person's vulnerable point. The tendon connecting the heel to the calf is also named after Achilles.

have I got what it takes to be a podiatrist?

Gerry believes there are three facets to being a good podiatrist. "There's skill, there's personality, and there's commitment ," he says. "And while skills can be taught, commitment and personality cannot."

A high level of commitment is required for success both in school and in a career, according to Gerry. "You've got to have the want and the desire to do it. If you don't have that, you won't make it," he says. "Residency is tough. When it's 3:00 in the morning and you're just getting off your shift, and you have an early paper to present, you've got to be determined."

Being able to work well with people is also high on Gerry's list of necessary qualities. "You need to be good with people. You need to be caring and empathetic," he says. "If a patient has a problem with his body, he wants someone who can help him understand what's going on and not make him feel dumb." Gerry enjoys the patient interaction. He says that the time he spends with his patients is the best part of his job.

What he does not enjoy about the job, however, are the paperwork and administrative duties. Because he is a private practitioner, he also functions as a manager—of staff, of supplies, and of finances. "The most difficult part is the red tape, the paperwork, the business aspects of medicine," he says. "When I went through med school, I imagined being the best doctor I could be. I did not envision or anticipate how much of a business person I would have to be." Since the vast majority of podiatrists work as private practitioners, Gerry cautions that anyone considering this field should be aware of the managerial aspects of the job.

how do I become a podiatrist?

From the time he entered high school, Gerry knew that he wanted to pursue some kind of medical career. Although he didn't settle on podiatry until he started his undergraduate study, he tailored both his high school and college curriculum to fit the requirements for medical school.

His advice for prospective podiatrists? "Science classes are going to be very important," he says. "Your undergrad studies are going to be the same as if you were going to medical school, and to get through that, you need a strong background in math and science."

To be a successful podiatrist, you should

- Enjoy working with people
- Have good manual dexterity
- Be caring and understanding of others
- Be self-motivated and confident in making decisions
- Have an aptitude for both science and business

education

High School

High school students who are considering a career in podiatry should have many natural science courses in their curriculum. Any courses that teach the workings of the human body, such as biology, physiology, and anatomy, will be especially helpful, both in college courses and in practice. Chemistry and physics are also helpful courses to take.

Courses that teach basic business skills will help provide the background needed for a podiatrist to run his or her own practice successfully. Among these courses are business math, accounting, computer science, and keyboarding.

Math courses will be important to the prospective podiatrist, both in postsecondary schooling and on the job. Finally, students should emphasize English classes to improve their written and oral communication skills.

Postsecondary Training

After high school, the prospective podiatrist should enroll in a four-year college program leading to a bachelor's degree. The majority of students choose to major in biology, although some major in other physical sciences. In order to be eligible for acceptance into a college of podiatric medicine, a student's undergraduate curriculum must include eight credit hours each of biology, general or inorganic chemistry, organic chemistry, and physics. Six credit hours of English are also required.

In rare cases, a college of podiatric medicine accepts a student who does not have a bachelor's degree, but who has completed at least ninety semester hours of college credit. Over 90 percent of students who enter a college of podiatric medicine do, however, have at least a bachelor's degree.

There are seven colleges of podiatric medicine in the United States; they are located in Florida, California, New York, Ohio, Pennsylvania, Illinois, and Iowa. They each offer a four-year course of study leading to a Doctor of Podiatric Medicine (DPM) degree.

During the first two years in such a program, students spend most of their time in the classroom and laboratory. They take courses in the basic medical sciences, such as anatomy, physiology, microbiology, biochemistry, pharmacology, and pathology. During the third and fourth years, students take clinical courses, such as general diagnosis, therapeutics, surgery, anesthesiology, and operative podiatric medicine. They also gain experience in the clinical sciences by spending time in college or community clinics and accredited hospitals.

certification or licensing

All practicing podiatrists must be licensed in the United States. As part of the licensing requirements for all states, podiatrists must pass a two-part National Board exam. These National Boards are taken during the second and fourth years of podiatric medical school. In addition, most states require written and oral examinations and a postgraduate residency of at least one year prior to licensing.

There are four categories of residencies: Rotating Podiatric Residency, Primary Podiatric Medical Residency, Podiatric Orthopedic Residency, and Podiatric Surgical Residency. There are also extended Podiatric Surgical Residencies, lasting from twenty-four to thirty-six months, for podiatrists who want to learn advanced surgical skills.

Residencies take place in accredited teaching hospitals, where residents from other disciplines may also be training. Rotations during the podiatric residency may include anesthesiology, internal medicine, radiology, general surgery, plastic surgery, orthopedics, emergency room, vascular surgery, biomechanics, and pediatrics.

In order to become certified in one of the three specialty areas of podiatry, a podiatrist must pass additional written and oral examinations and demonstrate experience in his or her specialty area.

scholarships and grants

There are several federal and private loan programs available to students considering a podiatric medical education. Interested students should contact the American Association of Colleges of Podiatric Medicine for information on loan programs; the association's address, phone number, and website are given later in this article, in the section titled "how do I learn more?"

In addition to loans, there may be scholarship or grant money available through private sources, such as community groups, corporations, or churches. Students should check with local libraries for information on scholarship and grant possibilities.

who will hire me?

There are more than 13,000 practicing podiatrists in the United States. Most of them work independently in their own practices. Gerry is no exception; he has been in private practice since he finished his surgical residency.

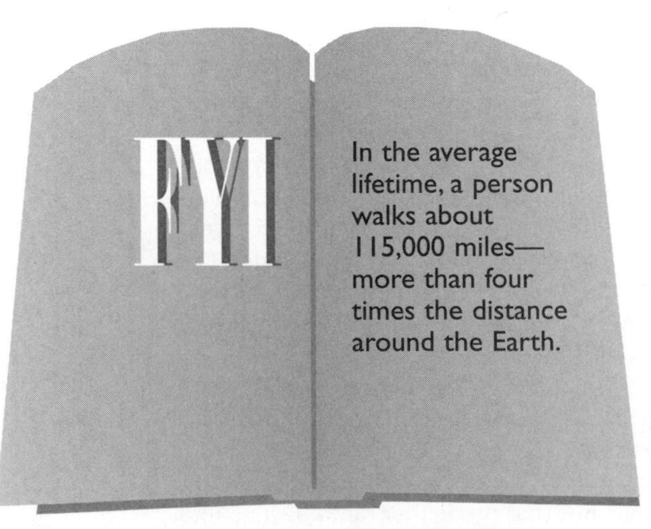

"It is very expensive to set up a practice," he says. "It's going to take anyone who's new three to five years to get established. Anyone who wants a get-rich-quick scheme isn't going to find it here."

Although most podiatrists work as solo practitioners, there are some who join partnerships or multispecialty group practices. Others are employed by hospitals, nursing homes, clinics, health maintenance organizations (HMO's), and public health departments.

Because most of these organizations are unlikely to advertise openings, podiatrists looking for positions should contact them directly. Talking with someone in an organization's personnel office might be a way to begin. In addition, a podiatrist may have made valuable contacts during his or her education and residency. Some of these contacts may be able to offer guidance in the job search or even help locate potential employers.

Podiatrists also work in the Armed Forces, the U.S. Public Health Service, and the Department of Veterans Affairs. The Veterans Omnibus Health Care Act of 1976, which launched an expanded VA podiatric medical program, greatly increased the number of podiatrists in federal service. Podiatrists interested in working for the Department of Veterans Affairs should contact a local VA office for more details.

where can I go from here?

The most common way that podiatrists advance their careers is by pursuing specialization. Gerry is following that path by specializing in surgery. Currently, his goal is to increase the amount of time he spends performing surgeries.

"Right now, I do one whole day of surgery each week," he says. "If that's your interest, then hopefully, you'll start doing a day and a half or two days of surgery. Some who start out doing general podiatric medicine eventually do all surgery." Gerry doesn't want to do surgery exclusively, however. "I'd like to spend maybe 30 percent of my time doing surgery and 70 percent with my patients," he says.

There are other areas of specialization for podiatrists. Some focus on caring for diabetic patients. Others might focus on foot diseases common in children or elderly patients. Still others specialize in sports medicine, treating athletes who have sustained foot or ankle injuries.

A podiatrist can also advance his or her career by becoming a professor at a college of podiatric medicine or the head of a hospital's podiatric department.

what are the salary ranges?

The earnings of podiatrists who work in private practice depend on the location and size of the practice and on the length of time the podiatrist has been in the field.

The average net income for a beginning podiatrist, after practice expenses, is about $35,000 per year. Those who have spent five to ten years in practice might expect to earn $85,000 to $95,000 annually. After fifteen or more years, the average podiatrist's salary is more than $100,000.

Podiatrists who work independently in their own offices must arrange for their own health insurance and retirement planning. Podiatrists who are employed by hospitals, nursing homes, and public health departments are typically provided with benefit packages that include insurance, paid vacations, and pension plans.

what is the job outlook?

Job opportunities in this profession are expected to grow about as fast as the average for all occupations through 2005. This expected growth is due in part to the increasing number of elderly people in our society. Elderly people—after years of standing, walking, and bearing weight on their feet—are especially prone to foot and ankle disorders.

Another reason for the expected growth in podiatry is the increasing number of people who are sustaining injuries related to sports and exercise. As more and more people become exercise-conscious, the number of foot and ankle injuries increase.

Finally, the demand for podiatric services is expected to grow as health insurance coverage for such care becomes more common. Currently, Medicare and private insurance plans often cover acute medical and surgical foot care; increasingly, HMO's and other prepaid plans are providing coverage for routine foot care as well.

Job openings that arise because of podiatrists leaving the field are expected to be relatively few, however. The turnover rate is low in this field.

The number of job opportunities available for a new podiatrist will depend largely upon where he or she hopes to practice. For example, the states containing the seven colleges of podiatric medicine—California, Florida, Illinois, Iowa, New York, Pennsylvania, and Ohio—have few available openings. In the south and southwest, where there is a shortage of such practitioners, the opportunities should be considerably better.

how do I learn more?

professional organizations

Following are organizations that provide information on podiatric careers, accredited schools, and employers.

American Association of Colleges of Podiatric Medicine
1350 Piccard Drive, Suite 322
Rockville, MD 20850
TEL: 800-922-9266
WEBSITE: http://www.aacpm.org

American Podiatric Medical Association
9312 Old Georgetown Road
Bethesda, MD 20814
TEL: 301-571-9200
WEBSITE: http://www.apma.org

bibliography

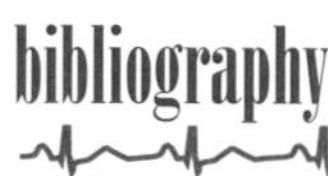

Following is a sampling of materials related to the professional concerns and development of podiatrists.

Books

Aldred, Heather, editor. *Podiatric Care Sourcebook.* Detroit, MI: Omnigraphics, 1997.

Alexander, Ian J. *The Foot: Examination and Diagnosis,* 2nd edition. New York, NY: Churchill Livingstone, 1997.

Harkless, Lawrence B., and Steven M. Krych, editors. *Handbook of Common Foot Problems.* New York, NY: Churchill Livingstone, 1990.

Levy, Leonard A., and Anne K. Thompson, editors. *Podiatric Medical Assisting,* 2nd edition. New York, NY: Churchill Livingstone, 1992.

Robbins, Jeffrey M., editor. *Primary Care Podiatry.* Philadelphia, PA: W.B. Saunders Co., 1994.

Tollafield, David R., and Linda M. Merriman. *Clinical Skills in Treating the Foot.* New York, NY: Churchill Livingstone, 1997.

Periodicals

American Podiatric Medical Association Journal. Monthly. American Podiatric Medical Association, 9312 Old Georgetown Road, Bethesda, MD 20814-1698, 301-571-9200.

Foot and Ankle International. Monthly. Focuses on new approaches to foot and ankle disorders and surgical treatment for orthopedic surgeons and podiatrists. American Orthopaedic Foot and Ankle Society, Inc., Williams & Wilkins, 428 E. Preston Street, Baltimore, MD 21202, 410-528-4000, 800-638-6423.

Foot and Ankle Quarterly. Quarterly. Data Trace Medical Publishers, Inc., 110 West Road, Suite 227, Baltimore, MD 21204, 410-494-4994.

Podiatric Products. Bimonthly. Product news releases and articles related to the profession. Novicom, Inc., 20000 Mariner Avenue, Suite 480, Torrance, CA 90503, 310-793-4138.

psychiatric technician

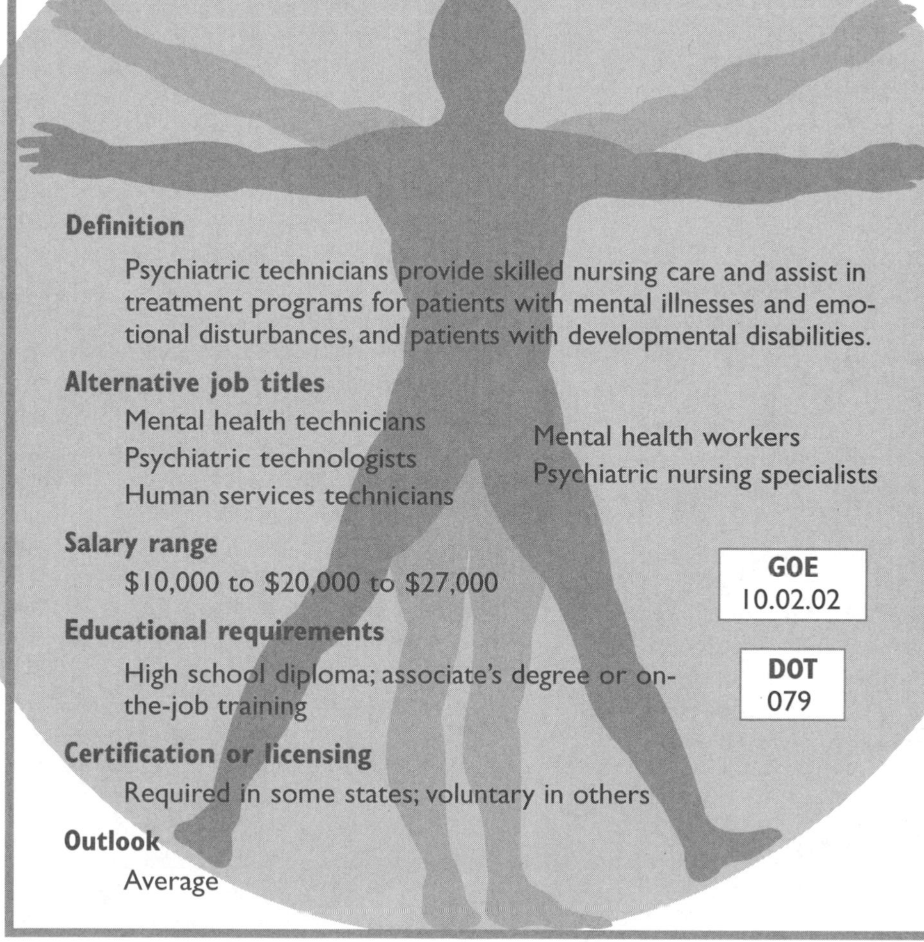

Definition

Psychiatric technicians provide skilled nursing care and assist in treatment programs for patients with mental illnesses and emotional disturbances, and patients with developmental disabilities.

Alternative job titles

Mental health technicians
Psychiatric technologists
Human services technicians
Mental health workers
Psychiatric nursing specialists

Salary range

$10,000 to $20,000 to $27,000

Educational requirements

High school diploma; associate's degree or on-the-job training

Certification or licensing

Required in some states; voluntary in others

Outlook

Average

GOE
10.02.02

DOT
079

High School Subjects

Psychology
Health
Biology
Social sciences
Political science
Mathematics
English
Speech

Personal Interests

Peer counseling
Tutoring
Helping others deal with traumas or emotional issues

A young boy charged through the adolescent psych ward, raging, his words choked in screams and tears. Powerful with fury, he lashed out at the walls with his fists. The boy had just been told he was being discharged from the hospital that day. Sue Jones, a psychiatric technician stood in the same ward with a junior technician.

"Should I take him down?" the junior technician asked Sue.

"No," Sue answered, "He's having a feeling. Let him work it out."

It was a calculated risk.

Sue had worked with the boy. She knew that he came from the streets, out of control, neglected by a mother who sold her body for drugs right in front of him. After four months in the ward, he'd made little progress. But this was only his first time in treatment. Given time . . .

The boy stood there, screaming. The staff moved between him and the other patients, ready to restrain him if he turned violent.

But it was better to do it this way, Sue thought. Let him feel his anger. For the first time in his life he'd found a structured environment, and now they were sending him away. And in this anger, there was hope, a chance to heal.

what does a psychiatric technician do?

People with mental illnesses and emotional disturbances, and those with developmental disabilities, require special care to prevent them from becoming a danger to themselves or others, and require treatment toward the possibility of functioning to the fullest extent possible in mainstream life. Whether in a psychiatric hospital or clinic, a residential halfway house or at a school for the mentally retarded, the health professional with whom these patients most often interact is the *psychiatric technician*.

Psychiatric technicians work intensively with patients in a variety of duties, including participating in prescribed treatment programs, such as group therapy, administering oral and hypodermic medications; and taking basic health measurements, such as blood pressure and temperature readings. Psychiatric technicians are also responsible for maintaining patient hygiene and assisting in other routine activities, including feeding and bathing patients and keeping their clothing and living areas clean; when possible, the psychiatric technician encourages and trains patients to perform these activities for themselves.

One of the most important roles of the psychiatric technician is to observe patients and to provide written and oral reports on their observations to the patients' medical and psychiatric physicians. A psychiatric technician spends a great deal of time with patients, speaking with them, playing cards, chess and other games with them, and escorting patients to medical appointments, church services, or to movies, museums, sports events, and other trips. The psychiatric technician also facilitates patient-to-patient interaction, encouraging them to participate in social and recreational activities, as a means of promoting the rehabilitative process. By developing a relationship with patients, psychiatric technicians provide regularity and trust in a structured environment, which may be beneficial and necessary to the patient's progress.

Under the supervision of psychiatrists, psychologists, and other mental health professionals, the psychiatric technician participates in the planning of treatment strategies, and is chiefly responsible for their implementation. Activities may include physical and mental rehabilitation exercises in recreational and occupational settings designed to build social and mental skills, modify behavior, and to encourage a sense of personal responsibility and confidence often lacking in psychiatric patients.

Because of their direct association with patients, psychiatric technicians are an important component of the psychiatric team. Their observations provide insight into the effectiveness of treatment strategies, so that each patient will receive the most appropriate care possible. Close contact with a patient also allows the psy-

lingo to learn

Neurosis A mental and emotional disorder that affects only part of the personality. A neurosis does not disturb the use of language, and is accompanied by various physical, physiological, and mental disturbances, the most usual being anxieties or phobias.

Obsessive-compulsive A neurosis that results in the patient's compulsion to carry out certain acts, no matter how odd or illogical or repetitive they are. This sort of neurosis is evident once the obsession or compulsive act interferes with normal life. For example, a person obsessed with cleanliness might take a dozen or more showers a day.

Paranoid schizophrenic The most common and destructive of the psychotic disorders, characterized by departure from reality, inability to think clearly, difficulty feeling and expressing emotions, and a retreat into a fantasy life.

Psychosis A more complete disintegration of personality and a loss of contact with the outside world than with neuroses.

Phobias Irrational or overblown fears that prevent a person from living a normal life.

chiatric technician an important awareness into the patient's behavior and state of mind, allowing the psychiatric staff to recognize times of stress, and possible harmful behavior. Timely intervention may prevent the patient from becoming a danger to himself or others.

Psychiatric technicians may also be responsible for maintaining contact with the patient's family, arranging family meetings, and conducting initial admission interviews and psychological testing. In a hospital setting, psychiatric technicians become involved in every part of their patients' lives. In other settings, such as clinics, halfway houses, and day centers, the psychiatric technician sees many patients who have left the hospital and are making the transition to everyday life. These patients require special attention from the psychiatric technician who, while working with families, government services, and other mental health agencies, will help to coordinate the many realities of life, such as housing, finance, and employment. The psychiatric technician will also establish continuing psychiatric and medical treatment.

Community mental health is another area that employs psychiatric technicians. In this particular setting, patients generally do not require hospitalization, but nonetheless need help in dealing with such problems as drug and alcohol abuse. Sometimes called *human services technicians,* the patients of these psychiatric technicians may also include the elderly, victims of spousal and sexual abuse, and clients of social welfare programs, child care centers, vocational rehabilitation workshops, and schools for people with learning disabilities and emotional and mental handicaps. Psychiatric technicians may also receive specialized training to work with the mentally disabled.

what is it like to be a psychiatric technician?

Sue Jones has been a psychiatric technician for five and a half years. She is a senior member of the nursing staff, working with adolescent inpatients at a private psychiatric hospital in New Hampshire. "The unit I work on is very violent at times. But not all are like that. It's quieter to work with adults, because many of them have been in the system a long time, and they're often depressed," Sue Jones says. "I prefer to work with adolescents because you seem to have more of a chance to help them. There's still a chance to get them out of the system and back into normal life."

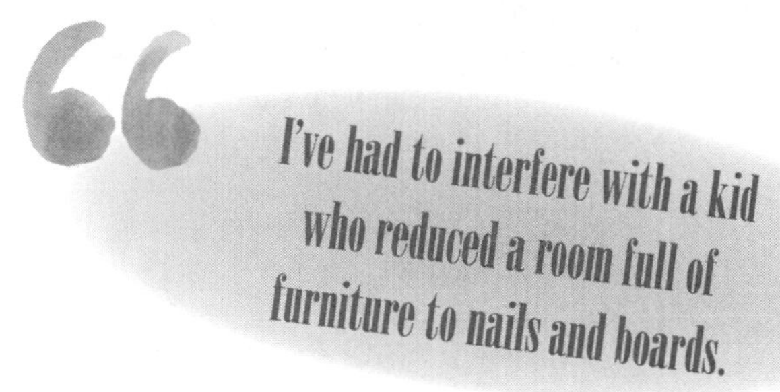

Typically, there are thirty patients in Sue's unit, ranging in age from twelve to seventeen, with varying degrees of emotional and mental disabilities, and with varying levels of functional ability. Assigned to this unit are ten or more staff, including nurses, psychiatric aides, and psychiatric technicians. The high ratio of staff to patients allows intensive supervision, observation, and interaction, which are key elements to psychiatric treatment.

"We keep patients on a highly structured schedule, from the moment they wake up to the time they go to sleep," Sue explains. "Their day begins at 8:00 AM, when they're expected to have prepared their rooms, made their beds, cleaned, showered and dressed. We call this 'milieu' therapy, which is an important part of their treatment. By holding them responsible for their own behavior, we encourage them to function at the highest level possible for them."

Patients are divided into two groups, according to their functional level. Throughout the day, Sue and the other psychiatric staff lead patients through a variety of group and individual activities, each designed to coordinate therapeutic and rehabilitative skills that may allow the patient to leave the hospital setting and return to the community. The typical day for these patients includes group therapy and individual counseling sessions, schooling, group and individual activities, and therapies such as art therapy. Sue also leads "life school" classes, in which patients are exposed to and taught skills they will need in the community, such as handling money, grocery shopping, and other facets of everyday life. Decreasing the stress of these activities may be an important factor in a patient's successful return to the community.

As a senior member of the staff, and because she is continuing her studies, Sue is considered a psychology intern. As such, she leads group counseling sessions under the supervision of a staff psychologist. "By talking about their problems, patients can help each other feel better. In group, they can talk through their problems, and maybe learn to avoid the behavior that brought them here in the first place."

Sue is also responsible, along with the other members of the staff, for maintaining a safe environment in her unit. "Things can get physical two or three times a shift," Sue says. "Often, I eat lunch on the fly. If there's a crisis, for example, if one of the patients begins to attack someone on the staff, or themselves, or one of the other patients, I have to be ready to help intervene. But a big part of my job is observing my patients, recognizing when things are going badly for them, figuring out where they are in an emotional cycle and at what point to intervene. I try to get to them before they turn violent, to talk it through, and help them resolve an emotional crisis themselves."

"It's part of what we call MAP, or Managing Aggressive Patients. By first recognizing anxiety and working with patients to create an alliance, we assist them in verbalizing their conflict instead of acting it out," Sue explains.

Although her work is stressful,Sue finds being a psychiatric technician very rewarding. "For me, it's exciting watching these kids grow, seeing the things that happen in the course of the day that make them feel better or worse about themselves. Although I've had many traumatic experiences here, I do have the reward of seeing a few people heal."

have I got what it takes to be a psychiatric technician?

Psychiatric technicians work with people who, because of their illnesses, may exhibit extreme forms of behavior. Often they may be unpleasant or disagreeable to work with, or even abusive to themselves and others. The job of psychiatric technicians requires them to work closely with these patients; compassion, sensitivity, and a strong motivation to help others are necessities. Sue Jones agrees. "I really care for my patients, and I love the work I do. It's very hard work, and I had to grow a lot to do it."

Patience is often required on the job, especially with patients whose disabilities allow for only slow, often insubstantial, improvement. What may outwardly appear to be a minor event may, for these patients, be a major moment of progress. Through encouragement, empathy, and an awareness of the patient's condition, the psychiatric technician is instrumental in motivating patients to reach these accomplishments and encouraging them to continue. A keen sense of observation allows the psychiatric technician not only to recognize times of stress in the patient, but to recognize the activities, events, and situations that bring progress to the patient's condition, and to build on them. Being able to relate to their patients and to present their observations to the patients' psychiatric and medical doctors, allows the psychiatric technician to function as an important bridge in the therapeutic process.

This field also requires physical prowess, if not strength. Restraining individuals who become violent can be a traumatic experience. "I've had to rescue one boy who tried to hang himself. Another girl tied her neck off with a strip of cloth she tore off her shirt. I've also had to interfere with a kid who reduced a room full of furniture to nails and boards," Sue says. "We diffuse situations like that as a team. We also process and debrief traumatic events as a team, and we'll discuss them informally with each other, too. Some of us have also had individual sessions to overcome traumatic events." But, at 5' 6'' and 125 pounds, Sue says that she is stronger than she looks. "I'm very active physically, anyway, and I've developed physically as a result of the job. And I know what I'm doing—I know when to ask for help. I would say that my strength is as much in my honesty and consistency as in my physical preparedness. I don't hesitate. And I don't bargain."

Sue finds the work very challenging. But there are frustrations too, Sue says. "Before we dispose—that is, transfer a patient to another facility—sometimes, the best we're able to achieve is to function as a sort of bandage. We have to work within the patient's insurance requirements," she explains, "which often means we can only provide the lowest level of care. Their insurance won't pay for anything more."

Sue's work as a psychiatric technician is never boring. "There's never a dull moment. I go in each morning knowing that I have to deal with what happens or has happened in the shift before, and that I will deal with it no matter what. I've amazed myself by doing this. I do what has to be done. It's the ultimate internship, and I have very little fear about the work I do."

how do I become a psychiatric technician?

The educational requirements for becoming a psychiatric technician can vary widely from state to state and from facility to facility. In some cases, no specialized schooling is required, and training is given on the job. Elsewhere, a psychiatric technician may be required to have a two-year associate's degree or even a four-year bachelor's degree from a psychiatric technician program. These schools will also feature clinical field work, in which a student participates in on- the-job training at a variety of facilities requiring psychiatric technicians. Sue Jones, for example, has continued her studies while working, and expects to receive her bachelor's degree shortly. "It's because I'm still studying that I've received more and more responsibilities, and now I'm considered one of the senior staff in my unit," Sue says.

To be a successful psychiatric technician, you should

- Be patient, compassionate, and mature, with a strong sense of responsibility
- Enjoy working with and relate well to people
- Be motivated to help others achieve their highest potential
- Be observant and articulate
- Be in good physical condition

education

High School

Students considering this field should plan to continue their education in either a two-year or four-year academic program. This will allow them greater growth in the field, increasing their responsibilities as they gain experience, with corresponding increases in pay. While in high school, students should focus on courses in psychology, if available, and biology, as well as mathematics and other science-related subjects. Developing good communication skills is important, too, so taking English and other courses that will build strong written and verbal skills is highly recommended. Because a psychiatric technician becomes intimately involved in the lives of his or her patients, subjects that prepare you for human interaction, such as social sciences courses, peer counseling, and tutoring programs, will also be an asset as you begin your career.

"Looking back," Sue reflects, sighing, "I wish I had concentrated more on biology, because that is the basis of much of psychiatric work. But one course I had in high school really helped—government. We're part of a system here, and it's helped me to understand why certain things like the insurance system are the way they are. And I deal with a lot of governmental agencies on behalf of my patients. I think it's important to understand the structure of our society."

Postsecondary Training

For those students pursuing postsecondary education as a psychiatric technician, two-year programs leading to an associate's degree, and four-year programs leading to a bachelor's degree, will usually include courses in human development, personality structure, and the nature of mental illness; anatomy, physiology, and basic medical science; and training in nursing techniques. Social science courses give the prospective psychiatric technician understanding into family and community relationships, and programs will also offer an overview of the mental health and medical system.

An important element of all programs is the practical and clinical phase of study, in which students will receive training and experience in the actual work of psychiatric technicians. Student's field experience may comprise as much as one-third of their study program.

Other postsecondary courses a psychiatric technician can expect to take include English, psychology, and sociology, and mental health-related courses including early childhood development, general and abnormal psychology, classes in family and social welfare institutions, psychopathology, general nursing, community mental health, and techniques of therapy.

Apart from field experience, many programs will offer training in interviewing and observation skills. Students may be trained in recognizing meanings behind certain tones of voice, ways of speaking and behaving, and in what people say and do. Because psychiatric technicians often administer psychological tests, students may also be trained in the proper administration of such tests, which are often in the form of questionnaires and have been designed to give health professionals insight into a patient's state of mind. Psychiatric technician students will also receive training in crisis intervention, group counseling, behavior modification, child guidance, and family therapy, as well as training in consulting and working with the variety of agencies, both public and private, concerned with mental health and the public welfare.

Prospective psychiatric technicians may also enter the field through military service. Military personnel may request secondary schooling as a Hospital Corpsman, and choose to specialize as a psychiatric technician. The Navy, for example, offers a fifteen-week general course at a Hospital Corpsman school, followed by two six-week training periods in psychiatric technology. The first of these periods features classwork; the second period is the clinical phase.

certification or licensing

Several states require that psychiatric technicians receive at least a two-year program in psychiatric technology at a state-approved training facility. Graduates of these programs are then expected to pass a state-administered certification test to achieve licensed status as a psychiatric technician. Certification in other states is voluntary. You will need to check the requirements for the state in which you intend to practice.

The AAPT offers four levels of national certification. According to the AAPT, first level certification is achieved by passing a comprehensive test, but requires no postsecondary training or practical experience. Level II requires thirty hours of college course work and one year of practical experience; level III requires sixty college course credits, or an associate's degree, and two years of field experience. Level IV certification is available to psychiatric technicians with at least three years of experience and a bachelor's degree in psychiatric technology or a related psychology major. AAPT certification at any level may be helpful in entering the field, and in increasing responsibility and salary levels.

internships and volunteerships

It is possible to find work in the field during high school, either part time or during the summer. Students may apply for positions as psychiatric aides or trainees, or find work in housekeeping, maintenance, or administrative positions, or as orderlies. These positions generally do not require formal education or training, and are an excellent opportunity for gaining experience and insight into the field.

Prospective psychiatric technicians may also gain practical experience by applying for jobs as a nurse's aide at a local hospital or clinic, or participating in volunteer programs related to this field. Many schools also offer peer counseling experience, and schools with developmentally delayed students may have need of student volunteers or tutors. This kind of work will help you decide if the field is right for you.

In addition, offering to help in local mental health and community service organizations, or job experiences in playgrounds, swimming pools, and summer camps, are all ways a prospective psychiatric technician can gain both experience and insight into the field and the nature of the work involved.

Students interested in these opportunities should talk to their school guidance counselor, or contact local hospitals and mental health clinics.

who will hire me?

Apart from state mental institutions and private psychiatric hospitals and clinics, there are a great many facilities that have need of skilled psychiatric technicians. For example, nursing homes, family service centers, public housing programs, public schools, prisons and courts-of-law are all places that employ psychiatric technicians.

A growing number of psychiatric technicians are finding employment in the community, rather than in the hospital setting. The trend is toward treating psychiatric patients in the home or school, allowing them to continue to be a part of the community. A psychiatric technician may work in the school, itself, or participate in half-day programs where patients can receive therapy and specialized attention without disrupting their daily life. Psychiatric technicians specializing in patients with developmental disabilities may find employment in training centers devoted to teaching these patients job and life skills.

In addition, a growing number of psychiatric technicians are working as part of privately funded "family stabilization teams." Much like social workers, these psychiatric technicians are assigned to specific patients and the family, and are available to intervene in periods of difficulty

Advancement Possibilities

Senior psychiatric technicians supervise and instruct junior psychiatric technicians, help coordinate schedules, and serve as the liaison between management and the technicians.

Psychiatric technician instructors work in hospitals and at technical schools to train psychiatric technicians according to the different levels. They may also teach certification courses, voluntary or otherwise.

Psychologists teach, counsel, and work in research and administration to help understand people, their capacities, traits, and behavior and to explain their needs. They normally hold doctorates in psychology, but they are not medical doctors and cannot prescribe medication.

Psychiatrists are physicians who treat patients with mental, emotional, and behavioral symptoms. They have completed all of the training required to become licensed medical doctors (M.D.s) and then have taken additional training to specialize in psychiatry.

or crisis, working with the entire family to resolve personal relationship issues, coordinate their access to community support services, such as welfare, medical treatment, and housing, and helping to resolve financial and legal issues. This work involves visiting patients in their own homes and communities, where living and social conditions may vary widely. Many members of family stabilization teams are required to carry beepers and to be on call twenty-four hours a day. Their intervention can often make a great difference in resolving a situation before it reaches a crisis point.

where can I go from here?

For Sue Jones, her work is a part of a career path that will eventually result in her receiving a Ph.D. in clinical psychology. "Although, looking back on it," she says, "if I had started early enough, I would have gone to medical school to become a psychiatrist."

Apart from gaining practical experience that will help in future studies, many aspiring psychologists and senior nursing staff find that their work as a psychiatric technician combines well with continued educational efforts, allowing them an opportunity to study, as well as to see in practice many of the theoretical concepts included in their classwork. This is especially true of those psychiatric technicians who work on the night shift, when most patients are asleep.

For psychiatric technicians, the increase in experience will lead to increased responsibilities, and increased pay. With the proper experience, a psychiatric technician can also achieve positions with supervisory duties.

In general, continuing educational growth will greatly expand a psychiatric technician's advancement opportunities. A psychiatric technician may choose to enter other specialties in the psychiatric field, which may require more specialized training. With experience, education or additional training, psychiatric technicians may also choose to become instructors for other psychiatric technicians.

what are the salary ranges?

The salary of a psychiatric technician can vary enormously, from a minimum wage, or less than $10,000 per year, to $20,000 and as much as $27,000 per year. Salary depends on a variety of factors, including geographical location, the type of facility, and the level or education and experience. Technicians employed in the community generally receive higher pay than those in institutional settings.

Most psychiatric technicians work a forty-hour week, which may include at least one weekend shift. Many psychiatric facilities require trained staff twenty-four hours a day, and psychiatric technicians may have their choice of day, evening, night, or weekend shifts. Fringe benefits often include health insurance, paid sick days, and paid vacations. Some state institutions and agencies may also grant financial assistance for continuing study.

what is the job outlook?

The outlook for psychiatric technician positions is expected to grow as fast as the average for other professions into the next century. The need for trained psychiatric support staff will grow because of the recent trend toward community-based mental health services. As more facilities are created, they will require more and more psychiatric technicians to staff them. Legislation requiring public school systems to include students with developmental, emotional, and neurological disabilities also requires the addition of psychiatric technicians to the educational staff. Many schools are also recognizing the need for trained psychiatric personnel for the general student population as well.

An additional need for psychiatric technicians will result from the nation's aging and elderly. More positions will be created for psychiatric technicians specialized in care for the elderly. The advancement in technology that allows more disabled infants to survive will also require the services of trained personnel to work with these children in order to help them develop to their fullest capabilities.

Finally, rising health care costs will encourage facilities to employ technicians and other paraprofessionals to take over some responsibilities and functions of higher-paid professionals. Concerns with the cost of welfare and other social service programs will generate positions for technicians who will be able to help their clients resolve personal, social, and financial issues and reduce their dependence on public support services.

how do I learn more?

professional organizations

Following are organizations that provide information on psychiatric technician careers, accredited schools, scholarships, and employers.

American Association of Psychiatric Technicians
1789 North Neltnor Blvd.
Suite 260
West Chicago, IL 60185
TEL: 800-391-7589
WEBSITE: http://www.niia.net/~aapt

American Psychiatric Association
1400 K Street NW
Washington, DC 20005
TEL: 202-682-6000
WEBSITE: http://www.psych.org

American Association of Psychiatric Services for Children
1200-C Scottsville Road
Suite 225
Rochester, NY 14624
TEL: 716-235-6910

bibliography

Following is a sampling of materials relating to the professional concerns and development of psychiatric technicians.

Books

Elliott, Gloria. *Nursing Attendants: Your Role Working in Psychiatry*. Bronx, NY: Good Sign, 1994.

Lazarus, Arthur, editor. *Career Pathways in Psychiatry: Transition in Changing Times*. Hillsdale, NJ: Analytic Press, 1996.

Periodicals

Psychiatric News. Semimonthly. General publication concerning all aspects of psychiatry. American Psychiatric Press, Inc., 1400 K Street NW, Suite 1101, Washington, DC 20005, 202-685-6250.

Psychiatric Times. Monthly. Magazine covering general topics of American psychiatry. CME, Inc., 1924 East Deere Avenue, Santa Ana, CA 92680, 714-250-1008.

psychiatrist

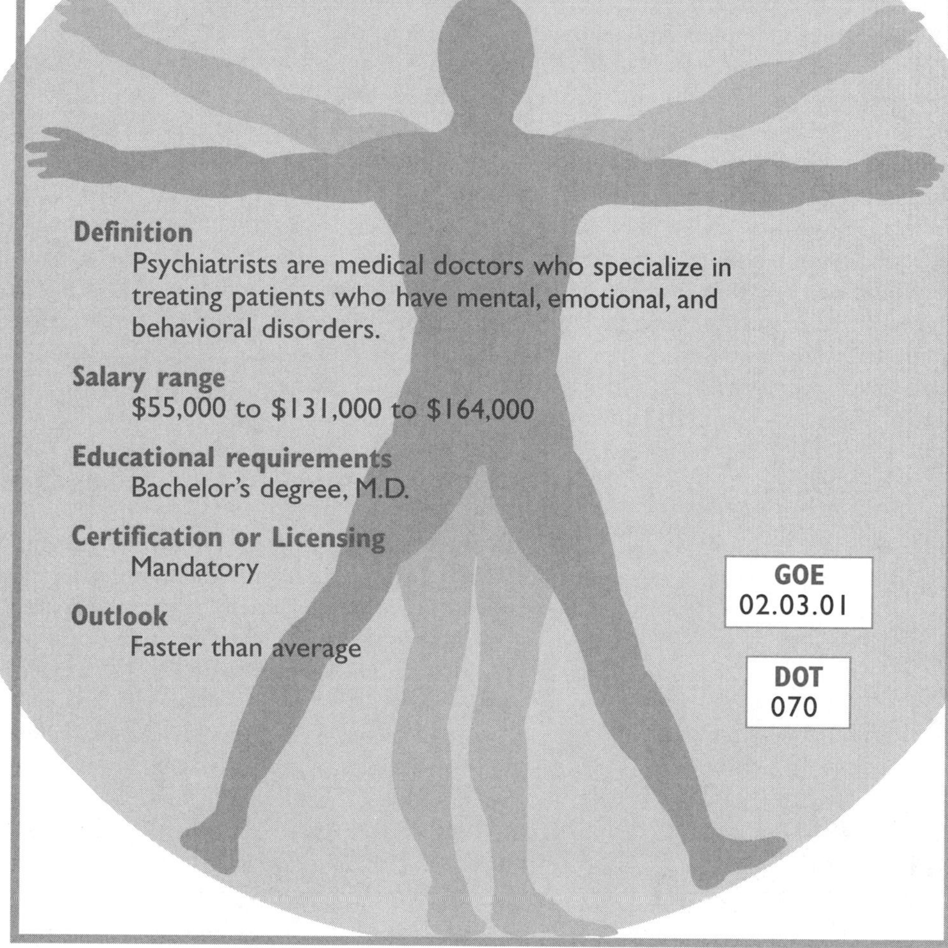

Definition
Psychiatrists are medical doctors who specialize in treating patients who have mental, emotional, and behavioral disorders.

Salary range
$55,000 to $131,000 to $164,000

Educational requirements
Bachelor's degree, M.D.

Certification or Licensing
Mandatory

Outlook
Faster than average

GOE
02.03.01

DOT
070

High School Subjects

Biology
Chemistry
Mathematics
Psychology

Personal Interests

Science
Medicine
Meeting a challenge
Helping people

Fidgeting uneasily in her chair in the patient lounge, Cheryl Vanden waits for Dr. Kane, her psychiatrist, to say something. Sunlight streams through the broad wall of windows. Sitting on the couch next to Cheryl, Dr. Jenny Kane looks over the notes she took during yesterday's session.

Cheryl is suffering from a depression severe enough to provoke a series of suicide attempts. She was admitted to the hospital four days ago, after overdosing on prescription painkillers. Although not antagonistic, she is very reluctant to talk about herself, and Dr. Kane has made little headway.

"Cheryl, this morning in group [therapy], you seemed very distressed when John talked about parents," Dr. Kane notes. After receiving no response, she continues. "Did you feel distressed by that?"

Cheryl picks at a fingernail, looks away. "I don't know," she finally says.

what does a psychiatrist do?

Just as cardiologists specialize in treating heart diseases and neurologists specialize in treating disorders of the brain and nervous system, *psychiatrists* specialize in treating mental and emotional disorders.

Psychiatrists treat patients whose emotional problems make it hard for them to function in society. These problems might stem from fairly common ailments—anxiety, stress, eating disorders, or addiction to drugs and alcohol—or less common disorders, such as schizophrenia or manic depression.

Doctors of psychiatry may work in private practice or for a private hospital. They also work in state mental hospitals, medical schools, community mental health centers, and in government agencies. Many psychiatrists combine a private practice with work in a clinic, hospital, or medical school.

Psychiatrists first evaluate their patients by examining them physically, talking with them about their problem or problems, and asking them questions designed to provide diagnostic information. They may order laboratory tests and X rays. If a patient's problem appears to be caused by a physical condition, the psychiatrist may refer the patient to another specialist, such as a neurologist, for treatment.

Once the doctor has obtained patient information, he or she sets up an appropriate treatment plan. The method of treatment depends upon the type of illness and the needs of the patient. Psychiatrists may prescribe medications, such as tranquilizers or antidepressants, which affect the patient's feelings and/or behavior.

They may also use psychotherapy. Psychotherapy is sometimes called "talking therapy." The psychiatrist spends several sessions talking with the patient to help him or her overcome emotional pain. By listening, asking questions, and pointing out important points, the doctor guides the patient through an exploration and interpretation of the feelings at the core of his or her problem. This type of therapy may be given to an individual in a one-on-one setting. It can also be used in groups of patients. It is often used with families.

Some psychiatrists use other forms of therapy. *Behavior therapists* use specific techniques to help patients learn how to change troublesome behaviors. These techniques might include the use of rewards or deterrents to bring about or eliminate behaviors. Some behavior therapists use meditation, biofeedback, and relaxation training to help their patients.

Psychiatrists try to help their patients uncover, understand, and deal with subconscious memories and emotions. They do this by encouraging the patient to express random thoughts, or "free associate." They may also analyze their patients' dreams for clues to the subconscious mind.

Some psychiatrists focus on a particular type of patient. *Child psychiatrists* work specifically with children and their parents. *Geriatric psychiatrists* work with elderly patients. *Industrial psychiatrists* are employed by companies to deal with employee problems that may affect their job performance, such as alcoholism or absenteeism.

lingo to learn

Psychotherapy The treatment of mental disorders by psychological, rather than physical, means.

Psychoanalysis A method of treating mental disorders by bringing unconscious fears and conflicts into the conscious mind.

Psychosomatic A physical illness caused or aggravated by a mental condition.

Neurosis An emotional disorder that arises due to unresolved conflicts, with anxiety often being the main characteristic.

Psychosis A major mental disorder, in which the personality is seriously disorganized and contact with reality is impaired.

Biofeedback The technique of making unconscious or involuntary bodily processes (such as heartbeats or brain waves) perceptible to the senses (through the use of an electronic monitoring device) in order to manipulate them by conscious mental control.

Phobia An obsessive, persistent, unrealistic fear of an object or situation.

Forensic psychiatrists combine a knowledge of law with a knowledge of psychiatry. They evaluate defendants and testify in court on their mental states. They may help determine whether defendants understand the charges brought against them, and whether they are able to help in their own defense.

Psychiatrists may also serve as mental health consultants to schools, day-care centers, and senior citizen's groups. In addition, they may work with courts, probation officers, police departments, and other community agencies.

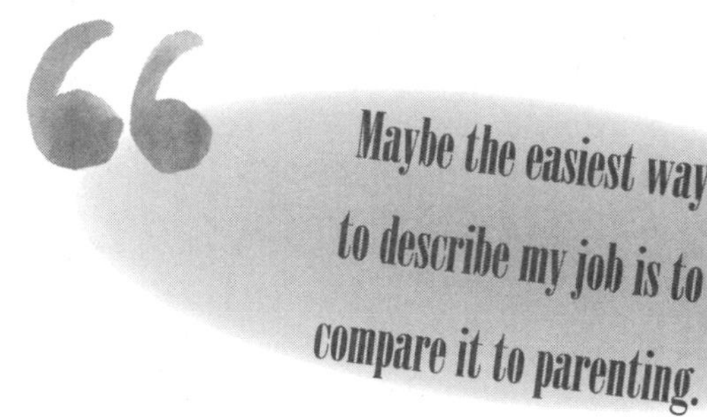

what is it like to be a psychiatrist?

Dr. Jenny Kane oversees the stress-care ward in the psychiatric unit of a hospital. Her ward is one of five in the unit; others include the crisis-care ward for patients who are extremely agitated; the med/psych ward for psychiatric patients who also require extensive medical treatment; the chemical dependency ward; and the adolescent ward.

Dr. Kane's ward usually houses twenty-three to twenty-four patients with disorders that vary in type and degree of severity. She is fully responsible for their psychiatric care during their stay on the ward.

"Maybe the easiest way to describe my job is to compare it to parenting," she says. "Whatever and whenever a patient needs me, it's my job to be there—or at least to make arrangements to have them taken care of."

For her, this means being on call practically all the time. "I can have another physician cover my ward for me, yes," Dr. Kane says. "But it's not uncommon for a patient to want to talk to me specifically. The patients on this ward are usually in very precarious mental health, and they sometimes really need stability and continuity." Because of this, even when another doctor is covering her ward, Dr. Kane remains available to answer questions or talk with patients.

The nature of her position also means that she does not have a set work schedule. She often spends time on the ward on Saturdays and Sundays. It's also not unusual for her to stop by in the evenings to check on patients. And, of course, she might be called in at any time if a patient is having a crisis severe enough to require her presence.

On an average weekday, Dr. Kane arrives on the ward between 7:00 and 8:00 in the morning. The first thing she does is make rounds. This involves talking with each patient and reviewing his or her chart to see what, if anything, occurred during the night.

Each patient is different, says Dr. Kane, so the nature of treatment is different. Most often, however, a patient's treatment involves some combination of psychotherapy and medication. "These days, medication is a very strong component of psychiatric care," she says. Dr. Kane is responsible for prescribing medication and for monitoring its level and effect on the patient.

Treatment also involves psychotherapy, or talking with the patients to help them work through their problems. This is done both one-on-one with individual patients, and in group sessions. Dr. Kane conducts four group sessions each week. The patients in the group are assigned to sessions that are appropriate to their problems. For example, one group session might focus on addictive tendencies, another on dealing with stress and anxiety.

While all patients on her ward are psychiatric patients, many of them have minor physical disorders as well. "For example, yesterday we admitted a patient who was diabetic. As her mental condition had worsened, she'd stopped taking her insulin and her blood sugar was way too high," Dr. Kane said. "Other times, patients come in off the streets. They may have frostbite, if it's in the winter. They may have infections because they haven't been capable of taking care of themselves."

Dr. Kane treats her patients' physical ailments as well. "I treat anything that a family practitioner would treat," she says. "If it's necessary, I call in a specialist."

In addition to dealing directly with patients, Dr. Kane also spends a considerable amount of time in various types of meetings.

The ward staff meets every morning to review patient cases.

"At least three to four times a week, we have treatment planning meetings," she says. "These meetings are multidisciplinary, so anyone who is involved with treating the patient is in attendance." This could include medical specialists, therapists, nurses, and representatives from outside agencies.

Dr. Kane also meets periodically with patients' families and with community mental health agencies to ensure that patients being released from the hospital will continue to receive the necessary care.

Another part of Dr. Kane's job is dealing with the justice system. She, along with the other hospital psychiatrists, treat inmates of the county jail. They may also be called upon to testify in competency or commitment hearings in court regarding the mental state of patients.

have I got what it takes to be a psychiatrist?

Not all psychiatrists' schedules are as irregular as Dr. Kane's. She is quick to point out that those doctors who work in a private practice usually set their own office hours. Although they may occasionally get phone calls at odd hours or see some patients on weekends or evenings, for the most part their schedules are more routine than hers.

Whatever type of practice they are in, however, psychiatrists must realize that they have a certain responsibility to their patients. "Some patients come to rely very heavily on their psychiatrists," says Dr. Kane. "And when you're dealing with emotionally and mentally fragile people, you must take that reliance very seriously."

Part of a psychiatrist's ability to form relationships with patients is his or her compassion for them. "You must be able to empathize with them, you must have a desire to help them," says Dr. Kane. "If that is lacking, I would imagine that you'd be constantly frustrated in your patient dealings."

To balance that empathy, however, a certain amount of detachment is needed. While the psychiatrist should have compassion for patients, he or she must not become emotionally involved with them. "It's sometimes very difficult not to become emotionally tangled up with the patients you care for," says Dr. Kane. "You grow to know them, you grow to care for them. But getting too involved can ultimately be hard on you emotionally. And it can get in the way of effective treatment as well."

Psychiatrists need to be good listeners and good interpreters. They need to be aware of what patients mean as well as what they say. An inquiring mind and good analytical skills are also important.

Finally, they should be emotionally stable themselves in order to deal with their patients, some of whom may be extremely depressed, hostile, or defensive. "Working with emotional disturbances on a daily basis can be draining and exhausting—even discouraging," says Dr. Kane. "Of course, the flip side is when you see people improve, when you know without a doubt that you've helped them. That's a real high."

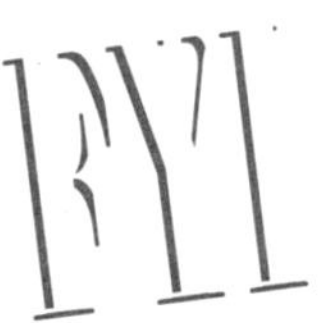

While in the past, emotional and mental disorders were often viewed with shame, society today is generally more enlightened. It is a commonly held view that emotional problems are medical problems, and should be treated as such.

how do I become a psychiatrist?

education

High School

High school students who want to become psychiatrists can begin early to tailor their course work. While psychology classes are an obvious and natural choice, students must remember that they are, first and foremost, aiming for admission into medical school.

A well-rounded college preparatory curriculum should include courses in English, natural and physical sciences, math, social studies, and a foreign language.

It will be particularly helpful for prospective psychiatrists to take as many science classes as possible. Biology, chemistry, physiology, physics, and, of course, psychology are all excellent choices.

The ability to comprehend quickly and communicate well is extremely important to being a successful psychiatrist. Advanced English classes and speech classes both offer good ways to develop and refine comprehension and communication skills.

In addition to making wise curriculum choices, there are other ways for high school students to explore their aptitude for a career in psychiatry. A summer job or volunteer work at a hospital might provide a taste of what a medical profession is like. It may even be possible to work or volunteer at a psychiatric hospital or community mental health clinic.

To be a successful psychiatrist you should

- Be able to analyze human behavior
- Have compassion, yet be able to be objective
- Be a good listener and a good communicator
- Be able to form positive relationships

Postsecondary Training

After high school, it takes between twelve and fourteen years of schooling and training to become a psychiatrist. These include four years of undergraduate school, four years of medical school, and three to four years of postgraduate residency training.

The first phase, undergraduate work, consists of four years of basic liberal arts classes. Most students who hope to attend medical school focus on science and math classes, often majoring in biology or chemistry. For a prospective psychiatrist, a concentration on psychology classes is also appropriate. In addition to these subjects, undergraduate students will take classes in English, arts and humanities, a foreign language, and social studies.

During their second or third year in college, students should take the Medical College Admission Test (MCAT), which most medical schools require. Medical schools have very high admission standards, so a good score on the MCAT is important, as is a good grade point average. Most medical schools also require letters of reference and a personal interview with applicants.

Medical school consists of four years' advanced training. During the first two years, students take such courses as anatomy, physiology, pharmacology, microbiology, psychology, pathology, medical ethics, and medical law. They learn how to examine patients and take medical histories.

The remaining two years of medical school involve hands-on learning. Students spend time in hospitals and clinics, working with patients under the supervision of practicing physicians. They get experience in various medical specialties, such as family practice, obstetrics and gynecology, pediatrics, internal medicine, surgery, and psychiatry. Upon completion of these four years, students receive their M.D. degrees.

At this point, however, the graduate is trained only in basic medicine, and not prepared to practice psychiatry. For this preparation, a residency is required.

In the first year of residency, the new physician works in several specialties, such as internal medicine, pediatrics, or family practice. The next three years are spent in either a psychiatric hospital or the psychiatric ward of a general hospital, learning how to diagnose and treat various emotional and mental disorders.

Some psychiatrists continue their professional training even beyond the four-year residency period. To become a child psychiatrist, for example, you must complete at least three years in general residency and two years in child psychiatry.

certification or licensing

At an early point in the residency period, all candidates are required to pass a medical licensing examination administered by the board of medical examiners in each state. At the end of an accredited residency training program, physicians must pass certification examinations in their field. The evaluation and examination program is directed by the appropriate specialty board (in this case, psychiatry) of the American Board of Medical Specialties.

scholarships and grants

Scholarships and grants are often available from individual institutions, state agencies, and special-interest organizations. The book *Dollars for College: Medicine, Dentistry, and Related Fields* by Ferguson Publishing Company is an excellent source for this information.

Many students finance their medical education through the Armed Forces Health Professions Scholarship Program. Each branch of the military participates in this program, paying students' tuitions in exchange for military service. Contact your local recruiting office for more information on this program.

The National Health Service Corps Scholarship Program also provides money for students in return for service. Another source for financial aid, scholarship, and grant information is the Association of American Medical Colleges. Remember to request information early for eligibility, application requirements, and deadlines.

Association of American Medical Colleges
2450 N Street, NW
Washington, DC 20037
TEL: 202-828-0400
WEBSITE: http://www.aamc.org
Specific information on financial aid programs can be found at:
WEBSITE: http://www.aamc.org/stuapps/finaid

Ferguson Publishing Company
200 West Madison, Suite 300
Chicago, IL 60606
TEL: 312-580-5480

National Health Services Corps Scholarship Program
U.S. Public Health Service
1010 Wayne Avenue, Suite 240
Silver Spring, MD 20910
TEL: 800-638-0824

who will hire me?

Dr. Kane's first position, which she was recruited for during her residency, was in a private practice. After seven years in private practice, she interviewed with the hospital where she now works.

Employment options for new psychiatrists, include private practice, general hospitals, state and private mental hospitals, medical schools, community mental health centers, and government agencies. Approximately one-half of practicing psychiatrists work in private practice; many others combine a private practice with work in a health care institution or community mental health center.

While still in their residencies, psychiatrists should start considering where they would like to practice. They may find positions through networking with other mental health professionals that they meet during their training. In other cases, the hospitals or agencies where they train may offer them permanent positions.

There are several professional journals for psychiatrists, and they may list job openings in their classified advertising sections. Also, members of the American Psychiatric Association have access to an online Job Bank which lists hundreds of available positions all over the nation.

where can I go from here?

Advancement for most psychiatrists takes the form of increased income. By building a reputation and expanding his or her patient base over time, the psychiatrist earns more money.

Psychiatrists who work in psychiatric hospitals, clinics, and mental health centers may work their way up to administrative positions. Those who go into teaching or research may eventually become department heads.

what are the salary ranges?

The average income for all psychiatrists is $131,300 per year, according to a 1994 survey by the American Medical Association. There are several factors, however, which can influence the level of these doctors' earnings.

Psychiatrists in private practice have higher incomes than those who are salaried employees of a health care institution. Salaried positions pay an average of $119,000, while a doctor in private practice averages $142,000.

Geographic location can also play a part in determining a psychiatrist's income level. Those in the south Atlantic states have the highest earnings—$144,000 on average—while those in New England earn the least—$116,600 on average.

Additionally, the type of institution for which one works is a factor. Psychiatrists working in medical schools start out at approximately $55,000 per year. Those just starting work in clinics, state hospitals, and veterans' hospitals may earn anywhere from $38,000 to $77,000. Experienced psychiatric doctors at these institutions may make between $46,000 and $93,000.

Psychiatrists who are employed by a health care institution are often given a benefits package in addition to their salaries. Benefits commonly include health insurance, paid vacation and holiday time, and a retirement plan of some kind.

what is the job outlook?

Employment opportunities for psychiatrists are expected to be excellent in the near future, both in private practice and in salaried positions. There are currently fewer than 25,000 psychiatrists in the entire United States, and the need exceeds the supply.

One reason for this demand is simply that the population is growing rapidly. The increased number of people leads naturally to the need for more medical care, including psychiatric care. Also, it is becoming increasingly common for people who need psychiatric treatment to actually seek it. As a society, we are becoming more aware of the importance of good mental health.

While in the past emotional and mental disorders were often viewed with shame, today society is more enlightened. It is a commonly held view that emotional problems are medical problems, and should be treated as such. This enlightened viewpoint has encouraged many people to seek psychiatric treatment who might not have otherwise.

Psychiatry itself has made advances which make treatment more effective. Perhaps most significant is the increased use of drugs to treat various forms of mental, emotional, and behavioral disorders. In many instances, pharmaceutical treatments are replacing the more traditional forms of therapy.

Since pharmaceuticals can only be prescribed by a medical doctor, some patients who might otherwise be treated by a counselor or a psychologist are choosing see a psychiatrist instead.

The need for more psychiatrists in the field should promote the need for more teachers of psychiatry at the university level. Finally, these doctors are needed as researchers to investigate the causes of mental illness and continue developing and refining treatments.

how can I learn more?

professional organizations

For additional information on becoming a psychiatrist, contact the following:

American Psychiatric Association
1400 K Street NW
Washington, DC 20005
TEL: 202-682-6000
WEBSITE: http://www.psych.org

American Medical Association
515 North State Street
Chicago, IL 60610
TEL: 312-464-5000
WEBSITE: http://www.ama-assn.org

bibliography

Following is a sampling of materials relating to the professional concerns and development of psychiatrists.

Books

Coles, Robert. *Mind's Eye: a Psychiatrist Looks at His Profession.* Boston, MA: Little, Brown, 1996

Keyes, Fenton. *Opportunities in Psychiatry.* Lincolnwood, IL: VGM Career Horizons, 1994.

Klitzman, Robert. *In a House of Dreams and Glass: Becoming a Psychiatrist.* New York, NY: Ivy Books, 1996.

Lazarus, Arthur, editor. *Career Pathways in Psychiatry: Transition in Changing Times.* Hillside, NJ: Analytic Press, 1996.

Nadelson, Carol C., and Carolyn B. Rabinowitz, editors. *Training Psychiatrists for the '90s: Issues and Recommendations.* Washington, DC: American Psychiatric Press, 1987.

Perry, Philip A. *Opportunities in Mental Health Careers.* Lincolnwood, IL: VGM Career Horizons, 1996.

Sternberg, Robert J. *Career Paths in Psychology: Where Your Degree Can Take You.* Washington, DC: American Psychological Association, 1997.

Periodicals

American Academy of Child and Adolescent Psychiatry Journal. Monthly. Presents original papers in psychiatric research and the treatment of children and adolescents. Williams & Wilkins, 428 E. Preston Street, Baltimore, MD 21202, 410-528-4000, 800-638-6423.

American Journal of Psychiatry. Monthly. Presents clinical research and discussion on current psychiatric issues for psychiatrists and other mental health professionals. American Psychiatric Association, 1400 K Street NW, Washington, DC 20005, 202-682-6020.

Child Psychiatry and Human Development. Quarterly. Serves allied professional groups of specialists in child psychiatry, social science, pediatrics, psychology, and human development. American Association of Psychiatric Services for Children, Human Sciences Press, Inc., 233 Spring Street, New York, NY 10013, 212-620-8000.

Directions in Psychiatry. Biweekly. Publishes scholarly, jargon-free articles on developments in psychiatry. Hatherleigh Company Ltd., 520 E. 51st Street, New York, NY 10022, 212-355-0882, 800-367-2550.

General Hospital Psychiatry: Psychiatry, Medicine, and Primary Care. Bimonthly. Emphasizes a biopsychosocial approach to illness and health, and provides a forum for communication among professionals with clinical, academic, and research interests in psychiatry. Elsevier Science, Inc., 655 Avenue of the Americas, New York, NY 10010, 212-989-5800.

Harvard Review of Psychiatry. Bimonthly. Examines a wide variety of subjects, emphasizing the integration of research findings with clinical care. Articles cover the diagnosis and treatment of a full range of psychiatric disorders. Mosby, Journal Subscription Services, 11830 Westline Industrial Drive, St. Louis, MO 63146-3318, 314-453-4351, 800-325-4177.

International Journal of Psychiatry in Medicine: an International Journal of Medical Psychology and Psychiatry in the General Hospital. Quarterly. Contains articles which apply the methods of psychiatry and psychology to the further understanding of disorders which are primarily psychiatric in nature. Baywood Publishing Co., Inc., 26 Austin Avenue, Box 337, Amityville, NY 11701, 516-691-1270.

Psychiatric Clinics: Annual of Drug Therapy. Annual. Summarizes the year's developments in the pharmaceutical treatment of psychiatric disorder. W.B. Saunders Co., Curtis Center, 3rd Floor, Independence Square West, Philadelphia, PA 19106-3399, 215-258-7800.

Psychiatric News. Biweekly. Delivers current information on everything from legislative activities to the latest developments in the drug and therapy fields. American Psychiatric Association, 1400 K Street NW, Washington, DC 20005, 202-682-6210.

Psychiatric Quarterly. Quarterly. Includes articles on the social, clinical, administrative, legal, political, and ethical aspects of mental illness care. New York School of Psychiatry, Human Sciences Press, Inc., 233 Spring Street, New York, NY 10013-1578, 212-620-8000.

Psychiatry: Interpersonal and Biological Processes. Quarterly. New and controversial issues in psychiatry and related social and biological science disciplines. Washington School of Psychiatry, Guilford Publications, Inc., 72 Spring Street, 4th Floor, New York, NY 10012, 212-431-9800.

psychologist

Definition

Psychologists study human (also sometimes animal) behavior and the mental, social, and biological processes that are involved in behavior. They evaluate and counsel clients, teach, administer programs, and conduct research.

Salary range

$24,000 to $50,000 to $100,000+

Educational requirements

Master's degree required; doctoral degree necessary for employment in most fields of psychology

Certification or Licensing

Mandatory in certain fields of psychology

Outlook

Average

GOE 11.03.01

DOT 045

High School Subjects

English
Science
Mathematics
Psychology

Personal Interests

Curiosity about behavior
Helping people
Doing research

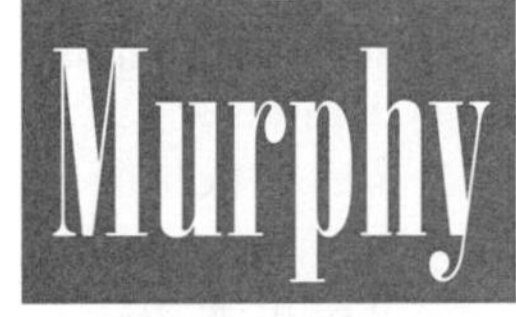

Thomas stepped into the attractive nineteenth-century house in Murfreesboro, Tennessee, that had been converted into an office. He had come in early this morning to work on a report about a murder case.

A clinical psychologist, Murphy began going through his interview notes. For a number of years, he had been doing consulting work in forensic psychology for both civil and criminal cases. The case at hand involved a young man accused of murder whom Murphy had been asked to examine.

The accused's lawyer wanted an expert opinion as to whether the prisoner was competent to stand trial. Or should the lawyer present an insanity defense? It looked like a difficult case.

what does a psychologist do?

Psychology as a scientific discipline has not been in existence for much longer than a century, though, of course, people have been interested in human behavior and mental processes for thousands of years. In the late nineteenth century, the field of psychology developed dramatically under the leadership of such pioneers as Wilhelm Wundt, William James, and Sigmund Freud.

Psychologists are specialists in human behavior. Some focus on research into the mental, social, and biological aspects of behavior, while others apply this knowledge as mental health service providers who work directly with clients. Many psychologists are involved in both research and the treatment of clients.

lingo to learn

Developmental tasks The achievements and skills considered necessary for a person to acquire at each stage of life in order to function well.

Experimental variable A condition or factor that is systematically manipulated by the experimenter in order to observe and assess its influence on behavior.

MMPI Minnesota Multiphasic Personality Inventory—one of the most widely used psychological tests.

Psychoanalysis The method of psychotherapy developed by Sigmund Freud.

Self-image A person's view of himself or herself, which may be quite different from an observer's perception of that person.

Stimulus Any object, action, or situation that causes a person or animal to respond in some way.

Survey research The gathering and assessing of data from large numbers of people by the use of questionnaires and sampling methods.

Transference The client's transferral to the therapist of past emotional attachments to parents or other significant figures.

People often confuse psychologists with psychiatrists. A *psychiatrist* is a medical doctor (M.D.) who specializes in psychology. Psychologists are not medical doctors, although they usually have a doctorate in psychology (a Psy.D.) or philosophy (Ph.D.).

The field of psychology is divided into many specialties (with some overlap in subject matter and methodology), all of which address mind and behavior in some way. Students typically choose their area of specialization early in their graduate school years.

Clinical psychology is the largest single specialty. About 36 percent of psychology doctoral students become clinical psychologists.The *clinical psychologist* works with clients who have mental, emotional, or behavioral disorders. They interview clients and administer diagnostic tests; they also provide psychotherapy sessions, behavior modification programs, and other forms of treatment.

Some clinical psychologists serve as directors of community mental health programs. Some specialize in work with children or the elderly. Other specialists within the clinical psychology field include *neuropsychologists* (who work with people undergoing rehabilitation after strokes or head injuries) and *health and rehabilitation psychologists* (who work with medical and surgical patients in overcoming such problems as chronic pain or illness).

Most clinical psychologists are in individual or group practice. Others work at hospitals, clinics, or universities.

Counseling psychologists work with clients who are usually not mentally ill but have problems dealing with the stresses in their lives, such as family crises, interpersonal conflicts, or vocational decisions. They help people to make decisions and develop better problem-solving skills. Like clinical psychologists, counseling psychologists provide individual, family, and group therapy.

Social psychologists make use of the insights of psychology, psychiatry, sociology, and cultural anthropology to study the different ways individuals and groups influence each other in their interactions. They analyze group structures, attitudes, and leadership patterns.

Developmental psychologists study behavioral and psychological developments from infancy through old age. They seek to identify and explain typical age-related patterns of behavioral and emotional change in the personality as a whole and in specific areas such as language comprehension and moral reasoning. Many developmental psychologists concentrate on research or teaching, but some work in programs for children or the elderly.

School psychologists work with children, teachers, parents, and educational administrators to identify and treat children's learning and behavioral problems. They test children who are thought to have special educational needs or who have been referred for evaluation because of their behavioral problems.

In cooperation with teachers and other educational experts, school psychologists design remedial and preventive programs to help all children develop their fullest potential. Sometimes school psychologists also work with parents and children to address problems in family relations.

Educational psychologists do research on the processes of teaching and learning. They evaluate learning outcomes and seek ways to make both teaching and learning more effective.

Experimental psychologists do research on human and animal behavior. (Rats, pigeons, and monkeys are common experimental animals.) They study such areas of behavior as motivation, thinking, learning and retention, sensory and perceptual processes, genetic factors, and the effects of substance abuse.

Industrial/organizational (I/O) psychologists apply psychological knowledge to the workplace. They work with the personnel department and management in screening job applicants. They also help train employees to improve both productivity and the quality of life in the workplace.

Consumer psychologists study consumer attitudes to products and services. They give advice on consumer preferences and effective advertising and marketing techniques.

Quantitative and measurement psychologists design, administer, and evaluate intelligence, personality, and aptitude tests. These psychologists also design the research tools used in gathering and analyzing psychological data.

Other fields of psychology include *correctional psychology* (working with inmates of correctional institutions) and *sports psychology* (working with athletes to help them overcome anxiety and become more motivated and competitive).

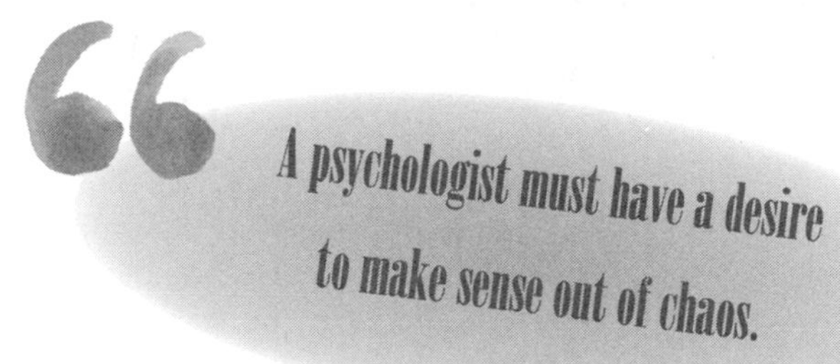

what is it like to be a psychologist?

After reviewing his notes on the murder case, Dr. Murphy Thomas glanced through his calendar of appointments for the week that was just beginning. It would be a typical week of ten- to twelve-hour work days. His first patient would be here any minute for his 9 AM appointment. After that session, the entire ten-member professional staff would gather for their weekly two-hour meeting to discuss their cases with a senior consulting psychologist who was not a member of the practice. Murphy believed strongly in the importance of collegiality. It was all too easy for a psychotherapist to become isolated and overwhelmed.

After the group meeting, he would go out for lunch. Although the next client was not scheduled until 2 PM, Murphy intended to return to the office early to do paperwork and return phone calls from insurance companies. He had calculated recently that he was averaging an hour a day on the phone with insurance companies as a result of the advent of managed care. It was the hardest part of his job these days. (The goal of managed care is to contain health care costs by tightly regulating authorizations for treatment and reducing or eliminating reimbursement for treatment plans considered unnecessary or cost-ineffective.)

Murphy would be seeing clients in individual hours that afternoon. He averaged twenty-five to thirty direct-contact hours weekly with patients in his office. Since he had a very active consulting practice, he also spent many work hours out of the office—another twenty to twenty-seven a week. Much of this time was devoted to work with various community training programs. Later that week, for instance, he would be advising the police department on their performance evaluation system. (Could the system be improved to offer greater motivation, and if so, how?) Next week, he would start a new project that would take him out of the office for two entire mornings a week for a month. He would be working with the city's management training program; it sounded exciting.

Murphy also did consulting at area hospitals, clinics, and hospices. Tomorrow he was scheduled for a consultation at a sleep-disorders clinic, he remembered. Other clients included organizations that wanted his advice on health benefits and disability claims. There was also the criminal- and civil-court work. Courts and attorneys often request input from psychologists on matters ranging from custody disputes to insanity pleas. As a member of the American Psychological Association's ethics panel, Murphy was sometimes called on to testify as an expert witness in professional malpractice suits. A recent case he had dealt with concerned a psychologist accused of having sexual relations with a client.

When Murphy Thomas started his undergraduate work at Emory University, he had been planning to become a doctor. He had always been drawn to the helping and healing professions. To his disappointment, however, he found premed coursework unrewarding. Then he registered for a course in psychology—and was fascinated. He became a psychology major.

FYI

In the late nineteenth century, the field of psychology progressed dramatically under the leadership of such pioneers as William James, Sigmund Freud, and Wilhelm Wundt.

Dr. Kathleen Hoover-Dempsey's introduction to psychology was less promising. "It was the heyday of behavioral psychology," the developmental psychologist at Vanderbilt's Peabody College recalled over thirty years later. "I had a miserable psych course about rats, pigeons, and snakes." (An equivalency between animal and human behavior had been assumed.) Kathleen concluded that she was not interested in studying psychology.

After graduating as a political science major, she became an elementary school teacher and soon found herself wanting to learn more about how children learn, how they change over the course of their education, and how their family situations affect their development. She enrolled in graduate school to study developmental psychology.

After completing her Ph.D. at Michigan State, Kathleen remained in the academic world, teaching undergraduate and graduate students and conducting research. Her current activities include directing Peabody's undergraduate major in child development and working with a team of faculty colleagues and graduate students on a long-term research project on parent/school/child relationships. She interviews parents about what they do (or don't do) to help their children succeed in school.

The project addresses such questions as how parents' views of their roles develop over their children's school years and how children's understandings of parental roles change. The evidence strongly suggests, Kathleen reported, that parents continue to be important to their children's school achievement and psychosocial development all through adolescence, contrary to some previous assumptions on that question.

have I got what it takes to be a psychologist?

The most important personal qualities for a successful career as a psychologist depend, in part, on which field of psychology one has chosen to specialize in. Clinical and counseling psychologists (and others involved in direct patient care) must have emotional stability, patience, and excellent communication skills. They need to be people-oriented individuals who enjoy helping others. School psychologists need to enjoy working with children of all ages.

Psychologists who focus on research must have logical minds and the ability to analyze data. They must also have patience for detail and precision. Computer skills are becoming increasingly important in psychological research. It is important for researchers and teachers to have good speaking and writing skills for communicating with both students and professional colleagues.

Since a master's degree is the minimal educational requirement—and a doctorate is strongly recommended—psychologists in all fields need to be above-average students who enjoy academic work and scientific inquiry.

A psychologist should be good at asking the "how and why questions," said developmental psychologist Kathleen Hoover-Dempsey. "How does environment influence people's development? Why are some people more effective than others?"

A strong curiosity about "what makes people tick" is basic for all psychologists, whether they are in applied or research fields, summed up Kathleen.

"A psychologist must have a desire to make sense out of chaos," was the way clinical psychologist Murphy Thomas put it. "You need to have respect for scientific theory and empirical research." He advises that psychology is not the right career for people who want to help others but lack an interest in scientific research and analysis.

To be a successful psychologist you should

- Have emotional stability and patience
- Be good as asking "how and why" questions
- Have excellent speaking and writing skills
- Be able to analyze complicated data
- Be curious about what makes people tick

how do I become a psychologist?

education

High School

A high school student thinking of a career in psychology should take a well-balanced college preparatory course. High school science and mathematics courses are an essential preparation for the scientific and quantitative work you will be doing later. English and communications courses are also important for developing verbal abilities. If your high school offers an introductory psychology course, that would be a good choice. Since Ph.D. programs generally require that students demonstrate a reading knowledge of two modern foreign languages, high school would be a good time to get started on French, German, or Spanish.

High school students who want some hands-on experience with the work that psychologists do might find volunteer opportunities or part-time jobs at hospitals, nursing homes, day care centers, or social service organizations.

Postsecondary Training

In a 1993 survey, 75 percent of psychologists polled said that a doctorate was either essential or recommended for their current job. Psychologists with only a master's degree are much more limited in their career options and have few opportunities for advancement. They are qualified for positions as industrial/organizational psychologists, school psychologists or counselors, and psychologist's assistants at community mental health centers. They may also be employed to do survey research or other forms of data collection for businesses, government agencies, or academic institutions.

People with only a bachelor's degree will find very few opportunities in the psychological field. They might be able to find work assisting psychologists at community mental-health centers, vocational rehabilitation programs, or correctional institutions. Government agencies are also a possibility. Although a bachelor's degree in psychology does not qualify a person to be a professional psychologist, the psychology major's communication and analytical skills and knowledge of the principles of human behavior are a good preparation for employment in many fields, including business, sales, service industries, and administrative support.

Nearly all colleges and universities offer a psychology major. Psychology is actually the second most popular undergraduate major (second only to business administration). In 1996, fewer than 10 percent of persons graduating with a psychology major chose to go on to graduate school to become professional psychologists.

A bachelor's degree in psychology is the most obvious way to prepare for graduate work in that discipline. As both Murphy Thomas and Kathleen Hoover-Dempsey pointed out, however, it is not necessary to major in psychology at the undergraduate level to become a psychologist. Some graduate programs require that applicants be psychology majors, but others welcome applicants with any major provided that they have had some undergraduate psychology courses, along with work in the social, biological, and physical sciences, mathematics, and statistics. Getting into a good graduate program is competitive.

A master's degree program typically lasts two years and usually includes supervised practical experience in a school or health-care setting and a master's thesis based on an original research project. Persons wanting to become school psychologists must do a year of supervised internship at a school after receiving the master's degree.

Doctoral degrees require two to five years of graduate work beyond the master's degree (or a total of four to seven years of graduate work if one enters a Ph.D. program without a master's degree). Most psychologists with doctoral degrees have a Ph.D. During the Ph.D. program, the student does course work and research in psychology (including work in quantitative research methods), passes comprehensive examinations, and writes a dissertation based on original research. If you are going to be a clinical, counseling, or school psychologist, a year of supervised internship is also required. Students focusing on research often do a postdoctoral fellowship year.

The Psy.D., offered at professional schools of psychology and some universities, is also an option for persons wanting to work as clinical, counseling, or school psychologists. The Psy.D. is less research-oriented than the Ph.D. and puts more stress on clinical work. It usually does not require a dissertation. Instead, the degree is awarded on the basis of the successful completion of course work, supervised clinical/practical work, and examinations. About 16 percent of doctoral degrees currently being awarded in psychology are Psy.D.s.

If you are going into clinical, counseling, or school psychology, it is important to choose a doctoral program that is accredited by the American Psychological Association (APA). The APA also accredits internship programs in school and clinical settings. APA accreditation is not relevant for doctoral programs that focus on preparing students for research and teaching at the college and university level.

certification or licensing

All states and the District of Columbia have licensing or certification requirements for clinical, counseling, and school psychologists who are involved in direct client care. Other psychologists in private practice, such as social psychologists, must also meet licensing or certification requirements. About one-third of states require that industrial/organizational psychologists be licensed.

The precise requirements vary from state to state. Licensing as a clinical or counseling psychologist requires a doctorate in psychology, successful completion of an approved internship, and a year or two of professional experience. There is usually a state licensing examination, which may have oral as well as written questions. School psychologists can usually be licensed with a master's degree and an internship year. Teachers of psychology at the high school level need to meet their state's educational certification requirements for public school teachers.

For psychologists working in research or teaching in colleges or universities, the doctoral degree is generally considered one's license.

scholarships and grants

There are many sources of financial aid for undergraduate and graduate students. Contact the financial aid office of the academic institution you plan to attend to learn about scholarships, fellowships, grants, work/study opportunities, loans, and other sources of financial aid. Be sure to allow plenty of time for the paperwork. Graduate students also need to contact their psychology department for information about research and teaching assistantships. Ethnic minority students should write to the American Psychological Association (APA) for information about the APA Minority Fellowship Training Program.

who will hire me?

When it becomes time to look for your first professional position as a psychologist, you should turn for assistance to your university placement office and the psychology professors you have worked with in your department (especially your dissertation adviser).

You can also seek assistance from your internship supervisors and other contacts in clinical and academic settings. Students can make useful connections by getting involved in professional organizations. The APA invites all undergraduate and graduate students in psychology to become APA student affiliates.

Professional publications list job openings in psychology. The *APA Monitor* is especially useful; it provides a very extensive monthly listing of available positions. Government agencies also publish job listings.

Psychologists are employed in a wide range of settings. In 1994, there were about 144,000 psychologists holding jobs in the United States.

About 40 percent of these were employed by educational institutions in nonteaching positions; they were testers, researchers, counselors, and administrators. Another 30 percent worked in clinical health settings, such as hospitals, rehabilitation centers, mental health clinics, and nursing homes.

About 15 percent were employed by government agencies (federal, state, and local) in hospitals, clinics, correctional institutions, and other settings.

About 80 percent of those working for the federal government were employed by the Department of Veterans' Affairs (VA) and the Department of Defense. (As a doctoral student, Murphy Thomas worked as an apprentice fellow at a large VA hospital that specialized in neuropsychiatric care.)

Some psychologists teach at high schools, colleges, or universities. Others are employed by social-service organizations, management-consulting firms, marketing-research organizations, or personnel departments in corporations.

After gaining some work experience, many psychologists go into individual or group private practice or set up research and consulting firms. About one-third of the psychologists employed by educational, clinical, or other institutions also see clients or do consulting on a part-time basis.

where can I go from here?

The definition of advancement depends, to a great extent, on the setting in which a psychologist is working. In academic institutions, one advances by being promoted from instructor to assistant professor to associate professor to full professor. Promotion is based on one's record of achievement in research and teaching.

Promotion to administrative positions is often the goal of psychologists working in business, industry, educational, or government agencies. School psychologists may be promoted to head pupil personnel services, special education programs, or a school system's psychological services.

For many psychologists, advancement means going into private practice as therapists or setting up consulting or research firms (on either a full-time or part-time basis). Clinical and consulting psychologists are especially likely to go into private practice, either as individuals or as groups.

For psychologists without doctorates, the recommended route to advancement is a return to graduate school to earn a Ph.D. or Psy.D.

what are the salary ranges?

Psychologists with doctorates consistently earn more than psychologists with master's degrees. A 1993 survey by the APA revealed that the median starting salary for a clinical, counseling, or research psychologist with a doctorate was $39,000 to $40,000; the median starting salary for a school psychologist with a doctorate was $45,000.

The median salary for all psychologists with doctorates is about $65,000. Those in academic teaching positions average $50,000, while those in academic administration average $74,000. Psychologists with doctorates employed in business and industry average $80,000 and can earn over $200,000. Clinical psychologists average $60,000, but those in private practice often earn much more.

Starting salaries for psychologists with a master's degree are about $20,000; in school psychology, the average beginning salary for the holder of a master's degree is $25,000. Experienced school psychologists with a master's degree can earn $60,000 or more, though the median is $35,000. Salaries are higher in business and industry, where the median is $58,000. In other fields of psychology, however, the median annual salary for those with a master's degree is only in the $20,000s.

what is the job outlook?

Overall, the job outlook for psychologists over the next few years is expected to be about as fast as the average for all occupations. Competition will be keen, however, for the limited number of positions open to applicants with only a master's degree.

Employment prospects look best for psychologists with doctorates in the clinical, counseling, health, industrial, and educational fields. Those with strong preparation in quantitative research methods and computer technology may have an additional advantage. Opportunities for school psychologists should continue to expand, as school systems address the problems of children with special needs and disabilities. As the population continues to age, psychologists with special expertise in work with the elderly should also find opportunities. The continuation of government funding will be an issue that could affect employment in some areas of psychology.

The public demand for counseling, mental health care, substance abuse programs, and preventive health plans should continue, but the long-term impact of managed-care restrictions remains to be seen. Many psychologists, along with other health care providers, are experiencing the frustration of trying to work with managed-care plans.

Despite these emerging concerns, the field of psychology remains strong. According to a 1993 APA survey, only 3 percent of psychologists with doctorates were unemployed and seeking jobs.

how do I learn more?

professional organizations

For information on careers in psychology, contact the following:

American Psychological Association (APA)
750 1st Street, NE
Washington, DC 20002
TEL: 202-336-5707
WEBSITE: http://www.apa.org

bibliography

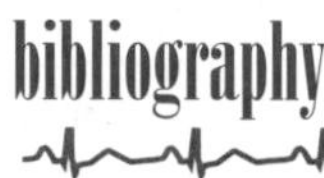

Following is a sampling of materials relating to the professional concerns and development of psychologists.

Books

American Psychological Association Staff. *Careers in Psychology.* Washington, DC: American Psychological Association, 1986.

Clayton, Lawrence. *Careers in Psychology,* revised edition. New York, NY: Rosen Group, 1996.

Coon, Dennis. *Essentials of Psychology,* 7th edition. St. Paul, MN: West Publishing Co., 1996.

Periodical

American Psychologist. Monthly. Publishes articles on current issues in psychology as well as empirical, theoretical, and practical articles on broad aspects of psychology. American Psychological Association, 750 First Street, NE, Washington, DC 20002, 202-336-5500.

public health worker

Definition

A health care professional in the public sector who is involved in the prevention and control of illness or disease and the promotion of health in the general population. Public Health incorporates virtually all health care jobs. Some jobs that are specific to public health include Community Health Administrator and Health Officer.

Salary range

Varies according to job

Educational requirements

The same requirements needed to practice your health care profession in the private sector are required for public health.

Certification or Licensing

Same as to practice your profession in the private sector.

Outlook

Faster than average

GOE
NA*

DOT
NA*

*Not Available. The classifications vary for different jobs.

High School Subjects

Biology
Chemistry
English
Health
Psychology
Sociology

Personal Interests

Helping others
Health
Working as part of a team

Time to go to school! Stumbling out of bed, you head for the shower, brush your teeth, gulp down a glass of milk and walk out to catch the bus. You arrive just in time for first period, with a little extra time to greet your friends whom you spy among the throngs of your classmates. Today is "career day." In the cafeteria at lunch, you see a booth about public health workers. "What has that got to do with me?" you wonder, munching on a fry from your lunch.

Consider this—the fluoridated water with which you brushed your teeth and showered, the pasteurized milk you had for breakfast, the immunization of all of your classmates, and the safety and nutrition of the food you eat for lunch, are all the result of the efforts of public health workers. You probably didn't realize that public health concerns affected you so closely! That is because public health is generally only recognized when there is a lapse in protection: occasional instances of water contamination or other ecological disasters; alarming statistics about teen pregnancy, domestic violence, and the spread of sexually transmitted and other infectious diseases; or overcrowded and understaffed public health clinics. When they are operating at their best, public health workers are hardly noticeable. They are the unseen force behind the health of the nation.

what does a public health worker do?

"Public health worker" is a blanket term, covering many different types of professionals with a variety of concerns, education, and goals. Most health care fields can have some application in public health: the difference is that public health workers are generally working for government funded institutions or departments instead of working in the private sector. The overall idea behind public health is preventative medicine—that a dollar of prevention is worth several dollars of cure. Public health workers interact with huge and diverse populations, using various methods to reach them.

According to the National Association of County and City Health Officials, the goals of *Public health workers* are to: prevent epidemics and the spread of disease by investigation, containment, and education; protect against environmental hazards; promote and encourage healthy behaviors and mental health; respond to disasters and assist communities in recovery; and assure the quality and accessibility of health services. Public health is part of the care provided by some private organizations.

There are several specific jobs which can be described under the heading of public health. *Health officers* act as chief administrative officers of local health departments. They create policies for the provision of health care in the community. Health officers are responsible for recognizing the needs of the community and advising residents and elected officials of ways to improve peoples' health. Other responsibilities include creating appropriate programs to service the community; seeing that those programs are carried out within budget; and being accountable to local governing boards for the allocation of funds and the results of programs. In about half of the states, health officers are required to be licensed medical practitioners for that state, and in the other half, non-physicians with administrative backgrounds may hold that position. A few states have no formal requirements.

Community health center administrators perform a similar function on a slightly larger scale. They coordinate efforts of public health and other health care workers in an entire state, as well as enforce state health regulations. Health center administrators are the link between the financial resources available for public health programming and the health officers who use this money to run their programs. They, too, evaluate the specific needs of the population whom they serve and help to distribute funds to programs whose goals are most in keeping with those needs.

lingo to learn

Accessible care refers to the ease with which a patient can initiate interaction with a health care worker for any health problem. It takes into account efforts to eliminate barriers such as those posed by geography, administrative tasks, financing, culture, and language.

Botulism acute food poisoning caused by a toxic by-product of bacteria. Characterized by muscle weakness and paralysis, disturbances of vision, slurred speech, or difficulty swallowing.

Communicable disease a disease capable of being transmitted from one person to another—diseases may be airborne, blood-borne, distributed through direct contact, sexually transmitted, or through contamination.

Epidemiology the study of diseases affecting many people at one time, how they spread, and their origins.

Reportable diseases a list of approximately thirty communicable diseases whose outbreaks in the community must by law be reported to local health officials. This list includes rabies, typhoid, hepatitis, and tuberculosis.

Public health nurses, physicians, dentists, and *medical assistants* all work in the same capacity as private members of their professions, serving the medical and dental needs of their clients. However, they add an element of community-based prevention to their focus. For instance, public health physicians may be assigned to a specific population which is underserved by the medical community. Or, they may concentrate on a specific problem which faces their community, such as sexually transmitted diseases. They are involved in primary care and the health education of their patients.

Part of the job for a public health worker is providing counseling and referrals: they must learn about each client's situation, determine a cause or perpetuating factor for the client's illness, ensure that the client has access to the proper care, and then address the problem within the larger framework of the community. *Public health dentists* meet the dental needs of residents of state institutions or of patients at local clinics. *Public health nurses* are often responsible for the immunization of school children and the neonatal training of expectant parents. *Public health medical assistants* carry out various tasks, from scheduling patients in community clinics to giving routine physicals to general office workers.

Public health nurse practitioners provide evaluations and treatment plans for clients and ensure that the plans are followed by regular check ups and counseling. *Public health nurse midwives* assist with childbirth and provide care for newborns. *Public health nutritionists* provide the population with information on proper diet and nutrition. They oversee some institutional food preparation areas, and educate food service workers. Nutritionists also act as advisors to other health care workers as well as to populations with specific nutritional needs, such as pregnant women, infants, children, and those without access to adequate or nutritional food.

In addition to medical programs, public health as a profession also deals with environmental health. There are many types of careers involved in maintaining safe water, air, and food. *Environmental specialists* conduct surveys, inspections, and investigations to ensure compliance with environmental safety guidelines and laws. Environment, in this instance, can mean the water in a fishing area or community pool; it can mean the air and building materials in an office building or school, or the soil in the park across the street.

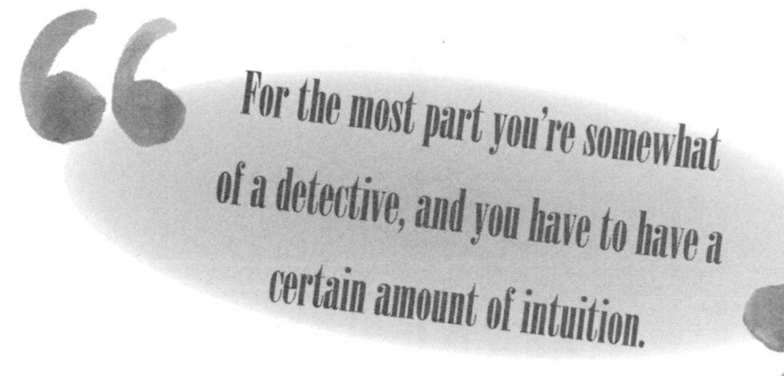

Epidemiologists, or *public health investigators,* work with those exposed to outbreaks of certain diseases, including typhus, hepatitis, botulism, lung cancer, and rabies. They work to control the spread of a illness that is known to be present in a population, and to give assistance to people affected. Epidemiologists develop policies and procedures for investigations, analyze incidents of outbreak, and advise other health care professionals about public health concerns. *Registered sanitarians* regularly inspect restaurants, grocery stores, and any other place food is sold to the public. They may also inspect new septic systems and new water wells.

Most public health providers are involved in some form of public education. Many create programs to emphasize good health in their community, such as sponsoring a wellness day or a mobile blood-pressure testing booth. Public health workers may also speak to schools and civic groups to educate large numbers of people about the dangers of unhealthy behaviors, or the benefits of regular health screenings. *Community health educators* coordinate these programs and use the media to promote public health issues in their community. They provide health education materials, determine attitudes about health in their communities, identify and advertise available health resources, and train other people in health education.

Public health also includes many types of social workers. *Case workers* often help people determine their eligibility for support from government-assisted programs and the agencies that can most help them. *Case coordinators* help people apply for Medicaid, and may provide child care and transportation for clients needing public health assistance resources. They also target populations for outreach and intervention programs. *Social workers* work with state agencies as advocates for the mental and physical health of their clients. They interview clients and other people to determine the causes of mental, physical, emotional, economic and social problems in their communities. They may investigate cases of reported abuse, provide protective services for the abused or neglected, or counsel families on proper child care.

what is it like to be a public health worker?

Public health is a huge job and it takes many skilled and dedicated professionals to make it work. Where does it begin? One of the major concerns for public health workers is prevention of disease. Primary care doctors are in the business of prevention, as are public health nurses and educators. Janie Weller is a Public Health Nurse at the Delta Public Health Center in Delta Junction, Alaska. "It's not really a 'center', it's a nine by thirteen [foot] room!" she laughs. Janie serves a community of about 1,200 in the heart of Alaska, and she deals mainly with children and parents. "One of the things I do is immunizations—there is a big focus on children from birth to age five, because that's when they are developing so much, undergoing so much change. Along with that goes well-child check-ups and health screening. We look for illnesses, especially tuberculosis right now, or for exposure to Hepatitis A. I also work with pregnant teens and new moms; do testing and counseling, make sure people are plugged into the appropriate programs, and teach childbirth classes."

It seems like a lot of work, particularly since Janie works alone with only occasional volunteer support. "It really allows you to be pretty creative in the programs you set up and work on," she says, adding that she still hopes to hire a full time person to help her with clerical duties that consume much of her time. She likes the flexibility that being a Public Health nurse gives her. "I've recently really gotten into parenting, I've really enjoyed that, and have created a parenting group that is really more for moms' mental health than anything else."

FYI

Every dollar spent on vaccinations for measles, rubella, and mumps saves fourteen dollars in treatment.

In addition to providing flexibility and autonomy, working within a smaller community also allows Janie to keep track of her clients more closely, to see if what she has suggested is working, and to maintain contact with those she has treated. "In a large town you might see people and suggest something and never see them again. You don't know if it worked or if they tried it or anything. In Delta, I experience a lot of closeness with the people, I have the chance to establish a good working relationship with them." If Janie encounters something beyond her scope of practice, she refers clients to the local doctor. "He gets the emergencies. In fact, some people like to come see me instead for the easy stuff, because I'm not so hectic, I have time to talk to them and kind of get to know where they are."

Janie works mostly out of her office but also makes visits to the local schools and travels to workshops that may be held out of town. She visits a village called Dot Lake, about ninety miles away, once every month or so to provide health services for residents. In Alaska, many communities are severely underserved, and traveling nurses may move among many small towns that do not have enough money to support a full-time public health nurse.

Another job at the preventative end of the public health spectrum is that of registered sanitarian. One such professional, Mark Macchiano, works for the McHenry County Health Department in northern Illinois. He works with eating establishments, conducting routine inspections and advising them on their food preparation and storage methods. Mark is also responsible for inspecting septic systems and water wells which are being installed for homes not connected to the public sewage systems.

The typical day for Mark, if there is such a thing, usually begins with planning out the day. "You never really know where you will end up. We investigate complaints and do regular check-ups on the restaurants we are responsible for." In a regular inspection of a food service establishment, Mark will check the temperature at which food is stored; ensure the availability of hand-washing materials and the regularity with which the staff washes their hands; watch for unsafe practices such as using hand-washing sinks for food disposal; check for a correct Ph balance and cleanliness of washing water, and other routine investigations. "We do have a lab that does water testing, but we don't use much hard science out there. Most of it is common sense. Are people washing their hands? Are the employees sick?"

Mark finds that most places are pretty cooperative but mentions that many owners and workers see him as the enemy. "We're trying to change that," he says. "Personally, I try to educate people as much as I can as to why they need to do that, why this regulation is important, and so on. I take the inspection as an opportunity to let people know that we're working with them, not trying to close them down."

Despite the watchful eyes of Mark and his co-workers, episodes of contamination still occur. When that happens, Mark's job becomes more intervention-oriented. "If they score a sixty or below on a regular inspection, they must be shut down by the Director of the Department. Most owners will close down when we ask them to . . . then we try to identify the cause. If ten people got sick here, what made them sick? We might take food samples to the lab for testing; we might have them throw out all of their open food; we might have them clean everything. We would also interview the cooks, ask them questions about meal preparation and storage."

Mark recalls one incident in particular. "I remember one restaurant where there was a party and over seventy people became ill. We didn't know at first what was going on. Was it in the water, maybe in the ice? Was the contaminated food still being served? It's hard to locate one source of bacteria, though. We tried to contact all the people that had been there, find out their symptoms; we basically tried to paint a picture of what most likely happened. It appeared finally like it had been the way the food was cooled down, combined with some poor personal hygiene and cross-contamination of bad chicken and lettuce."

It is important while Mark is working that he set a good example for the workers of the establishment. "If I'm going to be taking temperatures of their meat, I make sure I wash my hands well before I handle their food. We have to watch ourselves, see what message we're sending as regulators."

Mark's office also fields many questions. "We answer what we can, and refer some to other agencies like OSHA [Occupational Safety and Health Organization] or the EPA [Environmental Protection Agency]. The office also provides some instructions on how to keep food safe in the home as well as ways to care for septic systems and wells." Mark sometimes attends wellness fairs, where he promotes general knowledge of public health issues and of the job he does for his community.

To be a successful public health worker you should

- Have a sincere desire to help others.
- Have good oral and written communication skills.
- Be a team player.
- Work well with a variety of people.
- Have patience.
- Have good problem-solving skills.
- Be flexible.
- Have good organizational skills.

If a sanitarian discovers an outbreak of a disease in Karen Moore's region of suburban Cook County, Illinois, chances are that she will be on the scene, too. Karen is an epidemiologist and public health investigator in communicable diseases at the Cook County Department of Health. Her job often takes her to restaurants and other sites of suspected outbreaks of disease. Her job is to identify the source of the illness and how it was spread, eliminate the cause, investigate those people who may have been exposed to the source, and provide treatment information to exposed persons or health care professionals who encounter cases of it. She might investigate outbreaks of lice in schools, or a case of typhoid reported by hospital workers. There are about thirty diseases, that by law must be reported to the county health department, including meningitis, hepatitis, and typhoid. Karen also investigates cases of botulism from food service establishments in her region.

"For food-borne diseases, outbreaks are defined as two or more people sick from the same establishment, who have not shared any other meals for the past seventy-two hours. If there is evidence of an outbreak, I'm the first one called out to go investigate. . . . I usually go with an environmental inspector and a health inspector. We interview ill persons: what did they eat, who were they with, how soon did you get sick, what kind of symptoms did you have, can you give me any information about anyone else who was there. I ask the manager if any of his employees were sick, look for hand-washing procedures that may or may not be in use, anything that might fill in the picture."

In cases that are not readily identified as restaurant contamination, the questions must be just as thorough, and sometimes more personal. "We ask, where do you work, where do you buy your groceries: because of confidentiality, we can't say did so-and-so down the block baby-sit for you this week, but we can ask 'Do you have small children. . . .' Stuff like that." Even though epidemiology involves a lot of phone work from the office, as well as substantial written documentation of events, it still requires investigative work and creative thinking. "For the most part you're somewhat of a detective, and you have to have a certain amount of intuition about asking the questions that will give you the whole picture."

How does Karen find out about an outbreak? Sometimes citizens call in complaints about an establishment; sometimes hospitals report cases of diseases; sometimes potentially contaminated establishments call if they have been hearing health complaints related to their business. After she knows about an outbreak Karen does what she can to intervene in the situation and prevent the further spread of the disease.

Karen, Mark, and Janie all find that the best part of their jobs is the satisfaction that they are truly helping to make a difference in the quality of life of their communities. Additionally, Karen likes to be able to relieve people's fears. "A parent might call and say they just found out their child had lice; it seems like a little thing but if you don't know anything about it, it can be very scary. I like being able to make people feel better, feel informed and safer." Each also expresses their approval of the amount of variety their jobs have. "It's never the same day twice," Mark says, and Karen agrees, saying, "my work is almost seasonal—summer for me is a busy food-born illness season, but fall will bring something else. It's always changing."

FYI

The fluoridation of water costs about fifty cents per person per year—the cost of filling a cavity is about forty dollars.

have I got what it takes to be a public health worker?

"Public health can be a thankless job sometimes," says Mark. "Some of the people who I've visited before recognize me and I can tell, they're like, 'Oh, God, not you.'" Mark believes that patience is very important for anyone who will be working with the public. "People tend to not like governmental agencies for whatever reason," says Mark, "and that can be tough to overcome." Working well with others and really hoping to make a difference are other attributes Mark cites as making an effective sanitarian. "Public health is really a team effort—even if you are mostly by yourself, you have the support of your office behind you. In our office everyone is pretty compatible, and it helps to have that."

Public health work involves a lot of problem-solving and can require a lot of creative thinking. "As a public health investigator, you have to be quick with information, be able to speak off the top of your head," says Karen. "You deal with professionals all day who are asking your advice—'how do I approach this situation,' or 'what are the guidelines for this disease?' Flexibility and self-motivation are huge. Also, I think that someone who can talk to somebody and make them feel better without actually being able to change their situation is very valuable." The ability to relieve people's fears with just information and tactfulness is a skill that requires excellent communication and listening skills, as well as sympathy.

Additionally, the medical aspects of public health can be difficult to handle. "I wouldn't recommend nursing in general to anyone who's very paranoid," notes Janie, adding that she required her friends to wash their hands before they came into contact with her children when they were first born. "I just knew what was out there, what the dangers were, and I was careful!" she states. Organizational skills will help with the paperwork that is required for documentation of public health records and, as with any health care career, the sincere desire to help people live better lives is a key characteristic in a public health worker.

how do I become a public health worker?

education

Some jobs, such as public health physician, require much more education than others. For educational requirements for specific careers, see also chapters pertaining to those careers in the private sector. Administrative positions generally require a master's degree or extensive experience in either administration or in the specialty under consideration. Technical aides or assistants may require less education initially, but in most cases it is difficult to move up without a four-year degree.

High School

Public Health is so varied that it is difficult to list all of the subjects that will provide a good basis of education. Certainly communication, written and oral, is a part of every public health job. Classes in biology, chemistry, health, and psychology will help students understand the nature of diseases and other problems that face communities and the nation at large. Volunteering while in high school is an excellent way to discover aspects of public health.

Postsecondary Training

Karen, Mark, and Janie all have their bachelor's degree, and agree that most positions in public health require at least that level of education.

Classes that future public health workers should focus on vary according to what specific job they are interested in. "I knew I wanted to be in health care," says Karen. "I took a health class and really liked it, and I knew that that's what I was good at—it just made sense to me." Karen recommends finishing required courses first and then sampling a bit of everything that you are interested in while taking electives. "I also took education classes, and my public health major included psychology, biology, sociology, and health. It's really important to follow your interests, and don't be afraid to ask questions about what's out there. Counselors are there to help you find your niche."

Janie thinks that it is harder to find a job with just a licensed practical nurse degree from a nursing school. "They want people with the four-year degree, though in remote areas with understaffing problems, that isn't strictly necessary to get a job."

Mark got his bachelor's degree in environmental health, which required him to take classes in air quality, food quality, and hard sciences like chemistry and biology. "Not everybody who does this job has the background that I do," he says. "I don't think that environmental health is the only way in, as long as you have some sort of health degree." Mark also comments that he has brought students along with him on his work route, letting them experience first-hand the nature of his job. "Most of what you learn for this job you learn while doing it. I think it's an excellent idea for high schoolers to go with us on our rounds—that way you find out exactly what we do." He suggests calling the local director of environmental or public health to find out if such a program is available.

certification or licensing

In general, you need to fulfill the same licensing requirements for your profession in public health as you would if you practiced in the private sector. For instance, physicians must be licensed by the state in which they practice. Likewise, if your profession, as practiced in the private sector, requires certification by a professional association, then you need that certification.

Mark, is a registered sanitarian and he must take continuing education courses in order to keep his license. The same is true for Janie and Karen, and for most workers in this industry. "You can take time off to have a family, or whatever," Janie explains, "and still come back because your continuing education has kept you current." In some professions, continuing education credits may be earned by teaching courses, as well as attending seminars or organized public health events.

scholarships and grants

A major source of financial assistance for careers in public health is the United States Public Health Service. They provide loans, fellowships, and scholarships for people pursuing a health care career in public health.

internships and volunteerships

Internships are usually required for public health. Karen wrote protection orders for a domestic violence clinic; Janie worked a nurse internship in a hospital, rotating among several units including intensive care, pediatrics, and emergency medicine. Though neither is directly involved in the area of their internship anymore, both believe it was invaluable for teaching them what they wanted out of a career in public health.

"Seeing all the sick people, I decided to be on the well-people end of things," Janie recalls. "The people who want to see me generally want my help, they're interested in learning. I find this pace much better for me than hospital nursing was. Also, when you're in a hospital, you have a lot of other nurses and doctors telling you what to do all the time; I'm pretty unsupervised here in Delta."

Karen found out about her first job by way of her position as an intern. She ended up working for the Sexually Transmitted Disease (STD) department of her facility, and her experiences with survivors of domestic violence as well as work in STD control gave her insight into how to deal with the public. In effect, experience is the best education after one has received a bachelor's degree.

who will hire me?

State and federal departments of health are the primary employers of public health workers. Numerous other facilities also exist to promote health among various populations and most of these facilities rely on grant money and other government funding to continue working. Calling local health departments will give applicants an idea of what jobs are available in their area, and can also be helpful in finding out the qualifications that each field or department requires. The United States Department of Health and Human Services will be able to provide a national overview of available jobs, and also has information on several operating divisions, including the Food and Drug Administration and the Centers for Disease Control and Prevention.

Interested applicants should contact state agencies of employment as well as call the agencies where they would like to work directly. Janie moved to Delta shortly after they had already hired a public health nurse. She then got to know the nurse and her supervisor. When the nurse left, Janie already knew the person who was in charge of hiring a new public health nurse. Similarly, Karen stepped into the epidemiology department as a volunteer while the regular epidemiologist took a maternity leave.

where can I go from here?

Though some public health workers find jobs as consultants in the private sector, many choose to stay in public health for the same reason they started there: to benefit the whole population. One route of advancement is in administration. Administrative positions generally require more school and experience. Administrators make health policies, such as the decision to focus on a particular disease that is showing signs of emerging as an epidemic. They are generally given responsibility for a whole region and the workers who contact the population there. They may write proposals for grant money, allocate funds for the development of projects, or identify a far-reaching goal of public health workers for a specific problem.

In general, education is the way to advance in public health. Karen points out that, though her employer does not offer tuition reimbursement, they do allow flexible hours for those who commit to extra schooling.

what are the salary ranges?

Salary ranges are as broad as the definitions of public health worker. All salaries are based on the relevant field, amount of education and experience, area of the country, and length of time in the same position. Salaries for jobs in public health are generally less than those for equivalent jobs in the private sector. The benefits, however, are usually competitive or better than those found in private sector health care jobs.

Technical assistants may earn from $12,000 to $17,000, while physicians may make up to $70,000 per year. Health inspectors and investigators make from $25,000 to about $50,000. For a complete listing of salaries, contact the United States Department of Health and Human Services.

what is the job outlook?

The U.S. Department of Health and Human Services has 59,000 employees and an operating budget of over $350 billion. This indicates that public health is a huge concern for this country. Public health careers are expected to grow faster than average for all careers throughout the next five to ten years. In addition to an increased emphasis on preventative medicine, there is a general lack of professionals who are dedicated to public health, especially in rural areas.

Many Americans believe that everybody has the right to good health, and it is also increasingly recognized that the availability of health care and health education are important factors in some of the social problems faced today. In response to this realization, public health is enjoying some attention that it had not traditionally received. "People might not know what an epidemiologist is, but if I say I am from the Public Health Department, they will recognize that. Most people are really cooperative and glad to see us," notes Karen.

Health care in general is experiencing some budget constraints, and public health is not excluded from the critical eyes of those who finance it. "It is sort of hard to justify what you do," Janic admits. "You say, 'I'm in the business of disease prevention,' well, what's that? You can't prove how many people you've prevented from getting a disease. There is a push now to promote ourselves, and the accomplishments of the field. We really do have to do that because nobody else will." Finding ways to support their work will be one of the major tasks of public health workers in the future. In general, though, the country acknowledges the need to keep its citizens free of disease and informed of possible hazards, so public health will be a strong career in the years to come.

how do I learn more?

professional organizations

The following provides information on careers in public health:

National Association of County and City Health Officials
440 First Street, NW
Suite 450
Washington, DC 20001
TEL: 202-783-5550
WEBSITE: http://www.naccho.org/

government agencies

The United States Department of Health and Human Services has a Public Health Service with several agencies and institutions devoted to public health. Most provide information concerning their specific area. For general information contact:

United States Department of Health and Human Services
200 Independence Avenue, SW
Washington, DC, 20201
TEL: 202-619-0257
WEBSITE: http://www.os.dhhs.gov/

Public Health Service
200 Independence Avenue, SW
Room 716G
Washington, DC 20201
TEL: 202-690-7694

Some of the agencies and institutions of the Public Health Service are:

Agency for Health Care Policy and Research
2101 East Jefferson Street
Room 600
Rockville, MD 20852
TEL: 301-594-6662
WEBSITE: http://www.ahcpr.gov/

Agency for Toxic Substances and Disease Registry
1600 Clifton Road, NE
Atlanta, GA 30333
WEBSITE: http://www.atsdr1.atsdr.cdc.gov:8080/atsdrhome.html

Centers for Disease Control and Prevention
1600 Clifton Road, NE
Atlanta, GA 30333
TEL: 404-639-3311
WEBSITE: http://www.cdc.gov/

Food and Drug Administration
5600 Fishers Lane
Rockville, MD 20857
TEL: 301-443-1130
WEBSITE: http://www.fda.gov/

Health Resources and Services Administration
5600 Fishers Lane, Suite 1405
Rockville, MD 20857
TEL: 301-443-2216
WEBSITE: http://www.hrsa.dhhs.gov/

National Institutes of Health
1 Center Drive, Building 1, Suite 126
Bethesda, MD 20892
TEL: 301-496-2433
WEBSITE: http://www.nih.gov/

Another federal agency that deals with public health concerns is the Environmental Protection Agency. Contact them at:

United States Environmental Protection Agency
401 M Street, SW
Washington, DC 20460
TEL: 202-260-4700
WEBSITE: http://www.epa.gov/

bibliography

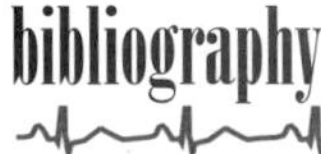

Following is a sampling of materials relating to the professional concerns and development of public health workers.

Books

Morgan, Bradley J., and Joseph M. Palmisano, editors. *Health Career Directory–Medical-Technical.* Detroit, MI: Gale Research, 1993.

Pickett, George, and Terry W. Pickett. *Opportunities in Public Health Careers.* Lincolnwood, IL: VGM Career Horizons, 1995.

Turnock, Bernard J. *Public Health: What It Is and How It Works.* Gaithersburg, MD: Aspen Publishers, 1997.

Periodicals

American Journal of Health Promotion. Bimonthly. Covers the science and art of helping people change their lifestyle to move toward a state of optimal health. Mosby, 11830 Westline Industrial Drive, St. Louis, MO 63146, 314-872-8370.

American Journal of Public Health. Monthly. Contains reports of original research, demonstrations, evaluations, and other articles covering current aspects of public health. American Public Health Association, 1015 15th Street, NW, Washington, DC 20005, 202-789-5600.

Healthline: Helping Keep Well People Well. Monthly. Offers current information on health and wellness, written in nontechnical language by health care professionals and medical journalists. Healthline Publishers, Inc., 830 Menlo Avenue, Suite 100, Menlo Park CA 94025, 800-325-4177.

The Nation's Health. 11 per year. Covers public health policy, including legislative and other federal action. American Public Health Association, 1015 15th Street, NW, Washington, DC 20005, 202-789-5600.

Public Health Reports. Bimonthly. Official journal of the U.S. Public Health Service. Reports on research and activities in areas of public health both nationally and internationally. U.S. Public Health Service, Department of Health and Human Services, J.F.K. Federal Building, Room 1826, Boston, MA 02203, 617-565-1442.

radiologic technologist

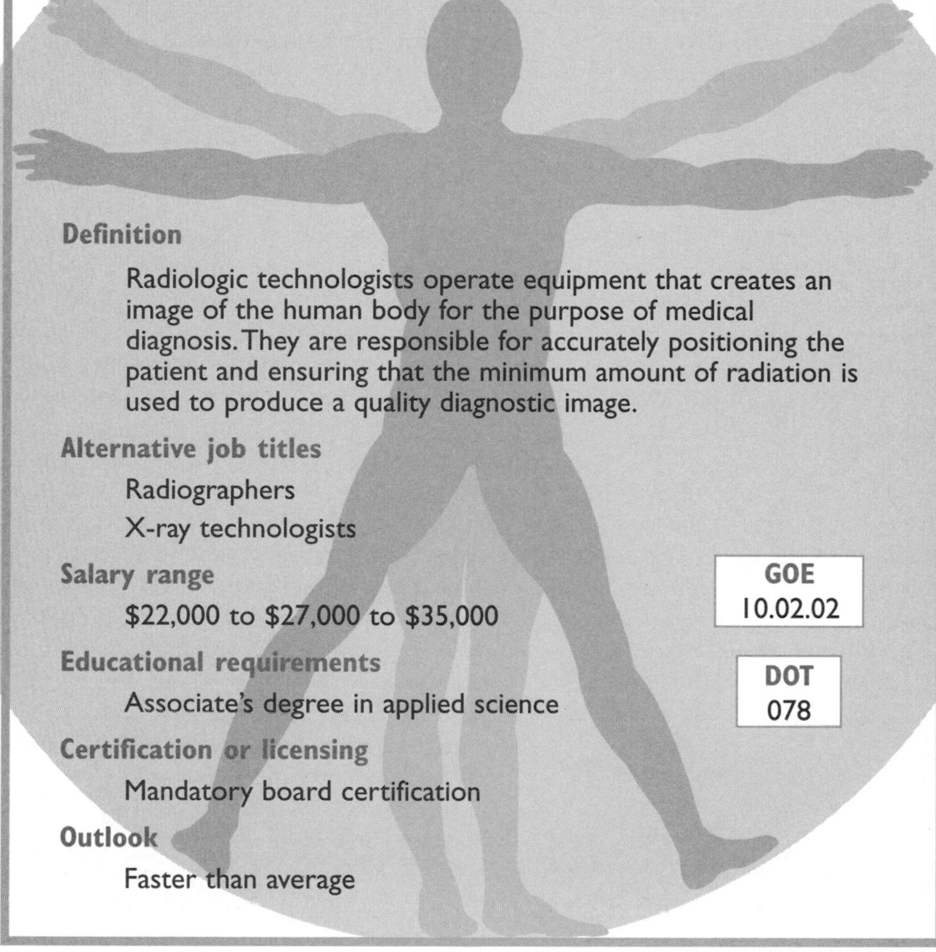

Definition

Radiologic technologists operate equipment that creates an image of the human body for the purpose of medical diagnosis. They are responsible for accurately positioning the patient and ensuring that the minimum amount of radiation is used to produce a quality diagnostic image.

Alternative job titles

Radiographers

X-ray technologists

Salary range

$22,000 to $27,000 to $35,000

Educational requirements

Associate's degree in applied science

Certification or licensing

Mandatory board certification

Outlook

Faster than average

GOE
10.02.02

DOT
078

High School Subjects

Biology
Chemistry
Human anatomy
Life science
Mathematics
Physics

Personal Interests

Science and medicine
Working with people

A boy, frightened and still wearing his baseball cap and uniform, is wheeled into Joanne Knock's work area. Joanne, who has significant experience in dealing with worried young children, instinctively knows that the best way to calm the boy and accomplish her job is to divert his attention from his throbbing leg.

With a smile and a few quick questions, Joanne learns the boy's name—Billy; the position he plays—pitcher and sometimes second base; and his team's record—not that great.

The boy grows more relaxed as Joanne explains the X-ray procedure. As she talks, she positions the boy beneath the X-ray camera for the optimum filming angle. She sets the controls of the X-ray machine so as to be able produce a picture of the correct density, contrast, and detail. She then adjusts a columnator, which is a knob that reduces the size of the X-ray area, therefore ensuring that the boy's leg will be exposed to the least amount of radiation for the shortest duration of time.

Joanne is acutely aware of the potential harmful effects of the radiation on both herself and the boy, and as a result, she wears protective clothing and a radiation badge as a matter of rule. Most importantly, she properly and professionally covers the boy with lead shielding before beginning the procedure. She makes the exposure, and removes the film so that it can be developed, then tells the boy the procedure is complete.

The boy is wheeled away and Joanne reloads the "bucky" with X-ray film and prepares for her next assignment. Before the day is over, she will have completed twenty to twenty-five X-ray procedures; among those are scans that reveal numerous broken bones, chest examinations, lung cancer and pneumonia, as well as scans to determine problems in the spinal column, IVPs, and upper and lower GI.

As a result of his fracture, the boy will be lost to his team for the rest of the season, but his leg will heal perfectly as the result of Joanne's competent imaging, which provided the physician with the precise view he needed to accurately set the broken bone and begin the healing process.

lingo to learn

Bucky The tray in which X-ray film is loaded.

Columnator A dial on the X-ray machinery which controls and adjusts the area of radiation exposure.

Contrast Medium A solution of barium sulfate that is administered orally or rectally to highlight organs such as the abdomen, which normally cannot be distinguished.

Diagnostic imaging Preliminary testing of the body tissues and skeletal structures through the use of X rays, sound waves, tomographic scans, and magnetic scans.

Fluoroscopy A procedure examining the upper or lower gastrointestinal areas.

Pigastat A device used to hold children during an examination.

Radiographs X-ray films.

what does a radiologic technologist do?

Radiologic technologists, sometimes called *radiographers* or *X-ray technologists,* operate equipment that creates images of the human body for the purpose of medical diagnosis.

Since all work is done at the request and under the supervision of a supervisor, radiologist, or attending physician, radiologic technologists do not complete any procedures on their own.

To do their job, radiologic technologists must help prepare the patient by explaining the procedure and answering any questions the patient might have. In some instances, a radiologic technologist may administer, under the supervision of a radiologist, a substance called a contrast medium, which is usually barium sulfate given orally or rectally, so as to make specific body parts, such as the kidney or abdomen, better able to be viewed. They must also make sure that the patient is free of jewelry or any other metal that would obstruct the X-ray process. radiologic technologists position the person sitting, standing, or lying so that the correct view of the body can be radiographed. Technologists are also responsible for protecting the test subject from radiation, covering adjacent areas with lead shielding. Special attention and protection is given to the very young and women in their child-bearing years, since they are the most susceptible to the effects of radiation. Radiologic technologists are keenly aware of the welfare of the patient in relation to radiation, ascribing to the term "ALARA," which means, "as low as reasonably allowable."

The technologist is responsible for the positioning of the X-ray equipment at the proper angle and distance from the part to be radiographed, and determining exposure time based on the location of the bone or organ and the thickness of the body in that area. Universal formulas which relate to body weight, degree of sickness, and density of tissue and bone, exist to help the radiologic technologist in their settings. The radiologic technologist must set the controls of the X-ray machine in order to be able to produce pictures of the correct contrast, detail, and density, then place the photographic film on the far side of the patient's body to make the necessary exposures. The film is then developed for the radiologist or other physician to interpret.

Secondary duties for radiologic technologists may include the performance of routine administrative tasks such as maintaining patient files, and keeping detailed records of equipment maintenance and usage. radiologic technologists may also be responsible for managing a radiation quality assurance program and, with considerable experience, manage other technologists in terms of work schedules and assigned duties.

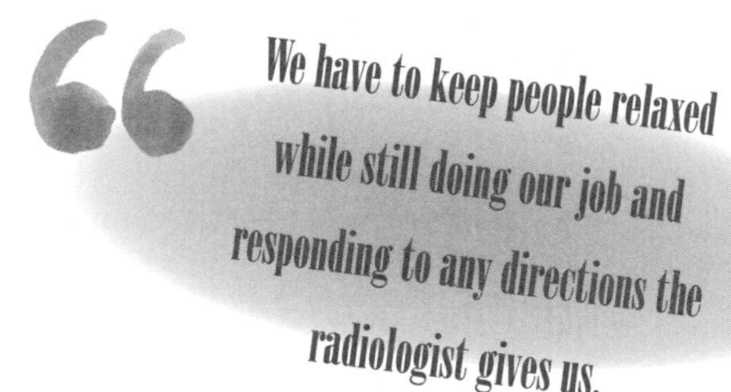

what is it like to be a radiologic technologist?

Joanne Knock has worked at Meyer Medical Clinic for the past two years. Her day begins at 7:00 AM and lasts till 4:00 PM, with overtime a frequent possibility. "In the morning," Joanne explains, "we do fluoroscopies (upper and lower GIs) and IVPs (kidney exams), in which we administer, under the supervision of a radiologist, barium as a contrast medium." This is where a personal touch and superior communication skills come into play between patient, radiologist, and radiologic technologist. "We have to keep the people relaxed while still doing our job and responding to any directions the radiologist gives us," she explains.

Working alone in the afternoon, Joanne takes mammograms and diagnostic X rays, which are basic X rays that examine the chest, skull, or extremities. On average, Joanne spends about ten minutes with each patient and individually sees about twenty to twenty-five patients daily. "Obviously, we spend less time on a broken bone as opposed to a lump on the spine," she explains. The most frequent radiologic tests that Joanne performs are chest X rays, then X rays of the extremities for broken bones. She is quick to add, though, that there are no typical days.

Joanne's secondary responsibilities at Meyer Medical Clinic include keeping patient files accurate and updated. "We keep three copies of each record, one for the patient's file, one for our own records, and one for the doctor." Each institution keeps X-ray files active for two years, and stores them up to five years. It is obvious that the proper preservation and notation of patient information is utterly important to radiologic technologists like Joanne. In addition, she is expected to check the machinery daily for fluctuations or malfunctions, and is responsible for the proper set-up of her equipment and film for each new patient. Joanne is also expected to maintain her certification in her off-hours in the form of continuing education courses, which requires the completion of twenty-four credit hours in a two-year span.

Joanne keeps up on the evolving technology in the radiologic field by reading trade magazines such as *Advance* and *RT Image*. "They keep you informed on new procedures or findings," she explains.

Joanne finds that the best part of her duties is the opportunity she gets to perform her job well and help people. She likes the idea that her professional abilities can assist a doctor in medical diagnosis, and that her work allows a disease or condition to be discovered and hopefully treated and healed.

have I got what it takes to be a radiologic technologist?

Radiologic technologists should be technically oriented and have a mastery of medical technology. They must enjoy helping and working with the sick who are sometimes worried or frightened. "People get nervous when taking G.I.s, or gastrointestinal examinations," Joanne says. "You have to keep them relaxed by talking to them, explaining to them what you are about to do."

Radiologic technologists need a lot of patience to be successful in this field, since patients are sometimes scared or worried, children are hard to position, and films are sometimes ruined by a patient's movements or other factors. Clearly, a personal touch is mandatory for success in the field, although one must learn to balance compassion and patience with a professional manner.

Communication skills, as previously mentioned, play a significant role in an radiologic technologist's daily duties. They must be able to relay information to radiologists and other technologists, and instruct patients into the proper position so a procedure can be completed. While being good communicators, radiologic technologists must also walk a fine line between affability and professionalism. They must always keep in mind their proper role when asked questions by the patient relating to the outcome of their tests, be it positive or negative. "We cannot give a diagnosis," Joanne states, "only a radiologist or other physician can report back to the patient the testing results." As a result, radiologic technologists must be able to deflect questions in a polite manner and be able to deal with any information they discover objectively and unemotionally so as to succeed at their job.

Joanne cautions prospective radiologic technologists to be aware of the repetitiveness of the job, that techs spend long hours on their feet, and are subject to frequent overtime. Other aspects which make the job demanding is the physical stress of lifting and moving patients and the emotional stress, especially in a hospital setting, of knowing a patient, sometimes a child, has a life-threatening illness.

Furthermore, she would like students to be aware of the dedication one needs to perform this job and follow through on continuing education requirements outside the workplace.

Finally, those pursuing a career in radiologic technology must be aware of the potential exposure to radiation and communicable disease. When confronted with the radiation issue, Joanne points out that, "the standards relating to radiation are quite high." Radiologic technologists wear lead aprons when performing fluoroscopies and other procedures. "We also wear a radiation badge," Joanne points to her collar, "that is checked once a month by a private firm for exposure levels." In terms of disease exposure, radiologic technologists prescribe to universal standards when dealing with diseases such as AIDS, hepatitis, and tuberculosis, wearing rubber gloves, gowns, and masks to maintain health and safety standards. Although radiation and disease pose a risk, radiologic technologists can be diligent and aware so as to avoid exposure in the fulfillment of their duties.

To be a successful radiologic technologist, you should

- Have compassion and a personal touch
- Have patience and a flexible personality
- Be extroverted and able to communicate in a clear and concise manner
- Have an understanding of medical terminology and procedures

how do I become a radiologic technologist?

Joanne earned an associate's degree in applied science from the radiology program at Moraine Valley Community College in Palos Hills, Illinois. Joanne always had an interest in science and, combining that with her love of helping people, found a career in the radiologic sciences to be a good fit.

After completing the requirements for her degree, Joanne found her job through word of mouth. She had the qualifications and educational experience necessary to be hired almost immediately out of school by Meyer Medical Clinic.

education

High School

Students who intend to pursue a career as a radiologic technologist should take courses in the sciences—namely, biology, anatomy, physics, and chemistry. They should also take courses in mathematics and take advantage of any technical writing, speech, and English classes, which will allow them to hone their communication skills. Unlike a few other technical careers, a high school degree is required for entry into radiologic technology training programs.

Postsecondary Training

Instruction in the radiologic sciences is offered at universities and colleges in the form of four-year baccalaureate programs and two-year associate's degree programs, in hospitals in the form of a two-year hospital certificate program, and also in the armed forces.

Joanne describes her education at Moraine Valley as, "time consuming and intense." A two-year associate's program consists of a mixture of theory and two thousand practical hours. Do to the intense nature of her education, Joanne found it necessary, like many other radiologic students, to take an additional year to complete the educational requirements.

The curriculum that aspiring radiologic technologists will experience includes instruction in anatomy and physiology, radiation physics and biology, pathology, medical technology instruction and procedures, principles and techniques of diagnostic imaging, patient care and medical ethics, and radiation safety and protection. Joanne counsels all prospective radiologic technologists to be sure that the program they invest their time and money in is accredited by the Joint Review Committee on Education in Radiologic Technology (JRCERT).

certification or licensing

All medical employers require certification by the American Registry of Radiologic Technologists (ARRT). Radiologic students, upon completion of their education, are expected to take and pass the National Registry Boards to allow employment.

Joanne is certified in X ray by the ARRT and describes the exam as intense. The Boards include a written test, consisting of two hundred questions in five categories: modality (equipment operation), patient care, radiation protection, radiation procedures, and image production and evaluation. All students must be registry-eligible, which means registered with the ARRT to take the test the next time it is offered. The Registry Boards are offered four times a year. Joanne is also certified by the Illinois Department of Nuclear Medicine (IDNM). Illinois is one of only twenty-six states that required state licensure by 1992.

In addition to standard certification, a vast degree of continuing education exists in the radiologic field. "This field is highly regulated and legislated, due to the use of radiation," comments Kathy Radcliffe, who is Joanne's supervisor and a department head at Meyer Medical. "The Illinois Department of Health, the Nuclear Safety Commission, and the Federal Drug Administration all have a role in regulating the radiologic industry."

Although she is not a member of a professional organization such as ASRT (American Society of Radiologic Technologists), Joanne does admit to their worth as a source of information and knowledge, and lauds their diligence in lobbying for universal standards for radiologic technologists relating to education and employment.

In order to maintain proper certification, Joanne and other radiologic technologists must take twenty-four hours of continuing education in the course of two years. These courses are offered by technical-type programs and also the Institute for Professional Growth (IFPG), which offers X-ray seminars at area hotels. "The state follows this very closely," Joanne says. "If you don't get credit, they suspend your license, and you could even lose it." Joanne's employer pays for her continuing education classes, although not all employers will do so.

internships and volunteerships

Radiologic technologists gain valuable internship experience in the course of the two thousand practical hours that are required to gain a degree. Those in a hospital certificate program will gain experience on-site throughout their education.

There is no direct way to gain radiologic experience without the appropriate qualifications. The medium of radiation causes strict legislation and regulation to be maintained.

For interested high school students, a school guidance counselor may be able to set up a meeting between students and a professional radiologic technologist at his or her place of work. In this way, students could observe the duties, facilities, and equipment used, as well as ask questions of the technologist. Another way to gain more information and make a good contact in the field is to speak with a teacher of radiology at an educational program.

who will hire me?

There are a wide variety of work environments in which a radiologic technologist may work. While most radiologic technologists work in hospitals, others may work in physician's offices, HMOs (Health Maintenance Organizations), mobile imaging clinics, or for a radiological group. Others may work in nursing homes or extended health care facilities.

Hospitals provide radiologic technologists with the best opportunity for employment. Three out of five radiologic technologists work in hospitals. Other potential employers include private physician's offices, HMOs, mobile imaging clinics, specialized imaging centers, industrial plants, research centers, and government agencies. Most cities have employment agencies which specialize in the health care field. Application through employment services, "headhunters," or through the personnel officers of potential health care employers will also prove successful.

Overall, rural areas and small towns will offer more opportunity for employment than cities will, while not offering the amenities or high pay and benefits an urban employer may be able to offer.

Joanne, although she found her job through word of mouth, is quick to point out that there are also job listings in radiologic trade magazines.

Related Jobs

Did you know that there are a number of jobs related to radiologic technologist? The U.S. Department of Labor classifies these technologists under the headings "Occupations in Medical and Dental Technology" and "Nursing, Therapy, and Specialized Teaching Services." Radiologic technologists can use their knowledge of sophisticated equipment to help physicians, dentists, and other health practitioners to diagnose patients. Others in this category are people who use different types of therapy, such as art, music, pet, and horticulture, to treat patients. Related jobs include nuclear medicine technologists, cardiovascular technologists, perfusionists, respiratory therapists, clinical laboratory technologists, diagnostic medical sonographers, and electroneurodiagnostic technologists.

where can I go from here?

Those interested in moving beyond a career in radiologic technology should be aware that advanced jobs can only be acquired through further education. This education may be provided in-house, at a teaching hospital, or a technical or college setting. Those obtaining a bachelor's degree will have the best chance for advancement. Further education will allow radiologic technologists to become certified in CT (cat scan), ultrasound, MRI (magnetic resonance imaging), nuclear medicine, and others, thereby gaining experience and flexibility to prosper in the work place.

With considerable experience, radiologic technologists can rise to teaching positions, or train new technologists in-house or at other locations. Other radiologic technologists may use their experience to work in sales and marketing, demonstrating new equipment for medically oriented businesses.

Radiologic technologists employed in hospitals have the opportunity to advance to administrative and supervisory positions. Those who gain their bachelor's degree, then a master's degree in health administration, may choose to seek a position as a hospital administrator or manage a business for radiologists.

Joanne enjoys the diagnostic part of her job and plans to broaden her capabilities and certification by taking the board exams for mammography later in the year. This certification will allow her to be more competitive and well-rounded if and when she decides to reenter the job field.

what are the salary ranges?

Starting salaries for entry-level radiologic technologists range from $22,000 to $29,000 per year. Technologists with experience may earn between $27,000 and $30,000 per year. Senior technologists with more responsibility and experience may earn up to $35,000 per year. On average, radiologic technologists that are employed by hospitals enjoy higher salaries than those that work for HMOs or private physician's offices.

Compensation and pay scales will vary based on the location of the employer—with urban areas more lucrative than rural and small towns—and on the level of education

Advancement Possibilities

Computed tomography technologists, working closely with physicians, are responsible for taking detailed cross-sectional pictures of the internal structures of the human body.

Magnetic resonance imaging (MRI) technologists use computers, radio waves, and powerful magnets to create images of specific parts of the body.

Diagnostic medical sonographers use high frequency sound waves, not radiation, to create images of internal body structures.

Chief technologists and **technical administrators** are radiologic technologists who have, through experience and further education, risen to supervisory positions in hospitals.

Radiologic instructors teach in university settings, teaching hospitals, and in two-year technical programs.

attained, the experience, and the responsibilities of the technologist.

what is the job outlook?

The field of radiologic technology is expected to grow faster than the average for all other occupations to the year 2005. This is due to the vast clinical potential of diagnostic imaging. New uses for radiologic technology will continue to be discovered, therefore increasing demand. Although enrollment in many radiologic education programs has increased, demand for qualified technologists in some areas of the country far exceeds the supply. Opportunities in small towns and rural areas exist for those flexible about location and compensation.

Another factor that will influence growth is the aging of the American population. As the median age rises, more attention will be focused on diseases that are prominent in older people. Many of these diseases require the use of imaging equipment and technologists. The southeast region of the United States offers significant employment opportunity due to its large population of retirement-age Americans.

The position of hospitals as a significant employer of radiologic technologists will be secure, yet a strong shift toward non-hospital settings such as imaging centers, HMOs, and private physician's offices will occur. This change will be caused by a cost-cutting trend by third party payers, possible government intervention in the health care system, and the rise of HMO-type systems. There will be little reduction in the number of procedures done in hospitals, though more will be done on an out-patient basis, and on weekends and evenings, therefore increasing the need for part-time technologists with flexible schedules.

A few major points offset these glowing predictions. The advent of new technology depends largely on cost and reimbursement considerations. The uneasy mood of the public and government concerning health care may cause some procedures, which might have brought new jobs and growth, to be deemed too expensive to be implemented.

It is also important to keep in mind the limited opportunity for employment for those who wish to remain in urban areas. "There is an overload in the field," Joanne admits. "There are very few full-time jobs." As hospitals downsize, more procedures are being performed as out-patient treatments, opening doors for part-time employees, while shrinking full-time opportunities. Kathy Radcliffe, Joanne's superior, agrees. "Our field, like others, is cyclical in nature. Yet, there will always be a need for imaging."

Although there will always be a need for imaging, prospective radiologic technologists must be aware that stiff competition exists for good jobs. One must be prepared to be flexible in order to prosper in the field. With the population continuing to age, and new technologies emerging, the saturation cycle gripping radiologic technology will end, creating new demand for qualified radiologic technologists. Education will provide the best means for advancement. Those technologists with advanced training in mammography, CT imaging, MRI, ultrasound, and other technologies, stand to prosper. A combination of flexibility, education, and awareness will help radiologic technologists succeed in the job field of the twenty-first century.

how do I learn more?

professional organizations

Following are organizations that provide information on radiologic careers.

American Board of Radiology
2301 West Big Beaver Road, Suite 625
Troy, MI 48084
TEL: 810-643-0300

American Healthcare Radiology Administrators
P.O. Box 334
Sudbury, MA 01776
TEL: 508-443-7591

Radiological Society of North America
2021 Spring Road, Suite 600
Oak Brook, IL 60521
TEL: 630-571-2670
WEBSITE: http://www.rsna.org

American Registry of Radiologic Technologists (ARRT)
1255 Northland Drive
St. Paul, MN 55120
TEL: 612-687-0048
WEBSITE: http://www.arrt.org

American Medical Association
515 North Dearborn Street
Chicago, Illinois 60610
TEL: 312-464-5000

American Society of Radiologic Technologists (ASRT)
15000 Central Avenue SE
Albuquerque, NM 87123
TEL: 505-298-4500
WEBSITE: http://www.asrt.org

American Association for Women Radiologists
1891 Preston White Drive
Reston, VA 22091
TEL: 703-648-8939

bibliography

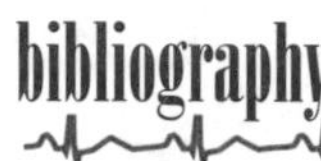

Following is a sampling of materials relating to the professional concerns and development of radiologic technologists.

Books

Bushong, Stewart C. *Radiologic Science for Technologists: Physics, Biology, and Protection*, 5th edition. St. Louis: Mosby, 1993.

Gurley, LaVerne T., and William J. Callaway, editors. *Introduction to Radiologic Technology,* 4th edition. St. Louis: Mosby, 1996.

Parelli, Robert J. *Radiation Technology Clinical Manual.* Delray Beach, FL: Saint Lucie Press, 1997.

Smith, Ronald R. *X-Ray Technologist.* San Jose, CA: R & E Publishers, 1993.

Torres, Lillian S. *Basic Medical Techniques and Patient Care for Radiologic Technologists,* 4th edition. Philadelphia, PA: Lippincott-Raven, 1993.

Periodicals

Radiologic Technology. Bimonthly. Aimed at professionals. American Society of Radiologic Technologists, 15000 Central Avenue SE, Albuquerque, NM 87123, 505-298-4500.

Radiology Management. Quarterly. Nonmedical topics involving healthcare radiology. American Healthcare Radiology Administrators, 111 Boston Post Road, Suite 215, Sudbury, MA 01776, 508-443-7591.

Radiology Today. Monthly. Newspaper with articles directed toward medical imaging personnel. Slack, Inc., 6900 Grove Road, Thorofare, NJ 08086, 609-848-1000.

radiologist

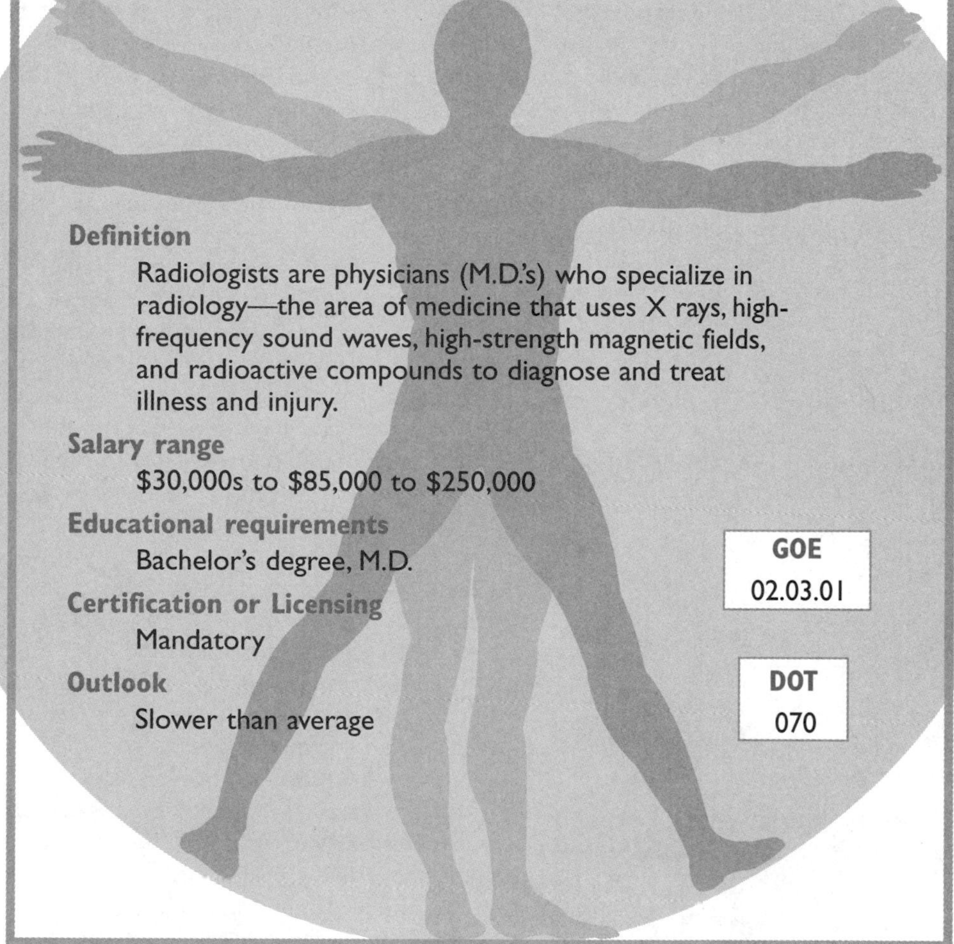

Definition

Radiologists are physicians (M.D.'s) who specialize in radiology—the area of medicine that uses X rays, high-frequency sound waves, high-strength magnetic fields, and radioactive compounds to diagnose and treat illness and injury.

Salary range

$30,000s to $85,000 to $250,000

Educational requirements

Bachelor's degree, M.D.

Certification or Licensing

Mandatory

Outlook

Slower than average

GOE
02.03.01

DOT
070

High School Subjects

Math
Biology
Chemistry
English

Personal Interests

Helping people
Solving problems
Scientific curiosity
Challenging oneself

Doctor Arildsen stepped into his office at Vanderbilt Medical Center's Radiology Department and checked the messages on his desk: a biopsy that had to be rescheduled, a colleague who wanted to arrange a consultation, and—this looked interesting—a request for a consultation with the sports medicine specialists concerning a football player's injured knee.

As a diagnostic radiologist specializing in work with body CT scans and MRIs, Ronald Arildsen was often called in on cases involving sports injuries. It was one of his favorite parts of the job.

Dr. Arildsen frowned intently at the MRIs of the athlete's knee. This knee had taken some serious damage, he concluded. There was no doubt about that.

what does a radiologist do?

Radiologists are physicians who specialize in the diagnosis and treatment of injury and disease by means of X rays, high-frequency sound waves, high-strength magnetic fields, and radioactive compounds. Radiologists read and interpret the images produced by radiological technologists and sonographers. The field of radiology is divided into several subfields, including *diagnostic radiology* (diagnosis through the use of various imaging techniques), *radiation oncology* (the treatment of tumors by various forms of radiation), and *nuclear medicine* (diagnosis and/or treatment by the introduction of radiopharmaceuticals [radioactive materials] into the body).

Radiology is slightly more than a century old. It came into existence in 1895 when the discovery of X rays by Wilhelm Roentgen revolutionized medicine by making it possible for doctors to see inside the body without cutting it open. In taking an X ray, streams of high-energy photons penetrate the body and produce images of internal structures that can be preserved on photographic film. Before the discovery of X rays, the only ways to study the body's bones and organs were 1) by touching the outside of the body (which gave very limited knowledge of the inside of the body), 2) through surgery, and 3) through autopsy of the body after the patient's death.

Diagnostic radiologists today still use X rays, but they also have many other more sophisticated imaging techniques that have been invented in recent decades. The CT (computed tomography) scan, developed in the early 1970s, makes use of computer technology to turn ordinary X-ray images into three-dimensional composite cross-sections. CT scans provide far more detailed information than ordinary X rays about the location, extent, and characteristics of the injury or disease. They are especially useful in planning reconstructive surgery or cancer therapy.

MRI (magnetic resonance imaging) is an advanced diagnostic technique in which the patient, who is lying inside a tube, is exposed to powerful electromagnetic fields. Computer technology turns the data obtained into two-dimensional images that enable radiologists to examine abnormalities of the spinal cord, abdomen, pelvis, brain, and other organs, bones, and tissues.

Ultrasound techniques use high-frequency sound waves (instead of radiation) to produce images. Because pregnant women should not be exposed to radiation, ultrasound images are obtained in order to discover the number, age, position, and condition of the fetus (or fetuses). Other ultrasound procedures are the echocardiogram (used to examine the heart) and Doppler ultrasound (used to study the blood flow in the veins and arteries).

Radiation oncologists are specialists in the use of various forms of radiation in the treatment of tumors. It is necessary to determine the location and extent of the tumor as precisely as possible, since the goal is to target the radiation (such as gamma rays, electron

lingo to learn

Angioplasty An interventional radiological procedure that uses a balloon-tipped catheter to open blocked or narrowed arteries.

CT scan Computed tomography scan—also known as a CAT (computed axial tomography) scan—a diagnostic procedure that uses computer technology to produce three-dimensional composite cross-sectional images of internal structures from X rays.

Echocardiogram An ultrasonic technique for examining a patient's heart.

Mammography X-ray examination of the breasts to detect cancer in its earliest stages.

MRI Magnetic resonance imaging: a diagnostic procedure that produces two-dimensional visual images of internal structures by placing the patient in a powerful electromagnetic field.

Oncology The branch of medicine that deals with tumors.

Pathology The branch of medicine that identifies and studies disease processes by examination of body organs, tissues, and fluids obtained during surgery or autopsy.

"Plain film" Ordinary X rays (as distinguished from more sophisticated radiological images).

Ultrasound The use of high-frequency sound waves to produce images of structures within the body.

beams, or other forms) to destroy the cancer cells without doing serious harm to the healthy cells that surround the tumor. Usually the radiation is administered by external beam, but sometimes radioactive sources (such as iodine or cesium) are inserted directly into the body at the site of the tumor. Cancer treatment often combines radiation therapy, surgery, and chemotherapy. Even when the cancer cannot be cured, radiation treatment often reduces pain and other symptoms.

Radiologists who work in the field of nuclear medicine produce images and treat disease by placing radiopharmaceuticals (radioactive materials) in the body. When radioisotopes are inserted into the circulatory system and tracked by special cameras, they yield information not obtainable by X rays. The PET (positron emission technology) technique, for example, is used to study blood flow and brain function and is an important tool in the diagnosis of Alzheimer's disease and cancer. SPECT (single photon emission computed tomography) is used to monitor heart function. Radioisotopes are also sent through the bloodstream to treat certain cancers.

Interventional radiological techniques are used to do biopsies, drain abscesses, and open blocked or narrowed arteries (balloon angioplasty). Through these high-tech minimally invasive procedures, radiologists often make it possible for patients to avoid having to undergo surgery.

what is it like to be a radiologist?

Like most radiologists, Ronald Arildsen spends the greater part of each day sitting in a darkened room reading and interpreting various kinds of images, preparing reports of his findings, and holding consultations with surgeons, internists, and other doctors. "Radiologists are often called doctors' doctors," he says, meaning that radiologists work more closely with other doctors than with patients.

"When doctors don't know what to do," explains Dr. Lisa Sheppard Boal, a diagnostic radiologist in basic community practice at Passaic-Beth Israel Hospital in Passaic, New Jersey, "the first people they consult are the radiologists and pathologists." (Pathologists are physicians who specialize in examining tissues, organs, and body fluids for clues to the diagnosis and prognosis of disease.) Because Boal is in community practice, she works in all fields of diagnostic radiology, although her special area of interest is neuroradiology (radiology of the head and spine). Dr. Arildsen is a specialist in body CT scans and MRIs. In addition to working with CT scans and MRIs, he also reads "plain film" X rays of the body.

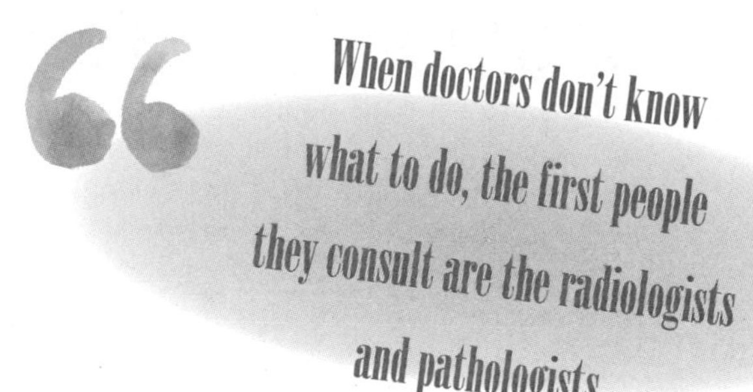

As the morning wore on, Ronald Arildsen studied one set of images after another, read the notes from the clinicians who had originally examined the patients, and formed his conclusions. This patient's problem was gallstones, painful but not life-threatening. And this one had a compound fracture of the tibia and a torn ligament. Here was some encouraging news, thought Dr. Arildsen as he examined new film of a tumor that was currently under treatment. He could see definite evidence that the tumor had shrunk, which meant that the treatment strategy was working.

Dr. Arildsen checked his watch. This year, he was teaching the basic radiology course for second-year medical students, and he needed to take time to go over his lecture notes before class. He was also codirector of the fourth-year radiology elective, which gave him the pleasure of working with future radiologists. Since coming to Vanderbilt in 1991, he had found that he particularly enjoyed teaching at the medical school and working with radiology residents.

After class, he would take care of that rescheduled liver biopsy. Guided by radiological imaging, needles can be inserted into almost any part of the body with a high degree of precision, which makes it possible to do biopsies and drain internal abscesses without performing surgery.

Dr. Boal was having a busy day, too, at Passaic-Beth Israel. She had been sitting in the viewing room reading X rays, ultrasounds, upper GIs (images of the upper gastrointestinal tract), CT scans, and MRIs for several hours, when the emergency room called. A stroke patient had just been brought in and Dr. Boal, as a specialist in neuroradiology, was needed to evaluate the damage.

That afternoon Dr. Boal would be working at the outpatient center, interviewing women coming in for mammograms (X-ray examination of the breasts) and then interpreting the results for them. She would also be working with some pregnant women who were having ultrasounds. Reading ultrasounds was one of the parts of her job that she found especially enjoyable as a thirty-year-old mother of two small children (the younger only nine months old).

Being in community practice is always stimulating, Dr. Boal thought, because it offers the opportunity to be involved with diagnostic work in so many different areas of medicine. With the recent introduction of managed health care, radiologists are also becoming increasingly involved in helping to make decisions about how the hospital can provide the best possible care for the lowest price.

Dr. Boal likes the intellectual challenge involved in diagnosis and feels a deep satisfaction when she is able to hit on the right answer in a perplexing case. She has never forgotten the advice of one of her professors at Jefferson Medical School: "If you hear thundering hoofbeats in the distance (and you're not in Africa), they're probably horses, not zebras." In other words, *first* consider the most likely explanations for the patients' symptoms before you start exploring rare diseases.

FYI

Radiology was developed in 1895 when the discovery of X rays revolutionized medicine by making it possible to see inside the body without cutting it open.

have I got what it takes to be a radiologist?

The first question to aske yourself, of course, is: "Have I got what it takes to be a doctor?" Becoming a doctor is a long and gruelling process, requiring strong academic ability (especially in the sciences), commitment, and perseverance.

The next question is whether radiology is the right medical specialty for you. Diagnostic radiology would not be the right field for a doctor who would want to experience a large amount of direct contact with patients, since diagnostic radiologists spend most of their time examining film and consulting with medical colleagues. Radiation oncologists and those radiologists who specialize in interventional radiological procedures spend more time with patients than diagnostic radiologists.

Radiologists describe their work as intellectually stimulating and full of variety. "You must be very alert to detail," stresses Lisa Sheppard Boal. Another radiologist described the field as attractive for "cerebral types who like to think things through," while also having opportunities for performing procedures and working as part of a medical team. One radiologist mentioned a colleague who found radiology a very satisfying field after developing a hearing loss that made it difficult to have a lot of direct patient contact.

Radiology is one of the best-paid medical specialties. It is not physically draining like some fields, especially surgery. After radiologists complete their residencies, they can generally count on "normal" working hours. Dr. Boal, for example, works eight-hour days at Passaic-Beth Israel. When she is "on call," it is via computer hook-up at her home (a recent innovation that she welcomes). That means she is able to receive film images on a home computer screen instead of having to drive into the hospital.

Because they do so much of their work behind the scenes, radiologists have more job-security concerns than doctors in some other fields. Patients will often insist on having a particular internist or obstetrician, but no one demands that a particular radiologist interpret their X rays. One result of this anonymity is that cost-conscious hospitals and HMOs are tempted to save money by replacing experienced radiologists with less experienced—and therefore lower-salaried—colleagues.

how do I become a radiologist?

education

To be a successful radiologist you should

- Have a good foundation in the sciences
- Enjoy intellectual challenges
- Have strong powers of concentration and an eye for detail
- Have the ability to work well with physicians in other fields of medicine

High School

Prospective radiologists, like all persons hoping to be doctors, should take a good college preparatory program in high school. The sciences—biology, chemistry, and physics—are especially important, as is a solid foundation in mathematics. You also need to take English, foreign languages, history, and other humanities courses. Future physicians should work on developing effective study habits and communication skills.

Postsecondary Training

In college, a future physician should enroll in a liberal arts program with a strong emphasis on the sciences. Biology and chemistry are the most obvious choices for a major. Many colleges offer a premed course of study for students planning on applying to medical school; this is the most appropriate track to follow if it is available at your college. Whatever your major, you need to take as many courses as possible in biology, chemistry (both organic and inorganic), and physics. Humanities and social sciences (psychology, sociology, economics, anthropology) are also important in providing a well-rounded education. High grades are essential.

Students should begin planning for medical school well in advance. Examine the admissions requirements for the medical schools to which you intend to apply and plan your undergraduate program accordingly; this information is available in the publication called *Admissions Requirements of American Medical Colleges Including Canada*. You should make arrangements to take the Medical College Admission Test (MCAT) *before* your senior year. This is a standardized test required by all U.S. medical schools, and your score is an important factor in admissions decisions. The test covers verbal ability (language skills), quantitative ability (mathematics), and the humanities and social sciences, in addition to biology, chemistry, and physics.

When it is time to apply to medical school, the American Medical College Application Service (AMCAS) is available to assist with the application process. You should apply to at least three medical schools to improve your chances of acceptance. (Sometimes students are able to enter medical school after only three years of college, but the usual practice is to complete the four-year undergraduate program first.) About half of all qualified applicants are accepted in medical school each year. If you are not accepted the first year you apply, consult your adviser about how to become a stronger candidate for the following year (by doing a year of graduate work in biology, for example).

Medical school is four years of rigorous study. When medical students feel overwhelmed, however, they should remind themselves that nearly everyone who starts medical school really does complete the program and graduate. The first two years of medical school are generally devoted to basic science work—human anatomy and physiology, biochemistry, microbiology, pathology, pharmacology, and human behavior. During this period, the student attends lectures and seminars and does laboratory work. The first two years may also include actual experience with patients and early instruction in giving physical examinations, interviewing, diagnosing, and counseling.

The last two years of medical school concentrate on the clinical sciences (the various medical specialties)—internal medicine, surgery, pediatrics, obstetrics, gynecology, psychiatry, and family medicine. While remaining closely supervised, the student is actively involved in patient treatment as part of a hospital medical team. The student also continues to do course work. In addition to the clinical sciences, there may be work in such areas as medical ethics and decision analysis cost containment. During these years, students begin zeroing in on a future specialty. A prospective radiologist at Vanderbilt Medical School, for example, could take the fourth-year radiology elective, currently being taught by Dr. Ronald Arildsen.

certification or licensing

After finishing medical school and receiving the M.D., students go on to do hospital residencies. At an early point in the residency period, all students are required to pass a medical licensing examination administered by the board of medical examiners in each state. The length of the residency depends on the specialty chosen. Radiologists spend four to seven years gaining advanced training as resident physicians. As all doctors warn, the residency years are tough—long hours of demanding work and intensive study that are physically draining and often put a severe strain on family and personal life. At the end of an accredited residency training program, physicians must pass certification examinations in their field. The evaluation program is directed by the appropriate specialty board of the American Board of Medical Specialties.

scholarships and grants

Becoming a physician is expensive, but strongly committed students should not be deterred by the financial obstacles involved. Consult the financial-aid office of the academic institution that you plan to attend to find out about scholarships, grants, loans, work/study programs, and other possible sources of assistance. Ronald Arildsen attended Columbia Medical School on a Navy scholarship. In return, he spent five years working as a general practitioner in the U.S. Navy after graduation. Then he returned to Columbia for his radiology residency.

Over 80 percent of medical students need to take out loans, and many graduate deeply in debt. Students must keep in mind, however, that physicians can expect high earnings after they complete their medical school and residency training. Residents' salaries are generally in the $30,000s.

internships and volunteerships

Students considering careers in medicine may find opportunities to test that interest through part-time or summer jobs or volunteer work at hospitals, clinics, or physicians' offices.

who will hire me?

About 90 percent of radiologists are in group practice. Some groups are composed exclusively of diagnostic radiologists or radiological oncologists, while others have members from both areas. New members generally need to belong to a group for several years before becoming full partners. The American College of Radiology (the professional association for radiologists and radiological physicists) defines a radiology group as any practice with at least two radiologists—this includes private groups, the radiology units of multispecialty groups, academic groups, and groups on the staffs of government facilities.

A job-listing service for radiology groups and a job-placement service for radiologists seeking employment are provided by the American College of Radiology, but relatively little use is made of these services. Professional contacts and recommendations play a much more important role in recruitment and placement.

where can I go from here?

Advancement for a radiologist, as for other medical specialists, means gaining the respect of one's colleagues and progressing in professional skill, knowledge, reputation, and income. Radiologists who are interested in research and teaching advance through involvement with university medical schools and teaching hospitals. A radiologist with an interest in administration might have the goal of becoming a hospital's director of radiology or chair of a medical school's radiology department.

Radiologists typically report a high level of satisfaction with their work. "I wouldn't be happy doing anything else," declared Dr. Lisa Sheppard Boal.

what are the salary ranges?

Residents in radiology earn salaries in the $30,000s. After completing their residency and joining radiological groups, they can eventually anticipate very high incomes. In 1993, the average income for a radiologist (after expenses and before taxes) was nearly $260,000. As was recently pointed out, however, there may be a trend toward cost-cutting by replacing high-paid experienced radiologists with radiologists who are just finishing their training. Data from the mid-1990s indicates that radiology groups prefer to hire recent graduates instead of radiologists with 10 or more years of experience.

what is the job outlook?

The job outlook for radiologists has been the subject of considerable research in recent years. In the late 1980s, a serious shortage of radiologists was predicted. In 1992, supply and demand in the field seemed to be balanced. Over the last few years, there have been signs that the job outlook for radiologists is weakening as a result of oversupply.

About 50 percent of radiology training program directors surveyed by the American College of Radiology in 1994 reported that the job market for radiologists completing their residency that year was "about the same" as in the last few years. Twenty-five percent said that the market was "somewhat more difficult," and 18 percent characterized it as "much more difficult" or "most difficult in many years." In early 1995, it was reported that new radiologists were having a harder time finding positions than in the previous year.

These comments should not taken out of perspective; 96 percent of graduating residents in 1994 already had job commitments by late spring when the survey was taken. The 1994 unemployment rate for all radiologists was only 0.5 percent. Nevertheless, the fact that 1994 hiring levels were only 70 percent those of 1991 should give cause for some concern that the outlook for radiologists is weakening.

Long-term predictions are difficult. The U.S. health care industry is in a period of change and transition. New developments, such as managed care, may result in an overall weakened job market for physicians, especially specialists.

how do I learn more?

professional organizations

For additional information about becoming a radiologist, contact the following:

American Medical Association
515 North State Street
Chicago, IL 60610
TEL: 312-464-5000
WEBSITE: http://www.ama-assn.org

American College of Radiology
1891 Preston White Drive
Reston, VA 20191
TEL: 703-648-8900
WEBSITE: http://plsgroup.com

bibliography

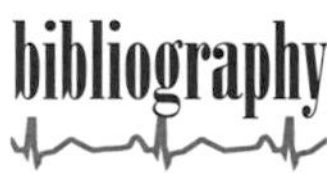

Following is a sampling of materials relating to the professional concerns and development of radiologists.

Books

Callaway, William J. *Mosby's Comprehensive Review of Radiology*. St. Louis, MO: Mosby, 1995.

Chen, Michael Y., Thomas L. Pope, and David J. Ott, editors. *Basic Radiology*. New York, NY: McGraw-Hill, 1995.

Mettler, Fred A., Jr. *Essentials of Radiology.* Philadelphia, PA: W.B. Saunders Co., 1995.

Periodicals

Radiation Research. Monthly. Scientific articles discussing radiation effects. Academic Press, Inc., 1250 6th Avenue, San Diego, CA 92101, 619-699-6646.

Radiational Health Bulletin. Monthly. Information on the prevention of unnecessary exposure to radiation. BRH Bulletin, FDA, 5600 Fishers Lane, Rockville, MD 20852, 301-443-5860.

Radiation & Imaging Letter. Semimonthly. Newsletter which includes radiation therapy topics. Radiology Letter, Quest Publishing Co., 1351 Titan Way, Brea, CA 92621, 714-738-6400.

recreational therapist

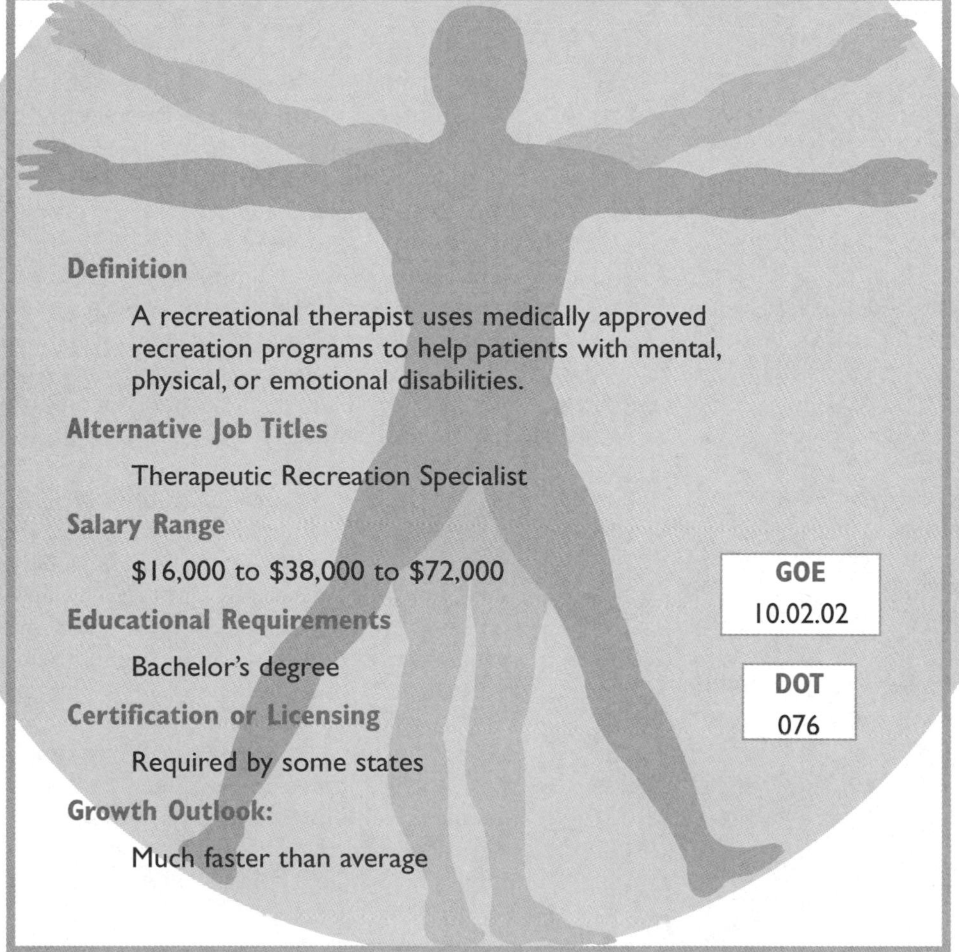

Definition

A recreational therapist uses medically approved recreation programs to help patients with mental, physical, or emotional disabilities.

Alternative Job Titles

Therapeutic Recreation Specialist

Salary Range

$16,000 to $38,000 to $72,000

Educational Requirements

Bachelor's degree

Certification or Licensing

Required by some states

Growth Outlook:

Much faster than average

GOE
10.02.02

DOT
076

High School Subjects

Biology
English
Psychology

Personal Interests

Exercise
Games
Helping people
Sports

Four people show up at a restaurant five minutes before their dinner reservations. They are talking, sometimes laughing as they wait. Two of them appear to be a little nervous, perhaps, but they are smiling and enjoying themselves just the same. They order, snack on appetizers, and then eat, taking time to savor the food and the evening out. When the meal is over, they pay and leave.

Sound ordinary? For thousands of people with cognitive or physical disabilities, a night like this one might rarely happen. This is not because they are unable to go out to dinner and enjoy themselves—it is because nobody has shown them the skills they need to take part in everyday life and to enhance their well-being. A recreational therapist is trained to assess the recreational needs of a disabled person, and to help find leisure activities that will be fulfilling, interesting, and accessible.

During dinner at the restaurant, one of the party leaves the table to find the rest room. Coming back she is beaming. In her wheelchair she has successfully navigated the tables and chairs in her way, and she receives the congratulations of her therapist and other dinner companions.

what does a recreational therapist do?

Recreational therapists, often referred to as *therapeutic recreation specialists,* work with people who have mental, physical, or emotional disabilities. They plan, organize, direct, and monitor recreation programs for patients in hospitals, clinics, and various community settings. These therapists use sports, games, music, arts and crafts, and other activities to assist clients in developing, improving, or maintaining functional skills.

Some clients need help in recovering from a recent injury or in learning how to stay active despite a disability. Therapists might design seniors' programs that use leisure activities to improve general health and well-being. Therapists who work with developmentally disabled people may use recreation to introduce clients to social interaction in a non-threatening, supportive, and fun environment. Among substance abusers or people in prison, recreational therapists use recreational activities as a way of stimulating acceptable social behavior and interests, and to raise self-awareness and self-esteem. Other clients use recreational therapy as a way to relax and to manage stress to maintain mental and physical health.

Some recreational therapists work in a clinical setting, where the emphasis is on recovery or rehabilitation from a specific illness, disease, or disability. They work as part of a team with other health professionals and develop recreational activities as a form of treatment. Clinical recreational therapists may work in hospitals, outpatient clinics, rehabilitation centers, and long-term care facilities. Other therapists work in a community setting, where the emphasis is on outreach and continuing education. Community recreational therapists work with people in public and private schools, adult day care centers, community agencies, and neighborhood and county parks.

Recreational therapy often groups people with similar interests or similar abilities. Even pursuits such as reading or sewing encourage interaction when they are set up as group activities, such as a reading club or sewing circle. Recreational therapists help their clients find meaningful ways to participate in society. In doing so, they promote health, adjustment, growth, and independence.

It is commonly known that stress can lead to mental instability and breakdown. Stress has also been implicated in the weakening of the immune system, which protects the body from infections and other physical ailments. Imagine how much added stress a person is under when faced with chronic illness or long-term interruption of the abilities they rely on—walking, seeing, memory retention. For people in this predicament, realizing that

lingo to learn

Geriatrics and Gerontology The medical study of the physical processes and problems of old age. Either of these terms may be used in hospital departments with elderly patients.

Leisure Education The use of sports, hobbies, and other activities to acquire skills and abilities to lead an independent lifestyle.

Orient To acquaint with an existing situation or environment. For example, to indicate obstacles for a blind person in a place he or she frequents so that they may make a mental "map" of the area and be able to guide themselves.

Recreation The opportunity to participate in leisure activities that improve health and well-being.

Special Olympics A program of physical fitness, sports training, and athletic competition for children and adults with mental retardation.

they can still be independent and enjoy themselves is as beneficial to their physical rehabilitation as are the skills they learn from their therapeutic program. Therapists in this situation are instrumental in getting their clients to taking the first step in that rehabilitory process, by encouraging them to press past the barriers they encounter as a result of their disability or illness.

For people with paralysis or other disabilities, sports has become a hugely popular and successful recreational therapy. People with limited mobility and skill can play basketball and rugby, go skiing, and race in marathons. Professional wheelchair athletes may obtain corporate sponsorships and train year-round for national and international competitions. Being physically active is a way these athletes express their competitive spirit and earn appreciation for their athletic abilities. The success of wheelchair athletes in high-profile events, such as the Boston Marathon, has gone a long way towards establishing acceptance and opportunities for all people with disabilities.

Recreational therapists who specialize in sports educate people with disabilities and limitations about activities that are available to them. The therapist may also be a part of developing adaptive equipment for a particular individual based on their knowledge of that person's abilities and goals.

what is it like to be a recreational therapist?

Therapists in hospitals and clinics generally have regular forty hour weeks, though they may need to be involved with special events that occur after hours or on weekends. The kinds of programs that a therapist initiates depend on the people with whom they work. The clinical recreational therapist first consults with other medical professionals to determine the therapeutic needs of the client. They may work with several other therapists—speech pathologists, occupational therapists, physical therapists—to achieve a common goal for a particular client. Then they will interview the client to discover his or her activities and interests.

After determining the therapeutic needs of a client, the recreational therapist plans a program that uses levels of accomplishment as steps in measuring progress. For instance, a person who has nerve damage may go through a physical therapy program to develop dexterity in the hands. This client may also take part in a recreational therapy group that engages in gardening. Progress may be measured by the recreational therapist in terms of the increasing levels of confidence with which the client repots plants, or the the length of time the client can hold pruning scissors. Therapists evaluate the client's interests to create a program that will not only fulfill therapeutic requirements but also will be enjoyable. The recreational therapist also periodically evaluates these programs for their effectiveness, and may restructure the therapy if a client does not respond as expected.

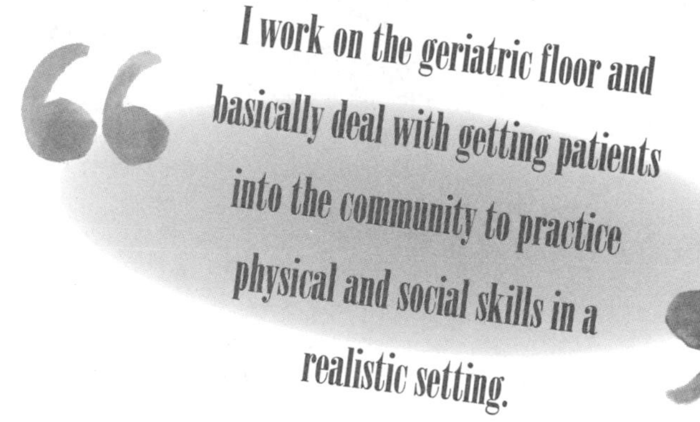

Cynthia Kowalski works with elderly hospitalized patients at the Ravenswood Hospital Medical Center in Chicago. "The trend in hospitals these days is to have a rehab department with speech therapy, recreational therapy, occupational therapy, all under one roof. I work on the geriatric floor and I basically deal with getting patients into the community to practice physical, cognitive, and social skills in a realistic setting." What works for one person may not work for another, so programs are as individually oriented as they can be, given the limitations of working within a hospital.

"First I do a planning session with the patient. Then once a week we put the program into effect—usually with other skilled co-workers like a physical therapist or occupational therapist. For instance, we might plan to go out to eat with someone who has a new disability, to focus on increased awareness. Now that they have a disability, they

Related Jobs

The U.S. Department of Labor classifies recreational therapists with other therapists concerned with the treatment and rehabilitation of persons with physical or mental disabilities or disorders. Their goal is to develop or restore functions, prevent loss of physical capacities, and maintain optimum performance. Among these workers are dance, art, and music therapists.

Dance therapists plan and conduct dance and body movement exercises to improve physical and mental well-being. *Art therapists* work with patients in various art methods, such as painting and ceramics, as part of their recovery program. *Music therapists* plan programs that can involve solo or group singing, playing in bands, listening to music, or attending concerts.

need to think about accessibility—does the restaurant have ramps? How much time will we need to give ourselves to get there? We also start them thinking about things like safety and judgment." All of these issues may seem simple, but they are things that a person with a disability might never have thought through before. The goal of the recreational therapist is to eliminate the uncertainty that might prevent their clients from continuing to live as well as they did before the disability or illness occurred.

To be a successful recreational therapist, you should

- Be comfortable working with elderly and disabled people
- Be creative, patient, and flexible
- Have good organization and communication skills
- Enjoy group activities

Cynthia also works with cognitive disabilities, like those which may be incurred from a head trauma or stroke. In a program called Advanced Reality Orientation, she gathers a group of such patients for a one-hour newspaper reading group. This serves several purposes for its participants. "We work on different cognitive functions," Cynthia relates. "Do they remember what they've read? Can they follow the thread of the conversation, and do they contribute? For this group, I really focus on the people who liked reading in the past. Sometimes, speech therapy will want [a client] there so they can practice taking part in a conversation group, but I usually suggest this program for people who are interested in current events and reading." Such a group also makes clients aware that there is a world outside the hospital, and that they can still actively participate in it.

If a reading group is not something that a client is interested in, Cynthia may suggest other therapeutic recreational programs. "I usually have a one-on-one evaluation for people who were active before; I may give them community resources on older adult programs. This kind of community re-entry depends on the functional level of the client, though." In this way, the clinical and community aspects of recreational therapy can overlap and be mutually supportive. Cynthia knows of programs in her area that will help her clients once they are out of her care, and can suggest them as a means of continuing therapy.

Other recreational therapists might have days that are completely different from Cynthia's. They might work at summer camps for disabled children, and live at the camp with their clients seven days a week. Their work might be seasonal, or oriented around events like the Special Olympics or sporting seasons. Therapists who work within community settings often spend time creating outreach programs and other social events in which disabled members of the community can voluntarily participate. Because there is less contact with participants than in hospitals, the focus of the community recreational therapist is on creating general events or activities, such as games or day trips, that can be enjoyed by any member of a specific group. Because of this, recreational therapists are sometimes called "quality of life professionals" by the National Recreation and Park Association.

do I have what it takes to be a recreational therapist?

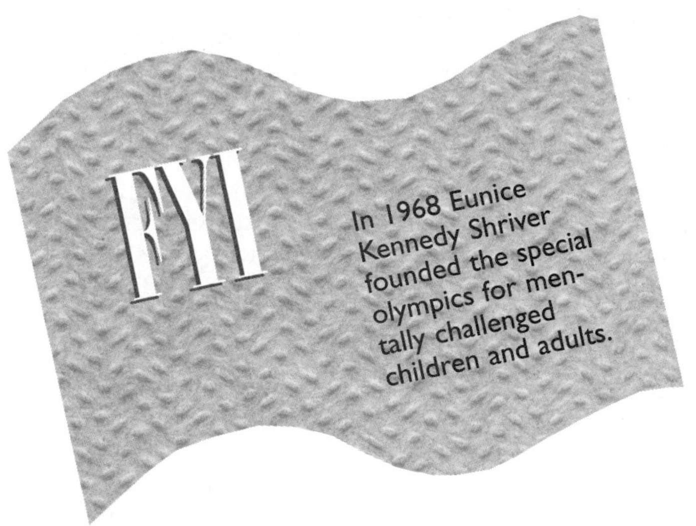

To be a recreational therapist, you must have a strong desire to help people live independently and meet their personal goals. Interest in recreational and leisure activities is also a requirement. Therapists come into contact with segments of the population, such as disabled or elderly people, who are often neglected or forgotten by traditional recreational programs. It is important to be able to recognize the value of these people as individuals, and to believe in their right to live active, healthy, and full lives. Working with other therapists and clients can be very stressful, and patience is very important when considering any job in therapy.

One of the most rewarding things about working with people in recovery and adjustment is seeing how the programs designed to help them do help. Because this kind of therapy is designed around what a client already likes to do, it can be fun to participate in the activities along with the clients. Leadership skills help the recreational therapist run programs efficiently and well. Open communication is critical to the success of the therapist-client relationship. A good therapist is willing to listen to the concerns of a client and incorporate the individual into the therapeutic goals.

A therapist with an aptitude for analysis and evaluation makes therapeutic treatment plans which are best designed for each client, and therefore most effective. An ability to focus on both short- and long-term goals allows the therapist to continue with programs that will be optimal for each client. Finally, the ability to see when a program is not working is key to helping speed recovery and adjustment.

how do I become a recreational therapist?

education

High School

While in high school, the future recreational therapist should be taking biology, sociology, and psychology, as well as developing interests in sports and other leisure-time activities. Anatomy and kinesiology are also valuable; therapists can more readily understand common dysfunction of the body if they understand common functions. Communication skills are very important to the success of the therapist, so speech and writing classes are also suggested.

While still in high school, it is possible to get some clinical experience by volunteering in hospitals or retirement communities. Duties may include bringing newspapers or magazines to patients, visiting with them, and generally being supportive of their rehabilitation efforts.

Cynthia has noticed that employment opportunities are based on the kind of volunteer work one has done. "For some reason it's hard to get a job in the park districts [community settings] if all your experience is clinical, and vice versa. So I would recommend getting as much experience in both settings as you can." Some examples of community settings include park district programs, day care facilities, summer camps, and independent programs organized by parents of children with developmental disabilities. Clinical experience might come from volunteering in hospital, a residential facility for seniors or mentally disabled, or a correctional facility in which therapy might be part of an inmate's social rehabilitation.

Postsecondary Training

More than 170 academic programs in recreational therapy are offered at colleges and universities in the United States. Course work includes natural sciences (anatomy, biology, and behavioral science) as well as social sciences (psychology, criminology and sociology). Cynthia's major course work included classes in recreation programming. These taught her how to evaluate clients to determine their course of therapy, how to develop goals, and understand the activity needs of various populations. Academic programs also require a minimum of 360 hours of internship under the supervision of a Certified Therapeutic Recreation Specialist.

Since the primary purpose of recreational therapy is to take into consideration and use the clients' needs and interests to help them take an active part of their therapy, it might be valuable to target a group with whom you are interested in working and include classes which provide information that group might find interesting.

certification or licensing

Certification is not required in most states. It does, however, indicate that the holder has met requirements set by the National Council for Therapeutic Recreation Certification. There are two standards of recognition: Therapeutic Recreational Specialist (professional level certificate), and Therapeutic Recreation Assistant (paraprofessional level certificate). There is only an exam for the professional level certificate, which earns the therapist who passes it use of the designation "Certified Therapeutic Recreation Specialist" or "CTRS."

FYI

Park districts in many communities provide special activity programs for developmentally disabled people as well as for senior citizens. The National Therapeutic Recreation Society is part of the National Recreation and Park Association. The NRPA campaigns to recognize the link between recreation and good health for everybody.

who will hire me?

The most pressing need for recreational therapists is expected to be in nursing homes and senior retirement communities, because of the increasing number of older Americans. Check with facilities in your area to see if they have recreational therapists on staff and what they expect from their therapists. How many hours of internship do they prefer? Do they look for a certain specialty more than others? How many therapists do they employ? Do they accept interns or volunteers?

Rehabilitation centers hire recreational therapists to work with the physically disabled and to develop adaptive sports programs, such as wheelchair basketball and marathon racing. Similarly, park districts, mental health facilities, and group homes use recreational therapists to teach and encourage participation in sporting events, such as the Special Olympics, for mentally or physically disabled people.

Correctional institutions hire recreational therapists to coordinate activities for inmates in order to reduce stress and depression, and to develop skills that will allow them employment opportunities when they are reassimilated into society.

General hospitals, veterans' hospitals, children's hospitals, and psychiatric hospitals provide a large number of recreational therapy jobs. Other potential employers include camps or day care centers that serve the needs of disabled or elderly people.

where do I go from here?

Therapists with three or four years of experience and a master's degree may advance to supervisory or administrative positions. Continuing education is another path to advancement. Approved classes are offered by numerous recreational therapy associations, including the American Therapeutic Recreation Association (ATRA) and the National Therapeutic Recreation Society (NTRS). Earning continuing education credits may increase a therapist's responsibility and salary levels. Some therapists teach or conduct research.

what are the salary ranges?

A newly certified recreational therapist can expect to make somewhere between $16,000 to $38,000 per year, depending on experience, educational background, and place of employment. Salary increases with experience and education. Therapists with six to ten years' experience earn between $18,000 and $50,000; those with master's degree earn between $18,000 and $72,000. Consultants and educators average $40,000 a year.

what is the job outlook?

According to the U.S. Department of Labor 1995 study, "Employment of recreational therapists is expected to grow much faster than average for all occupations through the year 2000." The number of recreational therapists, estimated at about 32,000 in 1995, is expected to reach 45,000 or more by 2005. This increase is mainly due to the growing number of older people in the U.S. population and to the increased life expectancies of the elderly and disabled people. Most job openings will be in nursing homes, retirement communities, adult day care programs, and social service agencies.

Additionally, the cost of health care will create a large demand for community-based care programs to supplement therapeutic programs in hospitals and other health care facilities. Community activity directors will most likely see an increased number of people taking part in community programs for their therapeutic, rather than leisurely, benefits.

how do I learn more?

professional organizations

Following are organizations that provide information on recreational therapy careers.

American Therapeutic Recreation Association
P. O. Box 15215
Hattiesburg, MS 39402
TEL: 601-264-3413
WEBSITE: http://www.atra-tr.org/educat.html

National Council for Therapeutic Recreation Certification
P. O. Box 479
Thiels, NY 10984
TEL: 914-947-4346

National Therapeutic Recreation Society
2775 South Quincy Street, Suite 300
Arlington VA 22206
TEL: 703-578-5548

bibliography

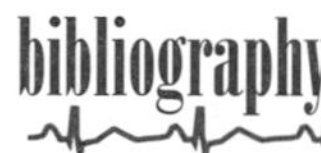

Following is a sampling of materials relating to the professional concerns and development of recreational therapists.

Books

Austin, David R., and Michael E. Crawford. *Therapeutic Recreation: an Introduction*, 2nd edition. New York, NY: Allyn & Bacon, 1996.

Carter, Marcia J., Glen E. Van Andel, and Gary M. Robb. *Therapeutic Recreation: a Practical Approach*, 2nd edition. Prospect Heights, IL: Waveland Press, 1995.

Hart, Robyn H. *Therapeutic Play Activities for Hospitalized Children*. St. Louis, MO: Mosby, 1992.

Hoey, Bernadette. *Who Calls the Tune? a Psychodramatic Approach to Child Therapy*. New York, NY: Routledge, 1996.

Periodicals

ATRA Newsletter. Bimonthly. American Therapeutic Recreation Association, Box 15215, Hattiesburg, MS 39404, 601-264-3413.

Employment Update. Monthly. Features employment and internship opportunities for therapeutic recreation professionals. American Therapeutic Recreation Association, Box 15215, Hattiesburg, MS 39404, 601-264-3413.

Recreation...Access in the 90's. Bimonthly. Provides information on integrating people with disabilities into community-based recreation programs. National Recreation and Parks Association, 2775 S. Quincy Street, Suite 300, Arlington, VA 22206, 703-820-4940.

Therapeutic Recreation Journal. Quarterly. Provides information on research in therapeutic recreation services for individuals with disabilities. National Recreation and Parks Association, 2775 S. Quincy Street, Suite 300, Arlington, VA 22206, 703-820-4940.

registered nurse

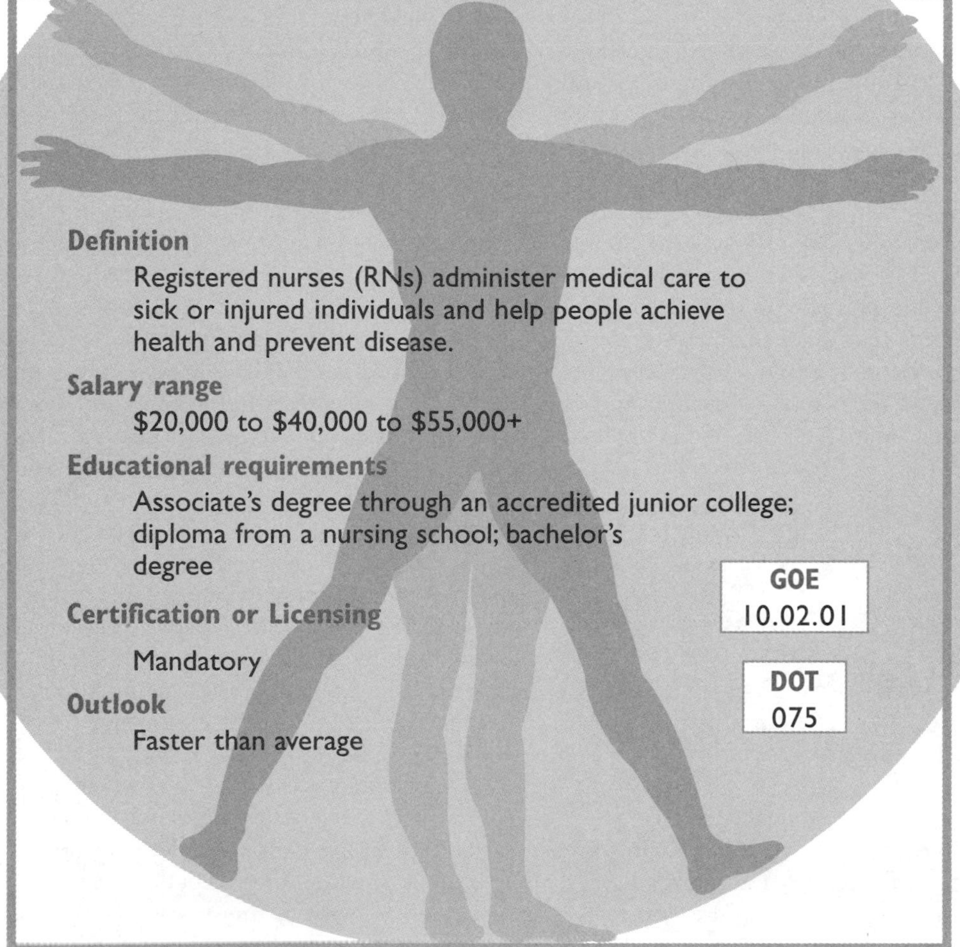

High School Subjects

Biology
Math
English

Personal Interests

Working with people
Health and fitness
Medicine

It is three in the morning in the intensive care unit. Nurses on the night shift are making their rounds, listening to the instruments that monitor their patients, changing IV bags, or giving medicine. In the emergency room it has been a slow night; only a few cases have come all at once. The flurry of activity there involves quick thinking and decision-making that could make the difference between life or death. This is quite a bit to ask of the trauma nurses who are seven hours into their shift.

Meanwhile, at a retirement community, a live-in nurse assists her client to the bathroom, walking slowly to help her navigate the long hallway from her bedroom safely. It is eleven o'clock at night. People need help at all hours, not only from nine to five. Nurses are there to provide the support, the medicine, the regimen prescribed by the doctor, to analyze a patient's progress. They also offer suggestions and emotional support to the friends and families of their clients.

what do nurses do?

Just as the title "doctor" encompasses numerous specialties and branches of study, the title *registered nurse* is an umbrella term, covering many different aspects of nursing. Although nurses work in various health-care facilities, they have three basic goals: to assist the ill, disabled, or elderly in the recovery or maintenance of life functions; to prevent illness and relapse of illness; and to promote health in the community. Most nurses come into contact with patients more frequently than other members of the health-care community. Doctors are busy with diagnosis and the creation of treatment plans, and often do not have time to carry out the plans themselves. Because of this, nurses often provide a human element in a patient's treatment. They observe a patient's symptoms and evaluate progress or lack of progress. Nurses are also responsible for educating their patients and families on how to cope with a long-term illness or disability.

The field of nursing is broken down by the setting in which a nurse works. A registered nurse typically works under the guidance of a physician, who will develop a care plan for a patient that the nurse helps to administer. But the specific work of each nurse can take many forms. About two-thirds of all nurses work in hospitals, where they are assigned to different areas. *General duty nurses* offer bedside nursing care and observe the progress of the patients. They may also supervise licensed practical nurses and aides. *Surgical nurses* are part of a logistical team in the operating room that supports the surgeon. They sterilize instruments, prepare patients for surgery, and coordinate the transfer of patients to and from the operating room. A *maternity nurse* looks after newborn infants, assists in the delivery room, and educates new mothers and fathers on basic child care. A *head nurse* directs and coordinates the activities of the nursing staff. Other hospital staff nurses are trained to work in intensive care units, the emergency room, and in the pediatrics ward.

Registered nurses work in varied settings. *Home health nurses* provide nursing care, prescribed by a physician, to patients at home. They assist a wide range of patients, such as those recovering from illnesses and accidents, and must be able to work independently. *Private duty nurses* may work in hospitals or in a patient's home. They are employed by the patient they are caring for or by the patient's family. Their duties are carried out in cooperation with the patients physician.

Office nurses work in clinics or at the private practice of a physician. Their duties may combine nursing skills—taking blood pressure, assisting with outpatient procedures, patient education—with administrative or office duties such as scheduling appointments, keeping files, and answering phones. Nurses in this field may work for a Health Maintenance Organization (HMO) or an insurance company.

Nursing home nurses direct the care of residents in long-term care facilities. The work is similar to that done in hospitals; however, a nursing home nurse cares for patients with conditions ranging from a hip fracture to

lingo to learn

Intubate To insert breathing apparatus into the throat of a patient who is unable to breathe satisfactorily.

Crash cart The cart which carries medicines, equipment, and machines that may be needed in an emergency situation in an intensive care unit or emergency room.

Case manager A nurse or administrator who coordinates the medical care of a patient.

Nursing Home A long-term care facility that provides the elderly and chronically ill with health care and assistance with daily activities, such as bathing, eating, and dressing.

Skilled Nursing Facility A facility that provides round-the-clock medical care by registered nurses and other licensed health care professionals.

Vital Signs The pulse rate, breathing rate, and body temperature of a person.

Parkinson's disease. *Public health nurses*, or *community health nurses*, work with government and private agencies to educate the public about health care issues. Their work might include creating a community blood pressure testing site, speaking about nutrition and disease, and providing immunizations and disease screenings for members of their community. Many school children are screened by public health nurses for such conditions as poor vision and scoliosis.

Occupational health nurses, or *industrial nurses*, provide nursing care in a clinic at a work site. They provide emergency care, work on accident prevention programs, and offer health counseling.

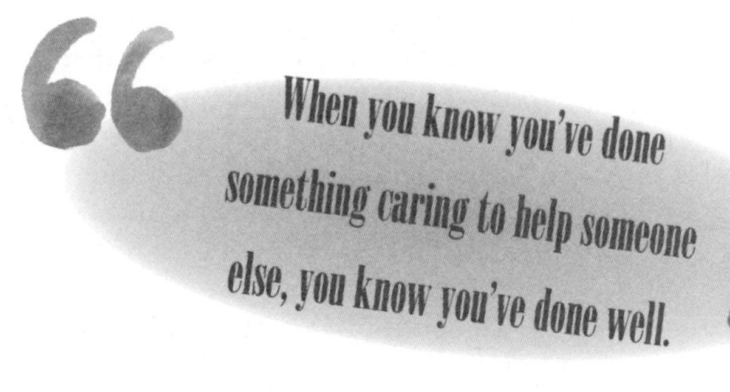

what is it like to be a nurse?

"A lot of people see nursing as bedpans and sponge-baths, but that isn't the case anymore." Jen Macri works in an intensive care unit (ICU) on second shift at Christ Center and Medical Hospital in Oak Lawn. Her workday runs from about 3:00 to 11:00 PM, four days a week. Although she acknowledges that new nurses often get night and evening shifts, she points out that that isn't necessarily a bad thing. "I like second shift because it doesn't interrupt my sleep patterns. Some people like the rush of first shift—there's always a lot going on then. Some people really like nights, and wouldn't give them up for anything. Night staff are a special breed." Because most of the hospital administrative staff goes home at the end of the first shift, hospitals usually quiet down during second shift; fewer nurses are assigned to night and evening duty.

Jen's regular duties in the ICU include administering medicines that patients are supposed to receive. "Any kind of patient care—bathing, changing linens, monitoring support systems—that is also our responsibility. We do all the things nurses in other parts of the hospital do for their patients." What makes the ICU different is its uncertainty. Jen's patients are stable but monitored. "If a patient becomes unstable, we address the problem ourselves—we can't just call for a doctor and wait for him to show up. We have to begin dealing with the situation ourselves."

Nurses often provide a human element to hospital stays. Because of the life-threatening conditions of her patients, comfort and support for concerned family members is a significant part of Jen's day. "Sometimes you'll end up doing part of the doctor's job. The doctor might sit the family down and explain a condition to them and they nod their heads, 'Yes, Doctor,' and have no idea what he was talking about. You kind of have to interpret what the doctor meant for people; you are more accessible to the patient and to the family than the doctors usually are."

Jen also finds that ICU nurses are allowed a certain freedom that is not usual on the other floors. "The doctors rely on us pretty heavily to keep track of patient status," she notes, and with the added responsibility comes an added amount of independence. Additionally, some ICU nurses may find that the restrictions placed on other hospital nurses by insurance companies or administrative staff are lessened for them, because of the immediate and critical nature of the care they provide.

Jen works with about ten other nurses per shift, and in her ICU there are twenty-two beds, so the nurse-to-patient ratio is about 1 to 2. In other parts of the hospital, this ratio can be 1 to 5 or as high as 1 to 25, depending on the type of care that is required and on the shift that is being scheduled. The general trend in hospitals is towards a higher nurse to patient ratio, which makes nurses responsible for more patients at a time. Jen works overtime if she is in the midst of a situation that has occurred on her shift. "You don't just go home when the shift is over. If somebody goes unstable in the last half hour of your shift, it is still your responsibility to handle it."

Nursing demands alertness, education, and a certain amount of mental and physical stamina. "Intensive care can be stressful physically, because you are moving people who aren't able to move themselves. And it can be mentally tiring, too, because you see a lot of sickness and death. Not everybody dying is eighty, either; I have seen twenty- and thirty-year olds in ICU." Occasionally, nurses in Jen's unit will have a debriefing to help them cope with a traumatic event or a death in their unit. "The people that you work with are so supportive—it's kind of the nature of the job. You really have to be there for each other."

Like other aspects of health care, nursing has become increasingly cost-conscious and somewhat political in recent years. Some nurses have a difficult time adjusting to the requirements of insurance companies and administrators, and resent the fact that they are allowed less contact with their patients than before. Because Jen is new to nursing, she was trained with the current health care issues in mind, and finds that she is not as critical about some requirements as some of her older co-workers.

have I got what it takes to be a nurse?

To be a successful nurse, says Jen Macri, you have to be adept at problem-solving. "You have to be pretty organized, especially now that [hospital administration] is laying more and more in your lap and you have less time to do everything." More than anything else, nurses must be genuinely concern for the people with whom they are working. "Ultimately, you're there to do good for the people," Jen summarizes. "People who aren't into that don't last very long."

Bunny Sendelbach, a nurse of almost 20 years, agrees. Bunny currently works in a retirement community where she provides care to elderly residents. "A nurse should be someone who has an aptitude in science, psychology, and who knows how to get along with a huge team. Most of all, you have to be able to inspire confidence and make your patients feel secure and good about themselves. That's the key to good health." Bunny feels that nursing is really still a calling, though this has gotten lost in the increasingly technical and financial aspects of the work. "To be a good healer, you have to be able to put aside your own ego, and give the patient the best environment you can so they can heal themselves. Nurses have to have heart, but they have to have brains as well."

The benefits of nursing are not limited to patients. Asked what made nursing worth the emotional stress and responsibility, both Jen and Bunny answered immediately. Jen appreciates the gratitude of patients and family; she also appreciates being able to contribute. "It's the people that get well and come back to say thank you, even if you only did a little smidge of something. You feel like you contributed by helping somebody. That's well worth everything else. When you know you've done something caring to help somebody else, you know you've done well." Patience, tact, and efficiency are qualities that make a good nurse. A strong sense of purpose and courage are qualities that will keep a good nurse in the career for years to come.

FYI

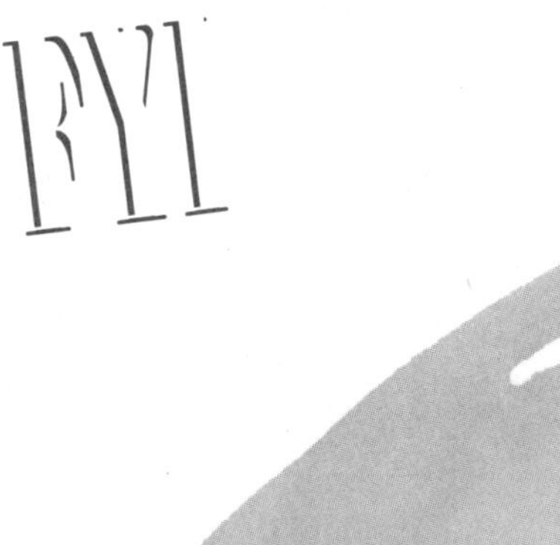

The first U.S. school of nursing was established in 1872 at the New England Hospital for Women and Children in Boston.

how do I become a nurse?

education

High School

While still in high school, students interested in nursing should take core science and math classes, including biology, chemistry, and physics. Other classes to take include psychology and sociology. Communication skills are vital to successful nurses, so English and speech courses will be useful.

It is possible to volunteer in many of the places nurses work, in order to decide if nursing is the career you want. Hospitals will take on high school volunteers as candy stripers or assistants, delivering mail and flowers, visiting with patients, and doing routine office work. While volunteerships at this level are not really concerned with patient treatment, they enable the prospective nurse to understand the way the hospital works and who is responsible for what duty.

While volunteering, you may be given more opportunity as a technician or as an aide to contribute to patient care. In many cases, according to Macri, if hospitals know you are seriously considering a career in nursing, they will give you better opportunities for hands-on involvement and experiences. "They'll say, come in here and help intubate Mr. So-and-so. One of the great things about being a volunteer is that it can be a direct line into a job at that hospital." Hospitals have a vested interest in training people to be nurses, especially if it means they will be able to hire somebody who is already familiar with the workings of their administration and setup.

Postsecondary Training

There are three training programs for registered nurses: associate's degree programs, diploma programs, and bachelor's degree programs. All three programs combine classroom education with actual nursing experience. Associate's degrees in nursing usually involve a two-year program at a junior or community college that is affiliated with a hospital. Many Associate's Degree Nurses (ADN) seek further schooling in bachelor's programs after they have found employment, in order to take advantage of tuition reimbursement programs.

The diploma program is conducted through independent nursing schools and teaching hospitals. This program usually lasts three years, and is the type that Jen went through and heartily recommends. "There are big differences in the programs. I think the best ones are done from big teaching hospitals, where you have the opportunities to see things that you wouldn't see in community hospitals or in associate's degree programs. I saw things at Rush (Presbyterian in Chicago) that I would never have seen in a suburban hospital, and will probably never see again."

A bachelor's degree (BSN) is recommended for nurses who must compete in an era of cutbacks and small staffs. Additionally, bachelor's degree programs are recommended for those who may want to go into administration or supervision. It is also required for jobs in public health agencies and for admission to graduate school.

To be a successful registered nurse, you should

- Have keen observational skills
- Be able to work under pressure
- Follow orders precisely
- Be well-organized
- Be caring and sympathetic
- Handle emergencies calmly

certification or licensing

Those who pass an accredited nursing program are known as nurse graduates, but must still pass the licensing exam to become a Registered Nurse. Licensing is required in all fifty states, and license renewal or continuing education credits are also required periodically. In some cases, licensing in one state will automatically grant licensing in reciprocal states.

Additional training is inevitable for those wishing to advance into specialized practices, administration, and teaching. This may include further clinical training within the hospital in an area such as pediatrics or gerontology, or entering a master's level program.

scholarships and grants

Scholarships and grants are often available from individual institutions, state agencies, and special-interest organizations. The book *Dollars for College: Nursing and Other Health Fields* by Ferguson Publishing Company is an excellent source for this information. Many students finance their medical education through the Armed Forces Health Professions Scholarship Program. Each branch of the military participates in this program, paying students' tuitions in exchange for military service. Contact your local recruiting office for more information on this program. The National League for Nursing publishes information on financial aid. Another source for financial aid, scholarship, and grant information is the Association of American Medical Colleges. Remember to request information early for eligibility, application requirements, and deadlines.

Ferguson Publishing Company
200 West Madison, Suite 300
Chicago, IL 60606
TEL: 312-580-5480

Association of American Medical Colleges
2450 N Street, NW
Washington, DC 20037
TEL: 202-828-0400
WEBSITE: http://www.aamc.org
Specific information on financial aid programs can be found at:
WEBSITE: http://www.aamc.org/stuapps/finaid

National League for Nursing
350 Hudson Street
New York, NY 10014
TEL: 212-989-9393

who will hire me?

Jen believes that belonging to an association makes you more marketable to employers because it increases your awareness of what is happening in the nursing community. "I joined an association to put it on my resume, but the magazines they sent me ended up being really helpful and interesting. They keep you up to date with new practices, and also advancements in the medical community and what that means to nursing. They have articles about medicine written for the lay person; they aren't written like medical trade journals. And managers love to see that stuff on applications—they know it keeps you aware and informed."

As with most jobs, persistence pays off, and special education can be a key element in winning specific jobs. "Right out of school I started knocking on doors. I wanted to work in the Surgical Heart Unit (SHU). I had extra cardiac training in watching monitors that other grads didn't. I interviewed with them but I didn't have the experience. From there I just bugged them every three months or so. Finally, the recruiter had an ICU position come up and she called me because I had kept in touch, because she knew me." Jen suggests keeping in touch with the recruiters at desired locations, introducing yourself with a letter or by getting their names and calling them, and then making sure they remember that you are waiting for them. "Part of it is just luck; if they need you when you are looking, you might luck into something that you'd be waiting forever for otherwise."

The most obvious place to look for a nursing job is in a hospital. Nurses also are needed in retirement communities, in government facilities, in schools and in private practices. In fact, nursing in hospitals is not expected to grow as fast as other aspects of nursing, due to rising costs and a general trend away from inpatient care. The slack caused by fewer available hospital jobs will be taken up by increased opportunities in newer fields. Insurance companies now hire registered nurses to assist in case management and to ensure that insured patients are getting the correct kind of care from their health-care providers. One of the fastest-growing fields in nursing is home-health care. Nurses who care for people on a part-time basis in their homes are in great demand for a variety of reasons. Technology has enabled many people to live free of health care institutions, but these people may still require assistance with some of their treatments.

Many surgical centers and emergency medical centers are taking the place of hospital emergency rooms. This will provide work for nurses who require a flexible schedule but who do not wish to work in a hospital. The number of older people with functional disabilities is growing, and jobs will be available in long-term care facilities for specialized conditions such as Alzheimer's disease.

Registered nurses should look in local papers and on the Internet for positions, in addition to contacting a preferred employer to ask what they may have available. Knowing where you would like to work, achieving educational credits in that field, and making sure those in charge of hiring know you are available are the key steps to finding a desirable nursing position.

where can I go from here?

Experienced registered nurses can advance in many ways. Those who want challenges beyond direct patient care may become teachers or administrators. Others continue their education and become clinical nurse specialists, nurse practitioners, certified nurse midwives, or nurse anesthetists. Master's degrees and doctorates are required for many of these positions.

what are the salary ranges?

Salaries can range from $20,000 to $40,000 to $55,000 per year, depending on the level of responsibility, the length of time spent working in one institution, experience, training received, and educational degrees earned. In 1994, the median income for full-time nurses was $35,400. This was true of staff nurses in hospitals and in chain nursing homes. Clinical nurses and nurse practitioners made closer to $47,000, and nurse anesthetists made approximately $80,000, the most for any practicing nurse.

Most health care employers provide a good benefits plan for their workers, as well as flexible work schedules, child care, and bonuses. Educational incentives take the form of in-house training and tuition reimbursement, which can enable nurses to increase their skills and potential for advancement at no or little cost to themselves.

what is the job outlook?

As with most health care fields, nursing is expected to grow faster than average in the next ten to fifteen years. As the cost for medical specialists skyrocket, more general health care practitioners will be in demand for the services that they can provide at less cost. Nurse practitioners, for example, can diagnose, treat, and manage uncomplicated health problems.

Technological advances in patient care and the health care needs of an aging population have created a demand for skilled nurses in many areas. Ambulatory, home health, and outpatient care are expected to provide the most employment opportunities, while need for nurses in hospitals will grow less rapidly. Registered nurses will be in high demand in nursing homes and in facilities that care for critically and terminally ill patients.

There are also many part-time job openings for nurses with family responsibilities that prevent them from holding a full-time position.

Staying aware of trends in health care will give prospective nurses a good idea of the job market for their skills. Trade journals, association membership materials, and health-care laws all discuss the course that health care is taking today, and are a valuable source of information for predicting where the future demand in nursing will be.

how do I learn more?

professional organizations

Following are organizations that provide information on various nursing careers, accredited schools, and employers.

American Nurses Association
600 Maryland Avenue, SW Suite 100 West
Washington, DC 20004
TEL: 202-651-7000
WEBSITE: http://www.nursingworld.org/about/

Association of Operating Room Nurses
2170 South Parker Road, Suite 300
Denver, CO 80231
TEL: 303-755-6300
WEBSITE: http://www.aorn.org/

bibliography

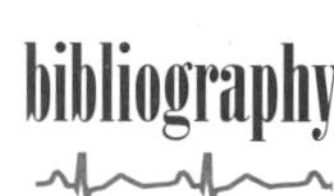

Following is a sampling of materials relating to the professional concerns and development of registered nurses.

Books

Anastas, Lila. *Your Career in Nursing*, 2nd edition. New York, NY: National League for Nursing, 1988.

Camenson, Blythe. *Nursing*. Lincolnwood, IL: VGM Career Horizons, 1995.

Cormack, Desmond, editor. *Developing Your Career in Nursing*. New York, NY: Chapman & Hall, 1990.

Fondiller, Shirley H., and Barbara J. Nerone. *Nursing: the Career of a Lifetime*. New York, NY: National League for Nursing, 1995.

Frederickson, Keville. *Opportunities in Nursing Careers,* revised edition. Lincolnwood, IL: VGM Career Horizons, 1995.

Heron, Jackie. *Exploring Careers in Nursing,* revised edition. New York, NY: Rosen Group, 1990.

Kelly, Lucie Y., and Lucille A. Joel. *The Nursing Experience: Trends, Challenges, and Transitions,* 3rd edition. Philadelphia, PA: Lippincott-Raven, 1996.

Newell, Robert, editor. *Developing Your Career in Nursing.* New York, NY: Cassell, 1996.

Sherman, Margie. *Your Opportunities in Nursing.* Salem, OR: Energeia Publishing Co., 1994.

Stanley, Linda, editor. *The Pfizer Guide: Nursing Career Opportunities.* Old Saybrook, CT: Merritt Communications, 1994.

Periodicals

The American Nurse. Monthly. Publication in a newspaper format, includes employment listings. American Nurses Association, 600 Maryland Avenue SW, Suite 100W, Washington, DC 20005, 202-682-5800.

Imprint. 5 per year. Practical journal for people interested in nursing careers. January issue is devoted to career planning. National Student Nurse Association, 555 W. 57th Street, New York, NY 10019, 212-581-2211.

Nursing and Health Care. 10 per year. Contains news, legislative updates, educational articles, service analyses, and editorials. National League for Nursing, 350 Hudson Street, New York, NY 10014, 212-989-9393.

Nursing: the World's Largest Nursing Journal. Monthly. Articles offer how-to, step-by-step approaches to clinical situations. Springhouse Corp., 111 Bethlehem Pike, Box 908, Springhouse, PA 19477, 215-646-8700, 800-346-7844.

rehabilitation counselor

Definition

Rehabilitation counselors help people with disabilities find employment and lead lives that are full and productive.

Alternative job titles

Case Manager
Job Placement Specialist
Substance Abuse Counselor
Vocational Rehabilitation Specialist

Salary range

$20,000 to $37,000 to $60,000

Educational requirements

High school diploma; a bachelor's degree in rehabilitation services or related field for employment in limited areas; a minimum of a master's degree in rehabilitation counseling is required for some employment.

Certification or Licensing

Mandatory

Outlook

Faster than average

GOE
10.01.02

DOT
045

High School Subjects

Business
Economics
Psychology
Social Sciences
Statistics

Personal Interests

Analyzing and solving problems
Helping people
Volunteering

Mario's life was changed forever in a split second. He had always been a hard-working man. In the mornings he worked as a short-order cook and in the evenings as a landscaper. But in one instant everything changed. Mario fell from a roof, struck his head, and sustained a disabling brain injury. Fortunately for Mario, there had been no other physical complications. He was soon eager to return to his job at the restaurant. However, now being disabled, he discovered there were new challenges he would have to face before he could begin working again. Mario had someone there to help him meet those challenges: his rehabilitation counselor.

Greg Cusick works for the Vocational Rehabilitation Services Department, an academic affiliate of the Rehabilitation Institute of Chicago. First, Greg put Mario through initial assessment testing to determine his functioning levels. Then he developed a work-trial program for him in the hospital's cafeteria. It only took a few days to see that Mario was ready to return to the restaurant. The restaurant owner agreed to let Mario return after Greg arranged for him to observe Mario working in the cafeteria. It was, as Greg describes it, ". . . one of the better success stories."

what does a rehabilitation counselor do?

Rehabilitation counselors help people with disabilities find employment and lead full and independent lives. Much of how people feel about themselves is influenced by their careers and their ability to contribute to society. Because of that, the services offered by rehabilitation counselors during a patient's transition back into the work environment play a crucial role in the rehabilitation process. Rehabilitation counselors develop programs that include client assessments, training programs, and job placement.

The majority of the clients Greg Cusick sees have physical disabilities and are outpatients of the Rehabilitation Institute of Chicago (RIC). Before clients can begin vocational rehabilitation therapy, an in-house psychologist must determine that they have adjusted psychologically to their physical disability. Though clients may still be involved in physical, occupational, or psychological therapy, most are ready to begin considering their vocational goals for the future.

Rehabilitation counselors first meet with other members of their client's treatment team to learn the client's medical history and current physical and emotional status. At RIC, the first time that clients and rehabilitation counselors meet face to face is during the initial consultation. During the consultation, rehabilitation counselors gather information regarding the client's employment and educational history, as well as any vocational goals the client may have for the future. Rehabilitation counselors may do a job analysis of a client's previous career to determine if it is possible to return to that career.

If it is impossible for clients to return to their former careers, rehabilitation counselors will discuss the possibility of clients entering new fields and beginning new careers. However, rehabilitation counselors do not force anything on clients. As Greg explains, "we don't have a bunch of jobs and try to fit people into those jobs. I'm not going to tell clients what to do, the clients are going to tell me what they are interested in doing and then I'm going to see if that's appropriate, and, if so, then try and help them reach that goal."

Clients must go through extensive testing. After the tests are completed, rehabilitation counselors have an understanding of the clients' vocational goals and their current level of skills and abilities. Furthermore, the results of the testing will determine if any additional training may be needed before clients can return to work.

One of the first tests clients must complete is an interest test. This will give rehabilitation counselors direction as they try to find areas of employment that clients may find interesting. Abilities testing assesses the clients' verbal and numerical skills, as well as their gen-

lingo to learn

Caseload management The ratio of clients to counselors, takes into account characteristics of each case.

Disability management The process of returning a person with a disability to work.

Peer Counseling Guidance and support given to a person by a person who has had similar experiences.

Prevocational services The evaluation, training, and assessment that a rehabilitation counselor uses prior to training a person with a disability a vocation.

Rehabilitation engineering Encompasses many disciplines including engineering and medicine with the aim of improving the quality of life for persons with disabilities.

Supported employment Competitive employment for persons with severe disabilities who require ongoing support.

Work adjustment Training designed to help persons with disabilities form work habits that will increase their productivity. Seeks to promote self-confidence, tolerance, and interpersonal communications.

eral learning potential. There are also additional tests for finger dexterity, motor coordination, and balance. Additionally, if appropriate to their interests, clients will undergo clerical tests, which assess office, computer, and keyboarding skills.

During a work-trial assessment, rehabilitation counselors try to place their clients in real work environments that simulate the field they are planning to enter. They are evaluated by their counselor on a daily basis. The program gives rehabilitation counselors an opportunity to assess their clients' skill levels, work behaviors, interaction with other people, and memory, in real-life environments. The work-trial program usually lasts from two to four weeks and the position is non-paying.

The next step is developing a tentative plan for employment. "Sometimes that means going and receiving some type of training," says Greg, "and we work with a lot of different training programs as well as community colleges."

In addition to working as vocational specialists, rehabilitation counselors can also work as job placement specialists. Job placement specialists help clients who have completed their training programs find jobs. The job placement specialists receive referrals describing the vocational goals of the clients, their level of skills, and their experience. Many job placement specialists work to cultivate strong relationships with the human resources managers of corporations in their area to learn of openings and potential employment opportunities for their clients.

However, even after clients become employed, the vocational rehabilitation counselors' responsibilities concerning the client still continue. They will check in regularly with both the employer and the client to see if everything is running smoothly. The counselor may need to make an on-site visit to observe clients at work. Rehabilitation counselors will arrange for any additional training if necessary.

The length of time a counselor may work with clients varies greatly. Each case is determined on a client-by-client basis. If a job placement fails, the rehabilitation counselor will work with the client to try again. It is not enough for a counselor to find the client a job, but to find the client a career. Because, as Greg explains it, the primary responsibility of the vocational rehabilitation counselor is ". . . to get people to work. That's what our goal is, that's our bottom line."

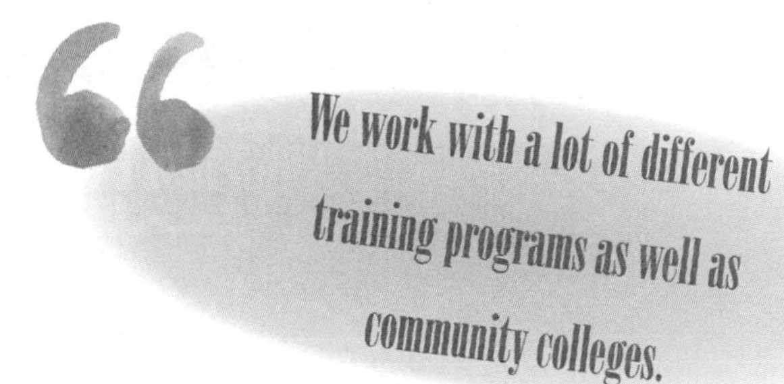

what is it like to be a rehabilitation counselor?

Although many people have earned a degree in rehabilitation counseling, their job titles can vary greatly. Some rehabilitation counselors, like Greg Cusick, work as vocational rehabilitation specialists, while others work as job placement specialists or case managers. Furthermore, even working as a vocational counselor, Greg's responsibilities change as his clients progress through therapy. First he works as a vocational evaluator. Then, once the clients begin working with job placement specialists, Greg's role becomes more of a case manager, overseeing their progress.

The number of clients rehabilitation counselors see during a week will depend on their specialization, as well as their place of employment. At the Vocational Rehabilitation Services Department for the Rehabilitation Institute of Chicago, Greg sees ten to twelve clients in a week. However, he may speak with as many as twelve more on the phone, checking on their status. Most rehabilitation counselors work a forty- hour week. To accommodate clients who may not be able to come in during the day, some rehabilitation counselors will work in the evenings or on weekends.

Some clients seek out the help of rehabilitation counselors on their own, after they have become disabled through an accident or illness. Others are referred to rehabilitation counselors by members of their treatment team, which may include a physician, psychologist, or social worker.

Rehabilitation counselors work with clients who face incredible challenges every day and are very vulnerable. Even though the clients Greg sees are there because of physical disabilities, they may also be struggling with psychological or emotional problems, like depression or anxiety. Often clients do not begin their vocational therapy immediately after they are released from the hospital. Some clients may have been discharged for up to six months before they begin their vocational therapy.

When asked to describe one of the major rewards of being a rehabilitation counselor, Greg replies, "Right here, this." He picks up a green form. "This is a placement notice for one of our clients. He just got a job today. . . . To see the client find the job that they want, to be happy, to stop receiving Social Security, to start receiving a wage, to start to become independent again. That's the fun part of the job."

On the other hand, the job of rehabilitation counselors can be very stressful. The job market is very competitive. And besides helping clients prepare for the job hunt, they also have to help potential employers see past a client's disability. However, vocational rehabilitation counselors have a great deal of confidence in their clients once their vocational therapy has concluded. Rehabilitation counselors do not expect special considerations for their clients. "We feel that we have clients that are just as competitive as anyone else . . ." Greg explains.

Working as a rehabilitation counselor can have its share of disappointments and frustrations. They may have worked several months to find the perfect placement for a client and still may not succeed. For various reasons, either the employer or the client may become unhappy in the situation and the rehabilitation counselor has to start all over again with the client. Greg recently placed a client in what he thought was the ideal environment, but it did not work out. Rehabilitation counselors cannot let their clients become discouraged. Instead they work just as hard to find their clients better placements the next time.

FYI

In 1990, Congress passed the Americans with Disabilities Act. This measure recognized the rights and needs of people with disabilities and developed federal guidelines and regulations aimed at eliminating discrimination and other barriers preventing people with disabilities from participating fully in school, workplace, and public life. Many government programs have since been created to aid people with disabilities.

have I got what it takes to be a rehabilitation counselor?

Successful rehabilitation counselors have strong problem-solving skills. When clients realize that they cannot return to their old jobs, it is the responsibility of rehabilitation counselors to give them direction toward new careers. They will have to answer any questions the clients may have about working with a disability. They will also have to explain to clients that they can begin new careers that will accommodate their disabilities and be just as exciting and fulfilling as their former careers.

It is important that rehabilitation counselors have strong interpersonal communication skills. They need to let their clients express their fears and disappointments. They need to know when they can encourage their clients to go a little further and when to leave them alone. Also, rehabilitation counselors need effective communication skills when they are interacting with the other members of the treatment team. Each member of the team needs to know how the client is progressing in their respective therapies to effectively treat the whole client.

Rehabilitation counselors must be sensitive people who generally care about the well-being of others. They must have an almost unending source of patience. Because placements sometimes fail, rehabilitation counselors have to be able to help clients until they find the right placement that will offer long-term employment. Most rehabilitation counselors are dedicated to their profession and believe that by helping people find employment and lead productive lives they are helping society, one person at a time.

Finally, successful rehabilitation counselors are often better salespeople than their contacts in the business community with whom they may place their clients. In some cases they must help potential employers overcome a reluctance to hire someone with a disability. Furthermore, because clients may become discouraged while trying to find employment, rehabilitation counselors have to help their clients keep their self-esteem high. A positive attitude is important. As Greg explains, ". . . they need a positive outlook and attitude if they're to go out and get a job. Because if they're not positive, no one is going to hire them."

To be a successful rehabilitation counselor you should

- Have strong problem solving skills
- Be adept at interpersonal communication
- Be sensitive to others
- Be able to persevere
- Understand organization of businesses
- Enjoy working with a variety of people
- Be a good listener

how do I become a rehabilitation counselor?

education

High School

While in high school, students interested in a career in rehabilitation counseling should take courses in psychology, sociology, economics, and statistics. These classes will provide useful insight into human nature. Also, they will begin to realize how different economic factors can affect the job market.

Speech and communication classes can help students develop the skills necessary to express themselves clearly and effectively, both to their clients and to potential employers. Additionally, because listening skills are so important, communication classes can teach students an understanding of both verbal and non-verbal communication.

Business classes are beneficial because rehabilitation counselors need to understand how businesses are organized and structured. When inquiring about potential job opportunities for their clients, they need to know who to contact in a business.

Finally, high school students should consider enrolling in anatomy and biology classes. To be effective rehabilitation counselors they will have to have a basic understanding of their clients' disabilities to understand how they affect vocational training and goals.

Postsecondary Training

In the field of rehabilitation counseling the level of responsibility and the place of employment will be determined by the degree held by the counselor. Counselors with only a bachelor's degree in rehabilitation counseling are usually employed as a counseling or rehabilitative aide.

Currently, there are more than fifty rehabilitation education programs across the country offering bachelor's degrees. Undergraduate coursework includes classes in sociology, psychology, history, and statistics.

A counselor with a master's degree in rehabilitation counseling will have many more employment opportunities in a wider range of areas. In fact, vocational and rehabilitative agencies will hire only applicants with master's degrees. Also, an advanced degree is required to apply for certification by the Commission on Rehabilitation Counselor Certification.

Most master's degree programs last for two years. At present there are more than eighty accredited master's programs across the country. Accreditation of rehabilitation counseling educational programs is granted by the Council on Rehabilitation Education (CORE). Some of the graduate course work includes classes in the medical and psychosocial aspects of disability and techniques of counseling, as well as training in vocational evaluations and job placement. In addition to course work, graduate students are expected to complete some form of supervised clinical training.

certification or licensing

The Commission on Rehabilitation Counselor Certification offers certification for counselors. Applicants need to have earned a master's degree from an accredited graduate rehabilitation counseling program to become a certified rehabilitation counselor (CRC). Also, the applicant must have completed an internship program and must have successfully passed a written examination. To retain their status, CRCs are required to complete 100 hours of continuing education within five years of receiving their certification.

Most states require some form of licensing for rehabilitation counselors. This usually involves passing a written exam and an evaluation by a state board of examiners. Also, most states require applicants to be CRCs.

scholarships and grants

The National Rehabilitation Counseling Association offers a $1,000 scholarship to a full-time student pursuing a master's degree in the field.

internships and volunteerships

High school students interested in gaining practical experience in the field of rehabilitation counseling should contact the volunteer office of the hospital in their area. Many hospitals have large volunteer programs. Volunteers are often placed in the department they are interested in; furthermore, the volunteer office may be able to arrange for the student to spend a day with rehabilitation counselors. Most rehabilitation counselors enjoy talking about their careers and are happy to answer any questions the student may have.

The Rehabilitation Institute of Chicago has several different programs that bring together professionals of different backgrounds to discuss one particular issue at area high schools.

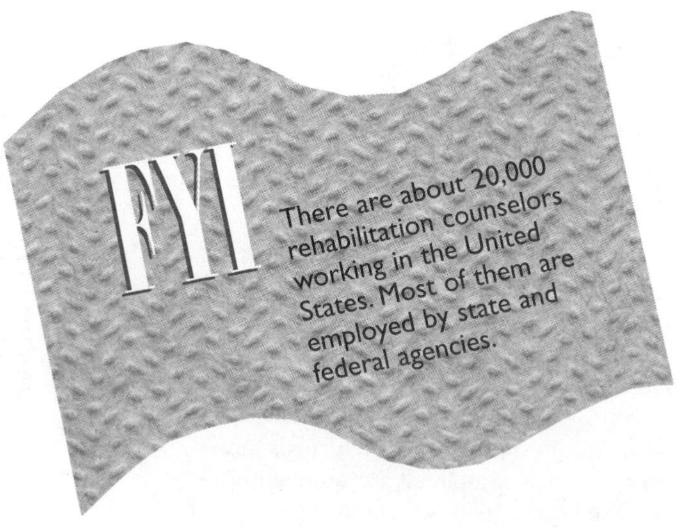

who will hire me?

Because rehabilitation counselors work with people of all ages and backgrounds who are looking for employment, their places of employment can vary greatly. Rehabilitation counselors who work with clients with physical disabilities may work for rehabilitation or vocational agencies. Some rehabilitation counselors work at halfway houses and correctional institutions with clients who are struggling with drug and alcohol addictions. Many licensed counselors have begun to work for HMOs and other insurance agencies.

Greg Cusick's first position as a rehabilitation counselor was for the student's center for disabilities at a community college in San Diego. Greg was supervised by a certified counselor. "So for a year and a half she would meet with me once a week and show me the ropes. We would go over cases and she supervised [me] very closely."

Counselors looking for employment can contact different professional associations that might be able to help them. The National Rehabilitation Counseling Association and the American Rehabilitation Counseling Association collect information regarding employment opportunities. Counselors should also take advantage of the placement office at the school from which they earned their degree.

The government, both state and federal, hire a large number of rehabilitation counselors to work for agencies that are funded with state or federal money. To assist disabled veterans, the Department of Veterans Affairs hires hundreds of rehabilitation counselors.

where can I go from here?

Students who earn their bachelor's degree in rehabilitation services may consider working in a supervised position to gain practical experience before committing the time and money required to earn a graduate degree.

However, to widen the scope of career possibilities, it is mandatory that counselors earn a master's degree. Counselors with graduate degrees have a wider scope of counseling areas that they can work in. After becoming certified, rehabilitation counselors can move into supervisory or administrative positions. However, as supervisors or managers, they may be required to work additional hours due to their increased responsibilities. Also, in some instances this may require additional training before they can move into managerial positions.

Often rehabilitation counselors decide to specialize and work in only one area of counseling. They may also chose to move into private practice.

Finally, many rehabilitation counselors find fulfillment as teachers, helping students become competent rehabilitation counselors. When rehabilitation counselors return to the academic environment to teach, they bring with them their real world experience, which helps their students gain a better understanding of the demands of the job.

what are the salary ranges?

Entry-level rehabilitation counselors can expect to earn between $20,000 to $23,000 a year. There are many factors that can influence the salary of rehabilitation counselors, including geographical residence, level of education, and years of experience. Highly experienced rehabilitation counselors can earn more than $50,000 annually. Furthermore, rehabilitation counselors who have moved into supervisory or administrative positions may earn as much as $60,000.

Counselors who have earned their master's degrees and are working for the federal government earned an average of $37,000 in 1995. Self-employed counselors earned the highest salaries. However, it should be pointed out that self-employed counselors have to pay for all of their own benefits.

what is the job outlook?

Recent congressional legislation has had wide ranging effects on the field of rehabilitation counseling. The passage of the Americans with Disabilities Act in 1990 increased the demand for rehabilitation counselors. Because several federal and state programs were developed to comply with the new law, the skills of rehabilitation counselors were needed, not only by the government but private companies as well.

Several government-funded programs that employ many rehabilitation counselors are threatened due to the changes caused by welfare reform. As Greg explains, "If money [available] to state and federal government programs decreases, due to welfare reform, it may affect some of the programs that fund governmental and other non-for-profit rehabilitation services. A lot of the job skills training programs for people with disabilities in the city are funded through the government." For that reason, Greg has begun investigating new ways of fund raising that will help programs continue even after their government funding is reduced.

Another factor affecting this field is the development of new technologies that continue to improve functionality for people with disabilities. These people need fulfilling jobs and rehabilitation counselors help them find that.

Finally, more and more health maintenance organizations and insurance companies are reimbursing rehabilitation counseling costs. This should increase the demand for certified rehabilitation counselors.

how do I learn more?

professional organizations

Following are organizations that provide information on rehabilitation counseling and possible sources of employment information.

American Rehabilitation Counseling Association (ARCA)
5999 Stevenson Ave.
Alexandria, VA 22304
TEL: 703-620-4404

Commission on Rehabilitation Counselor Certification
1835 Rohlwing Road, Suite E
Rolling Meadows, IL 60008
TEL: 847-394-2104

National Council on Rehabilitation Education (NCRE)
Administrative Office: c/o Dr. Garth Eldredge
Department of Special Education and Rehabilitation
Utah State University
Logan, UT 84322
TEL: 801-797-3241
WEBSITE: http://www.nchrtm.okstate.edu/ncre.html

National Rehabilitation Counseling Association (NRCA)
8807 Sudley Road, #102
Manassas, VA 22110
TEL: 703-361-2077
WEBSITE: http://www.ed.wright.edu/cehs/nrca/generalinformation/generalhome.html

bibliography

Following is a sampling of materials relating to the professional concerns and development of rehabilitation counselors.

Books

Garner, Geraldine O. *Careers in Social and Rehabilitation Services*. Lincolnwood, IL: VGM Career Horizons, 1994.

Parker, Randall, and Edna Szymanski, editors. *Rehabilitation Counseling: Basics and Beyond,* 2nd edition. Austin, TX: PRO-ED, 1992.

Pilling, Doria. *Approaches to Case Management for People with Disabilities*. Bristol, PA: Taylor & Francis, 1992.

Roessler, Richard T., and Stanford E. Rubin. *Case Management and Rehabilitation Counseling: Procedures and Techniques,* 2nd edition. Austin, TX: PRO-ED, 1992.

Rubin, Stanford E., and Richard T. Roessler. *Foundations of the Vocational Rehabilitation Process,* 4th edition. Austin, TX: PRO-ED, 1994.

Periodicals

Archives of Physical Medicine and Rehabilitation. Monthly. Provides original research and clinical reports to health professionals who work with the disabled, elderly, and handicapped. American Academy of Physical Medicine and Rehabilitation, 1 IBM Plaza, 25th Floor, Chicago, IL 60611, 312-464-9700.

Contemporary Rehabilitation. 8 per year. Includes calendar of events, listing of employment opportunities, chapter news, human interest stories, and practice information. National Rehabilitation Association, 633 South Washington Street, Alexandria, VA 22314, 703-836-0850.

Journal of Rehabilitation. Quarterly. Includes articles on rehabilitation research, new technology, and book reviews. National Rehabilitation Association, 633 S. Washington Street, Alexandria, VA 22314, 703-836-0850.

Rehabilitation Counseling Bulletin. Quarterly. Discusses psychological and social aspects of disability, psychiatric rehabilitation, developmental disabilities, career development, and job placement of persons with special needs. American Rehabilitation Counseling Association, c/o American Counseling Association, 5999 Stevenson Avenue, Alexandria, VA 22304, 703-823-9800.

Professional Report of the National Rehabilitation Counseling Association. Bimonthly. Membership activities newsletter which includes legislative news and listings of employment opportunities. National Rehabilitation Counseling Association, 8807 Sudley Road, Suite 102, Manassas, VA 22110, 703-361-2077.

respiratory therapy technician

Definition

Certified respiratory therapy technicians administer general respiratory care to persons with heart and lung problems. They work under the supervision of registered respiratory therapists or physicians.

Alternative job titles

Inhalation therapists
Respiratory care practitioners
Respiratory care workers

Salary range

$19,760 to $30,888 to $38,233

Educational requirements

High school diploma; one to two years of specialized training

Certification or licensing

Certification, registration, and licensing are mandatory in thirty-nine states. Seven states require at least certification; other states have title protection laws, or predetermined standards.

Outlook

Much faster than average

GOE
10.02.02

DOT
076

High School Subjects

Algebra
Biology
Chemistry
English
Physics

Personal Interests

Mechanical objects
Taking care of others
Working with your hands

At the bedside of an elderly woman, Scariakutty Thomas offers the woman his hand and a warm smile. "Mrs. Feldman? Hi, I'm Scariakutty." He can see that his new patient is anxious. "I'm a respiratory therapy technician. I'm going to check your vital signs and give you something so you can breathe easier."

Mrs Feldman smiles shyly but still seems nervous. Scariakutty continues trying to put her at ease.

"I understand you had an asthma attack last night. Pretty scary, huh?" Scariakutty knows that it's important to explain what he's doing so that his patient can relax and cooperate with the treatment. Soon Mrs. Feldman is telling him about her new grandson as he checks her blood pressure and pulse. As he is about to administer medication, Scariakutty hears the public address system.

"Code Blue—Room 736!"

He is on emergency call today and must respond to the distress code immediately.

"Mrs. Feldman," he explains, "I've got to respond to that call. I'll be back to see you as soon as I'm finished."

Scariakutty waves a signal to the nurse's station as he flies past the elevators to take the stairs.

In an emergency, there is no time to wait for an elevator.

what does a respiratory therapy technician do?

In extraordinary circumstances, it is possible to go without food for a few weeks, or without water for a few days. But without air, brain damage occurs within minutes; death follows after about nine minutes.

Respiratory care workers include therapists, technicians, and assistants (or aides). Assistants clean, sterilize, store, and maintain inventory, and care for equipment. They are usually beginners on their way to certification and registration, and have little patient contact. The duties of *registered respiratory therapists* (RRTs) and *certified respiratory therapy technicians* (CRTTs) are similar. They both treat patients with cardiorespiratory problems.

RRTs have more education, however. They apply scientific knowledge and theory to the practical problems of respiratory care under the supervision of doctors. They may be required to exercise independent clinical judgement. Sometimes they even advise doctors on appropriate therapy. Licensed RRTs can also order medication with a physician's approval. In addition, their responsibilities often entail training, teaching and supervising other workers, such as CRTTs.

CRTTs review clinical data, patient histories, and respiratory therapy orders. They interview and examine patients, and perform or recommend X rays and laboratory tests. CRTTs may evaluate patient information in order to determine the appropriateness of specific therapies. They perform and modify prescribed therapeutic procedures such as the administration of aerosol inhalants that confine medication to the lungs. They are also responsible for assembling, maintaining, and monitoring equipment, and for ensuring cleanliness and sterility. Equipment includes ventilators (respirators), positive-pressure breathing machines, or environmental control systems. The patients of CRRTs may be recovering from surgery and need respiratory care to restore full breathing capacity and to prevent respiratory illnesses. Other patients suffer from chronic conditions like asthma or emphysema. Victims of heart failure, stroke, drowning, or other trauma need life support. CRTTs observe patients' physiological response to therapy and consult with physicians if there are adverse reactions. CRTTs are often called to emergency rooms and intensive care units where their skill and devotion can mean the difference between life and death. Now that home care is becoming more widespread, CRTTs sometimes instruct patients and their families in the use of respiratory equipment at home.

An important aspect of the job is record keeping. CRTTs record critical information on patients' charts, make reports, and keep track of the cost of materials and charges to the patients. There is always a lot of paperwork.

lingo to learn

Bronchodilator Drug that aids expansion of the bronchial airway.

Cardiorespiratory Relating to the heart and lungs.

Clinical Involving direct observation of the patient.

Intubation Introduction of a breathing tube into the throat.

Pulmonary Relating to the lungs.

Ventilator A machine that maintains breathing for a patient who cannot breathe independently.

what is it like to be a respiratory therapy technician?

Tom Garcia reports to work at 7:00 PM at Northwestern Memorial Hospital, one of Chicago's major teaching hospitals. "Hey, Angie...Raymond, how's it going?...Evening, Dr. Katz."

He greets co-workers as he gets a cup of coffee and collects the reports of the day shift. When he sits down to read them over, he looks for important messages, patients who have undergone surgery that morning, and new admissions requiring evaluation. He makes notes of changes in therapy or medication. When Tom finishes scanning the last report, he realizes that one chart is missing. He sets down his coffee cup and dials the nurse's station on the pediatric floor.

"Hi, Joanie, it's Tom Garcia. Where's Jessica Brandon's chart?" Tom has been giving Jessica chest physiotherapy since she was admitted a month ago with complications of cystic fibrosis. There is a pause on the other end, then a sigh.

"Tom," Joanie says finally, "Jessica died this afternoon."

Tom covers his eyes with his hand and sits quietly for a moment. This is the part of the job Tom hates. He sees Jessica's smile as he left her room just last night. "You be sweet now," he told her, "and I'll see you tomorrow." Sometimes all the knowledge and skilled care in the world are not enough. The feelings of failure—however irrational—and having to witness the grief of survivors can be excruciating.

But right now Tom cannot indulge his feelings. It is going to be a tough night. Two other respiratory care workers are out with the flu, and Tom will have to work twice as hard, yet give each patient the same focused attention as he would on a slow day. Hastily, Tom drinks the last of his coffee and heads for the elevator.

In the intensive care unit, Tom inspects ventilators for recent surgery patients. Since these people are intubated and cannot speak, Tom asks *yes* or *no* questions that can be answered with hand squeezes. He takes a few moments to reassure these critical patients and let them know he is there for them. As he finishes up, the pager summons him to operating room seven. A young woman named Theresa Harper, the victim of a drunk driver, has just come out of emergency surgery. Tom connects her to a ventilator and confirms that the equipment is operating properly.

The surgeon, Dr. Susan Flannery, asks Tom questions about an oddity in the patient's blood gas analysis. This something Tom has seen before. He explains it to Dr. Flannery and makes a recommendation. Tom smiles to himself as he leaves the ICU, reflecting that only a few years ago, doctors did not ask the advice of lower-level professionals. But that is changing with specialization, the increasing sophistication of equipment, and new options in therapeutic technique.

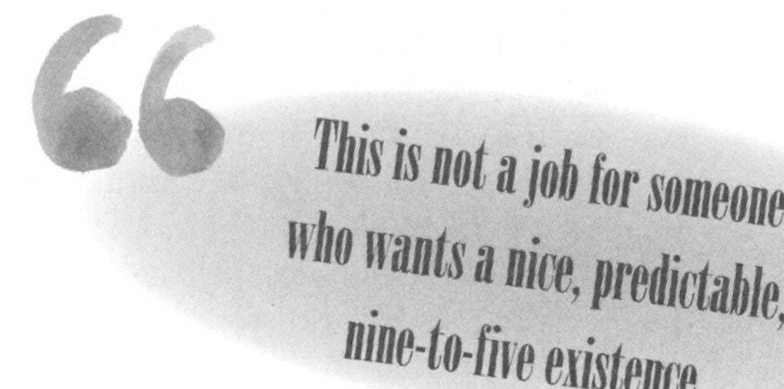

It is nearly midnight when Tom sits down to eat a quick lunch. After leaving the ICU, Tom administered bronchodilator aerosols to two pulmonary disease patients. He coached them on how to cough in order to clear their lungs. He also performed chest physiotherapy on a man recovering from pneumonia. This technique involves placing the patient in a posture to promote drainage, and thumping and vibrating the rib cage. As Tom munches a chicken salad sandwich, he expands the sketchy notes he made on his rounds. Finally, Tom writes out a to-do list for the remainder of his shift. He has to check on Theresa Harper again, and call the equipment manufacturer about a recurring problem with one of the ventilators. Since one of the aides is down with the flu, he will check to see that there are enough supplies for the next shift.

"This is not a job for someone who wants a nice, predictable nine-to-five existence," Tom says. "And you'll never get rich. On the other hand, you'll never be bored either. The rewards of a career in respiratory therapy are the constant challenge and knowing that you help people. You see results. What you do makes a difference."

have I got what it takes to be a respiratory therapy technician?

Because people can die so quickly if they stop breathing, respiratory care workers play a critical role in medical institutions. In cases of cardiac arrest, drowning, electric shock, and other kinds of trauma, they may literally hold people's lives in their hands. For this reason, CRTTs and RRTs need to develop maturity, the capacity to accept grave responsibilities, and a genuine desire to care for others.

"You can't be squeamish," says Tom Garcia. "Especially in a big city hospital, you see lots of bad injuries. You've got to keep your cool because the patient and the trauma team depend on you. And since you work with ventilators and other sophisticated machinery, it helps if you're good with your hands or have mechanical aptitude."

Scariakutty Thomas emphasizes the importance of a good character, a smiling face, and courtesy. "Sick people are anxious, vulnerable, and frequently depressed," Scariakutty says. "They need a lot of reassurance and kindness. This is not always easy, because sometimes fear is expressed as anger. You have to remember that angry, difficult patients need your compassion just as much as the easy ones," he stresses.

Pat Adney is Director of Respiratory Care and Rehabilitation Services at Chicago's Weiss Memorial Hospital. In addition to the qualities already described, Pat says having a natural curiosity and interest in the field is a plus. "A really good respiratory care worker possesses intellectual curiosity. Most of your education comes from the job; you constantly have to figure things out and learn on your own initiative because there's always something new." Pat also stresses emotional equilibrium. "You must strike a balance so you neither burn out nor become heartless and unfeeling."

Since respiratory care workers have to process a lot of paperwork, writing skills are a must. "You work with doctors and other highly educated people," says Tom Garcia. "In order to have credibility, you must be articulate and well read in your field. There's always so much to read because there are new things happening all the time."

To be a successful respiratory therapy technician, you should

- Have compassion, courtesy, and flexibility
- Be able to articulate your thoughts, ideas, and opinions
- Have a cool head under stress
- Be willing to follow instructions and be a team player
- Pay attention to details
- Have mechanical aptitude and good manual dexterity

Isabelle Orr, clinical coordinator for respiratory care at St. Augustine College in Chicago, emphasizes computer literacy. "It's an absolute must," she says. "The entire medical field is so dependent on computers."

Another factor to keep in mind is the necessity for shift work. Medical facilities operate twenty-four hours a day, so there are three shifts. Most respiratory care workers are expected to be flexible about shift changes, overtime, and holidays. Remember, too, that they are on their feet for most of the forty-hour week. They must also be able to take orders from superiors—even when they come from people who are not always pleasant. "You have to deal with professional egos," Tom Garcia comments, "and sometimes you're pulled in different directions because of great needs and a too-small staff."

Finally, one important factor to consider is safety. The pressurized gases used in respiratory therapy are potentially hazardous and every respiratory care worker runs the risk of contracting an infectious disease from a patient. Following safety precautions, regular maintenance, and equipment testing reduce the possibility of injury from pressurized gases, while strict adherence to proper procedure minimizes the risk of exposure to infectious disease.

how do I become a respiratory therapy technician?

Matthew Chirayil is the clinical coordinator of respiratory care at Ravenswood Hospital in Chicago. He began his medical career as a CRTT. Matthew remembers that as a child he wanted to be a doctor. "I always liked caring for people," he says, "and I get along particularly well with the elderly." After college, Matthew visited hospitals and did a lot of reading. He decided that he wanted a job that involved only partial patient care. "At that time, respiratory therapy was a growing field. I felt it would provide a steady job without too much hassle and emotional stress." Physiology, anatomy and lab work were his favorite subjects during training. "They provided perspective on what goes wrong with the human body." His least favorite courses? "I always hated math," Matthew laughs.

Tom Garcia's career grew out of two major boyhood interests. "I always liked fooling around with mechanical things, and I was interested in science. Applying mechanics to the human body is fascinating." Tom recalls his training period as being a tough two years. "There was a lot of memorization. Everything was very concentrated. In the second year you get thrown into patient care—you have to be an adult right away."

education

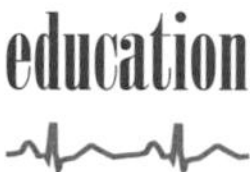

High School

Respiratory care requires a lot of fundamental mathematical problem solving. For instance, in their daily work, respiratory care workers must compute medication dosages and calculate gas concentrations. It is a good idea to take high school courses in algebra, physics, chemistry, and biology. English, health, computer classes as well as bookkeeping are also helpful.

A summer job in a hospital is a good way to see what the field is like. Although the job assignment may not relate to respiratory therapy, there will be chances to observe and get acquainted with respiratory care workers. If no part-time or temporary work is available, students may consider volunteer service.

Postsecondary Training

Formal training in respiratory care is provided in one-year programs leading to a certificate and two-year associate's degree programs that prepare students for the registry examination. There are some four-year bachelor's degree programs as well. A high school diploma or equivalent is required for all. Training is available through hospitals, medical schools, colleges and universities, trade schools, vocation-technical institutes, and the armed forces. It is imperative that the training institution be accredited by the Committee on Allied Health Education and Accreditation (CAHEA) of the American Medical Association (AMA).

More than 280 programs for RRTs were accredited by CAHEA in the early 1990s, and there were more than 180 accredited programs for CRTTs. These are mostly one-year programs that prepare the student for the certification examination. Two-year schools should include enough credit hours of clinical training (treating patients under supervision) to qualify the student to take both the certification and registry examinations. (Certification is required in order to sit for the registry examination.)

Course work consists of anatomy, physiology, medical terminology, chemistry, mathematics, microbiology, physics, therapeutic procedures, clinical medicine, and clinical expressions. Students learn to do procedures such as venous punctures, arterial blood draws, intubation, stress testing, and electrocardiograms. Social science classes in communication skills, psychology, and medical ethics support the basic science studies.

In respiratory care, as well as all other areas of medicine, education is ongoing. Constant improvements in equipment, medication, and therapeutic technique make continuing education a must. In addition to registry, a CRTT may pursue specialties in pulmonary function technology, pulmonary function therapy, pediatric neonatology, and many others. Frequent inservice training is usually done by supervising RRTs or equipment manufacturers. Good hospitals support additional training. Matthew Chirayil is certified to administer echocardiograms, for instance. His employer paid his tuition.

certification or licensing

Typically, a hospital hires uncertified new graduates providing that they pass the certification exam in six months to a year. Matthew Chirayil completed a two-year program in 1988 and became certified later that year. The following year, he passed the registry exam. Tom Garcia took the registry exam two years after certification. As an RRT, Tom is now a supervisor. "I enjoy teaching," he says. "I like to pass on knowledge, to help shape the careers of new people."

Certification and registry examinations are offered by the National Board for Respiratory Care. An applicant must have a diploma from a CAHEA-accredited program. In many states, a graduate from a one-year CRTT program can qualify for the registry examination with an additional sixty-two hours of college-level basic sciences and one to two years of on-the-job training.

scholarships and grants

The American Respiratory Care Foundation offers scholarships specifically for respiratory care education. Some hospitals may sponsor students on an as-needed basis. Individual states sponsor general scholarships.

labor unions

Some medical institutions are unionized, although not all departments in all institutions. In unionized departments, CRTTs and RRTs may find their job duties limited to specific tasks.

who will hire me?

When Matthew Chirayil finished his training, he applied to Sherman Hospital in Elgin, Illinois, where he knew that he would receive excellent training. While he was still in school, he asked lots of questions about outstanding employers of the teachers and professionals he met in his clinical work . "Your real education begins on the job," Matthew says. "I would encourage students to look for an institution with aggressive in-service education, a first-rate staff who will teach you and instill development." After several years at Sherman Hospital, Matthew had the confidence to apply to any hospital he chose.

Related Jobs

Did you know that there are a number of jobs related to respiratory therapy technician? The U.S. Department of Labor classifies these technicians under the headings "Therapists" and "Nursing, Therapy, and Specialized Teaching Services: Therapy and Rehabilitation." Also under these headings are people who rehabilitate victims of accidents and illness, train and instruct athletes, and work in various therapeutic modes. Jobs related to the respiratory therapist technician include corrective therapists, dialysis technicians, hypnotherapists, kinesiotherapists, medical assistants, medical technologists, music therapists, nuclear medical technologists, nurses, perfusionists, physical therapists, physician assistants, radiologic technologists, recreational therapists.

Respiratory care workers held around 74,000 jobs in 1992. Ninety percent of these jobs were in hospitals in departments of respiratory care, anesthesiology and pulmonary medicine. The remaining 10 percent were in home health care services, medical equipment rental companies, and nursing homes. Nevertheless, more and more respiratory care workers are now finding employment in skilled nursing and rehabilitation facilities, doctors' offices, companies that provide emergency oxygen services, and municipal services such as fire departments.

Many CAHEA-accredited schools have placement services to help graduates find jobs. The American Association for Respiratory Care publishes a monthly magazine, *The AARC Times*, which features classified job ads. Networking with people already employed in the profession is also a source of job referrals.

Like Matthew, many new graduates apply directly to potential employers. They do research by talking to respiratory care workers already working there. They ask about the quality of training and the general quality of health care available through the employing institution. It is a good idea to find out whether there will be support for additional training. Will the employer reimburse tuition expenses? Will it allow a flexible schedule to accommodate class time? Teaching hospitals are especially good places to begin a career. Equipment, technology, and training are likely to be first rate, with opportunities for varied duties and working with a range of patient needs.

Employers look for applicants who have made good grades and who have excellent attendance records. They evaluate personal qualities too, like courtesy, communication skills, enthusiasm, maturity, and a responsible, cooperative attitude.

where can I go from here?

Tom Garcia started out as a CRTT and later took the registry exam. "It's common to go into nursing or medical school or several ancillary fields once you acquire some technical skills," Tom says. "Many decide to stay in respiratory care, but usually a CRTT will want to become an RRT so that he or she can get into supervi-

Advancement Possibilities

Registered respiratory therapists perform the same duties as CRTTs, but have additional opportunities for supervisory and administrative work. RRTs take more responsibility for patient assessment, troubleshooting, and ventilator management.

Pulmonary function technologists use advanced techniques to diagnose pulmonary diseases.

Pediatric neonatal specialists work with premature newborns and newborns with respiratory problems. The needs of these infants are unique; since many more premature infants survive nowadays, this is a rapidly growing field.

sory or administrative levels. Still, it's not unheard of for a CRTT to do those things. Becoming a CRTT is a great place to start if you want to be in medicine but aren't quite sure which route to take. You go from a one- or two-year program right into a job. Then all kinds of possibilities open up."

Isabelle Orr started out as a CRTT. Today she teaches respiratory care at St. Augustine College. "There's so much you can do," she says. "I got into teaching because I want people to go into the profession with the same quality of training I got. But college isn't the only place to teach. There are supervisory jobs that require doing a lot of training. Most of your knowledge is acquired after you graduate and you're working. It's so important for newcomers to the profession to have supervisors who will nurture their development and set a good example." Regarding other career paths, Isabelle says, "After a few years on the job, you can switch to home health care—even start your own agency. This is a growing area, because insurance companies now demand it."

Pat Adney, who started her medical career as a physical therapist, says, "Many respiratory care workers go into home care after a few years. At first, you're on call on a rotating basis. You may have to go out on weekends or holidays, but eventually you get some options that allow more flexibility."

what are the salary ranges?

According to a survey by the American Association for Respiratory Care, the average entry-level salary for a CRTT was $19,760. According to a University of Texas Medical Branch survey, the median income for a respiratory therapy technician was $30,888. The average maximum salary was $38,233 a year. In addition, hospital workers usually enjoy excellent fringe benefits including health insurance, paid vacation and sick leave, and pension plans. Additional benefits may include parking, cafeteria discounts, uniform allowances, tuition reimbursement for job-related studies, and on-site day care.

what is the job outlook?

Employment in respiratory care is expanding rapidly in the nineties. It is expected to increase much faster than the average for all occupations through the year 2005.

Even though efforts to control rising health care costs have slowed down job opportunities in hospitals in recent years, this slow-growth trend is not expected to last. On the contrary, respiratory care professionals with credentials in neonatal care and pulmonary disease will be particularly in demand.

Several factors combine to make for this growing demand. One factor is the rapid increase in the middle-aged and elderly populations. The elderly are the most likely to suffer heart and lung ailments such as pneumonia, chronic bronchitis, emphysema, and heart disease. As the baby-boomers move from middle age into old age, the need for respiratory care workers will increase.

Another factor is the advances in the treatment of heart attack, traumatic injury, and premature birth. All these groups require respiratory care for some part of their treatment and this bodes well for workers in the field.

A third reason for an increased need is the AIDS epidemic. AIDS patients often have secondary lung ailments. Also, tuberculosis has made a reappearance in recent years. The increase in these disease populations will boost the demand for respiratory therapy professionals. The home care field, too, is expanding. This expansion has been fostered by the insurance industry's demand for less expensive alternatives to hospital care. Equipment manufacturers and rental firms, as well as companies that provide respiratory care on a contract basis, will also employ more respiratory care professionals.

how do I learn more?

professional organizations

Following are professional organizations that provide information on respiratory therapy technician careers and education.

American Association for Respiratory Care
11030 Ables Lane
Dallas, TX 75229
TEL: 214-243-2272
WEBSITE: http://www.aarc.org

American Medical Association
Division of Allied Health and Accreditation
515 North State Street
Chicago, Illinois 60610
TEL: 312-464-50000

American Respiratory Care Foundation
11030 Ables Lane
Dallas, TX 75229
TEL: 214-243-2272

National Board for Respiratory Care
8310 Nieman Road
Lenexa, KS 66214
TEL: 913-599-4200

Respiratory Health Association
301 Sicomac Avenue
Wyckoff, NJ 07481
TEL: 201-848-5875

Respiratory Nursing Society
437 Twin Bay Dr.
Pensacola, FL 32534
TEL: 904-474-8869

bibliography

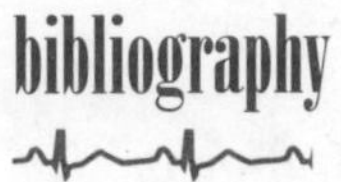

Following is a sampling of books and periodicals relating to both the professional concerns and the development of respiratory therapy technicians.

Books

Dantzker, David R., Neil R. MacIntyre, and Eric D. Bakow. *Comprehensive Respiratory Care*. Philadelphia, PA: W.B. Saunders Co., 1995.

Des Jardins, Terry. *Cardiopulmonary Anatomy & Physiology: Essentials for Respiratory Care,* 2nd ed. Albany, NY: Delmar Publishers, 1993.

Pryor, Jennifer A., editor. *Respiratory Care*. New York: Churchill Livingstone, 1991.

Springhouse Publishing Staff. *Providing Respiratory Care*. Springhouse, PA: Springhouse Publishing Co., 1995.

Periodicals

AARC Times. Monthly. This periodical features classified job advertisements for positions in the field of respiratory care. The American Association for Respiratory Care, Daedalus Enterprises, Inc., 11030 Ables Lane, Dallas, TX 75229, 214-243-2272.

Respiration. Bimonthly. Discusses scientific aspects of respiration and the respiratory organs. S. Karger Publishers, Inc., 26 West Avon Road, Box 529, Farmington, CT 06085, 203-675-7834.

Respiratory Care. Monthly. Inhalation Therapy, Daedalus Enterprises, Inc., 11030 Ables Lane, Dallas, TX 75229, 214-243-2272.

Respiratory Management. Bimonthly. Articles are directed toward respiratory personnel. Respiratory Therapy, Choices Publishing Group, 129 Washington Street, Hoboken, NJ 07030, 213-395-0234.

Respiratory Protection Newsletter. Bimonthly. Contains articles covering respiratory care in industrial and nuclear environments. RSA Publications, 19 Pendleton Drive, Box 19, Hebron, CT 06248, 203-228-0824.

social worker

Definition
Social workers help individuals, families and communities find solutions to personal and social problems. They address such issues as mental illness, family conflict, racism, poverty, and unemployment. Social workers do counseling and advocacy, link clients with public agencies that offer resources, and help develop social programs and policies.

Salary range
$20,000 to $30,000 to $50,000+

Educational requirements
Bachelor's degree; master's degree recommended

Certification or Licensing
Mandatory

Outlook
Faster than the average

GOE
10.01.02

DOT
195

High School Subjects

Social studies
Health
Psychology
Communications

Personal Interests

Helping people
Working with people
Social issues
Psychological issues

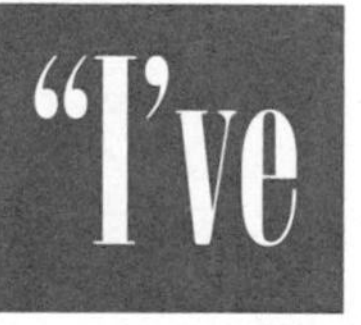

"I've got to catch up with my paper work before my first client comes in," remarked Carolyn Campbell. She and another social worker had just left the weekly staff meeting at the Lorene Replogle Counseling Center in Chicago. After briefly working on her records, Carolyn checked her watch and stepped out into the waiting room.

"Hello, Julie." She greeted the tired-looking young woman with a smile. "Please come in."

Ever since her marriage broke up, Julie has been having trouble sleeping. Through counseling, Carolyn hoped that she might help Julie lose some of her anxieties. It seemed to Carolyn that, despite her fatigue and discouragement, Julie's self-confidence was gradually returning.

Since this was staff meeting day, Carolyn had fewer counseling sessions scheduled than on her other work days. After meeting with Julie, she had a few minutes to write up her notes. Carolyn's record-keeping, like that of most health care professionals, had become more complicated over the last few years as a result of the stricter requirements of cost-conscious insurance companies. Of course, Carolyn had always written up detailed case notes on each of the clients she was counseling. Reviewing her notes helped her to see the client's personal situation and issues more clearly and to recognize the progress that was being made. She also kept notes on her conferences with the master's level social work student she was supervising at the center.

lingo to learn

Advocacy Defending the rights of individuals or communities.

Defense mechanisms Various mental processes, such as denial or displacement, through which individuals protect their personalities from guilt, anxiety, or unacceptable thoughts.

Empowerment The process of assisting individuals and groups to acquire greater effectiveness with the goal of enabling them to make positive changes in their lives.

Family therapy Therapy that focuses on the family group as a unit, rather than on the separate individuals of the family.

Grass-roots organizing Educating and mobilizing the people of a local community for action toward a common goal.

Intervention The social work equivalent of "treatment"; it includes all the professional activities through which social workers try to prevent or solve clients' problems.

Mediation Intervention in disputes between opposing groups with the goal of reconciling differences and/or achieving a mutually satisfactory compromise.

Norms The rules and expectations for appropriate behavior held collectively by any community, culture, or society.

Public assistance Government-provided financial aid for persons who are unable to support themselves.

what does a social worker do?

The social work profession grew out of the nineteenth-century realization that the problems of the poor could not be solved by the charitable efforts of well-meaning individual volunteers. The establishment of charitable organizations in the late 19th century and the settlement house movement (pioneered by Jane Addams at Chicago's Hull House) led to the creation of formal social work education programs.

Social workers in the 1990s serve human needs and work for social justice in a wide range of institutional and community settings. The National Association of Social Workers (NASW) has defined the profession's core values as commitment to service, social justice, the dignity and worth of the person, the importance of human relationships, integrity, and competence.

Most social workers are involved in what the profession calls "direct practice"—meaning that they work directly with clients in agency offices, schools, hospitals, outpatient clinics, prisons, and other settings. Some social workers have chosen to specialize in "indirect practice." Instead of working directly with clients, they work with institutional and social structures—developing, administering, analyzing, and evaluating programs and policies. Nearly 40 percent of all social workers are employed by government agencies. The others work in many parts of the private sector.

One of the most familiar areas of social work is child welfare and family services. The purpose of child welfare agencies is to protect the well-being of children. *Child welfare workers* counsel children and adolescents who have social adjustment problems. They also work with parents and teachers to help identify and address problems and locate appropriate resources. Social workers make home visits to investigate reports of child abuse, neglect, and abandonment. Sometimes they need to remove the children from the home and place them in shelters or find foster homes for them.

Social workers in child welfare and family services provide counseling on family relationships and teach parenting skills. They also counsel and evaluate potential adoptive parents and help families find the resources they need for disabled, ill, or elderly members. Parents may also need help obtaining child support payments or finding day care.

In recent years, social workers in child and family services have had to develop social services for children born with HIV-related conditions or congenital disabilities resulting from the mother's use of drugs like crack cocaine.

Clinical social workers specialize in providing mental health services to children, adolescents, and adults. They may offer individual and group therapy, crisis intervention, social rehabilitation, outreach services, marital counseling, stress management, and preventive mental health programs.

Health care social workers (also called *medical social workers*) help hospital patients and their families cope with serious medical problems, such as AIDS, cancer, or Alzheimer's. They help to educate the family about the illness and its treatment, as well as the changes it will bring to their lives. Health care social workers arrange for at-home services (visiting nurses, home oxygen equipment, or participation in a meals on wheels program, for example) that will be needed after the patient's discharge from the hospital. Sometimes they organize support groups for caregivers and other family members.

Gerontological social workers specialize in work with older people. They counsel the aged and their families and help make arrangements for housing, transportation, adult day care, and long-term care. Sometimes they organize support groups for caregivers or arrange respite services to give the principal caregiver some time off. They are also responsible for investigating reports that elderly persons are being abused or neglected.

School social workers are employed in school settings to provide counseling, education, and advocacy. They address such problems as teen pregnancy, the spread of AIDS and other sexually transmitted diseases, alcohol and drug abuse, racial discrimination, and conflicts related to multiculturalism. Since passage of the Education for All Handicapped Children Act, school social workers have also been helping to integrate children with disabilities into the mainstream of public education.

Other areas of social work include: working with the inmates of correctional institutions and their families; personnel department work for corporations; work with the homeless; community organizing at the grass-roots level.

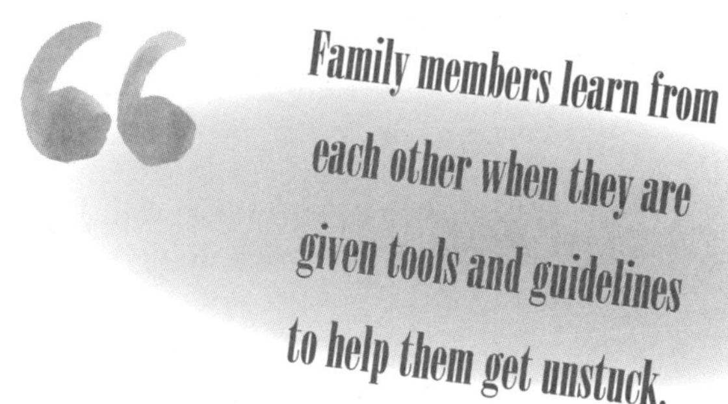

what is it like to be a social worker?

Carolyn Campbell had been a licensed clinical social worker on the staff of the Lorene Replogle Counseling Center for 19 years, yet every day continued to offer new challenges. Every client's situation was different. When she first came, she had no idea she would still be at the center nearly 20 years later. At that time, she was planning to concentrate on building up her private practice. As it turned out, she liked working at the center so much that she decided to make it the focus of her professional life, though she continued to maintain a small private practice out of her home office. One of the most positive features of the center's policies, Carolyn often thought, was its sliding-fee scale that made it possible for clients with low incomes to receive the benefit of individual counseling services.

Maria was her next client. Like Julie, she had been in therapy with Carolyn for about six months. Maria was dealing with interpersonal issues that went back to her childhood in a somewhat dysfunctional family.

As Carolyn was preparing to go out on an errand after her session with Maria, her telephone rang. It was the center's receptionist asking Carolyn to do an intake interview with a potential client who wanted to talk to a counselor. Usually the center director took care of the intake interviews, but he was leading a seminar on depression at another location that afternoon. Carolyn carried on a short conversation with the young man on the other end of the line and soon realized that the services offered by the center would not meet his needs. What he really wanted was to find a good drug-rehabilitation program, so Carolyn offered an appropriate referral.

Later that day, Carolyn met with Alan, one of the students who was doing supervised work at the center as part of Loyola University's Master of Social Work program. They discussed some of the frustrations that were making Alan wonder if counseling was really the right field of social work for him. Carolyn reminded him that one of the hardest truths for all counselors to learn was that they will not be able to "cure" all their clients or solve all their problems. "There are some circumstances in people's lives that cannot be changed, no matter how much we wish we could bring about those changes," she reflected.

Since most social workers enter the profession because they want to help people, having to acknowledge the limitations of intervention can be hard to accept. Fortunately, the occasional frustrations are usually balanced by the sense of satisfaction one gets from seeing individuals and families begin making positive changes in their lives.

"What drew me to social work was the opportunity it offered to combine my interests in psychology and sociology. I was interested in individuals *and* in larger groups," explained one licensed clinical social worker. Harrison Taylor, the clinical coordinator of the Adolescent Intensive Outpatient Program at the Tennessee Christian Medical Center in Madison, decided to specialize in family therapy after some early work experience with Children and Family Services in Nashville.

In his current position, Harrison is responsible for running a group therapy program for troubled adolescents between the ages of 13 and 17. The teenagers participate in adventure-based activities and the creative arts with the goal of learning problem-solving skills. Once a week, their parents come in to work on parenting skills. The purpose is to "rebuild the bridges between parents and teenagers," said Harrison. "Family members learn from each other when they are given tools and guidelines to help them get unstuck."

FYI

The social work profession grew out of the nineteenth-century realization that the problems of the poor could not be solved by the charitable efforts of well-meaning individual volunteers

have I got what it takes to be a social worker?

Social workers must be strongly committed to helping other people, but it is not enough simply to like people and enjoy working with them. The satisfaction experienced by social workers when they are able to help people improve their lives is great, but the work is not easy. Social workers need to develop excellent communication skills, especially listening skills. They must have patience, emotional maturity, self-control (even when confronted with tragic situations), and the ability to assess a client's circumstances with clarity and objectivity. It is essential for social workers to be able to demonstrate acceptance of their clients as people, even when they are not able to endorse the clients' actions.

Social workers are often responsible for making recommendations that will have a lasting impact on people's lives. Is there sufficient evidence to believe that this child is being abused and should be removed from his parents' home? Is this person still able to live alone despite her illness? Would this couple be suitable adoptive parents?

Despite the educational efforts of the National Association of Social Workers, many people still know little about the profession. One social worker cited the common misconception that social workers are just "people who bring food to the poor." Other misconceptions are that social workers are interfering busybodies or troublemakers who exaggerate social problems.

One licensed clinical social worker (LCSW) suggested that this situation may be changing with the advent of managed care (which stresses health care cost containment). Since services provided by LCSWs are less expensive than those offered by other mental health professionals, insurance companies and other organizations are turning more and more toward LCSWs as providers. At the same time, LCSWs are expressing frustration with the decrease of professional autonomy that results from these cost-containment measurements.

To be a successful social worker you should

- Be strongly committed to helping other people
- Have excellent communication skills
- Have patience, maturity, and self-control
- Have the ability to assess a client's circumstances with both compassion and objectivity

how do I become a social worker?

education

High School

High school students who are interested in the social work field should take a well-balanced college preparatory course. Classes that improve a student's communication skills (speech and writing courses) are especially helpful. Classes that provide an introduction to psychology, sociology, and the other social sciences are also good choices. A knowledge of history is important for developing an understanding of contemporary social problems.

High school students can also look for ways to gain experience in working with people. You might find part-time work or volunteer opportunities at a local social-service agency, the YMCA, summer camp programs, or tutoring programs. There may also be volunteer opportunities available through social-justice groups or religious organizations.

Postsecondary Training

Most social work jobs require a bachelor's degree, though the degree does not necessarily have to be a Bachelor of Social Work (BSW)degree. Sociology, psychology, or other social sciences are also appropriate majors. For many positions, especially those in health and mental health settings, a Master of Social Work (MSW) degree is necessary.

As an undergraduate, Carolyn had a double major in psychology and sociology, with a minor in history. One summer, she did an internship at a public-aid office; she spent another summer as a house parent in a children's home. After graduation, she worked at a small public assistance office in southern Illinois for three years.

This hands-on experience convinced Carolyn that social work was the right career for her, so she enrolled in the MSW program at Loyola University in Chicago. Harrison majored in sociology as an undergraduate and then earned an MSW at the University of Chicago. As an undergraduate, he worked part-time as a mental health assistant at an inpatient adolescent unit.

In 1994, there were 383 BSW programs and 117 MSW programs that were accredited by the Council on Social Work Education. There are also Ph.D. programs in social work and DSW (doctor of social work) programs. An accredited BSW program must include work in the following five areas: human behavior and the social environment, social welfare policies and services, social work practice, research, and a practicum (supervised field experience) of at least 400 clock hours.

MSW programs are generally two years in length and require at least 900 hours of supervised field experience. In their field work, most students focus on a specialized area of social work, such as child welfare, health or mental health, work with the elderly, or community organizing.

"I think social workers receive a greater amount of close supervision during their training period than members of any other profession," reflected Carolyn. "We had some really tough supervisors, but they gave us what we needed."

certification or licensing

All 50 states and the District of Columbia have requirements for the certification, licensing, or registration of social workers. The precise regulations vary by state. Becoming a licensed social worker (LSW) generally requires meeting certain educational and work-experience requirements, as well as passing a written examination.

Because Carolyn had decided to specialize in mental health (clinical) work, she had to gain additional experience and take the LCSW examination after becoming an LSW. Continuing education is also required for remaining licensed in Illinois.

In addition to the state licensing requirements, there are also various voluntary certifications offered by the National Association of Social Workers (NASW), such as School Social Work Specialist. Social workers who are accepted for membership in the NASW, have an MSW and two years of experience, and pass an examination may use the title ACSW (Academy of Certified Social Workers).

Professional credentials are especially important for social workers thinking of going into private practice, because many insurance companies require certain credentials for recognition as a provider of reimbursable services. In some cities and counties, it is also necessary for social workers in private practice to obtain local permits or registration certificates.

Social workers who want to be employed by federal, state, or local government agencies usually need to pass a civil service exam.

scholarships and grants

For information about scholarships, fellowships, grants, student loans, and other financial-aid possibilities, consult the financial-aid office of the academic institution that you plan to attend. Allow plenty of time for the paper work.

There are also a few scholarships and fellowships specifically targeted for women, African Americans, Hispanics, and Native Americans who want to study social work.

Contact the National Association of Social Workers for additional information on applying for financial aid.

who will hire me?

Social workers are employed by federal, state, and local government agencies in the following departments: social services, human resources, child welfare, health and mental health, housing, education, and corrections. In 1994, nearly 40 percent of all social workers worked for government agencies. If you would like to work for a government agency, you usually need to arrange to take a civil service exam. For most government jobs, the applicant's scores on the civil service exam are considered the most important factor.

In the private sector, social workers are employed by the following organizations: voluntary social service agencies, home health agencies, hospitals, clinics, nursing homes, community and religious organizations, businesses, and industrial corporations.

Some social workers teach and do research at colleges and universities; these faculty positions usually require a doctoral degree.

Some social workers choose to go into private practice after a few years at an agency. This seems to be a growing trend. Most social workers in private practice are clinical social workers who offer counseling and psychotherapy to individuals, families, and groups. Before venturing into private practice, a social worker must have an MSW and supervised experience. To succeed as a private practitioner, it is necessary to have a reliable network of professional contacts for client referrals.

Students looking for an entry-level social work position will receive assistance from their college or university placement service. It is also a good idea to ask for suggestions about job openings from your social work professors, field work supervisors, and other contacts made through your field work.

Information about job openings is also available through the local chapter of the National Association of Social Workers or your state's society for clinical social work. Professional journals and newsletters publish job openings. These publications should be available at your college or university library.

where can I go from here?

Harrison Taylor, who received his MSW eight years ago, is currently preparing to go into private practice as an organizational development consultant. He wants to do what he calls "change management" by moving beyond individual and family therapy to apply his knowledge to corporate and nonprofit organizations. As Harrison pointed out, family issues often get projected into the workplace. His potential clients would be organizations that have problems with conflict management, lack of teamwork, diversity issues, low morale, and high turnover. Harrison's change of focus was prompted in part by his desire to work for the benefit of the wider society and in part by his hope of regaining some of the professional autonomy he has recently lost through the coming of managed health care.

Carolyn Campbell is not planning any changes in her professional life at this time. She has long known that she does not want to move into administration—the traditional route of advancement in social work. Because she enjoys supervising clinical social work students, she sometimes thinks of teaching in a university social work program.

Social workers with a master's degree have better opportunities for advancement to administrative or supervisory positions in social welfare or health care. Some choose private practice as their route of advancement. Social workers who earn doctoral degrees have opportunities for teaching, research, policy analysis, and program development.

what are the salary ranges?

Social workers with the MSW earn more than those with only a bachelor's degree. Those with a doctoral degree have higher salaries than those with only the MSW.

A 1992 survey showed that BSW graduates were receiving starting salaries that averaged $18,025. Overall, social workers with only the BSW averaged $23,000. Those with an MSW were averaging $27,700.

Social workers employed by the federal government tended to earn higher salaries, as did school social workers and those in mental health or community planning and organization.

A 1993 survey revealed that hospital social workers averaged $33,300. Social workers in teaching, research, administration, and private practice generally have higher salaries than most social workers, but very few earn more than $60,000.

In general, salaries on the east and west coasts are higher than in the Midwest, while jobs in rural areas tend to pay less than those in the city.

what is the job outlook?

Social work positions are expected to increase faster than the average for all occupations through the year 2005 because of the population's growing need for social services, as well as the number of social workers leaving the field for other occupations. More gerontological social workers will be needed as the percentage of elderly persons in the population increases. The strong trend toward early discharge of hospital patients will increase the need for hospital social workers, who make arrangements for at-home medical services and social supports. The need for school social workers is also expected to grow, as schools will have to provide expanded social services for children with serious adjustment problems, as well as those with disabilities.

Employment opportunities in government agencies will depend on how much funding is available for social programs.

Although private practice is a growing field in social work, its viability will depend in large part on the willingness of vendors and insurance companies to pay for the services offered by clinical workers. Private practitioners who contract with businesses and corporations will probably do well.

The impact of lower budgets, combined with the need for more staff members, has resulted in some social-service agencies hiring less qualified human-services workers instead of professional social workers. This trend is a cause of concern to some social workers, who fear a decline in professional standards and the quality of service offered to clients.

how do I learn more?

professional organizations

For more information about the social work profession, contact the following:

National Association of Social Workers
Information Center
750 First Street, NE
Washington, DC 20002
TEL: 202-408-8600
WEBSITE: http://www.social.com

Council on Social Work Education
1600 Duke Street
Alexandria, VA 22314
TEL: 703-683-8080
WEBSITE: http://www.cswe.org

bibliography

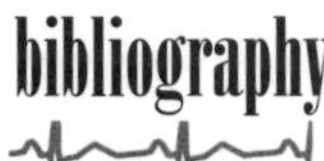

Following is a sampling of materials relating to the professional concerns and development of social workers.

Books

Calvin, Donna. *Good Works: a Guide to Careers in Social Change*. New York, NY: Barricade Books, 1993.

Garner, Geraldine O. *Careers in Social and Rehabilitation Services*. Lincolnwood, IL: VGM Career Horizons, 1994.

Ginsbert, Leon H. *Careers in Social Work*. New York, NY: Allyn & Bacon, 1997.

Morales, Armando T., and Bradford W. Sheafor. *Social Work: a Profession of Many Faces,* 7th edition. New York, NY: Allyn & Bacon, 1994.

Morgan, Bradley J., and Joseph M. Palmisano, editors. *Psychology and Social Work Career Directory*. Detroit, MI: Gale Research, 1993.

Simpson, Carolyn, and Dwain Simpson. *Exploring Careers in Social Work,* revised edition. New York, NY: Rosen Group, 1996.

Wittenberg, Renee. *Opportunities in Social Work Careers*. Lincolnwood, IL: VGM Career Horizons, 1996.

Periodicals

Health and Social Work. Quarterly. Examines health-related social problems and issues dealing with the client and the community. National Association of Social Workers, N A S W Press, 750 First Street, SE, Suite 700, Washington, DC 20002, 202-408-8600.

Social Service Review. Quarterly. Devoted to the professional interests of social work. University of Chicago Press, Journals Division, 5720 S. Woodlawn Avenue, Chicago, IL 60637, 773-753-3347.

Social Work. Bimonthly. Includes scholarly research and current information on social issues. National Association of Social Workers, N A S W Press, 750 First Street, SE, Suite 700, Washington, DC 20002, 202-408-8600.

special procedures technician

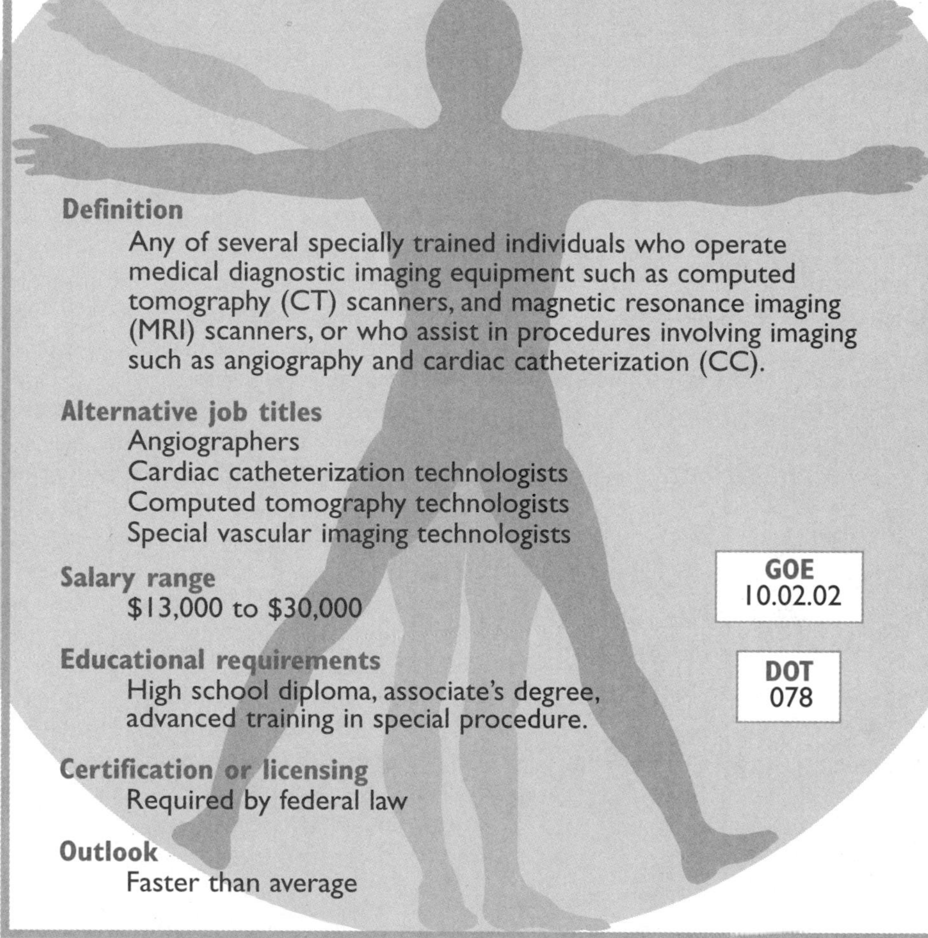

Definition

Any of several specially trained individuals who operate medical diagnostic imaging equipment such as computed tomography (CT) scanners, and magnetic resonance imaging (MRI) scanners, or who assist in procedures involving imaging such as angiography and cardiac catheterization (CC).

Alternative job titles

Angiographers
Cardiac catheterization technologists
Computed tomography technologists
Special vascular imaging technologists

Salary range

$13,000 to $30,000

Educational requirements

High school diploma, associate's degree, advanced training in special procedure.

Certification or licensing

Required by federal law

Outlook

Faster than average

GOE
10.02.02

DOT
078

High School Subjects

Algebra
Biology
Chemistry
English
Psychology
Sociology

Personal Interests

Communications
Health
Working with people

Something was wrong. Maybe David Brown felt it before he thought it. Maybe his years of training and experience as a cardiac catheterization technologist let him sense that "Mrs. Smith" was in trouble. She lay calmly, still under the anesthesia but disconnected from the EKG monitor now, as he transferred her from the table.

The other members of the cardiology team were in the second swing room, prepping for the next patient. The procedure had gone well, they'd found and removed significant blockage from "Mrs. Smith's" artery; she was stable. . . . But something was wrong.

David lifted her eyelids. Only the whites showed.

He called out: "She's crashed!"

He had her back on the table, hooked up again to the monitor, as the rest of the team rushed to his side. To the cardiologist he said, "Seizures. She's fibrillating."

The team's response was immediate. With the third shock from the defibrillator, "Mrs. Smith's" heart beat again. The cardiologist snaked the catheter through the artery to "Mrs. Smith's" heart. Studying the image on the fluoroscope, he said, "Vessel wall collapsed. Good catch, David. You just saved her life. Now, let's get a stent in there."

what does a special procedures technologist do?

Everyone is familiar with X rays. But, while X rays remain a valuable diagnostic tool, advances in technology have allowed medical staff to achieve even more precise images of the human body. Tools such as computed tomography (CT) scanners and magnetic resonance imagers (MRI), and techniques such as angiography and cardiac catheterization, allow physicians and specially trained technologists to pinpoint areas of medical concern. In some cases, intervention procedures may be performed right away, saving valuable time, and avoiding riskier surgical procedures.

This article will discuss four special procedures: cardiac catheterization, computed tomography, angiography, and magnetic resonance imaging. They are often grouped together, because each technique involves the making or use of visual images to assist physicians in treating their patients. Another link among these techniques is that they are often performed by *radiology technologists* who have received advanced training and education in their specialized area. Also, *special procedures technologists* are generally responsible for positioning the patient for examination, immobilizing them, preparing the equipment to be used, and monitoring the equipment and the patient's progress during the procedure.

Special diagnostic procedures may be grouped into two areas: invasive and noninvasive. CT scans and MRI scans are considered noninvasive, because the equipment does not enter the body. Angiography and cardiac catheterization are considered invasive techniques, because the imaging work is done from within the body. Sometimes patients will need to undergo more than one of these procedures.

Angiography

Blood vessels do not normally show up on X-ray photographs. Yet physicians need to be able to see the vessels of the circulatory system in order to detect and locate such life-threatening conditions as aneurysms, narrowing or blockage of the vessel, or the presence of clots in the vessel. Angiography accomplishes this by coating the vessels of the affected areas with a contrast medium, a substance that allows blood vessels to be seen because it makes the vessels opaque to the X rays. In patients with tumors or injuries to their organs, an angiogram can show any changes that have occurred to the pattern of the vessels. Studying the flow of the contrast medium through the vessels also gives the physician important information about the way the patient's blood flows. With this information, the physician can assess the extent of damage,

lingo to learn

Aneurysm A saclike bulging of a blood vessel, usually an artery. An extremely dangerous health condition.

Artery A vessel that carries blood away from the heart to the rest of the body.

Catheter A small, flexible, strong tube made of plastic, rubber, or metal, inserted into the body to inject medicines, drain fluids, and perform diagnostic procedures.

Catheterization The introduction of a catheter into the body.

Coronary stent A device inserted into a blood vessel in order to support a weakened or collapsed area of the vessel.

Diagnosis The determination, after examination, of the nature of the patient's health condition and extent of disease.

Electrocardiogram (EKG or ECG) A record of the electric current produced by the contractions of the heart. The EKG machine and monitor provide a graphic, real-time representation of this electric current.

or the progression of disease, and determine the necessary treatment.

In order to perform an angiography, a small tube, called a catheter, is inserted into the patient and moved through an artery to the area to be examined. The angiographer assists by operating and monitoring an X-ray fluoroscope. This device allows the physician to view the catheter while guiding it to the area of interest. The angiographer next prepares the contrast medium to be injected and is responsible for controlling the amount and rate of flow of the contrast medium into the patient's body. Using a video display, the angiographer adjusts the density and contrast of the image in order to obtain the highest possible quality image. The angiographer then takes a rapid series of X rays that will function as a movie of the vessel. This will allow the physician to study the blood flow within the vessel.

An angiography procedure can last from a few minutes to as long as three hours. Once the X-ray films have been exposed, the angiographer brings them to the hospital's dark room to be developed, and reviews the finished images for their quality to be certain that they properly record the area under examination.

Recent advances in technology make it possible to reduce the amount of contrast medium that needs to be injected into patients. Computers, in what is called digital subtraction angiography, enable the technologist to delete parts of the X-ray images that reduce the quality and visibility of the vessels. In some cases, this means that the contrast medium can be injected intravenously, eliminating the riskier catheterization procedure. Advances in intervention procedures, such as expanding a blocked artery or injecting medications directly into a tumor, mean that these can be performed while the catheter is still in place. In this way, surgery can often be avoided.

Cardiac Catheterization

Like angiography, the cardiac catheterization procedure is invasive. It involves the introduction of a catheter into the patient's body in order to examine and treat heart conditions. As part of a team assisting the cardiologist, the cardiac catheterization technologist performs one or more of several functions, including positioning the patients and explaining the procedure they will undergo; monitoring vital signs; documenting the procedure by typing data into a computer system used to control the amount, quality, and sequence for filming the X rays of the patient's heart; and assisting the cardiology team in preprocedure sterilization and by retrieving supplies and equipment necessary to the procedure.

During a cardiac catheterization procedure, a catheter is introduced through a small incision into a vein or artery and guided into the patient's heart. When the catheter is in position, it can be used for various diagnostic and intervention procedures, such as directly reading the heart's blood pressure, withdrawing blood to determine the amount of oxygen reaching the heart, injecting contrast medium for filming X rays, and for introducing tools and medications to repair damaged vessels. When these procedures are called for, the cardiac catheterization technologist will assist in preparing whatever tools and medications are needed.

When X rays are required, the technologist will enter data on the amount, quality, and filming sequence of the radiation beam, initiate the introduction of the contrast medium into the heart, and activate the fluoroscope that will film the heart. Technologists are also responsible for positioning the X-ray device and the table, raising and lowering them according to the cardiologist's request.

Finally, an important function of the cardiac catheterization technologist is to remain alert to changes in the patient's response throughout the procedure. Because patients undergoing this procedure generally suffer from life-threatening conditions, and because there remains a measure of risk in performing the procedure, the cardiologist and the other members of the cardiac catheterization team must be kept continually informed of the patient's progress.

CT (computed tomography) scan

CT scanning (also known as CAT—for computed axial tomography—scanning) represents an important breakthrough in diagnostic imaging. While invasive techniques such as angiography entail not only a degree of risk to the patient, but are also limited in their usefulness in highly complex organs like the brain, CT scanning combines X rays with computer technology to create clear cross-section images. These cross-sections, or slices, provide more detailed information than standard X rays, while the technique minimizes the patient's exposure to the X-ray radiation. First developed in the early 1970s for studying the brain, CT scanning has proven to be a useful technique for examination of much of the body.

A CT scanner is a large device consisting of a rotating scanner and a table that may be placed in a variety of positions as it enters the scanner. The CT technologist is responsible for positioning the patient on the table, making certain that the head and body are immobilized. The placement of the patient must be precise, and according to the radiologist's instructions, in order to achieve the necessary images of the area under examination. Contrast media are also used in CT scanning, and are either given orally or intravenously. The CT technologist enters data into the scanner's computer control, including information about the type of scan to be performed, the time required, and the thickness of the slice of the body to be imaged.

As the CT scan begins, large numbers of low dosage X rays are passed through the patient from a great many angles. These angles enable the computer to construct three-dimensional images of the parts of the patient's body. Different tissues in the body absorb X rays in different amounts; sensors allow the computer to gather this information and build the images. During the procedure, the CT technologist observes the patient through a window in the control room, and speaks to the patient over an intercom system. Because the CT scan can be an uncomfortable procedure, it is important that the CT technologist be able to provide reassurance to the patient.

more lingo to learn

Fluoroscope X-ray apparatus that uses a fluorescent screen of calcium tungstate to produce images of the varying densities of the body.

Imaging The creation of images of the parts of the body.

Intravenous Means within a vein. Refers to the injection of medicines, contrast mediums, and other drugs directly into a vein.

Stroke A condition, often accompanied by seizures, brought on by the collapse or rupture of a blood vessel in the brain.

Vascular Pertaining to or containing vessels.

Vein A vessel that carries blood from other parts of the body back to the heart.

X ray A type of radiation beam used to record on film shadow images of the portions of the body.

Magnetic Resonance Imaging (MRI)

MRI is the latest advance in imaging technology. Unlike the other procedures, it does not involve X rays, and therefore presents no risk to the patient. MRI scans also produce the most detailed and flexible images among the various imaging techniques. However, it is a relatively costly procedure.

As its name implies, MRI uses a strong magnetic field to affect the magnetic orientation of hydrogen protons (the nuclei of hydrogen)in the molecules in the body. Normally, hydrogen protons are randomly oriented; when subjected to the magnetic field of the MRI, however, the magnetic orientation of the protons becomes aligned. A pulse of radio waves is then used to knock the protons out of this alignment. As the protons return to their normal, random magnetic alignment, they produce radio signals, and the MRI scanner reads these radio signals to construct its images. Because the different tissues of the body contain different concentrations of hydrogen, each type of tissue will produce a radio signal of a different strength. The MRI computer interprets the strength of the signals as it builds the images of the section of the body under examination.

The MRI technologist first speaks to the patient, explaining the MRI procedure, and makes certain that the patient is not carrying any metal objects. These can be hazardous to the patient and can damage the equipment once the magnetic field is activated. The MRI technologist is responsible for positioning the patient on the table that is then inserted into the MRI scanner. Special coils, or receivers, are positioned on the patient over the area the radiologist wishes to examine. A microphone inside the scanner allows the patient and technologist to communicate throughout the procedure, which generally requires half an hour.

In the computer control room attached to the MRI scanning room, the MRI technologist enters data, such as the patient's history, the position for entry into the scanner, the part of the body to be scanned, and the orientation of the scan, into the computer. The MRI technologist initiates the scan and observes the patient through a window in the control room and on a closed-circuit video display, while maintaining voice contact. Thus, the MRI technologist can offer comfort and reassurance to the patient, while remaining alert to the patient's safety.

MRI scans are particularly useful for examining the brain, spinal cord, and the eyes and ears, and for determining the precise extent of tumors that may be present in the patient's body. MRI scans can provide detailed images of the heart, the circulatory system, as well as joints and soft tissues and organs such as the intestines. Continual refinements to MRI techniques are making possible the imaging of areas of the body that have previously resisted detailed examination.

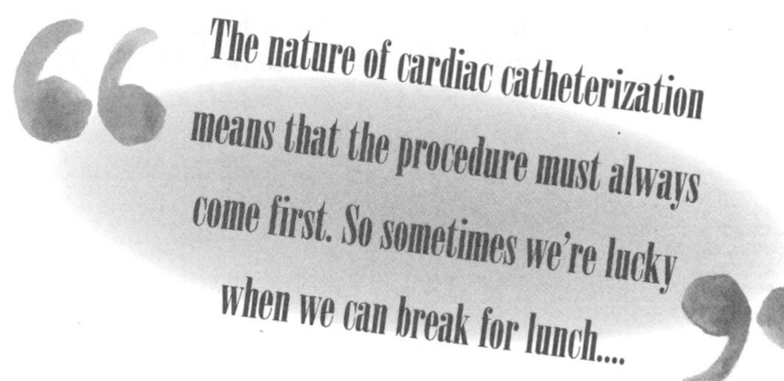

what is it like to be a special procedures technician?

Before the introduction of these special imaging procedures, physicians were dependent on X rays to give them an understanding of the conditions affecting their patients. X rays, however, are not usually precise enough to supply detailed images of many vital areas of the body. For some health conditions, exploratory surgery was the only way a physician could locate the source of a health problem. Yet even minor surgery can expose a patient to risk. Today, special imaging procedures have greatly enhanced the physician's diagnostic abilities; in some cases, these procedures allow the patient to avoid surgery altogether.

Special procedures have created a need for personnel trained to operate the equipment and assist the medical and nursing staff. The quality and precision of the images, and therefore their usefulness in treating the patient, depend highly on the technicians who make them.

David Brown is a cardiac catheterization technologist at the Texas Heart Center in St. Luke's Episcopal Hospital in Houston. "We're one of the premier cardiac centers in the world," David says. "We're a large facility, with eleven cath labs, which may be more than most places. But we remain involved in research, too. A lot of the procedures we perform are still experimental."

Typically David works in a team of four, including two nurses and two technicians, assisting the cardiologist. Teams are assigned to one of several different rooms, with each room set up according to the needs of its diagnostic specialty. Assignments to these rooms are rotated according to a daily schedule. In addition to these rooms, swing labs, which are really two rooms joined together, allow the cardiac team to perform more than one procedure. "That way, when we finish one procedure, one of us will manipulate the patient from the table while the others are already preparing for the next procedure."

"The nature of the room's specialty determines its schedule. A room set up for peripheral vascular work, for example, may only see one or two patients in the day," David explains. "In a swing lab, we'll work on eight to eleven patients a day. Compare that to an X-ray lab, where it's more like an assembly line—they'll do two hundred to three hundred patients in one day. Because what we do may be very intensive, our schedule operates according to a specific structure."

When David arrives at the hospital at 7:00 AM, he first meets with the other members of the cardiac staff to coordinate the day's schedule and receive his assignment. "There's a specific amount of time allotted for each procedure, based on how long they usually take. So I know at the beginning of the day what my schedule will be like." As part of the team, David is assigned to one of the four areas of the cardiac catheterization procedure described above.

"Each one is important, and I've been trained for all of the different fields of the procedure. Sometimes I drive the table, that is, position the patient, manipulate the X-ray camera. Other times, I do the procedural documentation, or I do what we call human dynamic monitoring, which means watching the EKG monitoring, reading the patient's blood pressure and other vital signs. Or I'll be the go-fer, running supplies, sterilizing the equipment, and scrubbing up the other members of the team."

"The nature of cardiac catheterization means that the procedure must always come first. So sometimes we' re lucky when we can break for lunch, if there's another team available to fill in for us," David says. "And I'd say we run late almost every day. But because I'm also in college, I can usually leave before 4:30."

The daily schedules of other special procedures technicians will vary according to the size of the hospital, their patient load, and the type of imaging technique they perform. An angiographer's day may be similar to David Brown's, as they too assist in an invasive procedure. MRI technologists and CT technologists may find their schedules to be much different. "Also," David says, "the other special procedures are generally assigned to the radiology department, while we're a part of the cardiology department. In fact, in our situation, I'd say there's not a strong rapport between us and the radiology department."

have I got what it takes to be a special procedures technician?

Special procedures technicians work with people experiencing extremely stressful times. "That can be a down side," says Kelly Yu, an MRI technician at a New Haven, Connecticut hospital. "Our job can be very stressful and full of hard situations. But the fact that I feel I am helping mankind helps balance the equation."

David Brown agrees. "We work with sick and dying people, and they are often pretty scared. I like it that I can interact with the patients, and I do my best to make them more comfortable. You really get to know your patients and there's an extra satisfaction when the intervention is successful. But when things don't go well, it can be pretty rough."

To be a successful special procedures technician, you should

- Have an interest in medicine
- Have an aptitude for science and math
- Work well with people, both independently and as part of a team
- Have strong communications skills and compassion for patients
- Have the ability to function under stress and emergency situations
- Be conscientious, responsible, and efficient
- Have good manual dexterity and stamina

Good communication skills are important not only when with the patient, but when working with other members of the medical staff as well. As a member of a cardiology team, David's contact with physicians, nurses, and other technicians is more intensive than Kelly's work in MRI. "But I like it that I'm allowed to interact with professionals on an equal level," says David, who is currently completing his premedical studies and expects to become a general surgeon. "I think being a cardiac tech allows me to prove myself to the others. There's more respect here than in other areas of radiology. They see me working; I'm part of the team, and really, the only thing that counts here is how well you perform your job. I think there's an attitude toward other radiology technicians that you're just a tech. I don't find that in cardiology."

For Kelly, the recent initiation of board certification for MRI technicians brings an added respect to her work. "Certification is a big step toward acknowledgment," she says. But Kelly finds a lot of satisfaction in the work itself. "I chose radiology, and MRI, because it's an up-and-coming career that's always taking steps toward being at the forefront of medicine in the years to come. Each year we get better upgrades, and we're able to do things that were never even imagined before, like magnetic resonance angiography, breast imaging, and imaging of heart, abdomen, and prostate. I like the fact that this career is always moving on, challenging me to become a better and more competent tech."

One of the exciting parts of David's work is the sometimes experimental nature of the procedures with which he assists. "A lot of the work we do is as part of major research studies into techniques and types of medication. For example, we pioneered the use of coronary stents. . . . I like being involved in new technologies. And I get to see procedures that never make it to being approved, too."

David, who began his radiology career as a radiologist technician in the army, finds his work in cardiology to be an important step in his future career. "I've dreamed of becoming a surgeon since I was young. And the work I do here is a lot like surgery. It's giving me a real exposure to what I hope to do in the future. I get to put in practice a lot of the things I'm studying in school, too. For that reason, I recommend this work to anyone considering a medical career."

Cardiology patients are often confronted with life-threatening conditions, and David must always be alert to signs that they are in trouble during the procedure. "I'm working with critical patients. I have to be able to see what can go wrong, and be prepared for it. If a patient crashes suddenly, or they can't tolerate the procedure, I have to know to call the anesthesiologist, or for respiratory support. That can be stressful, knowing that a person's life depends on what you do."

Patients undergoing these procedures may require extra sensitivity from the technicians and other health care personnel involved in their case. "You have to be able to inspire confidence in them," Kelly says. "That's a big factor in a patient's health, and whether they'll get better."

Hospitals are sterile, well-lighted work environments. However, working conditions may vary. A busy hospital, a critical care ward, or an emergency room may be a much more stressful environment than a health care clinic, a health maintenance organization, or a diagnostic imaging center. Hours may also vary. David Brown, for example, generally works eight hours a day, five days a week. "Although," David says, "they're considering adding a second shift, because of the increasing volume of patients we see." Other special procedure technicians may be assigned to night or weekend shifts, or they may be on-call, available to work twenty-four hours a day.

Related Jobs

Did you know there are a number of jobs related to special procedures technician? The U.S. Department of Labor classifies this job under "Occupations in Medical and Dental Technology" and "Nursing, Therapy, and Specialized Teaching Services: Therapy and Rehabilitation." Jobs related to special procedures technician include radiologic technicians, nuclear resonance imaging technologists, nuclear medicine technologists, electrocardiograph technicians, cardiovascular technologists, cardiac ultrasound technologists, cardiopulmonary function technologists, cardiology technologists, peripheral vascular technicians, and sonographers.

how do I become a special procedures technician?

Most special procedures technicians begin their careers in radiology as radiology technologists. Generally, they are required to hold an associate's degree in radiology, and then receive additional training and education in their special procedural area. In addition, federal legislation has directed states to require that radiologic technicians be licensed.

education

High School

"In tenth grade," David says, "I sort of fell into an advanced course—human anatomy and physiology—where we had to dissect a cat. Ever since I've dreamed of becoming a surgeon." Biology, chemistry, and algebra were also important classes for David. "Having good math skills makes everything go easier," he adds. "And I'd say that my English and social science classes were really helpful, especially when I'm relating to patients and the other members of the cardiology team."

Advanced courses were also a feature of Kelly Yu's high school curriculum. "I found taking advanced courses in anatomy, physiology, math, and physics to be very useful," she says. Classes in communication, such as speech, and classes that reinforce written and verbal skills will help the prospective special procedures technician throughout his or her career. Because most imaging specialties depend heavily on computer technology, students should gain a good understanding of the use of computers. Depending on where they will work, special procedures technicians, as with all health care professionals, will find themselves confronted with people from a great variety of cultural backgrounds and experiences. Students will do well to gain an awareness of, and respect and understanding for, issues confronting other cultures.

Postsecondary Training

A high school diploma or equivalent is a requirement for anyone interested in entering this field. After high school, most students will find it necessary to attend a two-year program and earn an associate's degree in radiology before employment. These programs are offered at community colleges, vocational and technical training schools, or in the military.

David, for example, began his career in the army. "Actually, I applied for the physical therapy program, but that was filled. So I went into radiography. It was a pretty extensive course, with twenty weeks in the classroom, and twenty-three weeks doing clinical practice. I was sent to a lot of different hospitals around the country for that part." After he left the army, David applied for his job in the cardiology department. "I was taught everything I needed to know about cardiac catheterization, as well as EKG monitoring, here at the hospital. The training program here usually lasts from three to six months, depending on how quickly you pick it up, and how much experience you've already had."

Kelly Yu received her associate's degree in radiology. "Then I was lucky enough to get into the Yale School of Medicine for a year to specialize in MRI."

Most radiology technicians receive training through a program accredited by the American Medical Association's Committee on Allied Health Education and Accreditation (CAHEA). Many of these programs are available at hospitals and clinics. They include classroom work, laboratory training, and clinical experience. Students can expect to study such areas as human physiology, medical terminology, radiation physics and protection, diagnostic imaging techniques and pathology, computer science, quality assurance, medical ethics and law, and patient care.

In all cases, special procedures technicians must complete additional training, usually offered through a hospital, medical center, college, or vocational or technical training school, in their specialty area.

certification or licensing

Graduates of accredited programs are eligible to take the four-hour certification examination offered by the American Registry of Radiologic Technologists (ARRT). In addition, recent federal legislation has made licensing for radiologic technicians a requirement. This requirement is usually satisfied by successfully receiving ARRT certification. Certification requirements and opportunities vary by state for the individual special procedures. However, where certification is available, technicians are strongly advised to complete those requirements. This will enhance your chances of finding employment.

internships and volunteerships

Any student interested in entering the health care field can begin his or her involvement while still in high school. Most hospitals have volunteer programs that will allow you to explore the hospital environment and gain valuable insight

Advancement Possibilities

Radiologic equipment specialists test, repair, calibrate, and assist in the installation of radiological and related equipment used in medical diagnosis or therapy. They apply their technical knowledge of computers test equipment, measuring instruments, hand tools, and power tools to a variety of electronic, radiological, and mechanical systems,

Chief radiologic technologists direct and coordinate activities of radiology or diagnostic imaging departments in hospitals or other medical facilities.

Radiologists diagnose and treat diseases of the human body using X ray and radioactive substances.

Radiology administrators plan, direct, and coordinate administrative activities of radiology departments of hospital medical centers.

into medicine and patient care. Many nursing homes, mental health centers, and other treatment facilities have need for dedicated volunteers to assist with patients. High school students may also be able to find part-time work in one of the lower-skilled medical fields, for example as a nurse assistant or as an orderly, or in other parts of the hospital, health clinic, or health care center, such as administration. Because careers in health care can be as stressful as they are rewarding, students considering a future in this area are advised to consider whether they are right for the field, and whether the field is right for them. Students can locate volunteer and employment opportunities by consulting with their high school guidance counselor, contacting local hospitals and health care facilities, or by searching job ads and other employment services.

who will hire me?

Special procedures technologists are employed in a variety of health care settings. Hospitals are the most likely source for employment, especially for techniques such as CT and MRI scanning, which require extremely costly equipment. Health maintenance organizations and health care clinics also need personnel trained to carry out the variety of testing procedures needed for medical care. There are also a great number of diagnostic imaging centers, often associated with hospitals, that perform a battery of special imaging procedures. Also, the United States government employs imaging personnel, most usually through the Department of Veterans Affairs or as members of the armed forces.

where can I go from here?

Advancement in special procedures fields is generally limited, as these specialties already represent advanced areas of radiology. With experience, however, a special procedures technician may advance to greater responsibilities and to supervisory positions. He or she may also choose to enter other areas of health care. For others, like David, special imaging procedures is a valuable bridge to becoming a doctor. David, in fact, credits his decision to pursue a medical career to his work as a cardiac catheterization technician. "It's prompted me to further my education. Right now I'm a freshman in the pre-medical program at the University of Houston."

Special procedures technologists will find demand for their skills throughout the country. Travel to other countries is also a possibility, as some countries, including Great Britain, South Africa, and Canada, recognize U.S. certification.

what are the salary ranges?

Salaries for the different branches of special imaging procedures vary by type of procedure, geographic location, type of employer, and experience level. Radiologic technologists in general averaged $566 per week, according to U.S. Department of Labor statistics for 1995. Nevertheless, the range can be wide. CT technicians in New Hampshire, for example, could be paid as little as $11.22 per hour, or as high as $20 an hour, while in Oregon, a cardiology technologist may receive an hourly wage in the range between $10.04 per hour to $18.89 per hour. The range of salaries for special procedures technologists spans from as little as $13,000 per year to as much as $30,000 per year.

what is the job outlook?

The outlook for employment in the special imaging procedures fields is considered to be excellent. Heart disease and cancer continue to be among the primary health concerns in the U.S. population, and there will continue to be a high demand for skilled technologists to assist in the diagnosis, prevention, and treatment of these and many other conditions. Also, because these procedures can reduce or even eliminate the need for riskier and costlier surgical interventions, their use can be expected to become more and more predominant in the health care industry. Health insurance companies, especially malpractice insurance underwriters, will also require more and more testing in order to limit physician and hospital liability.

As these procedures continue to gain in popularity and availability, and as new technologies become available, the demand for skilled technicians to carry out these procedures will continue to grow.

how do I learn more?

professional organizations

Following are organizations that provide information on special procedures technician careers, accredited schools and scholarships, and possible employers.

American Society of Cardiovascular Professionals/Society for Cardiovascular Management
120 Falcon Drive
Fredericksburg, VA 22408
TEL: 800-683-6728

Cardiovascular Credentialing International
4456 Corporation Lane, Suite 120
Virginia Beach, VA 23462
TEL: 804-497-3380

American Medical Technologists
710 Higgins Road
Park Ridge, IL 60068
TEL: 847-823-5169

American Registry of Radiologic Technologists (ARRT)
1255 Northland Drive
St. Paul, MN 55120
TEL: 612-687-0048
WEBSITE: http://www.arrt.org

American Registry of Clinical Radiography Technologists
710 Higgins Road
Park Ridge, IL 60068
TEL: 847-318-9050

Commission on Accreditation of Allied Health Education Programs
American Medical Association
515 North Dearborn Street, Suite 7530
Chicago, IL 60610
TEL: 312-464-4636

bibliography

Following is a sampling of materials relating to the professional concerns and development of special procedures technicians.

Books

Brant, William E., and Clyde A. Helms, editors. *Fundamentals of Diagnostic Radiology.* Baltimore, MD: Williams & Wilkins, 1994.

Daffner, Richard H. *Clinical Radiology.* Baltimore, MD: Williams & Wilkins, 1993.

Juhl, John H., and Andrew B. Crummy, editors. *Paul and Juhl's Essentials of Radiologic Imaging,* 6th edition. Philadelphia, PA: J.B. Lippincott, 1993.

Kreel, Louis, and Anna Thornton. *Outline of Medical Imaging.* 2 volumes. Boston, MA: Butterworth-Heinemann, 1992.

Mettler, Fred A., Jr., and Milton J. Guiberteau. *Essentials of Nuclear Medicine Imaging,* 3rd edition. Philadelphia, PA: W.B. Saunders Co., 1991.

Periodicals

Catheterization & Cardiovascular Diagnosis. Bimonthly. Wiley, 605 Third Avenue, New York, NY 10158, 212-850-6000.

Diagnostic Imaging. Monthly. Miller Freeman, Inc., 1515 Broadway, New York, NY 10036, 212-869-1300.

Diagnostic Imaging International. 7 per year. Miller Freeman Publications, 600 Harrison Street, San Francisco, CA 94107, 415-905-2200.

Diagnostic Imaging Scan. Biweekly. Discusses the business aspects of medical imaging. Miller Freeman, Inc., 1515 Broadway, New York, NY 10036, 212-869-1300.

Diagnostic Quarterly. Covers the diagnostic industry. Scientific Newsletters, RD 4, Box 7, Stapleton Court, Middletown, NY 10940, 914-355-9144.

Magnetic Resonance Imaging. Bimonthly. Technical articles about the development and use of MRIs. Pergamon Press, Inc., 660 White Plains Road, Tarrytown, NY 10591, 914-524-9200.

Magnetic Resonance Review. Quarterly. Reviews magnetic resonance literature. Gordon and Breach Science Publishers, 270 Eighth Avenue, New York, NY 10011, 212-206-8900.

Radiology and Imaging Letter. Semimonthly. Newsletter which includes radiation therapy and nuclear medicine topics. Radiology Letter, Quest Publishing Co., 1351 Titan Way, Brea, CA 92621, 714-738-6400.

sports physician

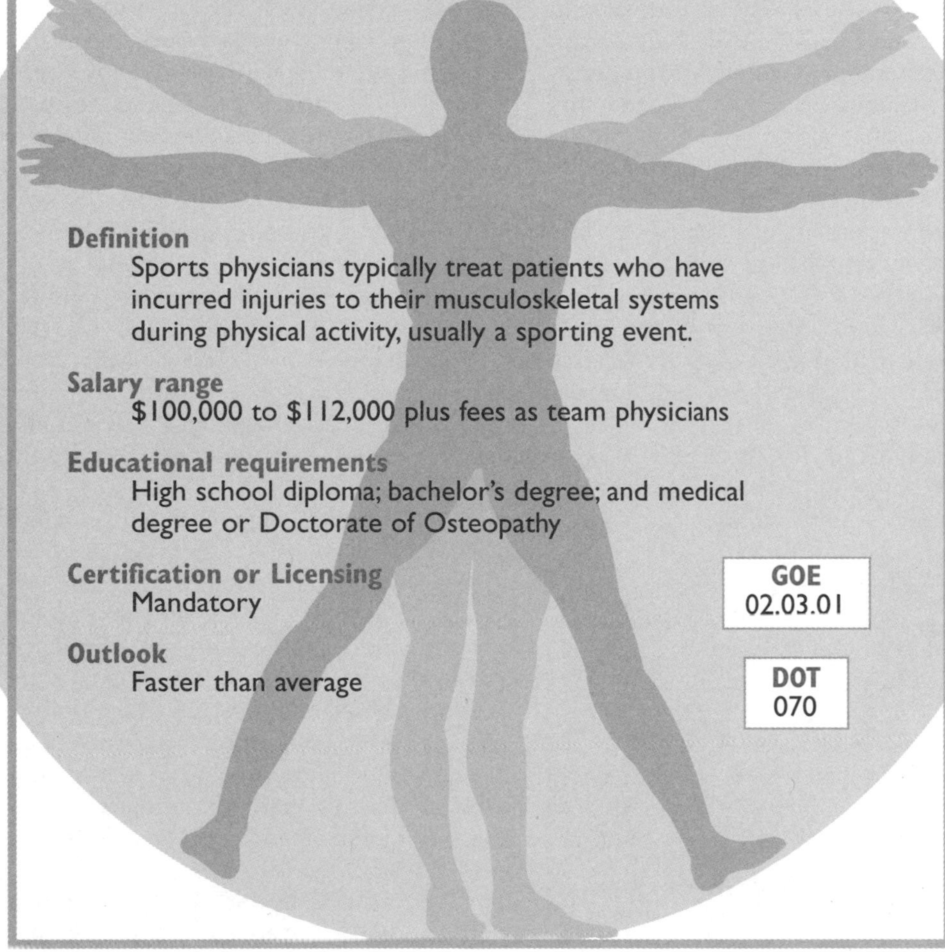

Definition
Sports physicians typically treat patients who have incurred injuries to their musculoskeletal systems during physical activity, usually a sporting event.

Salary range
$100,000 to $112,000 plus fees as team physicians

Educational requirements
High school diploma; bachelor's degree; and medical degree or Doctorate of Osteopathy

Certification or Licensing
Mandatory

Outlook
Faster than average

GOE
02.03.01

DOT
070

High School Subjects

Anatomy
Biology
Chemistry
Communications
Health

Personal Interests

Athletics
Coaching/teaching
Helping people

The injury hasn't completely healed yet. If the athlete returns to the field it might mean being in danger of further and more serious injury. But, if he doesn't play, the chances of the team winning aren't very good. This could mean the difference between a winning or losing season, advancement or elimination in post-season play, or earning or being passed by for an athletic scholarship. There is pressure from the coach, pressure from the athlete, and even pressure from the athlete's family to let him play. Sports physicians cannot let those pressures affect their decisions. In the end the athlete does not play. The team may lose the game, but the athlete may have won a healthy future.

what does a sports physician do?

The term *sports physician* refers to doctors who treat patients suffering from injuries to their musculoskeletal systems due to some form of physical activity, usually a sporting event. These injuries include broken bones, pulled or strained muscles, torn ligaments, and sprains. The majority of sport physicians are either general practitioners or orthopedic surgeons. The spectrum of clients they treat can range from professional athletes making millions of dollars a year to the weekend warrior who overdid it during a Saturday afternoon tennis game. Also, many general practitioners and orthopedic surgeons work as team physicians in addition to their duties in private practice.

For example, Dr. Rick Wilkerson, D.O., an orthopedic surgeon in Spencer, Iowa, treats patients with sports injuries, as well as patients in need of joint reconstructions or general orthopedic care. In addition to his work as an orthopedic surgeon, Dr. Wilkerson is the team physician and surgeon for Buena Vista University, at Storm Lake, Iowa. He is also responsible for the sports medicine care of nineteen area high school sports teams.

Team physicians are typically responsible for the health and well-being of athletes from pre-season training to post-season play. They develop and implement preventative programs that help athletes avoid injuries. Also, they develop specific rehabilitation programs that help injured athletes recover as quickly and as safely as possible. One of the most serious responsibilities of sports physicians is ensuring that athletes have completely recovered from their injuries before they return to the field.

Sports physicians often conduct pre-sports physicals of athletes. During the physicals, doctors learn the athletes' medical history as well as determine their fitness to participate in athletics.

Often, certified athletic trainers conduct performance testing that evaluates the speed, strength, and flexibility of athletes. The test results are used by both the athletes and the coaches to recognize the athletes' strengths and weaknesses. Conditioning programs are developed based on the results of the testing. The goal of conditioning programs is to increase the athletes' strength and endurance while minimizing their risk of injury. A general conditioning plan is also created for the entire team.

When an athlete does become injured, sports physicians conduct clinical examinations of the injury to determine the degree of damage. Orthopedic surgeons can use several different diagnostic tools to evaluate their patients' status. During a procedure called arthrography, physicians inject a dye into the injured joint. Then an X ray is taken of the joint that reveals the exact site and extent of the injury. During a procedure called arthroscopy, orthopedic surgeons insert a fiber-optic device, that acts as a video camera, into the injured area. The inside of the injured joint then appears on a monitor for the surgeon to evaluate. In some cases arthroscopy can also be used as a surgical procedure.

After athletes have become injured, sports physicians are responsible for developing and overseeing their rehabilitation program. The goal of the rehabilitation program is to return athletes to their normal performance level as quickly and as safely as possible.

lingo to learn

Arthrography is a diagnostic tool in which the physician injects a dye into an injured joint which then reveals in an X ray the exact site and extent of the injury.

Arthroplasty is an operation used to treat ligament injuries around joints. It can also be used to create new joints from plastic or metal materials.

Arthroscopy can be used as a diagnostic or surgical tool. As a diagnostic tool a tiny camera is inserted into the injured area to reveal the extent of the damage. As a surgical tool it is used to remove torn cartilage or bone fragments from an injured joint.

Computerized Tomography (CT) is a computerized diagnostic tool that combines X-ray images of the injured joint to create a detailed view of the injured area.

Magnetic Resonance Imaging (MRI) is a computerized diagnostic tool that measures the effects of a magnetic field on an injured area to determine the status of the injury.

The rehabilitation program may include a combination of surgery, physical therapy, and rest. Surgical procedures include arthroplasty. This is an operation often used to treat ligament injuries around the joint. In some cases during arthroplasty, artificial joints made of metal or plastic are fitted to replace damaged joints. As a surgical treatment, arthroscopy is used to remove torn cartilage or bone fragments from an injured joint.

The field of sports medicine is relatively new and research is constantly being conducted to discover better and more effective ways of preventing and treating injuries. The new discoveries help advance rehabilitation programs. As Dr. Wilkerson explains, "Over the years we have developed rehabilitation programs between myself and the physical therapists. These programs are continually being modified as new information becomes available in clinical and research studies in the area of sports medicine."

what is it like to be a sports physician?

Unlike most other medical specialties, sports physicians generally treat healthy people. They work with active people who have incurred an injury and may be in a great deal of pain, but usually are not suffering from a chronic or long lasting illness. There are tragic cases of athletes becoming permanently disabled due to a sports injury. However, there is a great deal of optimism in the field of sports medicine, mainly because the vast majority of patients are expected to recover completely.

For many sports physicians, treating sports-related injuries is just part of their job. Only half of Dr. Wilkerson's time is devoted to patients who have been injured during a sporting event. The other half of his time is concentrated on joint reconstructions or general orthopedics. Furthermore, the cases Dr. Wilkerson treats at the Sports Medicine Northwest Clinic, in Spencer, Iowa, are equally divided between sports-related injuries and general orthopedics.

Working in small towns, sports physicians may be responsible for the well-being of athletes from many different high schools. Team physicians may also be hired by large college athletic departments or professional athletic organizations and may be responsible for the medical care of the members of only one team.

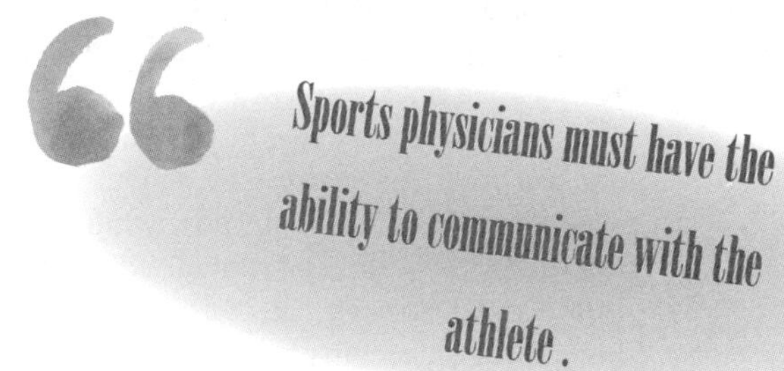

The actual responsibilities of team physicians vary. Some team physicians may be required to be on call or attend every game both at home and on the road. They can be hired to work on staff as team physicians or be hired as consultants. Many team physicians have staffs that include physical therapists and certified athletic trainers. Team physicians have to be aware of staff activities to ensure that athletes are being well-served.

One of the foremost responsibilities of sports physicians is the determination of athletes' eligibility to return to athletic events after they have recovered from an injury. If athletes return before they have fully recovered they are extremely vulnerable to injuring themselves again. As Dr. Wilkerson explains, "The most difficult portion of this career is basically the occasional conflict between trying to care for the patient's well-being, while at the same time being pressured by the athlete, coach, and possibly family, to get them back to playing sports at the earliest time possible."

The career of sports physicians can be incredibly exciting. They often get the opportunity to travel across the country. They may also treat professional athletes who are known throughout the world. Unfortunately, some athletes may not recover fully from an injury and that may mean they never play again. And often, it is sports physicians who have to tell the athletes that they have sustained a career-ending injury.

have I got what it takes to be a sports physician?

Successful sports physicians will have strong communication skills, an even temperament, good people skills, and a high level of dedication to their field. They need to understand the role of sports in society.

Strong communication skills are a necessity because physicians must be able to clearly express themselves to their staff, their patients, and coaches. For example, to effectively treat an athlete, trainers must know what parameters the physician has determined to be most important. Furthermore, it is very important that sports physicians be able to speak to athletes so they understand why they should not play. As Dr. Wilkerson explains, "[Sports physicians must have] the ability to communicate with the athlete and convey the physician's interest in returning them to the sport at the earliest and safest time."

Most successful sports physicians need to have an even temperament and the ability to interact easily with many different people. Throughout their careers, sports physicians coordinate projects with different members of their staff, different members of coaching staffs, and with athletes that may change every year. Sports physicians have to be able to take this diverse group of people and create a cohesive whole that acts as a support system for the athletes.

The field of sports medicine demands a high level of dedication. In addition to the time dedicated to their private practice, some sports physicians are required to put in additional time on the field and in the training room. Some sports physicians are required to travel with the team from pre-season to the playoffs. Furthermore, because research is constantly being conducted in the field, sports physicians must always be aware of new developments so they can best treat their patients.

Finally, effective sports physicians should have a clear understanding of the role of sports in today's popular culture. Sports physicians need to realize the objectives of the coaching staff, as well as the pressures on the injured athlete, so they can provide the best treatment.

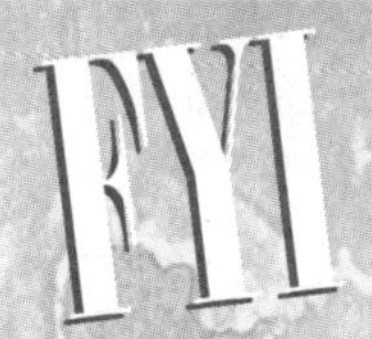

Sportsmed Profile

In 1960, as the team physician for the New York Titans (later the Jets), Dr. James A. Nicholas developed a keen interest in treating and preventing sports-related injuries. In 1973 he founded the Institute of Sports Medicine and Athletic Trauma at Lenox Hill Hospital, New York City. It was the world's first hospital-based sports medicine institute. Since then, Dr. Nicholas has gone on to work as a team physician for seven other professional teams and has worked with professional dancers. He also was a founding member of several sports medicine societies, including the Orthopedic Society for Sports Medicine.

In 1986 Lenox Hill Hospital changed the name of the Institute to the Nicholas Institute of Sports Medicine and Athletic Trauma. This institute has become a renowned center for the study of the treatment and prevention of sports-related injuries.

how do I become a sports physician?

education

High School

Acceptance into medical school is extremely competitive and it is never to early for students to begin preparing themselves. For that reason, high school students interested in entering the field of sports medicine should take as many science classes as possible. These would include biology, chemistry, and anatomy. It would be even more beneficial for students to take these classes at an advanced level, if possible.

If there are any communication classes available, students should consider taking them. Good communication skills will help throughout the students' academic and professional careers. Furthermore, good communication skills are a necessity to help physicians successfully interact with their staff, their patients, and with coaches.

While in high school, interested students should contact their athletic department to discuss the possibility of assisting the department's athletic trainers. If the high school has a team physician, the department may be able to arrange for an interview.

Postsecondary Training

Sports physicians must have a medical degree. Acceptance into medical schools is based on many things. Though an undergraduate degree is a requirement, not all medical schools require the applicant to have earned an undergraduate degree in premedical studies.

In fact, Dr. Wilkerson earned a degree in International Relations before beginning his medical career. Some people believe that a well-rounded, liberal undergraduate education is beneficial to a doctor. They believe that physicians with a fuller educational experience interact more effectively with their patients. Furthermore, it is not surprising for medical students to have worked a few years before deciding to enter medical school.

Many students wishing to pursue medicine do, in fact, follow a premed program for undergraduate studies. Typically, these programs require many courses in the sciences, including anatomy, biology, chemistry, and physiology. All medical schools in the country require applicants to take the Medical College Admissions Test (MCAT). Students usually take this exam during their third year of college. MCAT results are an important tool for medical schools in determining acceptance into a program. Admission to medical school is highly competitive and a superior grade point average is a must.

Medical students spend their first two years immersed in science classes. Their course work may include classes in anatomy, biochemistry, physiology, pharmacology, and microbiology. For the next two years medical students work in clinical environments, treating patients and developing their diagnostic skills.

After medical school, doctors will spend at least one year in an internship program. This will be followed by several years in a residency program, training in their specialty. In the case of a sports physician, this will usually mean a specialty in orthopedics or general practice.

To be a successful sports physician, you should

- Have the ability to communicate effectively with a variety of people
- Be a good listener
- Have an even temperament
- Be an effective motivator
- Enjoy working with athletes
- Be able to focus on patient's medical needs

scholarships and grants

Scholarships and grants are often available from individual institutions, state agencies, and special-interest organizations. The book Dollars for College: Medicine, Dentistry, and Related Fields by Ferguson Publishing is an excellent source for this information. Many students finance their medical education through the Armed Forces Health Professions Scholarship Program. Each branch of the military participates in this program, paying students' tuitions in exchange for military service. Contact your local recruiting office for more information on this program. The National Health Service Corps Scholarship Program also provides money for students in return for service. Another source for financial aid, scholarship, and grant information is the Association of American Medical Colleges. Remember to request information early for eligibility, application requirements, and deadlines.

Association of American Medical Colleges
2450 N Street, NW
Washington, DC 20037
TEL: 202-828-0400
WEBSITE: http://www.aamc.org
Specific information on financial aid programs can be found at:
WEBSITE: http://www.aamc.org/stuapps/finaid

Ferguson Publishing Company
200 West Madison, Suite 300
Chicago, IL 60606
TEL: 312-580-5480

National Health Services Corps Scholarship Program
U.S. Public Health Service
1010 Wayne Avenue, Suite 240
Silver Spring, MD 20910
TEL: 800-638-0824

certification or licensing

After completion of their residency programs, physicians apply for certification in their particular specialty. There are over twenty specialty boards that certify candidates based on their qualifications. The American Board of Family Practice will only consider certifying candidates who have three years of experience in postgraduate training. To become board certified by the American Board of Orthopedic Surgery, applicants must have completed five years of post-graduate training, three years of which must be in the area of orthopedic surgery.

To become licensed, sports physicians must pass the state board examination of the state in which they plan to work. A doctor cannot practice medicine without a license.

Continuing education is an important part of a sports physicians career. As Dr. Wilkerson explains, "the area of Sports Medicine is a fairly new area of medicine and new information regarding rehabilitation, training techniques, and injury prevention are continually being published."

The American College of Sports Medicine offers several opportunities for continuing education. Their annual meeting provides one such opportunity. It is a four-day event during which more than 1000 case studies and workshops are presented.

internships and volunteerships

High school students interested in gaining practical experience in the area of sports medicine should speak to the physical education teachers at their schools. They will be able to direct the student to either the athletic trainer or team physician. It may be possible for the student to volunteer to work as an assistant. Furthermore, the team physician or athletic trainer may be able to answer any questions the student may have regarding the field.

Another option is to contact a local hospital to someone in the volunteer department. Most hospitals have excellent volunteer programs and in some instances volunteers can work in the departments they are most interested in, including orthopedics or rehabilitation.

who will hire me?

After receiving certification and licensing, either as general practitioners or as orthopedic surgeons, most sports physicians begin to work in private practice. Although some recently licensed physicians open their own private practices, many doctors join partnerships with other physicians. This provides an opportunity to share the expenses of opening a new medical practice. Once physicians have developed a well-respected reputation and have successfully treated many patients, they may decide to open an office of their own.

To begin working as team physicians, doctors may contact their local school board, or the athletic department of local high schools and colleges to describe their qualifications and to determine if there are any employment opportunities. There are several thousand high schools, colleges, and universities across the United States. Most have athletic departments. Often team physicians can work for several high schools on a part-time basis. At any level, sports physicians may be employed as staff members, or on a consultative basis.

Sports physicians may also seek employment at sports medicine clinics, which are located throughout the country. Work at these clinics may be part-time or full-time. Established sports physicians may open a clinic themselves or in partnership with other sports medicine professionals.

Competition for positions with professional sports organizations is intense. Professional sports teams usually hire well-respected experts in their field with several years of experience. The salaries of professional athletes often run into the millions and organizations must ensure that these athletes have the best medical care and training that money can buy.

Finally, because research is so important, many sports physicians are hired by universities to conduct research and testing to develop new and better ways of preventing and treating athletic injuries. In addition, sports physicians at universities may also teach.

where can I go from here?

For sports physicians, like most doctors, advancement in their field consists of successfully treating their patients and building a highly respected reputation. Usually, sports physicians working as team doctors begin their career working for high schools and then move up to the college level. Professional athletic organizations and big-time college pro-

in-depth

Key's Miraculous Return

In July, 1995, New York Yankee pitcher Jimmy Key underwent surgery to repair a completely torn rotator cuff in his left shoulder. Though rotator cuff injuries are not uncommon for major league pitchers, Key's prognosis was grim. A complete return from a total tear had never been done before.

Advances in sports medicine allowed Key's surgeon, Dr. James Andrews, to use state of-the-art materials to create a strong repair that could withstand an aggressive therapy program. Key returned to pitching in the spring of 1996, a testament to his drive and the capabilities of his surgeon and physical therapist.

His problems, however, were far from over. He had a slow start in the 1996 season and was sent down to the minors to "work out the kinks." Many thought his career was over. Undaunted, Key and his rehabilitation crew made a spectacular comeback. He returned to the Yankees and finished the season with an 11-6 record. The Yankees went to the World Series and in game six, what would be the deciding contest, Key pitched five and a third innings as the Yankees defeated the Braves with Key getting the win.

grams usually only employ physicians who are highly regarded in their field and have many years of experience.

what are the salary ranges?

According to the American Medical Association, general practitioners and family practice physicians earn an annual net income of about $112,000. This does not include the fees paid to them by various athletic organizations for which they act as team physicians. These fees are determined on a case-by-case basis and can be affected by many factors including the level of athletic organization (high school, college or professional), their staff, and their scope of responsibilities. Typically the salary of team physicians is extremely low compared to their private practice income.

what is the job outlook?

The job outlook for sports physicians is very good. First of all, there will always be a demand for competent physicians who can treat injuries associated with athletic activity. It is the nature of competition that athletes are constantly trying to do better than their competitors. They try to push themselves to the limit to jump a little higher or run a little faster than their competition. The associated strain means there will always be a risk of injury.

Furthermore, the demand for sports physicians is increasing as professional organizations and collegiate athletic departments realize that sports physicians and that research in the area of sports medicine is helping athletes avoid injuries. It's common sense that a healthy athlete is more productive than an injured one and so more and more athletic organizations are utilizing sports physicians to prevent injuries before they happen.

how do I learn more?

professional organizations

Following are organizations that provide information on sports physicians and sports medicine.

American College of Sports Medicine
401 West Michigan Street
Indianapolis, IN 46202
TEL: 317/637-9200
WEBSITE: http://www.acsm.org

American Orthopaedic Society for Sports Medicine
6300 N. River Road
Suite 200
Rosemont, IL 60018
TEL: 847/292-4900
WEBSITE: http://www.sportsmed.org

bibliography

Following is a sampling of materials relating to the professional concerns and development of sports physicians.

Books

Edelson, Edward. *Sports Medicine*. New York, NY: Chelsea House, 1988.

Harries, Mark, Clyde Williams, William D. Stanish, and Lyle J. Micheli. *Oxford Textbook of Sports Medicine*. New York, NY: Oxford University Press, 1996.

Heinzmann, William R. *Opportunities in Sports Medicine Careers*. Lincolnwood, IL: VGM Career Horizons, 1995.

Kent, Michael, editor. *The Oxford Dictionary of Sports Science and Medicine*. New York, NY: Oxford University Press, 1996.

McLatchie, G., M. Harries, C. Williams, and J. King. *ABC of Sports Medicine*. Philadelphia, PA: American College of Physicians, 1995.

Sherry, Eugene, and Des J. Bokor, editors. *Sports Medicine: Common Problems and Practical Management.* New York, NY: Oxford University Press, 1997.

Periodicals

Journal of Orthopaedic and Sports Physical Therapy. Monthly. Clinical developments in sports medicine for practicing physical therapists, athletic trainers, and orthopedic surgeons. American Physical Therapy Association, Williams & Wilkins, 428 E. Preston Street, Baltimore, MD 21202, 410-528-4000, 800-638-6423.

Journal of Sport Rehabilitation. Quarterly. Investigates the process of rehabilitation of sport and exercise injuries regardless of age, gender, athletic ability, level of fitness, or health status. Human Kinetics Publishers, Inc., Box 5076, Champaign, IL 61825, 217-351-2674.

Medicine and Science in Sports and Exercise. Monthly. Research in sports medicine topics for exercise physiologists, physiatrists, physical therapists, and athletic trainers. American College of Sports Medicine, Box 1440, Indianapolis, IN 46206, 317-637-9200.

The Physician and Sportsmedicine. Monthly. A peer-reviewed journal on medical aspects of sports, exercise, and fitness. McGraw-Hill, 1221 Avenue of the Americas, New York, NY 10020, 212-512-2000.

Sports Medicine Digest. Monthly. Quest Publishing Co., Inc., 1351 Titan Way, Brea, CA 92621, 714-738-6400.

surgical technologist

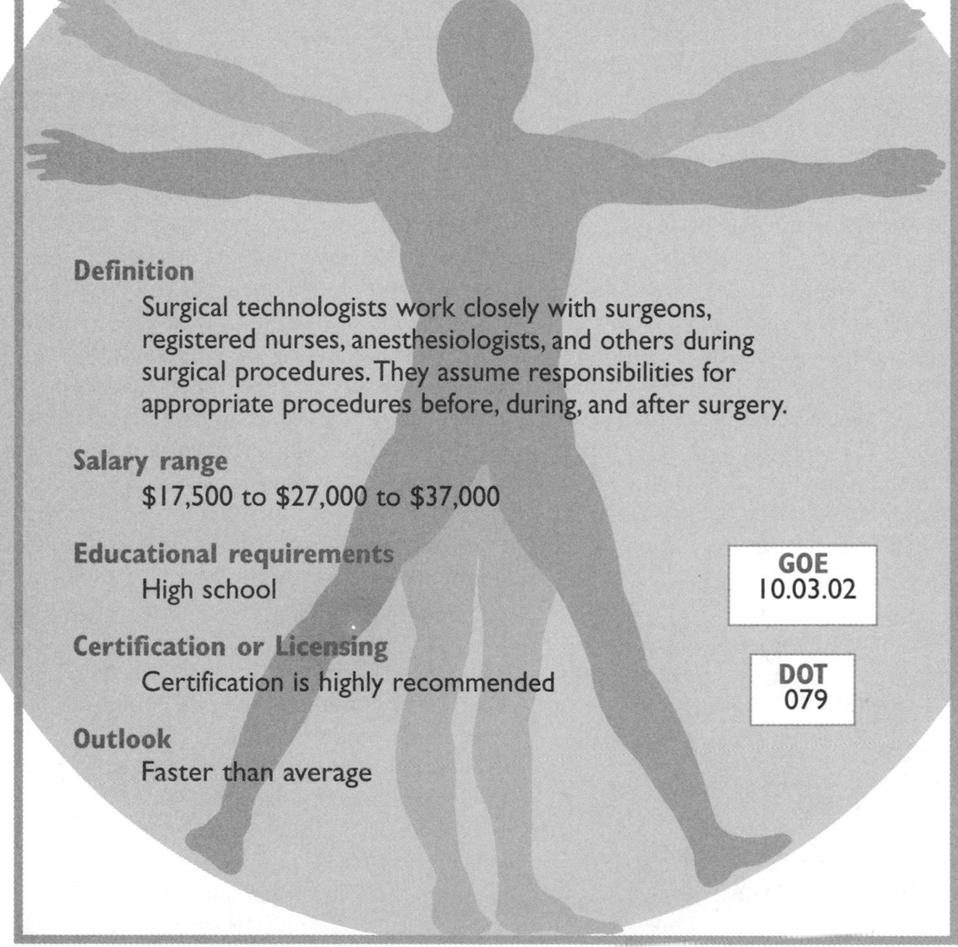

Definition

Surgical technologists work closely with surgeons, registered nurses, anesthesiologists, and others during surgical procedures. They assume responsibilities for appropriate procedures before, during, and after surgery.

Salary range

$17,500 to $27,000 to $37,000

Educational requirements

High school

Certification or Licensing

Certification is highly recommended

Outlook

Faster than average

GOE
10.03.02

DOT
079

High School Subjects

Anatomy
Biology
Physiology

Personal Interests

Helping people
Medicine
Science labs

Against a background of static, the words punch out a staccato beat: "Stab wound. O.R. Stat." The former quiet of the operating room lounge is instantly transformed. The three people who had been relaxing on a break scramble to their feet and hustle into action. John Houck, a surgical technologist, is already halfway down the hall to meet the patient coming in from the emergency room.

In an emergency like this, there is no time to set up for surgery. Houck has barely finished scrubbing when the patient, a woman in her mid-thirties, is wheeled into the operating room. "Boyfriend or someone really worked her over," the orderly says. "Got her in the chest and stomach." The woman is pale and unconscious. Her shirt and jeans have already been cut away in preparation for surgery and replaced by a surgical gown and drape.

Within minutes, a nurse, anesthesiologist, and surgeon arrive. Houck has to be doubly efficient in emergencies, not having had the time to organize the instruments, sutures, or sponges. He helps the other members of the surgical team to scrub and gown up. Surgery soon begins.

Houck deftly hands instruments to the surgeon as needed, counting the sponges, needles, and sutures used by the surgeon. He will help with the suturing, or stitching, at the close of the surgery. Once the initial frenzy is over, the surgery settles into a familiar rhythm, with everyone on the surgical team working together to ensure the survival of the patient on the table.

"I think we've got her," the surgeon says finally. Houck helps with the suturing, or stitching, to close the incision made by the surgery. "She's going to hurt for a while, but she'll make it."

An orderly comes to wheel the woman to the recovery room. The members of the surgical team pull off their gloves and pull down their masks, heading out to the locker room to change. Houck collects the instruments that need sterilizing, throws the disposables away, and begins prepping the operating room for the next surgery.

lingo to learn

Drape Sterile cloth used to surround and isolate the actual site or location of the operation on the patient's body.

Forceps Instrument Very similar in appearance to cooking tongs, used by surgeons to hold back skin or other soft tissue.

Scalpel A thin bladed knife that is used as a surgical tool.

Scrubbing Literally, the physical cleaning of the hands, wrists, and forearms of the surgeon and each member of the surgical staff. Scrubbing is performed prior to all surgeries in order to kill germs and harmful bacteria.

Sterilize A procedure in which living microorganisms are removed from an area or instrument.

Suture (s) The stitches used to close a wound or surgical incision.

what does a surgical technologist do?

Surgical technologists are an integral part of the surgery team, providing assistance to make operations run as smoothly as possible.

The role of a surgical technologist begins before the patient arrives in surgery and continues through surgery and after surgery. The operating room must be set up for the kind of surgery that will be performed. The tasks required range from organizing drapes and equipment to placing the necessary sterilized instruments on a sterilized tray and making sure nothing unsterilized touches them. The technologist scrubs and puts on a gown, cap, mask, gloves, and shoe covers, then helps the nurses and surgeons get gloved and gowned after they scrub. The most important role of the surgical technologist is creating and maintaining what is known as the sterile field around the operating table. The technologist is responsible for seeing that aseptic, or sterile, conditions and procedures are followed from beginning to end. "It could be so easy for a patient to get infected if someone's not monitoring the room," Houck says.

Preoperative duties include assembling, adjusting, and checking nonsterile equipment to ensure that it is in proper working order. Typically, surgical technologists operate sterilizers, lights, suction machines, electrosurgical units, and diagnostic equipment. Bob Caruthers, a surgical technologist and instructor, adds preparing medications to the list of the technologist's duties. "Depending on the surgery, the surgical technologist works with the nurse to prepare medications that will be administered within the sterile field." He elaborates. "The anesthesiologist, for example, isn't working in the sterile field, so the surgical technologist wouldn't prepare those medications. But if the medication will be handled by a member of the sterile team, and, say, administered into the wound, then the technologist would be the one to prepare it."

Once patients arrive in the operating room suite, the surgical technologist may assist in preparing them for surgery by checking charts and reading vital signs. Part of their training includes learning how to properly position the patient on the operating table, how to connect or assist other surgical personnel in connecting surgical equipment or monitoring devices, and how to prepare the incision site by cleaning the skin with an antiseptic solution and isolating the site with surgical drapes.

Once the surgery is underway, the technician pays attention to the needs of the surgeon, handing him or her instruments, sutures, and sponges, and perhaps holding back flaps of skin with forceps. "You are the surgeon's right-hand person," Houck says. "You have to be almost a mindreader. You definitely have to know your procedures."

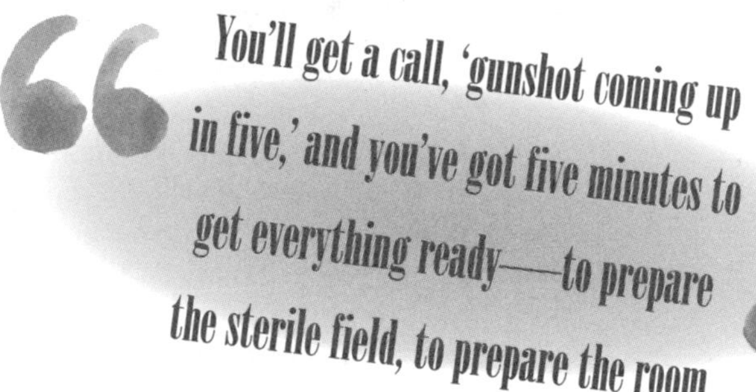

Caruthers agrees. "The job we're preparing students to do is to get to the point where they can predict what the surgeons are going to do before they do it, so they can prepare for it," he explains. "This is a very detailed job," Caruthers adds. Students need to observe everything the surgeon does in a surgery so that they can anticipate the surgeon's requests.

Technologists frequently count the sponges, sutures, and needles used in any given procedure, to make certain the nothing gets left inside a patient. A sponge left inside a patient could infect the patient and possibly lead to the patient's death. If there are specimens to be taken to the laboratory for analysis, it is the technologist who helps prepare, care for, and dispose of these specimens. Technologists help apply dressings to the patient and may be asked to operate sterilizers, lights, or suction machines.

Technologists are responsible for cleaning up after the surgery, including disposing of soiled drapes, disposable instruments and equipment, sterilizing nondisposable instruments and equipment, and restocking the operating room for the next operation.

what is it like to be a surgical technologist?

At most hospitals, surgeries are scheduled in the mornings or early afternoons. The surgical technologist who works the day shift is at the hospital by 7:00 AM, preparing the operating room for the scheduled cases. A morning technologist may have surgeries one after the other through his or her entire shift. "An average day for a surgical technologist," says Bob Caruthers, "means you spend the entire day within the operating suite."

No matter which shift is worked, surgical technologists are trained to work in every type of surgery. "Typically speaking, when you start out you're rotated through all the specialties," Caruthers says. "Trauma centers or smaller hospitals may just want surgical technologists who are generalists. Big hospitals, however, are concerned with efficiency. The most efficient way to process surgeries is to have everyone doing the same thing over and over again, from surgery to surgery. So," he explains, "many hospitals need surgical technologists who are more or less specialists. Most surgical technologists have one to two areas in which they work most of the time."

John Houck has worked as a surgical technologist since 1982. He works the 3:00 to 11:00 PM shift at Illinois Masonic Hospital in Chicago, Illinois. He likes to arrive early for his shift so that he can relax for a few minutes, hear about the morning from his coworkers, and organize himself for the evening. It is rare for there to be a lot of scheduled surgeries on John's shift. His shift involves simply finishing with the scheduled surgeries and then waiting for emergencies to come in. "The day-shift people don't get much emergency action," Houck says. "This shift, we see a lot of trauma cases—stabbings, shootings, accidents. We get at least three unscheduled cases a night, even during the slowest times."

In emergency situations, Houck says, a technologist has to move fast. "You'll get a call, 'gunshot coming up in five,'and you've got five minutes to get everything ready—to prepare the sterile field, to prepare the room. Sometimes you don't even get five minutes." He laughs. "One thing you get good at around here is fast set-up."

"You don't have a lot of awake contact with the patient," he says, "so it's not like you get to know them, but it's rewarding work. It's a good feeling when you hear that someone who was near death made it and is doing well."

have I got what it takes to be a surgical technologist?

"A good surgical technologist will be so familiar with a surgery that he or she will recognize the steps and know what to do next, what the surgeon is going to need. That can be hard when you're staring down into an open chest or brain," Caruthers states. "I tell my students, 'You need the ability to be focused and calm and creative.'" Technologists must be able to focus on their work in spite of the often hectic conditions of surgery, especially in a trauma center where more than one case may be in progress in the same room.

As a result, surgical technologists work under great pressure and tension. Each surgery, even the most routine procedure, carries with it some risk. People who work in this field must be prepared to make split-second decisions and have lightning-fast reactions, all the while remaining calm enough to carry out their jobs. Having nerves of steel doesn't hurt, either. "I used to get adrenaline rushes," says Houck. "And I'll admit, it gets crazy. But now I'm used to the pace. Now it's just part of my job." Not only do surgical technologists need to be able to react quickly and efficiently in high-stress emergency situations, but they also need to realize that flaring tempers are a part of the unique environment. They have to learn not to take anger personally. "This is a place where you need to stand up for yourself," says Houck. "You need to be confident and good at your job. No one has time for someone who doesn't know what they're doing. If you're meek and timid in this business, you get yelled at and walked all over."

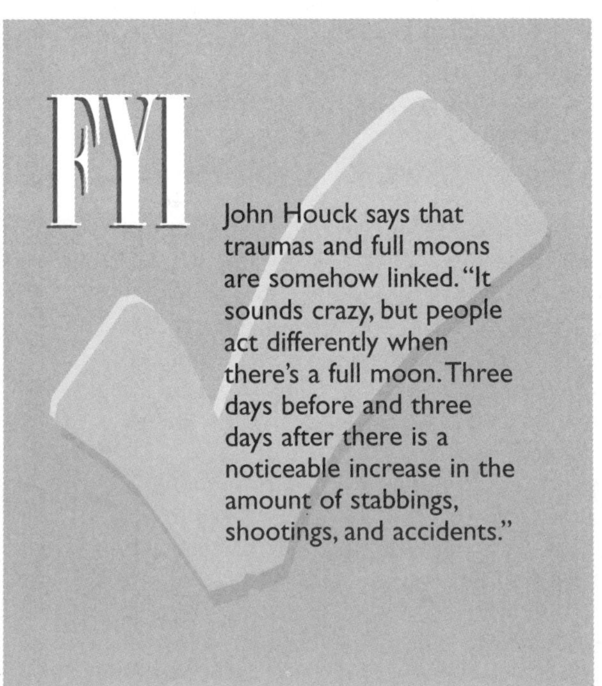

Surgical technologists must pay attention to details, have good organizational skills, and be very attentive during long surgeries, to both the surgeon and the procedure in progress. The intellectual demands are equalled by the physical demands; surgical technologists must stand for long periods of time, often without moving, while they hold a forceps or sponge in place. Good manual dexterity is also essential since surgical technologists are required to handle instruments and equipment with speed and precision. "There is a lot of responsibility here," Houck says. "But I like that there's a lot of variety to the work."

The operating room environment, whether in a hospital or a private clinic or office, is clean, brightly lit, cool, and fairly quiet. Even before managed care, many hospitals found that the most efficient way to handle a number of surgeries is to break them down by type. In these instances, the surgical technologist might specialize in one or two areas, say ophthalmological and cardiovascular surgeries. They might work all day in the operating suite and encounter nothing but these types of surgeries. On the other hand, in trauma centers or in smaller hospitals where there might not be more than one ophthalmological or cardiovascular procedure all day, the surgical technologist might be more of a generalist.

While most technologists work forty-hour weeks, schedules are not always fixed, and technologists may be expected to work different shifts as a part of that work week. Most technologists are expected to be available to work on-call from time to time. "The bottom line," says Caruthers, "if you want a job that is fast-paced, exciting, and allows you to help people—this is it."

how do I become a surgical technologist?

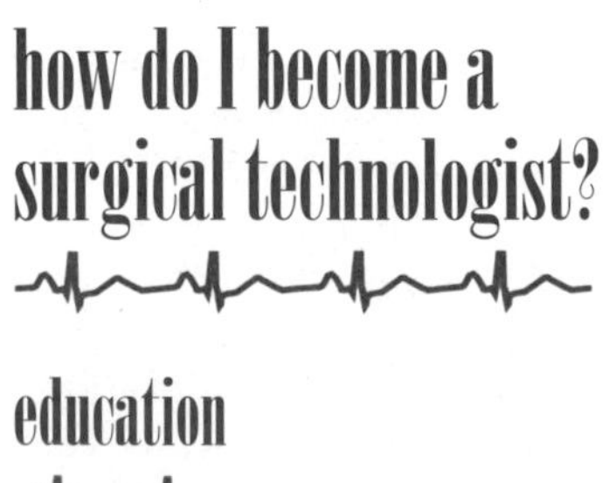

education

When in the army, John Houck decided that work as a surgical technologist would be interesting, and he participated in a training program on the Texas army base where he was stationed. He became certified and worked in the base's hospital. John was a fairly good student in high school. His favorite courses were science courses. According to Caruthers, "You should like science and anatomy if you want to do this job."

To be a successful surgical technologist, you should

- Be a fast learner
- Make decisions quickly
- React calmly and work efficiently in crisis situations
- Remain focused while working on several different tasks

High School

Surgical technologists are required to have a high school diploma or GED to enter a surgical technology program at a hospital or community college. High school courses in the basic sciences and in anatomy and physiology are important.

Postsecondary training

Surgical technologists receive their training in programs offered by community colleges, technical schools, hospitals, and the military. There are more than 130 accredited programs for surgical technology in the United States. "I became a surgical technologist the old-fashioned way," says Caruthers. "I was trained on the job. There weren't programs until later."

Training programs last from nine months to twenty-four months and can lead to a certificate, diploma, or associate's degree. Required courses included anatomy, physiology, pharmacology, microbiology, and medical terminology. During their training, students learn about surgical procedures and how to provide for the safety and care of patients during surgery. They learn how to sterilize instruments to prevent infection and how to handle drugs and equipment.

certification or licensing

Some states require certification, but even in those that do not, it is a good idea to become certified in order to advance in the profession. "Being certified is not the only way to work as a technologist," Houck says, "but it's smart. Employers look on it as a sign of commitment. You put time in to get certified, they think, 'this person is serious about his work.' Employers like that."

Certification is provided by the Liaison Counsel on Certification for the Surgical Technologist and it is national, which means that technologists can work in any state once they are certified. Recertification is required every six years, either in the form of an exam or by keeping up a required number of points by attending a certain number of conferences throughout the year. "Last month I went to a conference where we took gallbladders out of live pigs," Houck says. "It was really interesting. Going to conferences gives you points toward recertification and the conferences are a tax deduction." He laughs. "And it doesn't hurt that they're held in great places. Great warm places in the winter."

who will hire me?

After completing his training, and working as a surgical technologist for several years in the military, John returned home to Chicago, where he had no trouble finding employment. "There are always openings for qualified surgical techs," he says.

Most surgical technologists work in hospitals, and students who go through hospital training programs are often hired by those hospitals after graduation. Community colleges that offer programs have placement centers and work with area hospitals that like to hire technologists trained locally.

Within hospitals, surgical technologists may work in operating rooms, and central supply departments. In the private sector, surgical technologists are employed directly by surgeons instead of by hospitals. They may work in clinics or in the offices of physicians, or dentists. More and more technologists are working in home health care these days and will continue to do so well into the year 2005.

where can I go from here?

Surgical technologists have a broad range of advancement opportunities. A certified surgical technologist and instructor, Bob Caruthers recently accepted a management position at the Association for Surgical Technologists in Boulder, Colorado. He stresses the transitional nature of the profession. "Of the group of techs I worked with just out of school, we're all still in the medical field. One is a dentist, one's a cardiologist, and one's a gastroenterologist. Two others became teachers and paramedics, one became a certified registered nurse anesthetist, and one, a Ph.D." He pauses and smiles. "I'm the Ph.D. But you can see how it's really a transitional job." Caruthers became interested in the ethics of brain-death problems while working the respiratory machine in neurosurgery. He received his master's degree in theological ethics, but his interest in how people think about these ethical questions led him to a doctorate in developmental psychology. "The brain was the common thread," chuckles Caruthers.

"The great thing about this profession," he continues, "is that you really have the ability to advance both horizontally and vertically." Of the horizontal advancements, a surgical technologist can work in central supply or become a specialist in particular surgeries. On the other hand, it is equally possible for a surgical technologist to advance to the position of surgical first assistant by obtaining additional experience, training, and certification, or become a surgeon by gaining admission to medical school and continuing through the additional five years of surgical specialty.

Routinely, advancement begins in the form of salary raises, but once a surgical technologist has acquired some experience, he or she can be employed in a number of diverse areas. "The training we get is really broad," John Houck says. "It's a good thing, because you're able to adapt to different jobs from the start. And once you know what you're doing, there are a lot of possibilities." Among the diverse possibilities open to them are jobs as central service managers, surgery schedulers, and managers of instruments, equipment, or surgical supplies. Assistant operating room administrators order supplies and arrange work schedules. Assistant operating room supervisors direct and coordinate the efforts of surgical technologists in the operating room.

For those who would like to get out of the operating room atmosphere, there are positions available in sales and management with companies that sell medical operating room equipment, instruments, and supplies to hospitals and physicians. Some technologists find that they like to impart their knowledge and experience to others and they become instructors in surgical technology training programs.

Related Jobs

Did you know that there are a number of jobs related to that of surgical technologist? The U.S. Department of Labor classifies surgical technologists under the headings "Child and Adult Care: Patient Care" and "Occupations in Medicine and Health." Related jobs include people who deliver emergency medical attention to accident victims, care for the elderly, and exercise and rehabilitate patients with limited or impaired mobility. These jobs include surgical assistant, first-aid attendant, ambulance attendant, emergency medical attendant, medical assistant, nurse aide, occupational therapy assistant, orderly, orthotic and prosthetic technician, physical therapy aide, and psychiatric technician.

what are the salary ranges?

Surgical technologists are often hourly employees. Based on a recent survey of members by the Association of Surgical Technologists (AST), the average hourly rates range anywhere from a low of $10.18 per hour in Mississippi to a high of $14.51 per hour in Connecticut. Taking into account that the survey included entry-level and experienced technicians, both certified and non-certified, the average salaries for surgical technologists range from $17,500 to $27,000 to $37,000 per year. The highest hourly rate ($15.21 per hour) was reported in Hawaii.

Technologists working on the east and west coasts typically earn more than technologists in other parts of the country. "We don't make enough money in this business," admits Houck. "I think you could ask any surgical technologist and they'd feel the same way. Mechanics earn more than we do and they work on cars. We're dealing with life and death. It doesn't make sense."

Bob Caruthers agrees that the salaries could be higher. He recently became Manager of Pro-in-depth

Who's watching?—The Essentials of Surgical Technology

Has the surgical technologist working on your operation learned all he or she needs to know? As a student studying surgical technology, is your school preparing you for the real world? Who creates the standards and who's watching to make certain the schools are following those standards?

Well, the Essentials are minimum education standards adopted by the four collaborating organizations: the Association of Surgical Technologists (AST), the American College of Surgeons (ACS), the American Hospital Association (AHA), and the American Medical Association (AMA). Together, these four organizations jointly sponsor the Accreditation Review Committee on Education in Surgical Technology (ARC-ST). Each new program is assessed in accordance with the Essentials. Accredited programs in surgical technology are reviewed at least every sixth year to determine whether they remain in substantial compliance. The Essentials and Guidelines are available upon written request from the (ARC-ST).

fessional Development at the Association of Surgical Technologists. An instructor for seven years, he now spends his time promoting the profession, occasionally working to keep up his skills. "I love it," says Caruthers. "If they [hospitals] paid me what I'm making now, I would do craniotomies all day long. All you'd have to do is feed me, I wouldn't even need sleep!"

Technologists start at a base rate, explains Houck. "You get raises every year. Whatever the standard raise rate is." There are always ways to make extra income, though. Most technologists pick up on-call shifts, which means they are available to come in on days when they aren't normally scheduled to work. "You might make $52 for wearing a pager for eight hours," Houck says. "Call is the best money. When you have to go in for emergencies, you make time-and-a-half."

what is the job outlook?

Through 2005, job opportunities for surgical technologists are expected to experience better than average growth for all occupations. Surgical technology is listed as the seventh-fastest growing profession for the 1990s. Competent surgical technologists are in great demand. Population growth, longevity, and more advanced medical procedures have contributed to a growing demand for surgical services and therefore surgical technologists. As long as people continue to need medical assistance and surgery, there will continue to be a need for surgical technologists. While general economic conditions could affect the growth of this field, it is probable that the trend will continue for years to come.

Due to the rising cost of health care, more surgery is being done in hospitals on an outpatient basis. If this continues, there will be a great need for surgical technologists. But if more surgeries are performed in non-hospital settings, demand will drop because fewer technologists are hired full-time in those settings.

Some hospitals are discussing the employment of staff members who will handle a wider range of tasks than surgical technologists are qualified to do. Although this could limit the need for technologists, there are at present a lack of nurses in many hospitals, leaving more tasks available for surgical technologists. The more tasks technologists are allowed to perform, the greater number of technologists needed to perform those tasks.

In large cities, opportunities are especially good because there are more hospitals. Metropolitan areas with the largest number of hospital systems include: Los Angeles, Dallas/Fort Worth, Houston, Detroit, Tampa, Atlanta, Chicago, Philadelphia, New York, Minneapolis, Miami, Anaheim, and New Orleans.

To compete for the best positions for surgical technologists, students should pursue advanced training in anatomy and physiology and gain certification upon completion of their training programs.

how do I learn more?

professional organizations

Following are organizations that provide information on surgical technologist careers, accredited schools, and employers.

Association of Surgical Technologists
7108-C South Alton Way
Englewood, CO 80112
TEL: 303-694-9130
WEBSITE: http://www.social.com/health/nhic/data/hr0600/hr0687.html

Commission of Accreditation of Allied Health Education Programs
515 North State Street, Suite 7530
Chicago, IL 60610
TEL: 312-464-4636

bibliography

Following is a sampling of materials relating to the professional concerns and development of surgical technologists.

Books

Allmers, Nancy M. *Appleton & Lange's Review for the Surgical Technology Examination,* 4th edition. New York, NY: Appleton & Lange, 1996.

Association of Surgical Technologists Staff. *Core Curriculum for Surgical First Assisting,* 4th edition. Englewood, CO: Association of Surgical Technologists, 1993.

Boegli, Emily H. *Surgical Technology Review Book.* New York, NY: Prentice Hall, 1994.

Fuller, Joanna R. *Surgical Technology: Principles and Practices,* 3rd edition. Philadelphia, PA: W.B. Saunders Co., 1993.

Slagle, Thom. *Pharmacology for the Surgical Technologist.* Philadelphia, PA: W.B. Saunders Co., 1996.

Smith, Ronald R. *Surgical Technologist.* San Jose, CA: R & E Research Associates, 1993.

Periodicals

Surgical Technologist. Monthly. Emphasizing surgical procedures and equipment, legislative issues, aseptic techniques, and career development. Association of Surgical Technologists, Inc., 7108-C South Alton Way, Englewood, CO 80112, 303-694-9130.

thoracic surgeon

Definition
A surgeon who treats diseases and conditions of organs in the chest, including the heart, lungs, and esophagus.

Alternative job titles
Cardiothoracic surgeon
Cardiac surgeon

Salary range
$140,000 to $250,000 to $350,000

Educational requirements
Bachelor's degree; M. D.; five-year general surgery residency; two- or three-year thoracic surgery residency; optional one- to two-year fellowships.

Certification or Licensing
Mandatory

Outlook
Much better than the average

GOE
02.03.01

DOT
070

High School Subjects

Biology
Chemistry
English
Math

Personal Interests

Helping people
Problem solving
Research
Using your hands

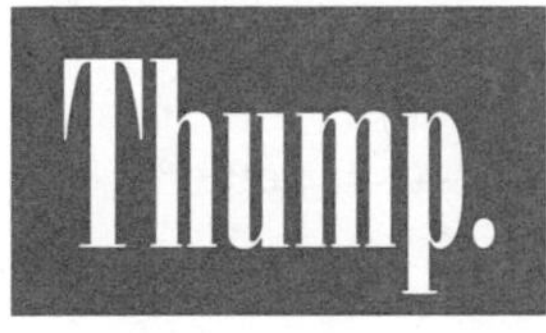

Thump. Thump. The nurse on intensive care duty looked up and down the hallway, but couldn't find the source of the noise. She went back to her paperwork, but an instant later, there it was again. Thump. Thump. Thump.

"Hey," she said softly but sternly. "Who's there?" No one answered. The hallway was deserted. The sound picked up, came a little faster. Thump. thump, thump, thump. It was close by.

The nurse came out from behind the nurse's desk and almost stumbled onto the boy who was sitting on the floor in front of her desk. The ball he was packing into his baseball mitt gave a dull thump as it fell from his glove and onto the floor. They both watched as it rolled down the smooth floor of the hall.

"Nice mitt," she said. "Can I see it?" The boy slid it off of his hand and gave it to her. She turned it over, admiring the smooth brown leather. She handed it back to him. "Are you visiting someone?" she asked. He nodded.

"It's his," the boy said in a whisper, "my grandpa's. He got it when he was ten." The boy stood up and stared in the direction his ball had rolled. "I'm ten, too. That's why he gave it to me." The boy's grandfather was recovering from a coronary bypass. They weren't too sure he would make it. It had been touch-and-go all day. The surgeon who'd done the bypass was in with him now.

"You're not supposed to be in here, you know," she said. Turning around, she looked him in the eyes. "Well, go on," the nurse said. "Go on. He's in the third room on the right."

"Thanks," he said. He found his grandfather with a woman in a long white coat. The woman was speaking in a low, quiet voice, but stopped talking when she saw the boy enter the room. The boy's grandfather smiled weakly at him, and touched the woman gently on the arm.

"It's okay, Doc. Since it's nothing but good news, I'd like to share it with my grandson." He motioned the boy over to his side. "Timmy, this woman saved my life. She's a heart surgeon."

lingo to learn

Echocardiogram A soundwave picture showing the structure and functions of the heart.

Electrocardiograph (EKG) A machine that constantly monitors the heart's activity.

Stress test A test to measure the heart's performance during exercise. It provides more information than a resting EKG.

Heart catheterization A test in which a small tube is placed in the heart in order to take X rays, measure blood pressure within the heart, and to determine if there are any deformities or defects in the heart.

Heart-lung machine A device that maintains circulation during open heart surgery. Blood is diverted from the heart and lungs, oxygenated, and returned to the body.

Lobectomy The surgical removal of a section, or lobe, of a lung. When the entire lung is removed the procedure is called a *pneumonectomy*.

what does a thoracic surgeon do?

The thorax is the cavity within the human body in which the heart and lungs lie. *Thoracic surgeons* treat diseases, repair injuries, and correct deformities of the heart, lungs, and other organs in the chest cavity. They are trained to diagnose and surgically treat coronary artery disease, irregular heart beats, abnormal heart valves, cancers of the lung and esophagus, and other conditions of the chest. Thoracic surgeons perform heart and lung transplants. They are concerned with pulmonary fibrosis, emphysema, cystic fibrosis, and other diseases of the lung.

A general thoracic surgeon is primarily concerned with diseases of the lungs, esophagus, and chest wall. Other surgeons operate on infants and children with congenital, or birth, defects of the windpipe, esophagus, or heart. Thoracic surgeons who perform heart operations—coronary bypass, pacemaker insertion, heart valve replacement—are often called *cardiothoracic surgeons.*

Thoracic surgeons are skilled in state-of-the-art diagnostic procedures, including X rays, computed tomography (CT), and magnetic resonance imaging (MRI). They are trained in oncology and in the use of chemotherapy, radiation therapy, other therapies used to treat thoracic diseases.

Patients with heart-and-lung disease are referred to thoracic surgeons when their primary care physicians believe that medication alone will not help and that surgery may be the best treatment for the condition. The thoracic surgeon reviews the patient's medical history and determines the best surgical procedure. The thoracic surgeon then discusses the case with the patient and other physicians, advising the patient of all the risks and benefits associated with the surgery.

The thoracic surgeon is responsible for working with a team of medical specialists and nurses to take the patient through the immediate evaluation prior to surgery, the final decision for surgery, as well as the recovery period following surgery. Usually, both the patient's physician and the thoracic surgeon see the patient in follow-up visits to make sure that the patient's recovery is progressing. Prior to a surgery, nurses and surgical technologists prep the patient for surgery. The thoracic surgeon heads the operating team that includes the anesthesiologist, assistant surgeons, nurses, and technicians responsible for the heart-lung machine that is required in many operations. Following the surgery, nurses will care for the patient in an intensive care unit.

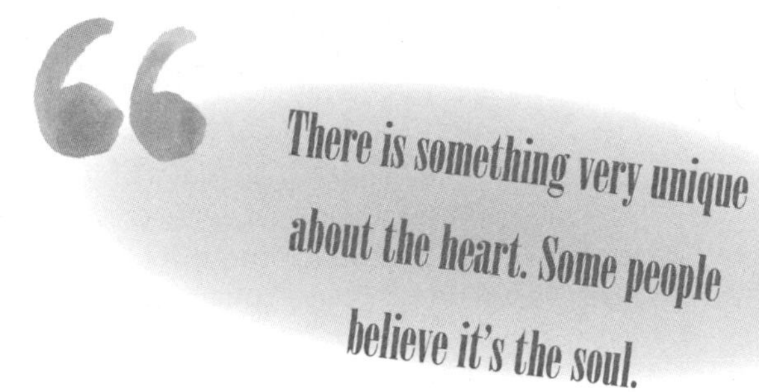

what is it like to be a thoracic surgeon?

"The ability to have somebody trust you with their life, to stop their heart, to fix it, work with it, repair it—and then start it again—that's an incredible responsibility," says Dr. Edward D. Verrier, speaking about his work as a thoracic surgeon from his office at the University of Washington in Seattle, where he is Chief of the Division of Cardiothoracic Surgery. "There is something very unique about the heart," Dr. Verrier says. "Some people believe it's the soul." In cultures across the globe, the heart symbolizes life. Someone who can hold it in his or her hand is often seen as something close to a god.

Thoracic surgeons themselves are not immune to the wonder and awe that surrounds them and their work. Most, in fact, vividly recall the very moment they first experienced the life-giving power with which they are entrusted. Dr. Paul S. Levy, a senior resident in cardiothoracic surgery at Chicago's Northwestern Memorial Hospital, will never forget his first encounter with a live heart. During college at Kalamazoo, students spent a semester focused on career development, working in and observing a profession of their choice.

"I spent four months working with five cardiothoracic surgeons in Arizona. To this very day, I remember it. I knew I wanted to go into cardiothoracic surgery when I was holding a beating heart in my hands. At that point, it was pure magic." Dr. Renee Hartz says, "I remember the day, I remember the patient. I was a junior resident in cardiac surgery and a young woman dying of a clot in her lungs was brought into the operating room. They were performing CPR on her as they wheeled her into the O.R. for pulmonary surgery. I saved her life. That was the day I decided to become a heart surgeon."

Just as unforgettable are the surgeon's experiences with patients that cannot be saved. "I remember a two-year old dying on the table unexpectedly," Dr. Hartz recalls. Currently the Chief of the Division of Cardiothoracic Surgery at the University of Illinois' Chicago College of Medicine, she says "It was very unsettling. I had seen a lot of children die when I was working in the emergency room, but for some reason this was different. I'd thought about going into pediatric cardiac surgery, but I knew then it wouldn't work. I couldn't, didn't, want to go through that on a daily basis."

These physicians are equally candid when sharing their reasons for entering medicine, in general. Says Dr. Hartz, "I'm not sure if I chose medicine, or it chose me. I came from a very poor family in small town where no one went to college. Even boys weren't counseled to go to college. Academics weren't emphasized. I only went to college because my friends were. I shocked myself by doing well."

"It's an evolutionary process, everyone has his own reasons," says Dr. Verrier of his decision to enter the field of medicine. "All the altruistic reasons, of course, hold true. But, also, I wanted to be successful. My father was an engineer. He built our house. But he didn't make a lot of money. I used to have to make a living and I had to caddy to earn money to help my father. And I caddied for successful people, a lot of whom were doctors. This profession gives you a good salary, a good security for your family. I very much wanted that security when I was growing up. And I wanted people to trust me and respect me," he says.

A typical case in which a cardiothoracic surgeon in private practice might see a patient is when the patient goes to the emergency room, complaining of chest pain. "A guy comes in with substernal chest pain to the E.R.," says Dr. Levy. "The E.R. calls his internist. With the cardiologist from the care unit, they determine he's got triple vessel coronary disease. They call us to come in and consult. They want to know, would he benefit from surgery?" Dr. Levy continues, "We'd look at the patient, talk to him, and if he's a good candidate for surgery, we explain the risk factors of surgery versus medical management of his condition. If he wants the surgery, we send him back to his internist to check him out, do bloodwork, see if he's in good enough health for surgery."

Thoracic surgeons in a university or teaching hospital see patients on a slightly different basis and their cases are used as the basis for instruction. For example, according to Dr. Levy, a typical patient in an urban teaching hospital might be a homeless man who's been referred to the attending physician. After an examination, it's determined that, in addition to having the risk factors for heart disease, the man is also a schizophrenic with vascular problems. The attending physician discusses the case with the resident or fellow. "Together, they review the results of the cardiac catheterization, which reveal single coronary disease; plus the guy's got an aneurysm in his arteries. As the fellow, I read up on the proposed procedure," says Dr. Levy. During surgery, they replace the ascending aorta and perform a bypass graft to the man's heart. Later, the thoracic surgeons provide postoperative care, and ready him for vascular surgery.

"There's lots of repetition—so you can see as much badness as possible, so you will be able to handle it the next time," Dr. Levy says about the work. "You're taking a lot of data and putting it all together."

FYI

The development of heart-lung machines in the 1950's launched the specialty of cardiovascular surgery.

have I got what it takes to be a thoracic surgeon?

"You have to learn a lot about death and dying," Dr. Verrier says. "It's very difficult to walk out to a mother and say, 'I'm sorry. I did all I could, but your child still died,'" he says. Dr. Levy agrees, the stakes are incredibly high, as is the pressure and responsibility. "There's no margin for mediocrity. When you get mediocre, people die."

Thoracic surgery is believed by most to be the most demanding surgical specialty. Physicians who enter this field will be challenged emotionally, physically, and intellectually. High levels of stress, long hours, and difficult, complex cases are among the drawbacks to working as a thoracic surgeon. Every case is a matter of life-and-death. While the surgical procedures are possible, they may not be successful."You can do everything right and the patient dies, anyway. Cardiothoracic surgery is a contact sport; it can go badly very quickly," explains Dr. Levy. "You'll be going along, and everything's perfect, and then all of a sudden, a suture breaks, or a tie on a vessel comes off and you either lose the patient, or have to start all over again."

Thoracic surgeons work long hours throughout the years of study, and these schedules can continue throughout their careers. Dr. Levy describes a typical year in thoracic residency, "You're on call all the time. We're talking about hundred-hour weeks, easily." On those days that they have surgeries scheduled, they usually spend the entire day on their feet. Surgeries can take an hour or two, or they can last for much longer. "Sometimes, the pathologist takes forty minutes trying to figure out whether or not the specimen is benign or malignant. Meanwhile, you've got this guy on the table with his chest opened up. It can be frustrating."

When it comes to their patients, thoracic surgeons are on call twenty-four hours a day. Like other physicians, they might be paged while eating dinner or watching a movie, or called while sleeping in the middle of the night. "You have to have a very understanding family," attests Dr. Verrier.

Dr. Hartz adds, "The work is labor-intensive. You have to want this very very badly, and you have to be able to focus—focus on a task and carry it to completion."

Thoracic surgeons, like all surgeons, must possess excellent manual dexterity skills and the ability to make and execute decisions promptly. "I'm an action-oriented person," Dr. Hartz says, "decisive and quick. I tried to talk myself out this profession, and did a year of pediatric residency; but I loved surgery, so I went back to it. It suits me." Although all surgeries are planned, the degree of planning will differ according to the situation, depending upon whether the procedure is an emergency procedure. In every surgery, however, the surgeon faces the unexpected—a sudden drop in blood pressure, an inexplicable reaction to anesthesia, complications in the surgery, itself. Surgeons must be able to cope with these crises, and others, always mindful of maintaining their composure in stressful situations.

Another essential quality in surgeons is a genuine concern for people. Surgeons treat the individual with a surgical condition, not merely the surgical condition, itself. Therefore, those who aspire to be thoracic surgeons must be able to deal compassionately with patients and their family, addressing any fears, questions, and needs they might have. A deep sense of responsibility should accompany a surgeon's compassion, as well.

To be a successful thoracic surgeon, you should:

- Be able to make lightning-fast decisions
- Function well in high-stress situations
- Have good hand-eye coordination and manual dexterity
- Be an effective communicator
- Be an effective surgical team leader, capable of giving orders calmly and clearly

how do I become a thoracic surgeon?

education

High School

High school students should prepare for a future in medicine by taking courses in biology, chemistry, physics, algebra, geometry, and trigonometry. Courses in computer science are a must, as well, since the computers are changing the way medicine is taught and shared by its professionals. Since colleges, universities, and medical schools are looking for individuals with a well-rounded background, students should not neglect the humanities, but take and perform well in English, history, literature, and psychology classes.

Postsecondary Training

Students interested in thoracic surgery must first earn a bachelor's degree from an accredited four-year college or university. Courses that may help prepare students for medical school are math, biology, chemistry, anatomy, physiology, and physics, as well as courses in the humanities, such as English composition.

After receiving an undergraduate degree, the student must apply to and be accepted by one of the 141 medical schools in the United States. Admission is competitive; applicants undergo an extensive admissions process which considers grade point averages, scores on the Medical College Admission Test (MCAT), and recommendations from professors. Most premed students apply to several schools early in their senior year of college. Only about one-third of the applicants are accepted.

In order to earn an M.D. degree, a student must complete four years of medical school. For the first two years of medical school, students attend lectures and classes and spend time in laboratories. Courses include anatomy, biochemistry, physiology, pharmacology, psychology, microbiology, pathology, medical ethics, and laws governing medicine. They learn to take patient histories, perform routine physical examinations, and recognize symptoms.

In their third and fourth years, students work in clinics and hospitals supervised by residents and physicians. They go through what are known as rotations, or brief periods of study in a particular area, such as internal medicine, obstetrics and gynecology, pediatrics, dermatology, psychiatry, and surgery. Rotations allow students to gain exposure to the many different fields within medicine and to learn firsthand the skills of diagnosing and treating patients.

Dr. Levy realized right away that he didn't enjoy the rotations in medicine. "It was so frustrating to keep dealing with chronic non-compliers," he says, referring to people who are told they have to quit smoking, drinking, or eating poorly and to start exercising. "I couldn't fathom myself doing that day in and day out."

After graduating from medical school, physicians must pass a standard examination given by the National Board of Medical Examiners. Most physicians complete an internship, usually one year in length. This helps graduates to decide what will be their area of specialization.

Following the internship, physicians begin a graduate program known as a residency. Physicians wishing to become thoracic surgeons, must first complete a five-year residency in general surgery. Then they begin a two- or three-year residency in general thoracic surgery and cardiovascular surgery. The residency years are as filled with stress, pressure, and physical rigor as the previous four years of medical school, perhaps even more so as residents are given greater responsibilities than medical students. Residents often work twenty-four-hour shifts, easily clocking in eighty hours or more per week. "You need a supportive environment to succeed," says Dr. Verrier. "You need to have the physical and intellectual skills, but you also need the discipline to get through this."

certification or licensing

To qualify for certification by the American Board of Thoracic Surgery, a candidate has been certified in general surgery by the American Board of Surgery; has completed the residency in thoracic surgery at an approved academic medical center; and has successfully completed both the written and oral examinations given by the American Board of Thoracic Surgery. Certification in thoracic surgery is valid for ten years, at which time the thoracic surgeon must apply for re-certification. While certification is voluntary, it is highly recommended. Most hospitals will not grant privileges to a surgeon without board certification. HMOs and other insurance groups will not make referrals or payments without certification. Licensing is required in all states before any doctor can practice medicine.

scholarships and grants

Scholarships and grants are often available from individual institutions, state agencies, and special-interest organizations. The book *Dollars for College: Medicine, Dentistry, and Related Fields* by Ferguson Publishing is an excellent source for this information. Many students finance their medical education through the Armed Forces Health Professions Scholarship Program. Each branch of the military participates in this program, paying students' tuitions in exchange for military service. Contact your local recruiting office for more information on this program. The National Health Service Corps Scholarship Program also provides money for students in return for service. Another source for financial aid, scholarship, and grant information is the Association of American Medical Colleges. Remember to request information early for eligibility, application requirements, and deadlines.

Association of American Medical Colleges
2450 N Street, NW
Washington, DC 20037
TEL: 202-828-0400
WEBSITE: http://www.aamc.org
Specific information on financial aid programs can be found at:
WEBSITE: http://www.aamc.org/stuapps/finaid

Ferguson Publishing Company
200 West Madison, Suite 300
Chicago, IL 60606
TEL: 312-580-5480

National Health Services Corps Scholarship Program
U.S. Public Health Service
1010 Wayne Avenue, Suite 240
Silver Spring, MD 20910
TEL: 800-638-0824

who will hire me?

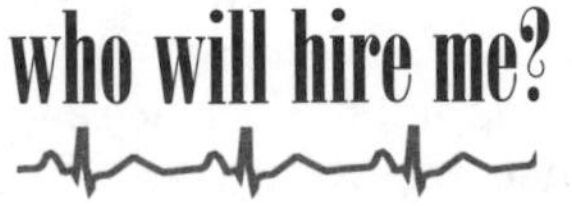

Many thoracic surgeons enter into private practice with a partner or a small group. Dr. Paul

Levy, for example, is finishing his last year of residency training in thoracic surgery, and has accepted an invitation to work in private practice with a much more senior surgeon in thoracic and cardiovascular surgery. At the moment, he doesn't envision pursuing research, but it remains an option. Private practice is an attractive option for many thoracic surgeons, as it provides a somewhat more stable routine. Patients will still need emergency care, but to some degree, the surgeon can try and aim for a more predictable schedule.

Many surgeons work at medical schools and in private hospitals. Dr. Verrier and Dr. Hartz, for example, practice in university hospitals so they can teach future generations of thoracic surgeons. "I've dedicated myself to teaching others about the responsibility of this work," says Dr. Verrier.

where can I go from here?

The field is competitive, but thoracic surgeons advance in the time-honored ways in which all physicians and surgeons advance: by doing their jobs extremely well, working to create and maintain a solid reputation among both peers and patients, and building up their practices. Many surgeons in private practice form single- or multi-specialty practice groups, which can lead to more referrals and greater income.

Thoracic surgeon who work as professors at universities and teaching hospitals usually advance to become department heads or heads of hospitals. Heading the Division of Cardiothoracic Surgery at a major medical institution is to reach the highest level.

what are the salary ranges?

The national average salary for first-year residents in the mid-1990's was approximately $31,000. That average increased to $41,800 by the final residency year. Salaries will vary depending on the kind of residency, the hospital, and the geographic area.

According to surveys by the American Medical Association, annual income for surgeons in the mid-1990's ranged from approximately $140,000 to $300,000, with the median income at about $200,000. These figures are for all surgeons, and incomes may vary from specialty to specialty. Annual income for thoracic surgeons ranges from $150,000 to more than $350,000. Other factors influencing individual incomes include the type and size of the practice, the number of hours worked per week, the geographic area, and the professional reputation of the surgeon.

what is the job outlook?

"We don't want to promote thoracic surgery when we're so worried about our specialty, as it is. There aren't enough jobs for graduates, and they're cutting programs," says Dr. Hartz, who goes on to say, "They're also telling medical students that 'if you don't go into primary care, you won't have a job in ten years.' I say, there's always room at the top. It's really desire." Dr. Verrier adds, "You pursue your career in a way that leads to success."

The health care industry, in general, is among the fastest growing in the United States. Although managed health care policies may curtail some higher-risk procedures, patients will continue to need the special skills and expertise of the thoracic surgeon.

how do I learn more?

professional organizations

Following are organizations that provide information on the field of thoracic and cardiothoracic surgery.

American Association for Thoracic Surgery
13 Elm Street
Manchester, MA 01944
TEL: 508-526-8330
WEBSITE: http://www.surgeon.org

Society of Thoracic Surgeons
401 North Michigan Avenue
Chicago, IL 60611
TEL: 312-644-6610
WEBSITE: http://www.sts.org/info

bibliography

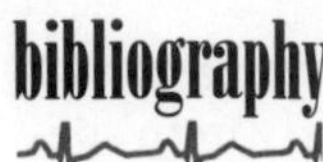

Following is a sampling of materials relating to the professional concerns and development of thoracic surgeons.

Books

Goldstraw, Peter. *Textbook of Thoracic Surgery.* Newton, MA: Butterworth-Heinemann, 1995.

Pearson, F. Griffin, editor. *Thoracic Surgery.* New York, NY: Churchill Livingstone, 1995.

Shields, Thomas W. *General Thoracic Surgery,* 4th edition. Baltimore, MD: Williams & Wilkins, 1994.

Waldhausen, John A., William S. Pierce, and David B. Campbell. *Surgery of the Chest,* 6th edition. St. Louis, MO: Mosby, 1995.

Periodicals

Annals of Thoracic Surgery. Monthly. Presents original papers on topics in thoracic surgery, featuring case reports, and current reviews. Society of Thoracic Surgeons, Elsevier Science Inc., 655 Avenue of the Americas, New York, NY 10010, 212-989-5800.

Seminars in Thoracic and Cardiovascular Surgery. Quarterly. Offers original articles on thoracic surgery. W.B. Saunders Co., Curtis Center, 3rd Floor, Independence Square West, Philadelphia, PA 19106, 215-238-7800

toxicologist

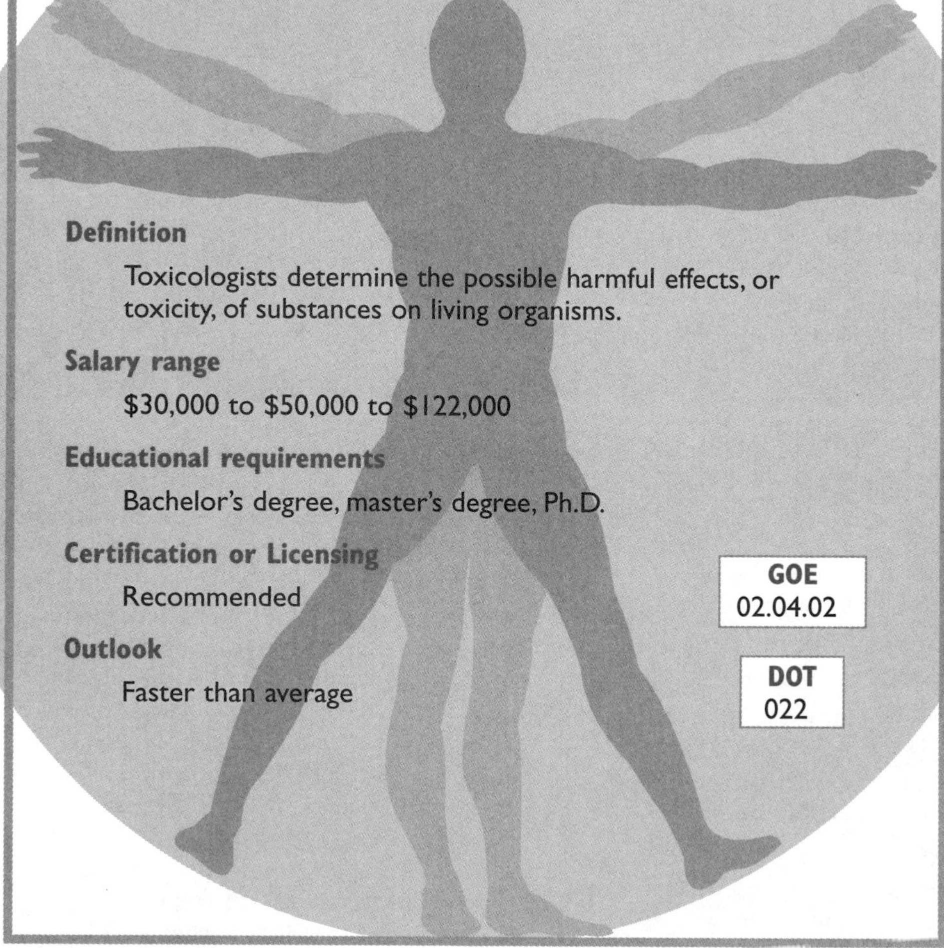

High School Subjects

Biology
Chemistry
Computer science
English
Mathematics

Personal Interests

Environmental issues
Governmental policy
Problem solving
Reading and continuous learning

A clue to the mystery was here somewhere, toxicologist Jim Bus was sure of it. He wandered through the neatly stacked cages in the animal lab and wondered what that clue was. For two years, he and his colleagues at Chemical Industry Institute of Toxicology (CIIT) had been exposing both male and female mice and rats to gasoline fumes to determine if they were harmful to living organisms. Throughout the study, the animals had demonstrated healthy behavior. Now the research team had begun dissecting the animals for examination and had been startled by what they found. All of the mice and all of the female rats had healthy organ tissue, but the male rats had developed kidney cancer. Suddenly the routine toxicology experiment had turned into a high-stakes puzzle.

If gasoline caused cancer in living organisms, millions of people each day were putting themselves at risk at the gas pump. Jim needed to determine how the gasoline fumes were causing cancer in the male rats and whether the same process could occur in human bodies. If it could, he would have to immediately alert the Environmental Protection Agency, the petroleum companies, and the public to the possible health threat. Measures would have to be developed to protect people from fumes at gas stations. The associated costs, in terms of both health care and new safety technology, would be staggering.

Jim opened a cage and drew out one of the remaining male rats. Gently stroking the animal's coarse fur, Jim considered several troubling questions. Why were the male rats getting sick when the mice and the female rats were not? Why were the rats able to live to their full expected life span despite the cancer? Was the kidney cancer somehow unique to male rats or did it indicate a potential health concern for humans?

After much research and hard work, Jim and his team were relieved to discover that the gas fumes causing cancer in the male rats would not have the same effect on humans. The toxicologists had quietly ensured society's safety for another day.

lingo to learn

Benign Referring to a tumor, it means noncancerous.

Carcinogen A cancer-producing substance.

Control group A group in an experiment that is not exposed to a procedure or chemical that the rest of the group is.

Dissect To expose, through cutting, the internal organs of an animal for scientific examination.

In vitro From the Latin, meaning "within glassware," referring to a biological process or experiment that takes place in laboratory equipment such as a test tube.

Malignant Tending to deteriorate or cause death. When referring to a cancer it means highly invasive and quickly spreading.

Metabolism The combination of chemical processes that take place in a living organism resulting in growth, body functions, distribution of nutrients, etc.

Toxin A poison produced by a living organism such as a plant.

what does a toxicologist do?

Toxicologists examine the way chemicals interact with living organisms. Their work enables us to use chemicals to improve the quality of our lives, without harming ourselves or our environment. Toxicologists are our protectors in a world that increasingly depends on manufactured chemicals to purify water, protect crops, cure diseases, and much more. It is the job of industrial and governmental toxicologists to help protect the public and the environment from harmful chemicals and to make sure that beneficial chemicals are used in safe and appropriate ways. One way they do this is by assisting in the creation of regulations governing the production and use of chemicals. Research toxicologists, many of whom work for universities or private research institutes, investigate the biochemical and cellular processes that take place in living organisms as a result of exposure to toxic substances.

Evaluating the safety of chemicals is a very complex process. Chemicals that are safe under some circumstances may be dangerous under others. In order to identify appropriate uses for chemicals, toxicologists must conduct extensive tests to determine if and how a chemical may harm living organisms, under what circumstances it might do so, and at what dosage. "In toxicology, we like to say that the dose makes the poison," says Jim. "Chlorine, for instance, can be dangerous in extremely high doses. The levels used to purify water, however, are not harmful." Thus, depending on the dose, a chemical may be beneficial or deadly.

Many of the tests toxicologists run are performed on laboratory animals. Toxicologists expose animals to a chemical by injecting it into their systems, by feeding it to them, or by surrounding them with fumes. To determine the dosage at which a chemical becomes harmful, toxicologists expose separate groups of animals to different amounts of the substance. The test results are measured by observing the animals' behaviors and by testing samples of their blood and tissue. At the end of a study, toxicologists usually dissect the animals to examine their organs for signs of damage or disease. To eliminate the possibility that something other than the chemical is causing the result, toxicologists also study one group of animals that is not exposed to the chemical.

"We are very careful to treat the animals in a humane manner," says Jim. "Whenever possible, we use in vitro, or test tube, studies, which do not involve animals. It is true, though, that toxicology experiments often cause disease in animals. We believe these tests are necessary because they enable us to prevent hazards to people. By testing animals," Jim explains, "science has been able to develop chemicals, medicines, and technologies that save lives."

Jim, who now works for Dow Chemical Company, is an industrial toxicologist. Before a company can commercially introduce a new chemical, industrial toxicologists must subject it to barrage of tests to ensure that the chemical will not harm humans or the environment. If a chemical company wants to introduce a new insecticide, for example, industrial toxicologists must first conduct tests to see if the product harms animals when applied to their skin or when ingested. Environmental toxicologists conduct studies to measure the residue the insecticide leaves in soil and water and to determine whether the residue is harmful to fish or wildlife. The results of these tests are then carefully scrutinized by toxicologists who work for government agencies, such as the Food and Drug Administration (FDA) and the Environmental Protection Agency (EPA). If the toxicologists at either of these agencies raise additional questions, the industrial toxicologist must run further studies.

"This is a very healthy process," says Jim. He explains, for example, that in the 1950's a chemical known as thalidomide was prescribed by doctors for some pregnant women to relieve anxiety and morning sickness. The results were disastrous. "Thalidomide caused birth defects in a large number of children. Thanks to toxicology, and to our system of checks and balances, the chance of a tragedy of that kind happening again are greatly reduced today. Toxicologists would discover a drug's potential to cause birth defects long before it could be approved for use."

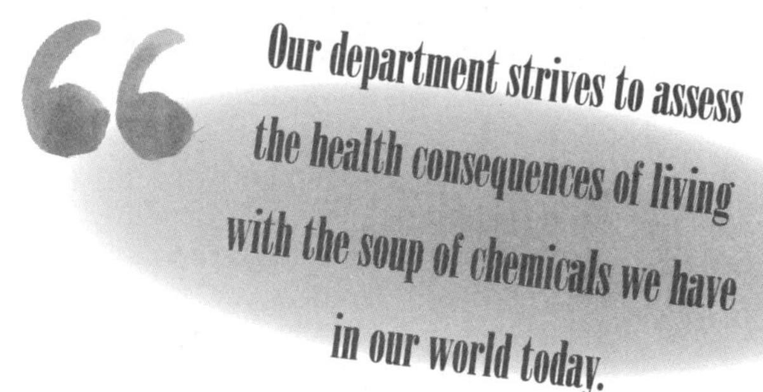

what is it like to be a toxicologist?

Jim describes his job in two words: terrifically exciting. "As a toxicologist," Jim says, "I can help ensure that chemicals are safely used to improve the quality of millions of lives. I can also have an impact on policies that protect the public."

In his work as an industrial toxicologist, Jim designs studies to test new chemical products for safety and regulatory compliance. These studies are typically conducted over a period of one to two years. Throughout this time, Jim supervises the toxicologists and laboratory technicians working on the study. These people implement the tests, observe the animals, and test the blood and tissue samples. Jim evaluates and interprets the results of the tests to determine how, and if, a product can be used safely. When an unexpected result occurs, Jim works with his research team to discover why that result occurred.

Once a study, or series of studies, has been completed, Jim presents the findings to the senior executives of Dow Chemical Company. These managers are extremely receptive to Jim's recommendations. "The last thing that this or any other chemical company wants to do is introduce a harmful product," Jim explains. "My job is to prevent that from happening. The company's management expects me to tell it the way I see it."

Because Dow Chemical Company does business all over the world, Jim also travels extensively to meet with regulatory agencies in other countries. "I've met with regulators in Russia, Japan, and many other countries to describe our testing procedures and to explain my evaluation of a product," says Jim. "These officials have a responsibility to make sure that we have thoroughly tested our products. Toxicology," he adds, "is not a huge discipline, but it is global in its impact."

In addition to meeting with foreign scientists, Jim occasionally must address the public. "Stories in the news may cause the public to feel inappropriate fear of certain chemicals. One special interest group put out a story that use of chlorine is dangerous. They neglected to explain that the chlorine levels used to purify water are harmless. Tragically, a developing nation in South America was alarmed and stopped chlorinating their water. Many people subsequently died of water-borne diseases. I try to counter these scare tactics by informing the public about our exhaustive testing procedures and about the stringent governmental regulations we observe."

Jim also makes time to attend professional conferences and seminars. "Science," he observes, "is constantly changing. Continuing education is absolutely essential to someone in this field."

Because Jim is employed by a major chemical company, the focus of his research is determined by the products his employer manufactures. Toxicologists who work for colleges and universities are usually able to exert more control over their research. Some engage in "basic" research. Basic research does not provide any immediate commercial or public use, but it does contribute to our understanding of basic life processes. Others conduct "applied" research. Applied research is expected to yield direct social or commercial benefit. Research toxicologists may also develop new testing techniques or suggest new mathematical models to check the validity of their tests. In addition to conducting research, toxicologist who work for colleges or universities usually have administrative and teaching responsibilities.

Toxicologists who work for the federal government have widely varied responsibilities. Some are responsible for establishing and enforcing regulations pertaining to the manufacture, distribution, and use of chemicals. Others conduct research to assess risks to the public. One such toxicologist is Linda Birnbaum, the director of experimental toxicology for the Environmental Protection Agency. "Our department strives to assess the health consequences of living with the soup of chemicals we have in our world today. We ask, for example, how air pollution affects the immune system and other body functions." As the director of a large department, Linda is rarely able to pursue her own research. Instead, she designs and supervises major studies while managing the department and coordinating efforts with other government branches.

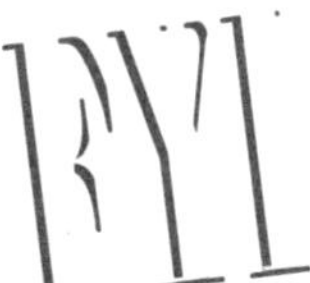

The Danger of Chemicals

In 1984 one of the worst chemical industrial disasters in history occurred in Bhopal, India, when a pesticide factory leaked toxic gas, killing at least 4,000 people. In order to protect US citizens from such a chemical disaster, the Congress in 1986 passed the Emergency Planning and Community Right-To-Know Act requiring industries, among other things, to immediately report to local and state agencies the release of hazardous substances.

have I got what it takes to be a toxicologist?

According to Jim Bus, toxicologists must be creative, intellectually curious, and insatiable readers. "I think it's important for people to realize that you don't have to be another Albert Einstein to be a successful scientist," he says. "I remember wondering if I would have enough good ideas to be a scientist. The truth is that you don't have to be a genius to come up with scientific ideas. You do have to read avidly, ask probing questions, and try to put things together."

Some toxicology studies may last up to two years, so a person who is considering toxicology as a profession must be persevering and patient. Extensive studies also require meticulous record-keeping, so toxicologists must be organized and disciplined. Jim also points out that many studies involve animal testing. "If a person would not be comfortable testing chemicals on animals," say Jim, "He or she should probably consider another field."

Studies in this field sometimes involve working with highly toxic chemicals. Toxicologists must be extremely responsible about taking every precaution to avoid exposing themselves or their colleagues to harmful substances. Because toxicologists usually work in research teams, strong interpersonal skills are also important. "Industrial toxicologists work closely with other scientists, with management, and with outside regulatory agencies," Jim explains. "You have to be able to communicate clearly about very complex issues."

To be a successful toxicologist, you should

- Be a responsible and detail-oriented worker
- Be able to interact with a variety of people and communicate clearly
- Enjoy problem solving
- Have patience
- Be able to perform experiments with animals
- Enjoy continuous learning

how do I become a toxicologist?

Students should be aware that there are a variety of ways to enter the toxicology profession. "There is no one straight and narrow path to becoming a toxicologist," Linda says. "Students do not have to decide in high school or even in college. I obtained a doctoral degree in molecular biology. I then completed postdoctoral fellowships in biochemistry and drug metabolism. While I was studying the way the metabolism reacts to foreign chemicals, I became interested in toxicology, so I pursued a third postdoctoral in toxicology."

education

High School

Although no definite educational route to becoming a toxicologist exists, if you believe you are interested in this career you need to begin by taking high school classes that are college preparatory. Courses in science, such as biology, chemistry, and physics, as well as courses in math, such as algebra and geometry, are not only necessary but will also allow you to discover the depth of your interest in these areas. English and speech classes will provide you with the opportunity to improve your research and communication skills. Social studies or government courses will give you an understanding of how society is structured, an understanding that will be necessary in your later career working with government agencies and government regulations. Finally, computer science classes are also beneficial to take, since much research and professional communication is done today using this technology.

Postsecondary Training

The next step on your educational path to becoming a toxicologist is to receive a bachelor's degree from an accredited college or university. Most students pursuing this career take a degree in a science-related field, such as biology or chemistry. College course work for this field usually includes classes in chemistry, biology, physics, statistics, and calculus. English courses continue to be helpful, providing you with the opportunity to develop your research and writing skills.

An additional way to gain skills and test your interest in the field is through summer work in research laboratories. The Society of Toxicology provides information on summer internship programs. Although you can enter the profession at this point, there are an extremely limited number of jobs for people holding only a bachelor's degree and advancement is quite difficult.

Most students, after receiving a bachelor's degree, choose to go into graduate programs, either for a master's or a doctoral degree. Again, professional advancement with only a master's degree is extremely difficult. Most students either complete a doctoral (Ph.D.) program in toxicology or receive a Ph.D. in a related field, such as molecular biology, and then complete postdoctoral training in toxicology. This second method is the educational route that Linda took. Studies at the graduate level vary, depending on whether the student is receiving a doctorate in toxicology or a doctorate in a related field and then postdoctoral training in toxicology. Courses at this level, though, generally include pathology, biochemistry, epidemiology, molecular biology, and environmental toxicology. Doctoral degrees usually take four to five years to complete, and postdoctoral training usually takes two to three years.

certification or licensing

Licensing is not required for this position. Certification is also not required, but it is recommended. Certification programs are available through the Academy of Toxicological Sciences and the American Board of Toxicology. The Academy of Toxicological Science bases its certification on the applicant's credentials, including published papers, research, and activities in the field of toxicology.

The American Board of Toxicology bases its certification on a 300-question examination. "The American Board of Toxicology exam offers a certification opportunity for industrial toxicologists who do not have as many opportunities to publish research papers as those employed by the government or by colleges and universities," says Jim. Toxicologists may apply to take this examination after practicing in the field for three to seven years.

scholarships and grants

A number of federal agencies, including the National Institute of Environmental Health Sciences, the National Science Foundation, the Environmental Protection Agency, and the Armed Forces provide financial support to students pursuing graduate toxicology degrees. Students should ask their guidance counselors for information or contact the following.

National Science Foundation
4201 Wilson Boulevard
Arlington, VA 22230
TEL: 703-306-1234
WEBSITE: http://www.nsf.gov

Society of Toxicology
1767 Business Center Drive
Suite 302
Reston, VA 22090
TEL: 703-438-3115
WEBSITE: http://www.toxicology.org

who will hire me?

Toxicologists work in industry (particularly for chemical and pharmaceutical companies), in government agencies, and in academia. Unlikely as it seems, Jim's first experience with toxicology occurred on a golf course. "I was studying science in college but didn't know what I wanted to do with it," he recalls. "By chance, I ended up in a golf foursome with a man who worked for Upjohn as a toxicologist. He told me about his job and said that toxicology was a great field for someone who wanted to do exciting things with science. Twenty years later I ended up at Upjohn in a very similar position to his."

Throughout his career, Jim has been involved in performing toxicological research for industry, and he is in good company. Approximately 37 percent of all toxicologists work for chemical, pharmaceutical, or related industries. Industrial toxicologist positions involve product development, product safety evaluation, and regulatory compliance.

The majority of toxicologists, 47 percent, are employed by academic institutions. Most of the academic opportunities are in schools of medicine and public health at major universities, though smaller institutions have recently begun hiring toxicologists to teach toxicology within basic biology, chemistry, and engineering programs.

Another 13 percent of toxicologists are employed by the government. Though these positions have historically been limited to federal regulatory agencies, many states are now beginning to employ toxicologists as well. A growing number of toxicologists are also working as consultants or joining research foundations to conduct research on specific problems of industrial or public concern.

where can I go from here?

Toxicologists who have organizational and administrative skills as well as excellent scientific credentials, like Jim and Linda, will find many opportunities for advancement in their careers. For example, toxicologists who work for private industry may be promoted to head a research unit. As highly visible and influential members of the corporate organization, they may also be asked to join the executive management team. Toxicologists in colleges or universities may advance by being promoted to full professor and asked to head a department.

Managerial advancement, however, can have drawbacks for toxicologists who enjoy the challenges and rewards of research. Although those with managerial responsibilities usually receive higher pay, they also have administrative and budgeting responsibilities that can detract from the time one is able to devote to research.

what are the salary ranges?

According to a 1995 survey conducted as a joint project by the American College of Toxicology and the Society of Toxicology, a toxicologist with a bachelor's degree typically receives a starting salary of $20,000. Those who have master's degrees can expect to begin at $24,000 to $30,000.

Toxicologists with doctoral degrees receive starting salaries that range from $30,000 to $40,000. A toxicologist who has a doctoral degree and two or three years of postdoctoral experience may earn $40,000 to $50,000. With more than ten years of experience and a doctoral degree, a toxicologist can earn from $75,000 to $122,000 annually. Most executive positions in toxicology pay more than $100,000. In general, research and government positions tend to offer lower salaries than those in industry.

what is the job outlook?

According to the Society of Toxicology, the demand for toxicologists has never been greater. In industry, agriculture, and health care, the world is becoming increasingly dependent on pharmaceuticals and chemicals to sustain its ever-increasing population. As the use of chemicals increases, so does the need for toxicologists who can develop, test, and regulate these substances.

Job opportunities for toxicologists should be most plentiful in large urban areas, near large hospitals, chemical manufactures, and universities. Toxicologists with the most education, training, and experience will receive the best positions. Toxicologists with only a bachelor's degree may have difficulty finding a position. Those who have only a master's degree may find positions as laboratory researchers, but their chances for advancement are minimal. Those with a Ph.D. will fair best in the job market.

how do I learn more?

professional organizations

Following are organizations that provide information on toxicology careers.

American College of Toxicology
9650 Rockville Pike
Bethesda, MD 20814
TEL: 301-571-1840
WEBSITE: http://landaus.com/toxicology/

American Board of Toxicology
PO Box 30054
Raleigh, NC 27622
TEL: 919-782-0036

National Science Foundation
4201 Wilson Boulevard
Arlington, VA 22230
TEL: 703-306-1234
WEBSITE: http://www.nsf.gov

Society of Toxicology
1767 Business Center Drive
Suite 302
Reston, VA 22090
TEL: 703-438-3115
WEBSITE: http://www.toxicology.org

bibliography

Following is a sampling of materials relating to the professional concerns and development of toxicologists.

Books

Bryson, Peter D. *Comprehensive Review in Toxicology for Emergency Clinicians*, 3rd edition. Philadelphia, PA: Lippincott-Raven, 1996.

Cheremisinoff, Nicholas P. *Health and Toxicology*. Houston, TX: Gulf Publishing Co., 1997.

Ellenhorn, Matthew J., Donald G. Barceloux, Seth Schonwald, and Jonathan Wasserberger, editors. *Medical Toxicology: Diagnosis and Treatment of Human Poisoning*, 2nd edition. Baltimore, MD: Williams & Wilkins, 1996.

Hodgson, Ernest. *Toxicology,* 2nd edition. New York, NY: Prentice-Hall, 1996.

Massaro, Edward J. *Handbook of Human Toxicology.* Boca Raton, FL: CRC Press, 1997.

Timbrell, John A. *Introduction to Toxicology,* 2nd edition. Bristol, PA: Taylor & Francis, 1995.

Periodicals

Clinical Toxicology. Bimonthly. For physicians, veterinarians, pharmacists, research scientists, and analytical chemists. Aims to provide information and to encourage the development of therapeutic methods and technology. American Academy of Clinical Toxicology, Pittsburgh Poison Center, 3705 5th Avenue, Pittsburgh, PA 15213, 412-692-6669.

Journal of Toxicology: Clinical Toxicology. Bimonthly. Correlates the various disciplines that deal directly with and contribute to the practical aspects of poisoning. American Academy of Clinical Toxicology, Marcel Dekker Journals, 270 Madison Avenue, New York, NY 10016, 212-696-9000.

Veterinary and Human Toxicology. Bimonthly. Contains contributions in the broad field of toxicology. Includes manuscripts of original research, scientific reviews, field observations in man or domestic and wild animals, and information of general educational value to toxicologists and related scientists. American Academy of Veterinary and Comparative Toxicology, Comparative Toxicology Laboratories, Publication Office, Kansas State University, Manhattan, KS 66506, 913-532-4334.

transplant coordinator

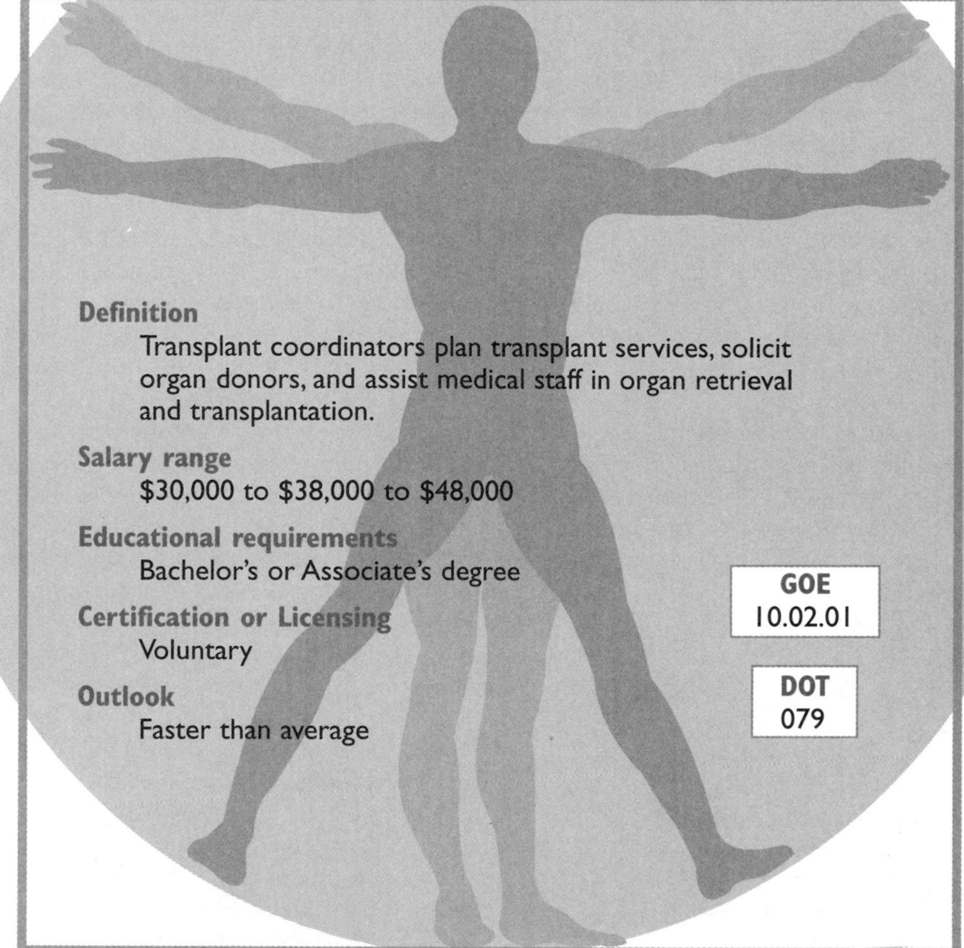

Definition

Transplant coordinators plan transplant services, solicit organ donors, and assist medical staff in organ retrieval and transplantation.

Salary range

$30,000 to $38,000 to $48,000

Educational requirements

Bachelor's or Associate's degree

Certification or Licensing

Voluntary

Outlook

Faster than average

GOE
10.02.01

DOT
079

High School Subjects

Biology
Chemistry
Math
Psychology

Personal Interests

Helping people
Planning
Science
Teaching

The beeper went off, waking Julie Petro, a transplant coordinator at a local hospital. She calls the organ procurement organization (OPO) where she works and learns of the death of a potential organ donor. The OPO gets over a hundred calls a day. Every death in the state is called in and then evaluated for the possibility of organ transplant. In this case, a heart, lung, and kidneys may save the lives of some very sick people in the state or somewhere else in the country.

On her way to the hospital Julie prepares herself emotionally to meet with the parents of the young man who has just died. Though she recognizes the importance of procuring the organs, she also feels that the parents must be comfortable with whatever decision they come to. Not only will she talk to them about organ donation, but she will also stay with them, as long as needed, to help them through the difficult time.

what does a transplant coordinator do?

In 1996 there were approximately 70,000 people across the country waiting for an organ transplant. They may have been waiting for a new heart, liver, kidney, or pancreas. Tissues, such as corneas, heart valves, and skin, and bone can be donated as well. Despite the efforts of transplant centers, the Red Cross, and other organizations promoting the importance of organ donation, nearly 4,000 people on this waiting list died without receiving the needed transplant.

In transplant centers (medical facilities where transplants are planned and performed) a number of professionals see to the needs of transplant recipients and the families of organ donors. A transplant center may be staffed by surgeons, nurses, operating room technicians, social workers, pathologists, psychologists, and transplant coordinators. A *transplant coordinator* is involved in practically every aspect of organ procurement (getting the organ from the donor) and transplantation; this involves working with medical records, scheduling surgeries, educating potential organ recipients, and counseling donor families.

Transplant centers have individual programs for specific organs—many of them have programs for kidney transplants, heart transplants, and pancreas transplants. In addition to the centers, there are separate organizations, such as organ procurement organizations and tissue typing laboratories, which deal with specific aspects of organ transplantation. Organ procurement organizations, or OPOs, focus on procuring the organ from a donor. The OPOs were developed to serve as links between transplant centers and hospitals.

There are two types of transplant coordinators: *procurement coordinators,* and *clinical coordinators*. Procurement coordinators help the families of organ donors deal with the death of a loved one as well as inform them of the organ donation process. Clinical coordinators educate recipients in how to best prepare for organ transplant and how to care for the new organ. Many coordinators, especially clinical coordinators, are registered nurses, but you are not required to have a nursing degree to work as a coordinator. Some medical background is important, however. Many transplant coordinators have degrees in biology, physiology, accounting, psychology, business administration, or public health.

Though procurement and clinical coordinators are actively involved in evaluating, planning, and maintaining records, an important part of their job is helping individuals and families.

For organs to become available, the donor patient must be declared brain dead, which means there is no brain function, no brain stem reflexes, no spontaneous movements, and the patient is no longer breathing on his or her own. Once this determination has been made by the physician, the procurement transplant coordinator approaches the donor's family about organ donation. If the family gives their consent, the coordinator then collects medical information and tissue samples for analysis. The coordinator also calls the United Network for Organ Sharing (UNOS), a membership organization which includes every transplant program, organ procurement organization, and tissue typing laboratory in

lingo to learn

Autotransplant A procedure in which an organ or tissue from one part of a patient's body is transplanted to another part of that patient's body.

CellCept A drug used to prevent the rejection of the transplant organ.

Crossmatching A test of compatibility between the blood of a donor and perspective recipient.

Graft A transplanted tissue or organ.

Hepatic Pertaining to the liver.

Heterotransplants A procedure in which an organ or tissue from one species is transplanted into the another species.

Homotransplants A procedure in which an organ or tissue is transplanted from one human to another.

Renal Pertaining to the kidney.

Tissue typing A blood test evaluating the match of tissues between the organ donor and the recipient.

the United States. UNOS keeps a waiting list of patients eligible for a transplant. This list is based solely on medical criteria, and there is a series of checks and balances to ensure this. A recipient must also match the donor's blood type and physical size.

UNOS attempts to match the organ with a recipient within the OPO's region. When no local match can be made, the coordinator must make arrangements for the organ to be delivered to another state. In either case, the procurement coordinator schedules an operating room for the removal of the organs and coordinates the surgery.

Once the organs have been removed and transported, a clinical transplant coordinator takes over. The clinical transplant coordinator has been involved in preparing the recipient for the new organ. He or she has arranged for the patient to be evaluated by transplant surgeons and has arranged for tests and procedures. The coordinator has also educated the patient about the transplant surgery, what to expect from transplantation, and how to care for the new organ. It is the clinical coordinator's job to see to the patient's needs before, during, and after the organ transplant. This involves admitting the patient, contacting the surgeon, arranging for an operating room, as well as contacting the anesthesiology department and the blood bank. After the transplant, the coordinator will help patients through their recovery and arrange for outpatient housing.

Another important aspect of the job of all transplant coordinators is educating the public about the importance of organ donation. Transplant coordinators speak to hospital and nursing school staffs and to the general public to encourage donation.

what is it like to be a transplant coordinator?

Julie Petro and Kathleen Ruping work for two different kinds of transplant centers. Julie is a procurement coordinator in Philadelphia and Kathleen is a clinical coordinator in Orlando.

Though Julie does spend time at her desk with paperwork and writing letters to donor's families, she says, "most of my time is not spent in the office; most of my time is spent in hospitals for procurement, or giving lectures." These lectures are to promote donor awareness among physicians, hospital administrators, and nurses.

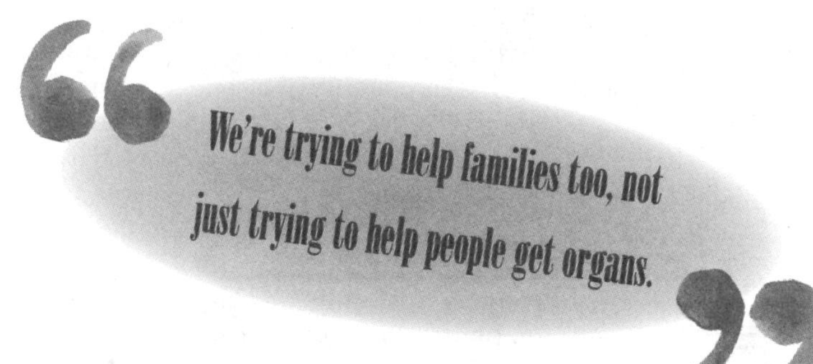

Julie emphasizes the importance of counseling families of organ donors. She says, "people don't understand how much of this job has to do with the families. Half of our training is in bereavement issues. We're trying to help families too, not just trying to help people get organs." Sometimes this involves staying in touch with the family long after the death of the organ donor and she remains available to answer the family's questions. Though she doesn't give out the actual names of the organ recipients, she does keep the donor families updated as to the recipient's health and progress.

After first talking to the family about donation and receiving the family's consent, Julie coordinates the organ donation. The patient, after being determined brain dead, stays on the ventilator so that blood and oxygen is still delivered to the organs. "I order the medications," Julie says, "the fluids, and all the tests necessary to determine if the organ can be transplanted." She then contacts UNOS for a list of patients in need of an organ. If a match is found in the local area, Julie calls the physicians of the recipient patient to offer them the organ. She then contacts the surgeons.

"Once I've placed all the organs," Julie says, "I set up operating room times and take the patient there." Sometimes there are five or six surgeons in the operating room at the same time, one for each donated organ. "I'm in charge of the OR, [operating room]...and of making sure they all do what they're supposed to do. I act as a liaison between the donor's family and the organ recipient. I make sure everything's done ethically, and arrange for optimal organ care."

After surgery, a technician who specializes in organ restoration will package the organ. Sometimes an organ is placed on a commercial airline; the life of a kidney is twenty-four to forty-eight hours outside a patient's body but a heart should be transplanted within four hours. Julie also responds to calls from OPOs across the country; if a patient in her area is to receive an organ from another state, Julie will schedule a jet and, with a surgeon, fly out to get the organ.

Kathleen Ruping works with the recipients of organs, preparing them for transplant surgery. She evaluates blood work and visits patients. She offers support and teaches patients how the transplant process works and how to care for a new organ. She also promotes donor awareness. "Transplants saves lives," she says. "We need more donors."

Kathleen usually arrives at the Translife clinic at 7:00 AM. She starts her day by typing up blood labels for patients before the clinic opens at 8:00 AM. "We have anywhere from two to twenty patients each day," she says. She draws blood from the patient, reviews medications, and discusses any problems that the patient may have. She then sends the blood to the lab.

At 9:30 AM, Kathleen completes the lab work. She puts the completed work in charts for the physicians, then goes with the physician to visit the patients. By noon the clinic is closed and Kathleen returns to her desk to do paperwork. At this time she may interview new patients to see if they fit transplant criteria.

There are two different settings for Kathleen's work: the office and the hospital. "In the office," she says, "I'm evaluating patients, and I'm responsible for getting a patient to see a physician. Any testing is done through us." It is in the hospital where she does the physical evaluation of patients. "And if they have a new transplant," she says, "I teach them how to care for their kidney."

Kathleen works more regular hours than Julie. Kathleen has a schedule of Monday through Friday, 7:00 to 3:30, and is on call every fifth weekend. Julie may work fifty to seventy hours a week.

FYI

There are 25 different organs and tissues in the human body capable of being transplanted.

have I got what it takes to be a transplant coordinator?

A transplant coordinator must pay close attention to many different details at once. Coordinators must be well-organized and efficient and also be able to work quickly. The work isn't just careful planning and scheduling. Because coordinators work with families suffering the loss of a loved one, or with sick patients needing an organ transplant, they must be caring and compassionate.

"You should be very detail-oriented," Julie Petro says, "but relaxed. You can't be stressed about everything. You're dealing with people's lives, so there's no room for mistakes." It's also important to maintain perspective. "If you're not dedicated to saving people's lives through transplant," she says, "you'll lose sight of what you're doing and why you're working so hard."

It's easy for Julie to keep a good perspective because she knows she's saving people's lives and helping families through difficult times. "I've been known to sit and talk with a family of a donor for six to seven hours to help them through things," she says. But this time commitment can also be frustrating. "You can be out all night, sleep for six hours, then your beeper goes off and you have to go back to work." This makes for a certain amount of unpredictability; Julie doesn't always know where she'll be going from day to day. "But it's nice to go to several different hospitals. You meet lots of people...CEOs, nurses, physicians."

A transplant coordinator must also be prepared to deal with death on a daily basis. "Every death in the area must be called into us," says Julie, "then we determine suitability. We may get a hundred calls a day."

Both Julie and Kathleen stress the importance of standing their ground with physicians. A procurement coordinator must make sure that orders are taken by the physicians who may have gone on to deal with their living patients. "They stop focusing on the donor patient," Julie says, though many things must be done to keep the organs working until surgery.

Kathleen Ruping also must make demands for her patients who are to receive the organs. "I'm not afraid to get yelled at by doctors at two or three in the morning," she says. "I stand up for my patients. The best care is my concern." But the stresses of the job are made easier by the people she works with. "There are always other coordinators available," she says, "so I can bounce ideas off them."

Kathleen emphasizes the importance of good organization skills as well as compassion and intelligence. "I learn new things every day," she says. "I'm always amazed at what the body can do."

To be a successful transplant coordinator you should

- Be able to pay close attention to details
- Have good communication skills
- Be well-organized and efficient
- Have a compassionate personality
- Be able to work quickly and accurately
- Be a persuasive speaker

how do I become a transplant coordinator?

Transplant coordinators come from a variety of backgrounds, though a medical background is most beneficial. Julie Petro received a bachelor's degree in nursing from the University of Delaware. She became familiar with transplants while working for four years in a children's hospital; she then worked for a year in Switzerland, helping a pediatric surgeon set up a hospital. Kathleen Ruping received her diploma in nursing from the Albany Medical Center, a teaching hospital. Neither Julie nor Kathleen are certified, but both plan to take the test in the coming months.

education

High School

The courses that will prepare you for a medical-based education will be the most valuable. Science courses such as biology and chemistry are important, as are courses in psychology or sociology. You should also take math courses and courses in health and physical education.

If you live near a transplant center, there may be volunteer opportunities available at the center or in an outpatient care home for transplant recipients. Your local Red Cross also needs volunteers for promoting donor awareness.

Postsecondary Training

There is no specific educational track for transplant coordinators. One transplant coordinator may focus on financing and insurance, while another on education and awareness. Another coordinator may perform physical tests and evaluations, while another counsels grieving families. The more experience and education with health care and medicine you have, the better your job opportunities. Though a nursing degree isn't required of all coordinators, it does give you a good medical background. A bachelor's degree in one of the sciences, along with experience in a medical setting, will also open up job opportunities for you. Some people working as coordinators also have master's degrees in public health, or in business administration, and other coordinators even hold doctorates in psychology or social work.

certification or licensing

Certification, though not required, is available through the American Board of Transplant Coordinators. To qualify for certification an applicant must have already completed a year of full-time work as a coordinator.

There are two separate tests given; one for clinical transplant coordinators and one for procurement transplant coordinators. The test covers all organs, and asks questions about analysis, treatment, and education of patients.

who will hire me?

A number of different institutions and organizations require transplant coordinators. In addition to the 281 transplant centers across the country, there are fifty-six independent organ procurement organizations and fifty-six independent tissue typing labs. There are also twelve organ procurement organizations and a hundred tissue typing labs within the transplant centers themselves. These organizations and centers may be hospital-based, independent, or university-based.

Positions for transplant coordinators are advertised nationally in medical publications and on the Internet. The North American Transplant Coordinators Organization (NATCO) also offers job referral information.

where can I go from here?

Kathleen Ruping is very happy in her current position, though she would like to become more involved in the transplantation of organs other than kidneys. Julie Petro would be interested in moving into a clinical coordinator position. "Being on call is a little easier to deal with," she says. However, within the OPO where she works, there is an internal clinical ladder. She could eventually move up into a senior coordinator position, which would involve less on-call duties and more internal education and mentoring. There are also different manager positions, and positions that focus entirely on education.

A coordinator may also head committees and special programs within a transplant center or professional organization. Some may also pursue degrees while working as a coordinator, either to help them in their work, or to move into another aspect of transplantation, such as surgery or hospital administration.

what are the salary ranges?

Your educational background, experience, and responsibilities as a coordinator will determine your salary. Someone with a doctorate may be responsible for directing and developing a program; someone with a master's degree may handle records or coordinate education and public awareness programs within the transplant center, or may work as an instructor. These people may have a higher salary than those working at the clinical end.

Most transplant coordinators are registered nurses and have average weekly earnings of $680. The average annual salary is about $30,000, with some nurses making more than $50,000 a year. Nurses working on the east and west coasts will make more money than those in the Midwest. Though transplant centers and organ procurement agencies are non-profit organizations, transplant coordinators receive very good health and retirement benefits.

what is the job outlook?

The medical community must become even more dedicated to finding organ donors. The UNOS national patient waiting list contains thousands of people who have been evaluated and determined ready recipients for new organs. On the list, as of April, 1997, there were 35,637 registrations for a kidney transplant; 8,178 for a liver transplant; 3,811 for a heart transplant; and 2,398 for a lung transplant. There are also people waiting for other organ transplants or multiple transplants. These numbers can be contrasted with the numbers of transplants actually performed. In 1995 there were 10,892 kidney transplants, 3,925 liver transplants, and 2,361 heart transplants.

The number of organ donations increased only slightly from 1995 to 1996. Because there is still a shortage of donors, a number of organizations have been developed to promote organ donation, particularly among minorities. These education and public awareness programs are often run by transplant coordinators.

Because the stress level can run high, transplant coordinators have a high burnout rate. Also, for a procurement coordinator, the hours can be long and irregular. On the average, procurement coordinators move on to other positions after only eighteen months. This means continued job opportunities for those looking to work as coordinators.

how do I learn more?

professional organizations

The following are organizations that provide information on a career as a transplant coordinator and the certification process.

in-depth

A Little History

Scientists have been researching human and animal organ transplantation since the 18th century. A technique for grafting human tissues was developed in 1875 by Jacques Reverdin, a Swiss surgeon. In 1905 Alexis Carrel, a French surgeon, developed a way to connect blood vessels that allowed a transplanted organ to function. That year also marked the first successful corneal transplant.

Greater research led to refinements in transplant technology and in 1954 the first successful human kidney transplant occurred, in Boston.

The 1960's brought many successes in the field of organ transplants, including successful human liver and pancreas transplants. A headline-grabbing transplant occurred in 1967, when Dr Christiaan Barnard, a South African surgeon, performed the world's first successful heart transplant in Cape Town, South Africa. His achievement became known throughout the world.

Despite these successes, many transplants eventually failed because of the body's immune system—its natural defense against foreign objects. The body of the organ recipient would eventually reject the new organ as a "foreign object." This was especially true of transplants that involved complex tissues, including hearts and kidneys. Early attempts at "overriding" the body's immune system, including high doses of radiation, had limited success.

Drugs that were designed to help the body accept transplanted organs were beginning to be developed in the 1960's. It was not until the early 1980's, however, with the introduction of *cyclosporin,* that a truly effective "immunosuppressant" drug was available. The new drug substantially improved the success rate of transplant surgeries. Also increasing the success rate was more precise tissue typing, or matching of donor and recipient tissues.

Though successful organ transplants have increased, some transplants still fail over time, despite modern drug treatments and closer matches of tissue. Research in this area continues to be done with the hope of continually increasing the rate of successful transplants.

American Board of Transplant Coordinators
PO Box 15384
Lenexa, KS 66285
TEL: 913-599-0198

North American Transplant Coordinators Organization
PO Box 15384
Lenexa, KS 66285
TEL: 913-492-3600

bibliography

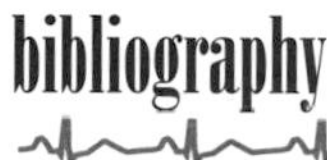

Following is a sampling of materials relating to the professional concerns and development of transplant coordinators.

Books

Hackel, Emanual, Sally Swenson, James AuBuchon, and Douglas Smith. *Advances in Transplantation.* Bethesda, MD: American Association of Blood Banks, 1993.

Kittredge, Mary. *Organ Transplants*. New York, NY: Chelsea House, 1989.

Schmitz, Cecilia, and Richard A. Gray, editors. *The Gift of Life: Organ and Tissue Transplantation: an Introduction to Issues and Information Sources*. Ann Arbor, MI: Pierian Press, 1993.

Sher, Linda, and Leonard Makowka. *Ortho Handbook of Organ Transplantation.* Austin, TX: R.G. Landes Co., 1995.

Youngner, Stuart J., Renee C. Fox, and Laurence J. O'Connell, editors. *Organ Transplantation: Meanings and Realities*. Madison, WI: University of Wisconsin Press, 1996.

Periodicals

Journal of Heart and Lung Transplantation. Bimonthly. Latest information on heart and heart-lung transplantation. International Society for Heart Transplantation, Mosby, 11830 Westline Industrial Drive, St. Louis, MO 63146. 314-872-8370, 800-325-4177.

Journal of Transplant Coordination. 3 per year. Includes clinical articles addressing transplantation issues. North American Transplant Coordinators Organization, Box 15384, Lenexa, KS 66285, 913-492-3600.

Liver Transplantation and Surgery. Bimonthly. Discusses surgical techniques, clinical investigations, and drug research in the subspecialties of liver transplantation and surgery. American Association for the Study of Liver Diseases, W.B. Saunders Co., Curtis Center, 3rd Floor, Independence Square West, Philadelphia, PA 19106, 215-238-7800.

Transplantation. Semimonthly. Publishes original papers and abstracts from pertinent specialities: immunology, hematology, endocrinology, and embryology. Transplantation Society, Williams & Wilkins, 428 E. Preston Street, Baltimore, MD 21202, 410-528-4000, 800-638-6423.

Transplantation Proceedings. Bimonthly. Includes reviews and original reports in current problems in transplantation biology and medicine. Transplantation Society, Appleton & Lange, Journal Division, 25 Van Zant Street, Box 5630, Norwalk CT 06856, 203-838-4400.

Transplantation Reviews. Quarterly. Contains review articles on the latest developments in both clinical and experimental transplantation surgery. W.B. Saunders Co., Curtis Center, 3rd Floor, Independence Square West, Philadelphia, PA 19106, 215-238-7800.

urologist

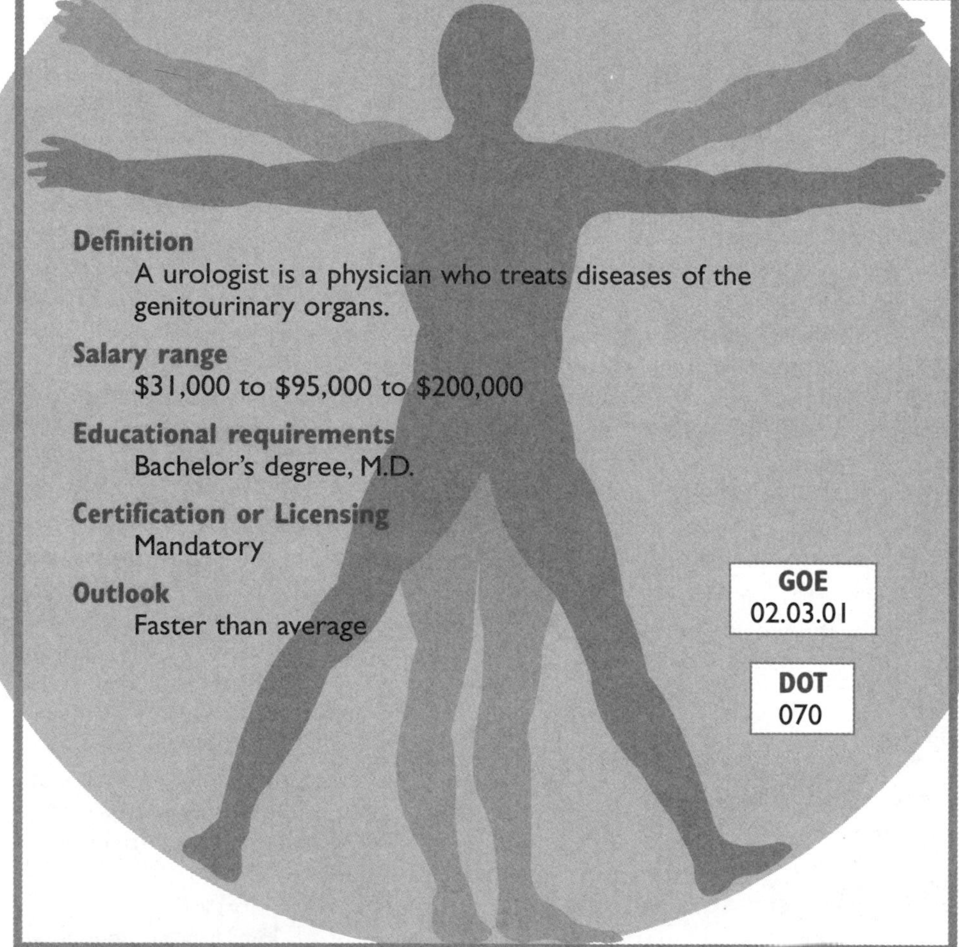

Definition
A urologist is a physician who treats diseases of the genitourinary organs.

Salary range
$31,000 to $95,000 to $200,000

Educational requirements
Bachelor's degree, M.D.

Certification or Licensing
Mandatory

Outlook
Faster than average

GOE
02.03.01

DOT
070

High School Subjects

Biology
Chemistry
Physics
Mathematics

Personal Interests

Scientific curiosity
Helping others
Solving problems

"Everybody ready?" the urologist asks the members of his surgical team. He walks over and looks down at the patient, whose tiny body is lying on the operating table. She is turned on her side to give the surgeon access to her kidneys, which are growing outside her body.

Her name is Heidi Lynn and she's three days old. The urologist is about to move her kidneys back inside her body where they belong. He glances over his shoulder at the room where Heidi Lynn's parents watch anxiously. "Okay, Heidi girl, let's do it."

Several hours later, the parents look in on their daughter. Sutures line her delicate, pink skin where it's not covered by bandages, and tubes seem to spring from all over her tiny body. But her parents are smiling as they hold onto each other.

what does a urologist do?

Urologists treat medical and surgical disorders of the adrenal gland and of the genitourinary system. They deal with diseases of both the male and female urinary tract and of the male reproductive organs.

Technically, urology is a surgical subspecialty, but because of the broad range of clinical problems they treat, urologists also have a working knowledge of internal medicine, pediatrics, gynecology, and other specialties.

Common medical disorders that urologists routinely treat include prostate cancer, testicular cancer, bladder cancer, stone disease, urinary tract infections, urinary incontinence, and impotence. Other, less common, disorders include kidney cancer, renal (kidney) disease, male infertility, genitourinary trauma, and sexually transmitted diseases (including AIDS).

The management and treatment of malignant diseases constitute much of the urologist's practice. Prostate cancer is the most common cancer in men, and the second leading cause of cancer deaths in men. In 1996, the Prostate Health Council estimated that more than 315,000 American men will develop prostate cancer, and more than 40,000 men will die of it. If detected early, prostate cancer is treatable, but once it has spread beyond the prostate, it is difficult to treat successfully.

Testicular cancer is the leading cause of cancer in young men between the ages of fifteen and thirty-four. Major advances in the treatment of this cancer, involving both surgery and chemotherapy, now make it the most curable of all cancers. Bladder cancer occurs most frequently in men age seventy and older, and treatment for it also has a high success rate.

Young and middle-aged adults are primarily affected by stone diseases, which represent the third leading cause of hospitalizations in the United States. Kidney stones, composed of a combination of calcium and either oxalate or phosphate, usually pass through the body with urine. Larger stones, however, can block the flow of urine or irritate the lining of the urinary system as they pass. What has become standard treatment today is called extracorporeal shock wave lithotripsy (ESWL). In ESWL, high-energy shock waves are used to pulverize the stones into small fragments that are carried from the body in the urine. This procedure has replaced invasive, open surgery as the preferred treatment for stone disease.

Urologists also consult on spina bifida cases in children and multiple sclerosis cases in adults, as these diseases involve neuromuscular dysfunctions that affect the kidneys, bladder, and genitourinary systems.

The scope of urology has broadened so much that the following are now considered subspecialties: *pediatric urology*, *urologic oncology*, and *female urology*.

lingo to learn

Bladder A membranous sac that serves as a receptacle for fluid or gas, often used to describe the urinary bladder in humans.

Endoscope An instrument used to examine the interior of a hollow structure, such as the bladder.

Extracorporeal shock wave lithotripsy High-energy shock waves that pulverize kidney stones into small fragments so they can easily pass through the urinary system.

Kidneys A pair of organs that filter the blood, excreting the waste products of body metabolism in the form of urine.

Percutaneous Performed through the skin, such as the removal of tissues for a biopsy.

Ureter A duct that carries urine away from the kidney to the bladder.

what is it like to be a urologist?

"As a urologist, you're involved with people, instead of staying in a lab all the time," says Dr. William Kennedy. Dr. Kennedy, who happens to be a talented chef as well as a urologist, originally intended to go to cooking school. As he tells it, however, he was destined for other things. "My parents convinced me to go to college, which I didn't want to do. I ended up enjoying school, especially the science courses. At the end of college, I knew I wanted to do something fulfilling, and helping people regain their health was a good way to accomplish that."

Dr. Kennedy is currently a Fellow in Pediatric Urology at Children's Hospital of Philadelphia, where he will spend one year in clinical practice and another year in research. Dr. Kennedy says he chose urology for a very specific reason.

"I wanted a specialty where I could enjoy the continuity of care for all of my patients—from surgery to follow-up care and, in some cases, long-term postoperative care. And I liked the fact that I could be working with both adults and children, in both medicine and surgery."

One of the reasons medicine may have been in the back of his mind all along has to do with his brother. "He had a Ewing sarcoma, a tumor of the leg," explains Dr. Kennedy. "He was a patient for ten years at Sloan-Kettering. I know my exposure to the doctors there had something to do with why I'm now in medicine. I saw the science being brought to the patient's bedside, and it was exciting and inspiring."

He describes his work in pediatric urology as covering a range of problems of the kidney, bladder, and the genitourinary system. "Pediatric urology deals with everything from simple infections to complicated cancers and reconstruction," explains Dr. Kennedy. "We treat cancer with medications or radiation, or we remove it."

"Reconstructive cases involve rebuilding. Children are often born with congenital abnormalities; their bladders are exposed to the outside skin, or there are blockages in the renal collecting system—the kidney's plumbing, so to speak."

Children can also have kidney stones, and a pediatric urologist uses sound waves to break the stones up. This process is the same as the one performed on adults, but special care must be given to the child with kidney stones.

The typical pediatric exam consists of an abdominal exam and a kidney exam, in which the urologist is feeling for lumps or bumps in the abdomen, pain or pressure when pressing on the bladder.

In treating children, urologists want to minimize radiation exposure, so they use more ultrasound than X rays in diagnostic procedures and treatments.

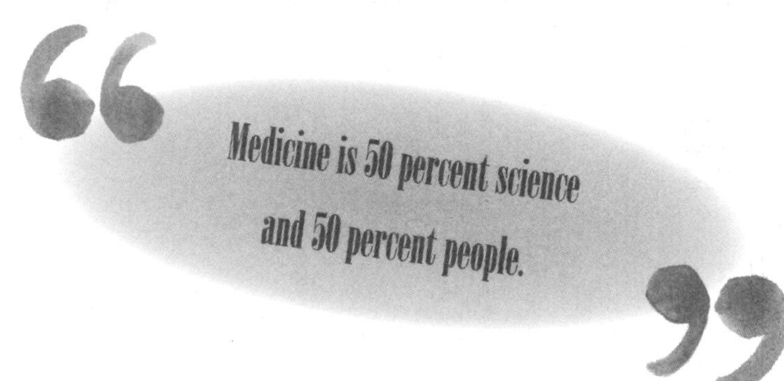

have I got what it takes to be a urologist?

Urologists should like working with people, and have a strong interest in promoting good health through preventative measures such as diet and exercise. "Medicine is 50 percent science and 50 percent people," says Dr. William Kennedy. "You have to maintain an active interest in the things people do. It helps you relate."

The urologist diagnoses and treats conditions of a very personal nature. Many patients are uncomfortable talking about problems relating to their kidneys, bladder, or genitourinary system. The urologist must show compassion and sensitivity to dispel the patient's fears and put him or her at ease.

Excellent communication skills are essential to patient-physician encounters. Urologists should be able to clearly articulate both the patient's problem and the recommended forms of treatment, including all of the options and their attendant risks and advantages.

Because of their frequent consultations with other physicians, urologists need to develop good working relationships with other medical specialists.

Urologists, like all surgeons, should be in good physical condition; they must remain steady and focused while standing for hours on their feet. Urologists who work in hospital trauma units should be prepared for the frenetic pace and tension of split-second decision making.

how do I become a urologist?

education

High School

High school students should take courses in biology, chemistry, physics, and mathematics. Courses in computer science are also recommended. Since colleges and medical schools are looking for individuals with well-rounded backgrounds, you should also take English, foreign languages, and history. Many colleges and universities that have medical schools offer special programs to high school seniors planning to attend medical school.

Postsecondary Training

In order to become a urologist, you must first graduate from an accredited four-year college or university. College courses that help prepare students for medical school are math, biology, chemistry, anatomy, and physics, as well as courses in the humanities.

After receiving an undergraduate degree, you must then be accepted by one of the 141 medical schools in the United States. Most premed students apply to several schools early in their senior year of college. Admission is competitive; only about one-third of the applicants are accepted. Applicants must undergo a fairly extensive admissions process which considers grade point averages, scores on the Medical College Admission Test (MCAT), and recommendations from professors.

In order to earn an M.D. degree, students must complete four years of medical school. For the first two years, students attend lectures and classes and spend time in laboratories.

Courses include anatomy, biochemistry, physiology, pharmacology, psychology, microbiology, pathology, and medical ethics. Students learn to take patient histories and perform routine physical examinations.

In their third and fourth years, students work in clinics and hospitals. They go through what are known as rotations, or brief periods of study in a particular area, such as internal medicine, obstetrics and gynecology, pediatrics, dermatology, psychiatry, or surgery.

Rotations allow students to gain exposure to the many different fields of medicine and to learn firsthand the skills of diagnosing and treating patients. In fact, many physicians credit the rotation program for helping them choose their area or specialty. "I know I would never have thought about urology if not for the rotations. I really enjoyed my rotation in urology," Dr. Kennedy says.

Upon graduating from an accredited medical school, physicians must pass a standard examination given by the National Board of Medical Examiners. Most physicians complete an internship. The internship is usually one year in length, and helps graduates decide what will be their area of specialization.

Following the internship, physicians begin what is known as a residency. Individuals wishing to pursue the surgical specialty of urology must complete a five- or six-year residency in urology, of which the first two years are typically spent in general surgery, followed by three to four years of urology in an approved residency program. Currently, there are 116 approved residency programs.

Many urologic residency training programs are six years in length, with the final year spent in either research or additional clinical training, depending on the orientation of the program and the resident's focus. The residency years, without a doubt, are filled with stress, pressure, and physical labor. Residents often work twenty-four-hour shifts, easily clocking in eighty hours or more per week.

FYI

Bladder cancer is the fourth most common form of cancer in men and the ninth most common in women. Each year, there are more that 50,000 new cases of bladder cancer, accounting for seven percent of all new cancers found in men and two percent in women. Nearly 10,000 Americans die each year of bladder cancer.

certification or licensing

At an early point in the residency period, all students are required to pass a medical licensing examination administered by the board of medical examiners in each state. The length of the residency depends on the specialty chosen.

Certification requires the successful completion of a qualifying written examination, which must be taken within three years of completing the residency in urology. The subsequent certifying examination, which consists of pathology, uroradiology, and a standardized oral examination, must be taken within five years of the qualifying examination. Certification by the American Board of Urology is for a ten-year period, with recertification required after that time.

scholarships and grants

Scholarships and grants are often available from individual institutions, state agencies, and special-interest organizations. The book *Dollars for College: Medicine, Dentistry, and Related Fields* by Ferguson Publishing is an excellent source for this information. Many students finance their medical education through the Armed Forces Health Professions Scholarship Program. Each branch of the military participates in this program, paying students' tuitions in exchange for military service. Contact your local recruiting office for more information on this program. The National Health Service Corps Scholarship Program also provides money for students in return for service. Another source for financial aid, scholarship, and grant information is the Association of American Medical Colleges. Remember to request information early for eligibility, application requirements, and deadlines.

Association of American Medical Colleges
2450 N Street, NW
Washington, DC 20037
TEL: 202-828-0400
WEBSITE: http://www.aamc.org
Specific information on financial aid programs can be found at:
WEBSITE: http://www.aamc.org/stuapps/finaid

To be a successful urologist, you should:

- Have good hand-eye coordination and manual dexterity
- Be a good clinician
- Be able to put patients at ease and comfortably discuss intimate areas of health
- Enjoy helping and working with people
- Be able to listen and communicate well

Ferguson Publishing Company
200 West Madison, Suite 300
Chicago, IL 60606
TEL: 312-580-5480

National Health Services Corps Scholarship Program
U.S. Public Health Service
1010 Wayne Avenue, Suite 240
Silver Spring, MD 20910
TEL: 800-638-0824

who will hire me ?

The vast majority of urologists enter into clinical practice after completing their residency program. However, fellowships exist in various subspecialties, including pediatrics, infertility, sexual dysfunction, oncology, transplantation, and others.

Academic medicine also offers opportunities. The American Urological Association (AUA) is fostering the development of AUA scholars, hoping to encourage residents to enter academic medicine.

what are the salary ranges?

The national average salary for first-year residents in the mid-1990's was approximately $31,000. That average increased to $41,800 by the final residency year. Salaries will vary depending on the kind of residency, the hospital, and the geographic area.

According to surveys by the American Medical Association, practitioners of internal medicine in the mid-1990's had a salary range of approximately $95,000 to $200,000. The median income was about $130,000. These figures are for all doctors of internal medicine, and income for urologists may vary from these numbers. Other factors that influence annual income include size and type of practice, hours worked per week, professional reputation of the individual, and the geographic location.

what is the job outlook?

Employment prospects for urologists are good. While an oversupply of all specialists is predicted through the year 2000, the rate at which new urologists are entering practice is decelerating—a clear indication that the projected oversupply is not as great in urology as perhaps it will be in other fields.

Finally, the demographics of American society illustrate that the increase in the aging population will increase demand for services that cater, in large part, to them. With baby boomers aging, the need for qualified urologists will continue well into and beyond the year 2000.

how do I learn more?

professional organizations

For additional information on becoming a urologist, contact the following:

American Medical Association
515 North State Street
Chicago, IL 60610
TEL: 312-464-5000
WEBSITE: http://www.ama-assn.org

American Board of Urology
31700 Telegraph Road, Suite 150
Bingham Farms, MI 48025
TEL: 810-646-9720
WEBSITE: http://www.surgeon.org

American Urological Association, Inc.
1120 North Charles Street
Baltimore, MD 21201
TEL: 410-727-1100
WEBSITE: http://www.auanet.org

bibliography

Following is a sampling of materials relating to the professional concerns and development of urologists.

Books

Bullock, Nigel, Gary Sibley, and Robert Whitaker. *Essential Urology,* 2nd edition. New York, NY: Churchill Livingstone, 1994.

Murphy, William M. *Urological Pathology,* 2nd edition. Philadelphia, PA: W.B. Saunders Co., 1997.

Rous, Stephen N. *Urology: a Core Textbook,* 2nd edition. Cambridge, MA: Blackwell Science, 1996.

Periodicals

Contemporary Urology. Monthly. For office- and hospital-based urologists. Includes news and features on solving clinical problems. Medical Economics, Five Paragon Drive, Montvale NJ 07645, 201-358-7208.

Journal of Urology. Monthly. Publishes clinical papers, commentary, research, and new techniques for the urologist. American Urological Association, Williams & Wilkins, 428 E. Preston Street, Baltimore, MD 21202, 410-528-4000, 800-638-6423.

Techniques in Urology. Quarterly. Provides expert guidance on the most advanced procedures for the treatment of urologic disorders. Lippincott-Raven Publishers, 227 E. Washington Square, Philadelphia, PA 19106, 215-238-4200.

DOT index

This index lists health care careers by their *Dictionary of Occupational Titles* (fourth edition, revised 1991) groups. The group number and title are given, followed by a description of the classification. Chapter titles are listed under the appropriate group in alphabetical order, followed by their DOT number (when applicable). Page references to *Exploring Health Care Careers* are given in bold, following the DOT number.

019 occupations in architecture, engineering, and surveying, not elsewhere classified

This group includes occupations, not elsewhere classified, concerned with the application of the theoretical and practical aspects of engineering and architecture.

022 occupations in chemistry

This group includes occupations concerned with research and development in the chemical and physical properties and compositional changes of substances. Specialization generally occurs in one or more branches of chemistry, such as organic chemistry, inorganic chemistry, physical chemistry and analytical chemistry. Chemistry specializations within the field of environmental control are also included here.

041 occupations in biological sciences

This group includes occupations concerned with research in the reproduction, growth and development, structure, life processes, behavior, and classification of living organisms and the application of findings to the prevention of disease in the maintenance and promotion of health in plant and animal life. Also includes investigations into economic utilization, environmental impact, or harmful aspects of specific animals and plants.

045 occupations in psychology

This group includes occupations concerned with the collection, interpretation, and application of scientific data relating to human behavior and mental processes. Activities are in either applied fields of psychology or in basic science fields and research.

070 physicians and surgeons

This group includes occupations concerned with diagnosis, prevention, and treatment of diseases and injuries; and research in the causes, transmission, and control of diseases and other ailments.

071 osteopaths

This group includes occupations concerned with the application of manipulative procedures in treating patients, in addition to the other accepted methods of medical care. Includes diagnosis, prevention, and treatment of diseases and injuries; research in the causes, transmission, and control of disease and other ailments.

072 dentists

This group includes occupations concerned with examinations, diagnosis, prevention, and treatment of ailments or abnormalities of gums, jaws, soft tissue, and teeth. Includes oral surgery.

074 pharmacists

This group includes occupations concerned with compounding prescriptions of physicians, dentists, and other practitioners; and the bulk selection, compounding, dispensing, and preservation of drugs and medicines.

075 registered nurses

This group includes occupations concerned with administering nursing care to the ill or injured. Includes nursing administration and instruction; and public health, industrial, private duty, and surgical nursing. Licensing or registration is required.

076 therapists

This group includes occupations concerned with the treatment and rehabilitation of persons with physical or mental disabilities or disorders, to develop or restore functions, prevent loss of physical capacities, and maintain optimum performance. Includes occupations utilizing means, such as exercise, massage, heat, light, water, electricity, and specific therapeutic apparatus, usually as prescribed by a physician; or participation in medically oriented rehabilitative programs, including educational, occupational, and recreational activities.

077 dietitians

This group includes occupations concerned with the application of the principles of nutrition to plan and supervise the preparation and serving of meals. Includes planning menus and diets for special nutritional requirements; participating in research; or instructing in the field of nutrition.

078 occupations in medical and dental technology

This group includes occupations concerned with the application of technical knowledge in fields of medicine or dentistry for examination and treatment of patients or for research. Occupations occur in a doctor's or dentist's office, hospital, or laboratory.

079 occupations in medicine and health, not elsewhere classified

This group includes occupations, not elsewhere classified, concerned with the health care of humans or animals.

120 clergy

This group includes occupations concerned with serving spiritual needs of congregation members, usually as a minister, priest, or rabbi. Includes delivering sermons, conducting services, administering religious rite, instructing prospective congregation members, and counseling members in need of spiritual advice.

141 commercial artists: designers and illustrators, graphic arts

This group includes occupations concerned with designing and executing artwork to promote public consumption of materials, products, or services; influences others in their opinions of individuals or organizations; or illustrate and adorn subject matter. Includes preparing animated cartoons.

Medical Illustrator 141.061-026, **397**

143 occupations in photography

This group includes occupations concerned with photographing people, events, fictionalized scenes, materials, and products with still or motion-picture cameras. Includes conceiving artistic photographic effects and arranging and preparing subject matter.

Medical Photographer 143.362-010, **397**

168 inspectors and investigators, managerial and public service

This group includes occupations concerned with examining the condition of person, plants, and animals; the quality of consumer products and services; and the operations of establishments, serving in the capacity of a governmental or private inspector or investigator in order to verify compliance with and enforcement of regulatory laws, health, and safety laws, or the establishment's quality standards.

Occupational and Safety Health Worker 168.167-062, **511**

187 service industry managers and officials

This group includes managerial positions concerned with hotels and other lodging places; establishments providing personal, business, repair and amusement services; medical, legal engineering, and other professional services; nonprofit membership organizations, and other miscellaneous services.

Health Care Manager 187.117-010, **305**

195 occupations in social and welfare work

This group includes occupations concerned with rendering assistance to individuals and groups with problems, such as poverty, illness, family maladjustment, antisocial behavior, financial mismanagement, limited recreation opportunities, and inadequate housing.

Human Services Worker 195.367-010, **351**
Social Worker 195.107-030, **813**

276 sales occupations, medical and scientific equipment and supplies

This group includes occupations concerned with selling dental, medical, veterinary, and ophthalmic equipment and supplies, such as surgical instruments, dental tools, eyeglasses, hearing aids, orthopedic appliances, artificial limbs, and related hospital supplies.

Pedorthist 276.257-018, **631**

299 miscellaneous sales occupations, not elsewhere classified

This group includes occupations, not elsewhere classified, concerned with sales transactions.

Dispensing Optician 299.361-010,**199**

334 masseurs and related occupations

This group includes occupations concerned with giving massages to patrons of public baths, beauty parlors, reducing salons, or health clubs, using hands or vibrating equipment.

Massage Therapist 334.374-010, **375**

354 unlicensed birth attendants and practical nurses

This group includes occupations concerned with bathing patients, taking and recording pulse and temperature readings, giving injections, assisting women in childbirth, caring for and feeding infants, giving first aid, and performing similar routine nursing tasks. Knowledge is acquired primarily through practical experience. Licensed practical nursing occupations are included in group 079.

Home Health Aide 354.377-014, **327**

355 attendants, hospitals, morgues, and related health services

This group includes occupations concerned with attending to the physical comfort, safety, and appearance of patients; performing routine menial tasks; and assisting in conducting occupational and physical therapy.

Nurse Assistant 355.674-014, **481**

359 miscellaneous personal service occupations

This group includes occupations, not elsewhere classified, concerned with personal services.

Child Life Specialist 359. 677-010, **75**

712 occupations in fabrication and repair of surgical, medical, and dental instruments and supplies

This group includes occupations concerned with fabricating and repairing dental, medical, surgical, ophthalmic, and veterinary instruments, apparatus, and supplies, other than electrical used by those in the professions, laboratories, and schools; orthopedic, prosthetic, and surgical appliances and supplies, such as arch supports and other foot appliances, fracture appliances, elastic hosiery, abdominal supporters, braces, trusses, bandages, surgical gauze and dressing, adhesive tapes and medicated plasters, and personal safety appliances and equipment; artificial teeth and dental metals, alloys, and amalgams.

Dental Laboratory Technician 712.381-018, **139**

Orthotic and Prosthetic Technician 712.381-034/038, **587**

716 occupations in fabrication and repair of engineering and scientific instruments and equipment, not elsewhere classified

This group includes occupations concerned with grinding, polishing, and coating optical lenses, reflectors, filters, and prisms and ophthalmic eyeglass sunglass, and contact lenses.

Optics Technician 716.382-018, **555**

GOE index

This index lists health care careers by their *Guide for Occupational Exploration* (1979) interest areas, work groups, and subgroups. The interest area number and title are given, followed by a description of the classification; the work group number and title are given, followed by a description of the classification; and finally, the subgroup number and title are given, followed by job titles listed in alphabetical order. Page references to specific chapters in *Exploring Health Care Careers* are given in bold, following the job title.

01 artistic

An interest in creative expression of feelings or ideas. You can satisfy this interest in several of the creative or performing arts fields. You may enjoy literature. Perhaps writing or editing would appeal to you. You may prefer to work in the performing arts. You could direct or perform in drama, music, or dance. You may enjoy the visual arts. You could become a critic of painting, sculpture, or ceramics. You may want to use your hands to create or decorate products. Or you may prefer to model clothes or develop acts for entertainment.

01.02 visual arts

Workers in this group create original works of art or do commercial art work, using such techniques as drawing, painting, photographing, and sculpting to express or interpret ideas or to illustrate various written materials. Some visual artists design products, settings, or graphics (such as advertisements or book covers), and oversee the work of other artists or craftsmen who produce or install them. Others teach art, or appraise or restore paintings and other fine art objects. Advertising agencies, printing and publishing firms, television and motion picture studios, museums and restoration laboratories employ visual artists. They also work for manufacturers and in retail and wholesale trade. Many are self-employed, operating their own commercial art studios or doing free-lance work.

01.02.03 commercial art

02 scientific

An interest in discovering, collecting, and analyzing information about the natural world and applying scientific research findings to problems in medicine, the life sciences, and the natural sciences.

You can satisfy this interest by working with the knowledge and processes of the sciences. You may enjoy researching and developing new knowledge in mathematics. Perhaps solving problems in the physical or life sciences would appeal to you. You may wish to study medicine and help humans or animals. You could work as a practitioner in the health field. You may want to work with scientific equipment and procedures. You could seek a job in research or testing laboratories.

02.02 life sciences

Workers in this group are concerned mostly with living things such as plants and animals. They conduct research and do experiments to expand man's knowledge of living things. Some may work on problems related to how the environment affects plant and animal life. Others may study causes of disease and ways to control disease. These workers are usually employed in the research facilities of hospitals, government agencies, industries, or universities.

02.02.01 animal specialization

02.02.03 plant and animal specialization

02.03 medical sciences

Workers in this group are involved in the prevention, diagnosis, and treatment of human and animal diseases, disorders, or injuries. It is common to specialize in specific kinds of illnesses, or special areas or organs of the body. Workers who prefer to be more general may become general practitioners, family practitioners, or may learn to deal with groups of related medical problems. A wide variety of work environments is available to medical workers ranging from large city hospitals and clinics, to home offices in rural areas, to field clinics in the military or in underdeveloped countries.

02.03.01 medicine and surgery

02.03.02 dentistry

02.03.04 health specialities

02.04 laboratory technology

Workers in this group use special laboratory techniques and equipment to perform tests in the fields of chemistry, biology, or physics. They record information that results from their experiments and tests. They help scientists, medical doctors, researchers, and engineers in their work. Hospitals, government agencies, universities, and private industries employ these workers in their laboratories and research facilities.

02.04.01 physical sciences

02.04.02 life sciences

05 mechanical

An interest in applying mechanical principles to practical situations using machines, hand tools, or techniques. You can satisfy this interest in a variety of jobs ranging from routine to complex professional positions. You may enjoy working with ideas about things (objects). You could seek a job in engineering or in a related technical field. You may prefer to deal directly with things. You could find a job in the crafts or trades, building, making or repairing objects. You may like to drive or operate vehicles and special equipment. You may prefer routine or physical work in settings other than factories. Perhaps work in mining or construction would appeal to you. Some have their own engineering firms, and accept work from various individuals.

05.03 engineering technology

Workers in this group collect, record, and coordinate technical information in such activities as surveying, drafting, petroleum production, communications control, and materials scheduling. Workers find jobs in construction, factories, engineering and architectural firms, airports, and research laboratories.

05.03.05 electrical-electronic

05.05 craft technology

Workers in this group perform highly skilled hand and/or machine work requiring special techniques, training, and experience. Work occurs in a variety of nonfactory settings. Some workers own their own shops.

05.05.11 scientific, medical, and technical equipment fabrication and repair

05.05.17 food preparation

05.09 materials control

Workers in this group receive, store, and/or ship materials and products. Some estimate and order the quantities and kinds of materials needed. Others regulate and control the flow of materials to places in the plant where they are to be used. Most have to keep records. Jobs are found in institutions, industrial plants, and government agencies.

05.09.01 shipping, receiving, and stock checking

05.10 crafts

Workers in this group use hands and hand tools skillfully to fabricate, process, install, and/or repair materials, products, and/or structural parts. They follow established procedures and techniques. The jobs are not found in factories, but are in repair shops, garages.

05.10.01 structural

06 industrial

An interest in repetitive, concrete, organized activities in a factory setting. You can satisfy this interest by working in one of many industries that manufacture goods on a mass production basis. You may enjoy manual work—using your hands or hand tools. Perhaps you prefer to operate or take care of machines. You may like to inspect, sort, count, or weigh products. Using your training and experience to set up machines or supervise other workers may appeal to you.

06.02 production work

Workers in this group perform skilled hand and/or machine work to make products, usually in a factory setting.

06.02.08 machine work, stone, glass, and clay

Optics Technician **555**

07 business detail

An interest in organized, clearly defined activities requiring accuracy and attention to details, primarily in an office setting. You can satisfy this interest in a variety of jobs in which you can attend to the details of a business operation. You may enjoy using your math skills. Perhaps a job in billing, computing, or financial recordkeeping would satisfy you. You may prefer to deal with people. You may want a job in which you meet the public, talk on the telephone, or supervise other workers. You may like to operate computer terminals, typewriters, or bookkeeping machines. Perhaps a job in recordkeeping, filing, or recording would satisfy you. You may wish to use your training and experience to manage offices and supervise other workers.

07.05 records processing

Workers in this group prepare, review, maintain, route, distribute, and coordinate recorded information. They check records and schedules for accuracy. They may schedule the activities of people or the use of equipment. Jobs in this group are found in most businesses, institutions, and government agencies.

07.05.03 record preparation and maintenance

Medical Record Technician **429**

08 selling

An interest in bringing others to a point of view by personal persuasion, using sales and promotional techniques. You can satisfy this interest in a variety of sales jobs. You may enjoy selling technical products or services. Perhaps you prefer a selling job requiring less background knowledge. You may work in stores, sales offices, or in customers' homes. You may wish to buy and sell products to make a profit. You can also satisfy this interest in legal work, business negotiations, advertising, and related fields found under other categories in the Guide.

08.02 general sales

Workers in this group sell demonstrate, and solicit orders for products and services of many kinds. They are employed by retail and wholesale firms, manufacturers and distributors, business services, and non-profit organizations. Some spend all their time in a single location, such as a department store or automobile agency. Others call on businesses or individuals to sell products or services, or follow up on earlier sales.

08.02.02 retail

Pedorthist **631**

09 accommodating

An interest in catering to the wishes and needs of others, usually on a one-to-one basis. You can satisfy this interest by providing services for the convenience of others, such as hospitality services in hotels, restaurants, airplanes, etc. You may enjoy improving the appearance of others. Perhaps working in the hair and beauty care field would satisfy you. You may wish to provide personal services, such as taking tickets, carrying baggage, or ushering.

09.05

Workers in this group perform services that make life easier and more pleasant for people. They do things that people can't or don't want to do for themselves, like opening doors, delivering messages, carrying luggage and packages, and dishing up food. They find employment in a variety of settings, such as hotels, airports, golf courses, theaters, reducing salons, and gymnasiums.

09.05.01

Massage Therapist **375**

10 humanitarian

An interest in helping individuals with their mental, spiritual, social, physical, or vocational concerns. You can satisfy this interest by work in which caring for the welfare of others is important. Perhaps the spiritual or mental well-being of others concerns you. You could prepare for a job in religion or counseling. You may wish to help others with physical problems. You could work in the nursing, therapy, or rehabilitation fields.

10.01 social services

Workers in this group help people deal with their problems. They may work with one person at a time or with groups of people. Workers sometimes specialize in problems that are personal, social, vocational, physical, educational, or spiritual in nature. Schools, rehabilitation centers, mental health clinics, guidance centers, and churches employ these workers. Jobs are also found in public and private welfare and employment services, juvenile courts, and vocational rehabilitation programs.

10.01.01 religious

Hospice Chaplain **343**

10.01.02 counseling and social work

Genetic Counselor **291**
Rehabilitation Counselor **797**
Social Worker **813**

10.02 nursing, therapy, and specialized teaching

Workers in this group care for, treat, or train people to improve their physical and emotional well-being. Most workers in this group deal with sick, injured, or handicapped people. Some workers are involved in health education and sickness prevention. Hospitals, nursing homes, and rehabilitation centers hire workers in this group, as do schools, industrial plants, doctors' offices, and private homes. Some sports also have a need for workers in this group.

10.02.01 nursing

Anesthesiologist Assistant **25**
Clinical Nurse Specialist **91**
Licensed Practical Nurse **365**
Nurse Anesthetist **473**
Nurse-Midwife **487**
Nurse Practitioner **495**
Physician Assistant **699**
Registered Nurse **789**
Transplant Coordinator **863**

10.02.02 therapy and rehabilitation

Creative Arts Therapist **109**
Dental Hygienist **131**
Dialysis Technician **175**
Hypnotherapist **357**
Nuclear Medicine Technologist, **465**
Occupational Therapist **519**
Occupational Therapy Assistant **527**
Physical Therapist **683**
Physical Therapy Assistant **691**
Psychiatric Technician **731**
Radiologic Technologist **765**
Recreational Therapist **781**
Respiratory Therapist and Technician **805**
Special Procedures Technician **821**

10.03 child and adult care

Workers in this group are concerned with the physical needs and the welfare of others. They assist professionals in treating the sick or injured. They care for the elderly, the very young, or the handicapped. Frequently, these workers help people do the things they cannot do for themselves. Jobs are found in hospitals, clinics, day care centers, nurseries, schools, private homes, and centers for helping the handicapped.

10.03.01 data collection

Cardiovascular Technologist **65**
Electroneurodiagnostic Technologist **207**
Ophthalmic Technician **539**

10.03.02 patient care

Dental Assistant **125**
Emergency Medical Technician **217**
Medical Assistant **383**
Nurse Assistant **481**
Perfusionist **637**
Surgical Technologist **839**

10.03.03 care of others

Child Life Specialist **75**
Home Health Aide **327**

11 leading-influencing

An interest in leading-influencing others by using high-level verbal or numerical abilities. You can satisfy this interest through study and work in a variety of professional fields. You may enjoy the challenge and responsibility of leadership. You could seek work in administration or management. You may prefer working with technical details. You could find a job in finance, law, social research, or public relations. You may like to help others learn. Perhaps working in education would appeal to you.

11.03 social research

Workers in this group gather, study, and analyze information about individuals, specific groups, or entire societies. They conduct research, both historical and current, into all aspects of human behavior, including abnormal behavior, language, work, politics, lifestyle and cultural expression. They are employed by museums, schools and colleges, government agencies, and private research foundations.

11.03.01 psychological

11.05 business administration

Workers in this group are top level administrators and managers who work through lower level supervisors to direct all or a part of the activities in private establishments or government agencies. They set policies, make important decisions, and set priorities.These jobs are found in large businesses, industry, and government. Labor unions and associations also hire these workers.

11.05.02 administrative specialization

11.07 services administration

Workers in this group manage programs and projects in agencies that provide people with services in such areas as health, education, welfare, and recreation. They are in charge of program planning, policy making, and other managerial activities. The jobs are found in welfare and rehabilitation agencies and organizations, hospitals, schools, churches, libraries, and museums.

11.07.02 health and safety services

11.10 regulations enforcement

Workers in this group enforce government regulations and company policies that affect peoples' rights, health and safety, and finances. They examine records, inspect products, and investigate services, but do not engage in police work. Most workers find employment with government agencies, licensing departments, and health departments. Some are employed by retail establishments, mines, transportation companies, and nonprofit organizations.

11.10.03 health and safety

job title index

This index lists health care job titles as they appear in *Exploring Health Care Careers*. Page references to chapters are given in bold, following the job title.